# The Year in
# Hematology
## 1977

# The Year in Hematology

## 1977

Edited by

### Albert S. Gordon, Ph.D., F.R.S.M.

*Graduate School of Arts and Science*
*New York University*
*New York, New York*

### Robert Silber, M.D.

*New York University School of Medicine*
*New York, New York*

and

### Joseph LoBue, Ph.D.

*Graduate School of Arts and Science*
*New York University*
*New York, New York*

SPRINGER SCIENCE+BUSINESS MEDIA, LLC

Library of Congress Cataloging in Publication Data

Main entry under title:

The Year in hematology, 1977.

    Includes bibliographies and index.
    1. Hematology. 2. Blood—Diseases. I. Gordon, Albert Saul, 1910-     II.
Silber, Robert, 1931-     III. LoBue, Joseph. [DNLM: 1. Hematology—Period, W1
YE395]

| RC633.Y4 | 616.1'5 | 77-8412 |
|---|---|---|

ISBN 978-1-4899-6690-2     ISBN 978-1-4899-6688-9 (eBook)
DOI 10.1007/978-1-4899-6688-9

© Springer Science+Business Media New York 1977
Originally published by Plenum Publishing Corporation in 1977
Softcover reprint of the hardcover 1st edition 1977

# Contributors

**John W. Adamson,** M.D., Associate Professor of Medicine, Division of Hematology, Department of Medicine, University of Washington School of Medicine; and Chief, Hematology Section, Veterans Administration Hospital, Seattle, Washington

**Israel F. Charo,** M.S., M.D., Ph.D. Candidate, Department of Biochemistry, State University of New York Downstate Medical Center, Brooklyn, New York 11203

**W. Cieplinski,** M.D., Ph.D., Research Associate, Department of Cell Biology, Albert Einstein College of Medicine, Bronx, New York 10461

**Martin J. Cline,** M.D., Bowyer Professor of Medical Oncology, and Chief of Hematology–Oncology, Department of Medicine, University of California School of Medicine, Los Angeles, California 90024

**Harvey J. Cohen,** M.D., Ph.D., Associate, Division of Hematology–Oncology, Children's Hospital Medical Center; and Assistant Professor of Pediatrics, Harvard Medical School, Boston, Massachusetts 02115

**Neville Colman,** M.B., B.Ch., Ph.D., Research Associate, Veterans Administration Hospital, Bronx, New York 10468; and Assistant

Professor of Medicine, State University of New York Downstate Medical Center, Brooklyn, New York 11209

**Maryrose Conklyn,** B.S., Graduate Student, Department of Biology, New York University Graduate School of Arts and Sciences, New York, New York 10003

**Maria da Costa,** M.D., Associate Professor of Medicine, Division of Hematology/Oncology, Department of Medicine, New York Medical College, New York 10029

**Thomas C. Detwiler,** Ph.D., Professor of Biochemistry, Department of Biochemistry, State University of New York Downstate Medical Center, Brooklyn, New York 11203

**Alfred G. Ehlenberger,** M.D., Ph.D., Resident, Department of Psychiatry, Stanford University Medical Center, Palo Alto, California 94304

**Michael L. Freedman,** A.B., M.D., Professor of Medicine, Department of Medicine, New York University Medical Center, New York, New York 10016

**Robert C. Gallo,** M.D., D.Sc. (hon.), Chief, Laboratory of Tumor Cell Biology, National Cancer Institute, Bethesda, Maryland 20014; and Adjunct Professor of Genetics, George Washington University, Washington, D.C. 20007

**David H. Gillespie,** Ph.D., Head, Nucleic Acid Hybridization Section, Laboratory of Tumor Cell Biology, National Cancer Institute, Bethesda, Maryland 20014

**David W. Golde,** M.D., Associate Professor of Medicine, University of California School of Medicine, Los Angeles, California 90024

**Ronald B. Herberman,** M.D., Chief, Laboratory of Immunodiagnosis, National Cancer Institute, Bethesda, Maryland 20014

**Victor Herbert,** M.D., J.D., Director, Hematology and Nutrition Laboratory, Veterans Administration Hospital, Bronx, New York 10468; and Professor of Medicine, State University of New York Downstate Medical Center, Brooklyn, New York 11209

**Elizabeth Jacob,** M.D., Assistant Professor of Medicine, Department of Medicine, State University of New York Downstate Medical Center, Brooklyn, New York 11209

**Simon Karpatkin,** M.D., Professor of Medicine, New York University Medical School, New York, New York 10016

**Sanford B. Krantz,** M.D., Professor of Medicine and Chief of Hematology, Departments of Medicine, Vanderbilt University School of Medicine; and Veterans Administration Hospital, Nashville, Tennessee 37203

**Mahin D. Maines,** Ph.D., Associate Professor, The Rockefeller University, New York, New York 10021

**Julia A. McMillan,** M.D., Assistant Instructor, Department of Pediatrics, State University of New York, Upstate Medical Center, Syracuse, New York

**Victor Nussenzweig,** M.D., Professor of Pathology, Department of Pathology, New York University School of Medicine, New York, New York 10016

**Frank A. Oski,** M.D., Professor and Chairman, Department of Pediatrics, State University of New York, Upstate Medical Center, Syracuse, New York

**Oscar D. Ratnoff,** M.D., Professor of Medicine, Department of Medicine, Case Western Reserve University School of Medicine, and University Hospitals of Cleveland, Cleveland, Ohio 44106; Career Investigator of the American Heart Association

**Sheldon P. Rothenberg,** M.D., Professor and Vice Chairman, Department of Medicine, and Chief, Division of Hematology/Oncology, New York Medical College, New York, New York 10029

**M. D. Scharff,** M.D., Professor and Chairman, Department of Cell Biology, Albert Einstein College of Medicine, Bronx, New York 10461

**Robert Silber,** M.D., Director of Hematology and Professor of Medicine, New York University School of Medicine, New York, New York 10016

**Thomas P. Stossel,** M.D., Chief, Medical Oncology Unit, Massachusetts General Hospital; and Associate Professor of Medicine, Harvard Medical School, Boston, Massachusetts 02114

**S. Donald Zaentz,** M.D., Assistant Professor, Departments of Medicine, Division of Hematology, Vanderbilt University School of Medicine; and Veterans Administration Hospital, Nashville, Tennessee 37203

# Preface

Scientists, physicians, or students cannot be considered educated unless acquainted with the important developments in their chosen discipline. Over the last decade there has been an enormous production of valuable experimental and clinical observations in hematology. The published information must be assessed as to how the new differs from the old, what can be discarded as of little use, and what should be avidly pursued in the hope of yielding significant answers to important questions. This review series will endeavor to provide a critical appraisal of some recent observations of the normal and abnormal functions in the hematopoietic system, the overall objective being to provide current information in fields rich in new concepts which point the way to future work.

The contributors to this first volume have attempted to present a summary of some high points of recent research against a background of historical perspective. Good reviews are not born from an instinctive ability for preparing compendia. Instead, they are the result of intelligent, patient, critical analysis which culminates in a scholarly labor of love. We thank our contributors for the generous gift of their time, and we trust that their efforts will be rewarded by the expert guidance provided to students of hematology. The readers' reaction is invited to guide us in the preparation of future volumes.

Albert S. Gordon
Robert Silber
Joseph LoBue

*New York*

# Contents

## Chapter 2

## Hemoglobin Synthesis in Normal and Abnormal States

Michael L. Freedman

## Chapter 3

## Clinical Significance of 2,3-Diphosphoglycerate in Hematology

Frank A. Oski and Julia A. McMillan

## Chapter 4
## The Interaction of Folate Ligands with Macromolecules
Maria da Costa and Sheldon P. Rothenberg

## Chapter 5
## Pure Red Cell Aplasia
Sanford B. Krantz and S. Donald Zaentz

## Chapter 6

## Neutrophil Function: Normal and Abnormal

Thomas P. Stossel and Harvey J. Cohen

## Chapter 7

## Phagocytosis: Role of C3 Receptors and Contact-Inducing Agents

Alfred G. Ehlenberger and Victor Nussenzweig

## Chapter 8

## Leukocyte 5'-Nucleotidase

Maryrose Conklyn and Robert Silber

## Chapter 9
# Metabolism and Functions of Monocytes and Macrophages
Martin J. Cline and David W. Golde

## Chapter 10
# The Production of Immunoglobulins by Mouse Myeloma Cells
W. Cieplinski and M. D. Scharff

Chapter 11

# The Origin of RNA Tumor Viruses and Their Relation to Human Leukemia

Robert C. Gallo and David H. Gillespie

Chapter 12

# Immunological Aspects of Leukemia

Ronald B. Herberman

## Chapter 13
## Antihemophilic Factor
Oscar D. Ratnoff

## Chapter 14

# Research on the Biochemical Basis of Platelet Function

Thomas C. Detwiler and Israel F. Charo

## Chapter 15
## Significance of Platelet Volume Measurements
Simon Karpatkin

## Chapter 16
## Mechanisms of Polycythemia
John W. Adamson

Chapter 17

## Nutritional Anemias Overview; Megaloblastic Anemias

Victor Herbert, Neville Colman, and Elizabeth Jacob

# Heme Metabolism: Factors Affecting the *in Vivo* Oxidation of Heme

## Mahin D. Maines

## 1.1. Introduction

The mechanism underlying the conversion of heme compounds to bile pigments has been extensively explored since the mid-1940s. Although the relationship between the formation of bilirubin and the catabolism of heme (hemoglobin) were noted as early as 1847 (Virchow), later studies by investigators such as Mann and co-workers (1926), conclusively showing that bilirubin is derived from hemoglobin, as well as later work by Fischer and Hess (1931) which identified the correct structure of bilirubin, led to a new era of investigation on heme metabolism. This chapter presents a summary of some major features of the older literature on bile pigment formation and compares and analyzes more recent developments in the field of heme oxidation and the factors influencing this process.

## 1.2. Heme and Bile Pigments

The porphyrins (Fig. 1) are derived from porphine, which is an essentially planar ring of four pyrroles joined by unsaturated carbon

MAHIN D. MAINES • The Rockefeller University, New York, New York 10021.

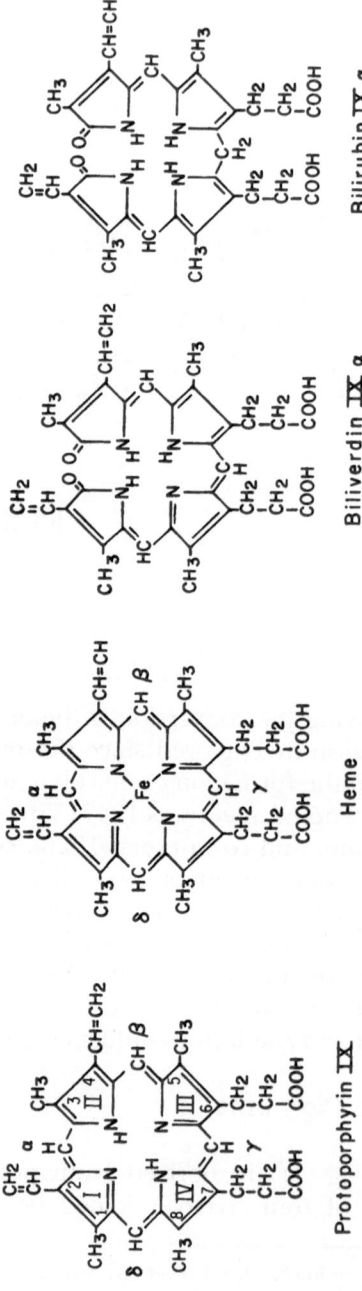

Fig. 1. Structures of protoporphyrin, heme, biliverdin, and bilirubin. The bridge carbons are designated as $\alpha$, $\beta$, $\gamma$, and $\delta$.

bridges referred to as the methene or meso bridges, with replacement of some or all hydrogens $\beta$ to the pyrrole nitrogens by various substituents. Metalloporphyrins, or hemes, are formed through displacement by a divalent metal (Fe, Co, Mg, Mn, Ni, Cu, Zn, Sn) of two protons from two pyrrole rings. The porphyrins of animal origin are fully substituted in positions 1 through 8 of the porphyrin nucleus and, depending on the spatial positions of different side chains, different positional isomers are possible. Protoporphyrin-IX has three different types of $\beta$ side chains: 4-methyl, 2-vinyl, and 2-propionate. Fe-protoporphyrin-IX, also referred to as protoheme, hemin (in HCl solution), hematin (in alkali medium), heme type $b$, or simply heme, is the most ubiquitous heme of the animal kingdom and constitutes the prosthetic moiety of such widespread hemoproteins as hemoglobin, myoglobin, catalase, mitochondrial cytochrome $b$'s, and the microsomal hemoproteins, cytochrome P-450 and $b_5$, in addition to the cytosol enzyme tryptophan pyrrolase. When the nature of the substituents of protoporphyrin-IX is changed, different types of hemes are formed; for example, in heme type $c$, which is the prosthetic group of cytochromes $c$ and $c_1$, the two vinyl groups are replaced by two cysteine groups; and heme type $a$, which serves as the prosthetic moiety of cytochrome $a$ and $a_3$ contains an isoprene side chain as indicated below:

$$\underset{\displaystyle CH_2-CH_2-\underset{\displaystyle |}{\overset{\displaystyle CH_3}{\overset{\displaystyle |}{CH}}}-CH_2-CH_2-CH_2-\underset{\displaystyle |}{\overset{\displaystyle CH_3}{\overset{\displaystyle |}{CH}}}-CH_2-CH_2-CH_2-\underset{\displaystyle |}{\overset{\displaystyle CH_3}{\overset{\displaystyle |}{CH}}}-CH_3}{}$$

bound through a formaldehyde group at ring I in place of a vinyl group. Heme type $a$ also contains a formyl group (—CHO) instead of the methyl group in ring IV.

Most studies concerning the oxidative degradation of heme have dealt with this process as it affects heme type $b$. In mammalian systems as well as in avian species, reptiles, and amphibians, heme is oxidatively degraded to form an open chain tetrapyrrole, biliverdin, with 1 mole of carbon monoxide being formed and the central metal being released. In all these animal classes the biliverdin formed is of the IX$\alpha$ isomer type— that is, the oxidation of the heme molecule takes place at the $\alpha$-meso carbon bridge. The formation of carbon monoxide as a result of heme degradation is also observed in other species including insects, as well as in hemolytic bacteria under aerobic conditions (Engel *et al.*, 1972). The biliverdin formed from degradation of heme in mammalian systems is converted to bilirubin. Biliverdin-IX$\alpha$, which is a bilatriene, contains four conjugated pyrrole rings and is reduced at the central methene bridge in a number of tissues by the action of a cytosol enzyme, biliverdin reductase, to form bilirubin. The latter is an isomer-specific enzyme which is reactive almost exclusively toward biliverdin-IX$\alpha$ isomer; other biliverdin isomers are not utilized to any significant degree as substrate for the reductase. Bilirubin is a biladiene in which the two unconjugated dipyrroles are joined by an electron-insulating methene bridge. Tetrapyrroles closely related to bilirubin have been identified through the plant kingdom and in lower animals. In many instances these pigments serve vital biological functions such as acting as photoreceptors in photosynthetic processes; however, in higher animals there is no known physiological role ascribed to bile pigments, though these pigments provide the source, as do porphyrins, for the pigmentation of egg shells and feathers.

Numerous studies have been carried out since the mid-1950s concerning the relationships between the degradation of heme and the formation of carbon monoxide and bilirubin. These studies have been carried out in man as well as in animals. The early work of Sjöstrand (1949) and that of Ludwig and co-workers (1957) and Gray et al. (1958) demonstrating that endogenously produced carbon monoxide in mammalian systems is derived only from the $\alpha$-methene bridge carbon of heme, and the subsequent findings by Sjörstrand (1952), Ostrow et al. (1962), and Coburn et al. (1964) demonstrating that carbon monoxide and bilirubin are produced on an equimolar basis from heme, opened a new chapter in the study of heme degradation.

Although bilirubin constitutes the only identified heme-related pigment of uncontaminated mammalian bile, there is evidence that heme compounds may be degraded to products other than bilirubin under certain conditions. These include occasions when exogenous heme is administered to animals in concentrations exceeding the binding capacity of plasma haptoglobin (Ostrow et al., 1962), or in patients with congenital Heinz body hemolytic anemia (a condition in which the urine contains dark pigments, tentatively identified as dipyrroles by Kreimer-Birnbaum et al., 1966), or in normal rats exposed to phenylhydrazine (to stimulate Heinz body hemolytic anemia), in which the heme moiety of the oxidatively denatured hemoglobin is degraded to metabolites exhibiting solubility and spectroscopic properties of mesobilifuscins (Goldstein et al., 1968). Moreover, when certain compounds such as the barbiturate analog allylisopropylacetamide are administered to animals, the molar ratio of carbon monoxide produced to bilirubin recovered exceeds 1.0, indicating the conversion of heme to metabolites other than bilirubin (Landaw et al., 1970). These metabolites, commonly referred to as "green pigments," were first observed by Schwartz and Ikeda in 1952; their exact chemical configuration is not as yet fully established.

Following the formation of bilirubin, this bile pigment—which is relatively insoluble in aqueous solution—is conjugated with 2 moles of glucuronic acid to form an ester diglucuronide. This activity is catalyzed by the endoplasmic reticulum-bound enzyme UDP glucuronyl transferase which is found in hepatocytes as well as in several nonhepatic tissues. UDP glucuronyl transferase has not been completely isolated and characterized and thus it is not fully established that there is more than one molecular species of glucuronyl transferase; however, the preponderance of recent evidence supports the idea of more than one distinct enzyme moiety. In addition, there is uncertainty concerning the formation of a monoglucuronide of bilirubin, since there are some findings which indicate that the monoglucuronide may be an artifact of the isolation procedure, being composed of a mixture of diglucuronides and unconjugated bilirubin. Arias and co-workers (1969) have studied this aspect of heme degradation extensively and have provided a great deal of insight into and knowledge of the field of bilirubin conjugation; therefore, this topic is not reviewed further here.

Bilirubin in plasma is bound mainly to albumin (Odell, 1959; Ostrow and Schmid, 1963). A small amount may also be found in the globulin fraction (Klatskin and Bungards, 1950; Cooke and Roberts, 1969). This globulin has been identified as a $\beta$-lipoprotein (Cooke and Roberts, 1969).

In the cytoplasm, although bilirubin is not bound to albumin, low molecular weight intracellular binding proteins for bilirubin have been identified and referred to as Y (or ligandin) and Z proteins (or protein A). These proteins are also capable of binding carcinogens and a number of organic anions (Ketterer *et al.*, 1967; Levi *et al.*, 1969a). Ligandin is the major organic anion binding protein of hepatocyte cytoplasm. The Z protein, or protein A, is present also in the mucosa of the small intestine. These cytoplasmic proteins have been extensively studied in the laboratories of Arias and of Ketterer and co-workers.

Conjugated bilirubin is excreted into the bile and subsequently into the intestine. It should be noted that the bilirubin in bile does not account for all sequestered heme—in the rat, for example, it has been demonstrated that bilirubin recovered in bile accounts for only 60–80% of sequestered heme (Ostrow *et al.*, 1962). The fate of the remaining fraction of heme is not known; it may be that there are other means of heme degradation which do not lead to the formation of bilirubin. In intestine, bilirubin remains in the conjugated form ("free" bilirubin is reabsorbed by intestinal mucosa) until it is converted, through a sequence of hydrogenation reactions by the action of intestinal bacteria, to urobilinogens. Urobilinogens are formed when two methene bridges and the two vinyl groups of bilirubin are reduced; urobilinogens are then partially dehydrogenated to form urobilins. Although there is substantial evidence that it is conjugated bilirubin which undergoes reduction in the intestine, Troxler *et al.* (1968) demonstrated that a membrane-bound component isolated from mixed human fecal bacteria could convert free bilirubin to urobilins, indicating that free bilirubin may be the form which is initially converted to urobilinogens and subsequently to urobilins in the gut.

A number of intermediates produced in the course of the conversion of bilirubin to urobilins have been isolated and identified from the intestinal contents. The structures and the sequence of formation of these fecal pigments are shown in Fig. 2. As depicted, there is first a sequence of hydrogenations followed by dehydrogenation reactions, all mediated by the enzymes of mixed intestinal bacterial flora, which leads to the production of urobilins, the orange-red pigments excreted in the feces. The intensive, intricate, and elegant studies carried out in the laboratories of such investigators as C. J. Watson, S. Schwartz, C. H. Gray, and D. C. Nicholson have greatly contributed to our knowledge of the structure and the formation of these bile pigments. A detailed and extensive review of bile pigments in the gastrointestinal tract has been published by Elder *et al.* (1972).

## 1.3. Mechanism of Heme Oxidation

The mechanisms by which heme compounds are degraded may be classified into two categories—enzymatic and nonenzymatic.

### 1.3.1. Nonenzymatic Heme Oxidation

The demonstration of nonenzymatic conversion of heme compounds to bile pigments dates back to the studies of Foulkes, Lemberg, and Pardom (1951) showing that the coupled oxidation of reducing agents, such as ascorbate, and hemoglobin leads to the formation of choleglobin, which upon hydrolysis yields biliverdin.

O'Carra and Colleran (1969) demonstrated that coupled oxidation of hemoproteins, including myoglobin, with ascorbate, under physiological pH and temperature, produced isomers of biliverdin which in the case of myoglobin had a composition consisting of 100% of the IXα type; hematin did not undergo oxidation in this system. Hemoglobin under the same conditions gave rise to 65–80% IXα isomer, with the remainder being of the IXβ configuration. The yields of biliverdin obtained from these coupled oxidations were very poor. Moreover, when myoglobin was denatured, all four possible isomers of biliverdin were formed. The X-ray diffraction studies of Kendrew *et al.* (1960) indicate that the α-methene bridge of heme in myoglobin is positioned at the bottom of a heme-

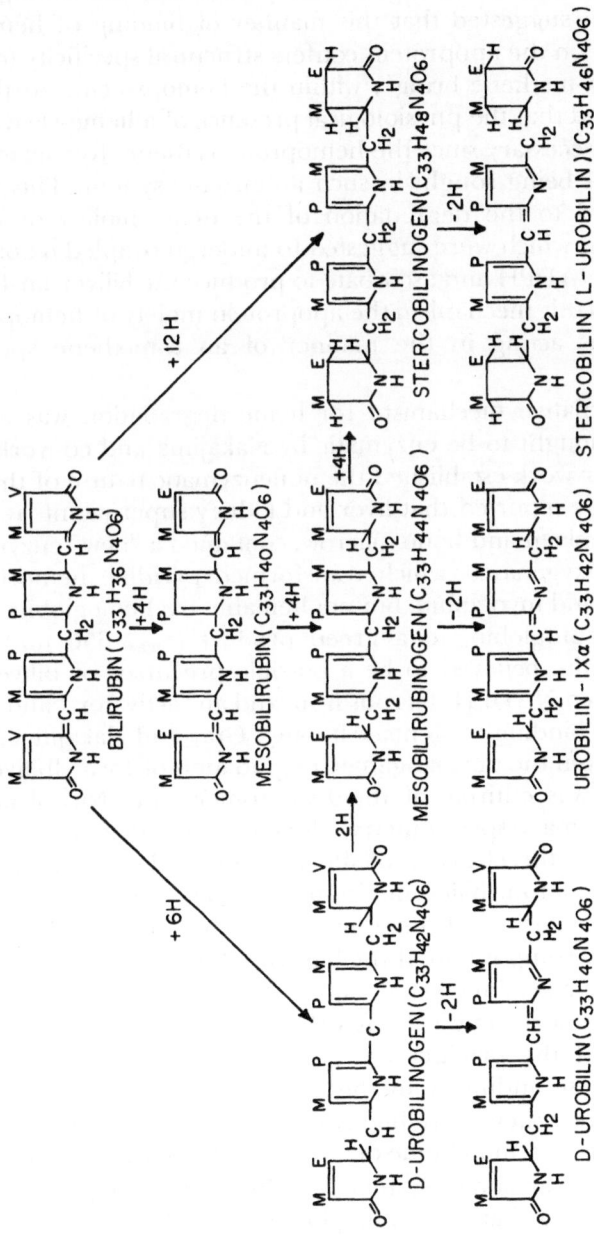

**Fig. 2.** Structure and classification of some bile pigments.

containing crevice, surrounded by hydrophobic amino acid side chains, leaving the $\beta$, $\gamma$, and $\delta$ bridges entirely accessible. Accordingly, O'Carra and Colleran suggested that this manner of binding of heme to heme binding sites on the apoprotein confers structural specificity to the oxidation of the $\alpha$-methene bridge, within the hemoprotein. Furthermore, it was concluded that the physiological presence of a heme-cleaving enzyme system is unnecessary since the hemoproteins themselves seem to have all the attributes being sought in such an enzyme system. This mechanism was extended to the degradation of the heme moiety of microsomal hemoproteins which were suggested to undergo coupled oxidation in the presence of NADPH and ascorbate to produce the biliverdin-IX$\alpha$ isomer. According to this mechanism the apoprotein moiety of hemoproteins was envisioned as acting in the manner of an $\alpha$-methene specific heme "oxidase."

An alternative mechanism for heme degradation was earlier proposed and thought to be enzymatic by Nakajima and co-workers (1963) although later work established the nonenzymatic nature of their system. These workers reported that liver and kidney supernatant fractions, but not those of spleen and bone marrow, contained a "new" enzyme—heme $\alpha$-methenyl oxygenase—which transformed pyridine hemochromogen, hemoglobin, and myoglobin, but not hematin, oxyhemoglobin, methemoglobin, or haptoglobin, to a green product ($\lambda_{max}$ 656 nm), allegedly formylbiliverdin, believed to be a possible precursor of biliverdin. The system required NADPH, ferrous iron, and an "activator," and was inactivated by thiol binding reagents. Although Gray and Nakajima (1967) had concluded, from the permanganate degradation of formylbiliverdin, that this product was entirely of the IX$\alpha$ isomer type, Nichol and Morell (1969), using mass spectrometry, demonstrated that in the system of Nakajima *et al.* the cleavage of all methene bridges occurred with the production of all four biliverdin isomers. Similarly, Colleran and O'Carra (1969), using a sensitive chromatographic technique, found no difference in the isomeric composition of the bilverdin formed from pyridine hemochrome by the Nakajima system and that produced by coupled oxidation of pyridine hemochrome with ascorbate. In both instances the isomeric composition of the product was that of the four possible isomers of biliverdin. These findings plus the fact that the organ and the substrate specificity of the system were highly unexpected ruled out any physiological role for this system in heme degradation. Rather it was postulated that the activity of Nakajima's system was due to the coupled oxidation of substrate, with ascorbate remaining loosely bound to the protein throughout the preparation process, thus conferring a nonenzymatic mode of action to the system.

Masters and Schacter (1976) have recently shown that heme is nonenzymatically degraded to biliverdin by proteolytically purified cytochrome *c* reductase when incubated with NADPH under physiological conditions of pH and temperature. However, it was observed that the rate of biliverdin reduction to bilirubin, by the action of biliverdin reductase—which as mentioned earlier is a IXα-specific enzyme—was less than 10% of the rate of biliverdin production in the system. One may infer from these differences in rates of biliverdin and bilirubin formation that production of a mixture of isomers of biliverdin by this system took place. This finding further suggests the necessity of a specific heme binding and catalytic site for the oxidation of heme—i.e., a specific enzyme protein—in the formation of the physiological IXα isomer of biliverdin.

## 1.3.2. Enzymatic Heme Oxidation

Several enzyme systems have been described which degrade heme compounds to biliverdin. One such system is that reported by Wise and Drabkin (1964). The source of enzyme was the light mitochondrial fraction of the hemophagous organ of dog placenta which, in the presence of NADP, NAD, ATP, boiled cell sap, and ascorbate, could aerobically convert hemoglobin or heme to biliverdin, which was 90% of the IXα configuration. This system was extremely unusual in the organ source, the subcellular distribution of the enzyme, and the cofactor requirement for enzymatic activity, particularly when compared with that subsequently described by Tenhunen *et al.* (1968) and referred to as "heme oxygenase." The latter had a microsomal membrane source and was identified in a number of tissues, e.g., liver, kidney, brain, spleen, and bone marrow. Moreover, a requirement for NADPH in the latter system was indicated. The widespread tissue distribution of the heme oxygenase complex was an important characteristic of the latter system since the limited tissue distribution of the enzyme described by Wise and Drabkin rendered their system of questionable physiological importance. The heme degrading system described by Terhunen *et al.* was an oxygenase, since the reaction depended on the activation of molecular oxygen; i.e., it was an oxygen-fixation reaction. Furthermore, it subscribed to the criterion of a monooxygenase type of reaction (Hayaishi *et al.*, 1955), also referred to as "mixed function" oxygenase (Mason *et al.*, 1955). In a series of subsequent studies this heme oxygenase system was further characterized and the conclusion was reached that the system contained cytochrome P-450 as the terminal oxidase and was dependent for activity on this hemoprotein (Schmid, 1972; Tenhunen *et al.*, 1972, 1969b). The latter conclusion was based on the findings that heme oxygenase activity was inhibited by carbon monoxide and that this inhibition could be reversed by monochromatic light (Tenhunen *et al.*, 1972) in a manner somewhat analogous to that seen with the microsomal mixed-function oxidase responsible for the hydroxylation of drugs and steroids. However, with the drug and steroid metabolizing system the inhibition by carbon monoxide of oxidation activity is reversed by monochromatic light in the 450-nm wavelength region (Cooper *et al.*, 1965), whereas light in a longer wavelength region (460–470 nm) was required to activate heme oxygenase. The discrepancy between the wavelength at which the inhibition by carbon monoxide of heme oxidation activity is reversed (464–468 nm) and the wavelength at which the inhibition of cytochrome P-450-dependent microsomal activities is reversed (450 nm) was questioned as early as 1973 (Maines, 1975). This discrepancy in the wavelength of the reversal of carbon monoxide inhibition was noted in conjunction with other facts such as the great difference existing between the tissue distribution of heme oxygenase activity and cytochrome P-450 content, i.e., activity of heme oxygenase in the splenic microsomal fraction was more than 10 times greater than in the liver, although the cytochrome P-450 content of spleen is less than 2–3% of that in the liver (0.7–0.9 nmol/mg protein for liver, 0.02–0.025 nmol/mg protein for spleen); the failure of inhibitors and substrates of cytochrome P-450-dependent systems to alter heme oxygenase activity; the lack of response of heme oxygenase to inducers of cytochrome P-450; and the failure of induction of cytochrome P-450 by inducers of heme oxygenase. In addition, several of the heme compounds that had been demonstrated to be substrates for the heme oxygenase system *in vitro* (Tenhunen *et al.*, 1969a), such as mesoheme, methemalbumin, and hematin itself, under the *in vitro* conditions described for the heme oxygenase system had potent degradative effects on cytochrome P-450 and on P-450-dependent activities of the mixed-function oxidase system (Maines and Kappas, 1974a, 1975a). The latter finding in particular raised serious doubts concerning the validity of the hypothesis that cytochrome P-450 was essential for heme degradation as had been earlier reported. Other investigators (e.g., Nichol, 1970, 1971), when studying heme degradation and biliverdin formation in cultured chicken macrophages (which do not have detectable cytochrome P-450 activity), were also unable to confirm an association of heme oxidation with cytochrome P-450 activity. Subsequently, the activity of heme oxygenase and cytochrome P-450 were totally dissociated in liver (which has a high content of cytochrome P-450 and relatively low heme oxygenase activity) by Maines and Kappas (1974b, 1975b), and in spleen (which has a very high heme oxygenase activity, with small amounts of cytochrome P-450) by Yoshida *et al.* (1974). Maines and Kappas in a series of subsequent experiments showed that the hepatic heme oxygenase could be induced markedly ($10\times$ or more) by treatment of animals with cobalt chloride, with the same treatment causing up to 60–70% reduction in microsomal cytochrome P-450 content. This finding together with earlier data showing discordant patterns of development of P-450 and heme oxygenase in liver (Maines and Kappas, 1975c) clearly indicated that this cytochrome could not be the terminal oxidase for hepatic heme oxygenase and that there was no direct correlation between the rate of heme oxidation and the microsomal content of cytochrome P-450. Some of the data on the dissociation of heme oxygenase activity from cytochrome P-450 are summarized in Table I.

It is known that treatment of microsomes with 4 M urea causes denaturation of cytochrome P-450 and its conversion to the inactive form, cytochrome P-420 (Mason *et al.*, 1964). Therefore, microsomes from cobalt-treated animals in which microsomal content of cytochrome P-450 had already been reduced to about 30% of control levels by cobalt were treated with 4 M urea (30 min, 25°C). As shown (Table I), this treatment reduced the spectrally measurable microsomal content of cytochrome P-450 to an undetectable amount; nevertheless, heme oxygenase activity of the microsomes remained highly elevated, at a level about 900% above normal. As expected by the complete loss of cytochrome P-450, the mixed-function oxidative activity of such microsomes was also totally eliminated. Although NADPH cytochrome *c* reductase activity of urea-treated microsomes from the cobalt-treated animals was decreased to only a fraction of the control (20–25%), heme oxygenase activity was still nine times greater than normal. This finding indicated that although the oxidation of heme requires reduced pyridine nucleotide and cytochrome

**Table I.** Dissociation of Microsomal Heme Oxygenase from Cytochrome P-450 Involvement and Evidence for the Existence of Two Distinct Microsomal Mixed-Function Oxidases

| Treatment *in vivo* | Treatment *in vitro* | Bilirubin formed (nmol/mg hr) | Ethylmorphine *N*-demethylation (nmol/mg hr) | Cytochrome P-450 (nmol/mg) | NADPH cytochrome *c* reductase activity (nmol/mg min) |
|---|---|---|---|---|---|
| Control | None | 1.01 | 205 | 0.61 | 56.6 |
| Control | Urea (4 M) | 0.18 | 26 | 0.07 | 9.4 |
| Co²⁺ | None | 15.66 | 18 | 0.22 | 52.3 |
| Co²⁺ | Urea (4 M) | 9.71 | 0 | 0 | 12.5 |

*c* reductase, the activity of the latter enzyme is not rate limiting in the heme oxidation process, as had been suggested (Schacter *et al.,* 1972). O'Carra (1975), on the assumption that apocytochrome P-450 is synonymous with heme oxygenase, interpreted the data of Maines and Kappas (1974b) and Yoshida *et al.* (1974) to support this notion. However, the hypothesis that apo-P-450 and heme oxygenase are identical seems untenable on the basis of direct and indirect evidence which has been accumulated in this laboratory and elsewhere. The view that the denatured apoprotein moiety of the cytochrome (P-420) is the heme-cleaving enzyme for exogenously added heme, would be acceptable if there were more than one specific heme binding site available on the denatured apoprotein, or if the affinity of the apo-P-420 for the added heme were greater than the affinity of albumin which is used as the heme carrier protein in heme oxygenase assays. There are no experimental data available defining the number of specific heme binding sites on apo-P-420, but there is experimental evidence indicating that apo-P-420 has multiple *nonspecific* heme binding sites (Maines and Anders, 1973a). Moreover, it can be presumed, since cytochrome P-450 has 1 mole of heme per mole of protein, that cytochrome P-420 also would possess one specific heme binding site. In addition, as already mentioned, a second criterion for the apoprotein of the cytochrome to serve as the specific heme-cleaving enzyme is that the apocytochrome have a higher affinity for heme than albumin does. However, this contention is not supported by the data of Maines *et al.* (1974) which show that the affinity of albumin for heme exceeds that of apocytochrome P-420. Aside from this indirect evidence for the existence of heme oxygenase as a separate entity distinct from apocytochrome P-450, there are more direct experimental data supporting the distinctiveness of these microsomal entities. Maines and Kappas (1975d) have shown that under experimental conditions in which excessive amounts of apo-450 were present in hepatocytes there was no observed increase in heme oxygenase activity in the liver. Correia and Meyer (1975) have reported that the treatment of animals for several days with phenobarbital (to increase the synthesis of cytochrome P-450 apoprotein and heme) followed by treatment with cobalt chloride (to decrease the heme content) causes an accumulation of apocytochrome in the hepatocytes. Such an apoprotein-rich microsomal preparation from the rat was utilized in this laboratory in the expectation of finding high heme oxygenase activity if the apoprotein of P-450 were, in fact, this enzyme. However, it was noted that the heme oxygenase activity of this microsomal preparation was actually somewhat less than that observed with cobalt treatment alone. The most direct evidence for the existence of heme oxygenase as a distinct heme-cleaving enzyme system comes from the most recent work in this laboratory (Maines *et al.*, 1977a) in which heme oxygenase was isolated from rat liver and purified to the point of exhibiting only one band on sodium dodecyl sulfate (SDS) gel electrophoresis. This preparation is totally free from cytochrome P-450 and heme contamination and has an absolute requirement for reduced pyridine nucleotide. Both NADH and NADPH, when present with NADH cytochrome $b_5$ reductase or NADPH cytochrome $c$ reductase, respectively, can serve as electron donor for the reaction, although the reaction rate with NADPH is approximately twice that with NADH. The presence of a flavoprotein, NADPH cytochrone $c$ reductase or NADH cytochrome $b$ reductase, is required for the enzyme activity. Moreover, when the oxidation of heme by the splenic microsomal fraction was reexamined the same ability of NADH as well as NADPH to satisfy the requirement for the reduced nucleotide was observed (Maines and Kappas, 1977a).

### 1.3.3. Substrate Specificity

Microsomal heme oxygenase has been studied with respect to its substrate specificity. In the solubilized hepatic preparation studied in this laboratory it has been demonstrated that in addition to heme and methemalbumin, methemoglobin is also a substrate for the enzyme (about 30–40% effective) although the reactivity of the latter is less than that of hematin or hemin bound to albumin. Other protein complexes of heme are also degraded by heme oxygenase; these include methemoglobin and isolated $\alpha$ and $\beta$ chains of hemoglobin (Tenhunen *et al.*, 1969a). Free porphyrins are not substrates *in vitro* for the enzyme.

*In vivo* experiments also indicate that free porphyrins are not substrates for the heme oxidation system. Coburn *et al.* (1967) noted that when dogs were injected with $^{14}$C-labeled protoporphyrin-IX (aqueous solution or complexed with albumin or globin), $^{14}$C-labeled carbon monoxide and [$^{14}$C]bilirubin were formed. The source of these $^{14}$C-labeled products was identified as cellular heme. When heme was isolated from the livers of the treated animals and analyzed for $^{14}$C activity the isolated heme had a rather high specific activity, particularly when [$^{14}$C]protoporphyrin had been injected complexed with protein. These studies support the idea that free porphyrin must be converted *in vivo* to heme before it is degraded to bile pigments.

The reactivity of a number of other metalloporphyrins and the effect of side chain constituents of the tetrapyrrole ring on the iron heme degradation have also been investigated. Tenhunen *et al.* (1969a) had demonstrated that substitution of the vinyl groups on rings 1 and 2 by less electronegative side chains, as is the case with mesohemin, deuterohemin, or "coprohemin," markedly decreases the effectiveness of these hemes as substrates for heme oxygenase. Schacter and Waterman (1974) investigated the effectiveness of manganese and copper protoporphyrin-IX, cobalt mesoporphyrin, and nickel, copper, and palladium deuteroporphyrin-IX, as substrates for heme oxygenase. They reported that none served as effective substrates for the splenic heme oxygenase system. Therefore, it was considered that microsomal heme oxygenase activity is specific for the iron protoporphyrin-IX complex. Accordingly, it has been asserted that the central iron of heme is essential for its oxidation by heme oxygenase (Tenhunen *et al.*, 1969a). This question was reexamined in light of the finding that cobalt heme (Co-protoporphyrin-IX) shared the heme oxygenase-inducing property of ionic cobalt (Maines and Kappas, 1975b), although in other studies no evidence had been obtained for *in vivo* formation of cobalt heme after administration of the labeled metal ion. In these studies animals were injected with $^{58}$Co and were killed at various intervals. Heme was isolated from liver and kidney and analyzed by thin-layer chromatography and measurement of $^{58}$Co activity of heme fractions (Maines, unpublished observations). No incorporation of isotope into heme was detectable in these studies. Therefore, it appears most probable that the induction of heme oxygenase produced by cobalt heme is mediated by the metal alone rather than by the metalloporphyrin. Thus it was inferred that cobalt heme must be subject to enzymatic oxidation so as to release the chelated cobalt which would then produce the observed enzyme-inducing action. Subsequent studies (Maines and Kappas, 1977a) showed that cobalt heme could indeed serve as substrate for the microsomal heme oxygenase system and that the product of the oxidation reaction with cobalt heme was the natural bile pigment, biliverdin-IXα isomer. The oxidative cleavage of cobalt heme by rat splenic microsomal preparations displayed typical characteristics of an enzyme-mediated reaction such as inactivation by heating (60°C, 5 min) or inactivity at 0°C, appropriate kinetics of the reaction with expected dependence on protein concentration, substrate concentration, and length of incubation (37°C). However, the apparent $Km$'s for cobalt heme oxidation by spleen and liver heme oxygenases were 8 to 10 times those for iron heme, indicating a low affinity of the enzyme for the substrate.

The apparent discrepancy between these findings, showing oxidative metabolism of cobalt heme by the splenic microsomal heme oxygenase, compared with the findings of Schacter and Waterman (1974) is likely due to the fact that in the latter studies Co-mesoporphyrin-IX—rather than Co-protoporphyrin-IX—was utilized as the test substrate. Moreover, the traditional spectrophotometric method of detection of bilirubin formation was used; this is less sensitive for the detection of small amounts of the pigment than the extraction of bilirubin formed with chloroform which was utilized in the studies from this laboratory. In the past, criteria such as the inhibition of heme oxidation by KCN, Na$_3$N, and carbon monoxide have been taken as evidence for the involvement of hemoproteins in heme degradation. However, studies from this laboratory (Maines and Kappas, 1977a) have shown that oxidation of cobalt heme is also inhibited by certain heme ligands (KCN, 0.1 mM, and carbon monoxide) as effectively as is that of iron heme. In addition, it was found that Fe-heme oxidation was also substantially inhibited (50–60%) by Na$_3$N (1 mM) whereas the oxidation of Co-heme was not inhibited even at high concentrations of this ligand (5 mM). This finding indicates that the observed inhibition of Fe-heme oxidation is a consequence of the ligand binding with the substrate rather than with a hemoprotein enzyme, and that the differential effect of Na$_3$N on the oxidation of the two heme compounds is attributable to preferential binding of the ligand to the iron, as compared with the cobalt moiety of the metalloporphyrin substrates.

### 1.3.4. Heme Oxygenase: Postulated Mode of Action

The data just discussed, including the utilization of a noniron metalloporphyrin as substrate by heme oxygenase, and the finding that purified hepatic heme oxygenase (Maines *et al.*, 1977a) and solubilized splenic heme oxygenase (Yoshida *et al.*, 1974) are not hemoproteins, permit certain inferences to be drawn concerning the characteristics and mode of action of this enzyme system in the oxidation of heme compounds. First, in contrast to earlier reports (Tenhunen *et al.*, 1969a; Yoshida *et al.*, 1974) that splenic heme oxidation activity utilizes NADPH as the sole source of reducing equivalents for the reaction, the splenic microsomal system (Maines and Kappas, 1977a) as well as the purified hepatic enzyme (Maines *et al.*, 1977a) can utilize either NADH or NADPH as an electron donor for heme degradation, although NADPH is more effective in this regard. In addition, the iron atom of the tetrapyrrole is not indispensable, as believed earlier (Tenhunen *et al.*, 1969a; Schacter and Waterman, 1974), for heme oxygenase activity and can be replaced, at least by cobalt; however, a central metal atom is undoubtedly necessary for heme oxidation. This conclusion is based on the finding from several laboratories that the free porphyrins, mesoporphyrin and protoporphyrin, are not oxidizable by the enzyme. Finally, it appears likely that lipophilic substituents on pyrrole rings I and II, e.g., of hemes, are an essential feature for oxidation of the heme molecule. This conclusion is based on experiments in this laboratory with copro- and uroporphyrin complexes of cobalt in which it was found that these metalloporphyrins were not oxidized, as well as the experiments of Tenhunen *et al.* (1969a) with "coprohemin." The view that such lipophilic side chains are necessary for the binding of the metalloporphyrin to the enzyme protein is consistent with the suggestion made earlier by O'Carra and Colleran (1969) concerning the mode of binding of porphyrins to proteins.

On this basis a plausible hypothesis for the degradation of heme compounds can be formulated which in part resembles that proposed by O'Carra and Colleran (1969), O'Carra (1975), and Kikuchi and Yoshida (1976). The active sites of microsomal heme oxygenase enzyme consist of hydrophobic "pockets" which can accommodate two rings of a tetrapyrrole molecule possessing lipophilic substituents on two adjacent pyrroles such as the vinyl groups on rings I and II of heme; at the center of this pocket there is a coordinating site for the central metal atom of the metalloporphyrin. The coordination may take place with a sulfur atom, as heme oxygenase is a —SH active enzyme (Maines et al., 1977a). In this form the substrate heme and the enzyme protein form a "transitory" hemoprotein. The binding site for heme must permit reactivity of both microsomal flavoproteins, NADPH cytochrome $c$ reductase as well as NADH cytochrome $b_5$ reductase, with the newly formed transitory hemoprotein thus allowing utilization of either nucleotide. Following the formation of the transitory hemoprotein, an electron transport chain is created with this hemoprotein serving as its own terminal oxygenase. It is evident that the transitory hemoprotein is not an obligatory Fe-heme hemoprotein since, as reported here, it may be a Co-heme hemoprotein as well. The function of the transitory hemoprotein would be to bind molecular oxygen, which is then utilized for the oxidative cleavage of the tetrapyrrole ring and the formation of water.

The idea that heme oxidation is a "mixed function" type of oxidative reaction is not novel; however, it had been previously considered that this oxidative reaction utilized a native microsomal hemoprotein as the terminal oxygenase for heme in a manner analogous to the mixed-function oxidation of drugs (Tenhunen et al., 1969b, 1972; Schmid, 1972). The mechanism formulated here differs from the latter type of reaction, however, in that the "oxygenase" is not a preformed microsomal hemoprotein, but rather the substrate heme–enzyme complex itself which serves to activate molecular $O_2$. The mechanism described also differs from that proposed by O'Carra and Colleran (1969) who, although suggesting that exogenous heme undergoes an autocatalytic oxidation, postulated that the apoprotein moiety of cytochrome P-450 serves as the binding site for the substrate heme—i.e., exogenous heme replaces the rapidly turning over heme moiety of P-450, obviating the need for a specific enzyme catalyzing heme degradation. However, the total dissociation of cytochrome P-450, apoenzyme or holoenzyme, and cytochrome P-420 from heme oxygenase activity does not substantiate O'Carra and Colleran's hypothesis.

Rather, the sum of the observations reviewed here supports the view that microsomal heme oxygenase is a discrete enzyme protein which in the native state may be considered an "apoenzyme" having a specific requirement for heme binding in order to become catalytically active. The "holoenzyme" thus formed becomes capable of binding molecular $O_2$ and acting enzymatically as a membrane-bound "oxygenase."

## 1.4. Factors Regulating Heme Degradation

### 1.4.1. Heme (Hemoglobin, Hematin, Methemalbumin)

As early as 1949 Sjörstrand noted that the percentage of carboxy-hemoglobin in blood is elevated in patients with increased rates of erythrocyte degradation. This finding suggested that the source of carbon monoxide in blood is hemoglobin, and permitted the inference that the rate of heme degradation is induced in the presence of hemolysis. The later observations of Coburn *et al.* (1966) that in these patients the rate of carbon monoxide production is also elevated further indicated that carbon monoxide is a degradative product of hemoglobin and in retrospect that endogenous heme serves to induce an enzyme system leading to increased heme degradation. The studies of Gray *et al.* (1958) established that the carbon monoxide produced from the *in vivo* breakdown of hemoglobin originates exclusively from the $\alpha$-methene bridge of the heme molecule. Coburn and co-workers (1967) provided more direct evidence for increased heme degradation activity in the presence of excess hemoglobin by showing that carbon monoxide production in experimental animals, following injection of damaged erythrocytes, is increased by 400% over the baseline value within 3 to 4 hr after treatment. Later in 1970 Tenhunen *et al.* showed that when rats were treated with hemoglobin or methemalbumin hepatic heme oxygenase activity was, in fact, increased by two- to sevenfold and experimental hemolytic anemia in rats also caused a three- to fivefold increase in hepatic heme oxidation activity. Pimstone *et al.* (1971a) studied the induction of heme oxygenase by hemoglobin in nonhepatic cells and demonstrated that the enzyme in kidney tubular epithelial cells, but not in glomeruli, is also substantially induced by hemoglobin. The induction of heme oxygenase in renal tissue by hemoglobin requires *de novo* synthesis of protein since this induction is minimized or blocked by actinomycin D or puromycin when administered prior to or shortly after administration of hemoglobin (Pimstone *et al.*, 1971a).

An interesting finding in reference to the induction of heme oxygenase in the kidney by hemoglobin was that of DeSchepper and Vander Stock (1971). These investigators showed that there was an apparent sex difference in the basal level of heme oxygenase activity in the intact dog, as indicated by the daily excretion of bilirubin in the urine—with that of the male dog being somewhat higher than that of the female. There was also a pronounced difference in the urinary excretion of bilirubin in the urine of animals following the injection of excess amounts of hemoglobin, with the urinary bilirubin excretion of the male animals increasing by nearly 30-fold, whereas that of the females increased only by one- to threefold. It was established that there was a true sex difference in the rate of conversion of hemoglobin to bilirubin in renal tissue by carrying out experiments in perfused dog kidneys, in the presence of high hemoglobin concentrations (>50 mg/100 ml). In this system they also found a marked increase in the rate of heme degradation in the kidneys of all male animals whereas in the kidneys from females the increase in bilirubin production was observed in less than 20% of the animals.

The induction of heme oxygenase by heme compounds has been observed in many cell types and tissues. It has been demonstrated that heme compounds, such as methemalbumin, also have inducing effects on the enzymatic activity of peritoneal macrophages (Pimstone et al., 1971b). There are indications that heme oxygenase is induced by heme compounds in the brain and in the arachnoid and choroid plexes (Roost et al., 1972). Maines and Cohn (1977) have demonstrated that such is the case with intact skin as well. In the latter studies it was interesting to note that the induction of heme oxygenase in skin by hemoglobin and by heme occurred locally at the site of injection and did not extend to the skin distant from the site of injection. Moreover, when skin was injured by bruising, which releases hemoglobin and myoglobin, there was most pronounced induction of heme oxidation activity at the site of injury. The induction of heme oxygenase activity of skin by factors such as hemoglobin and myoglobin may be partially due to the response of skin fibroblasts to the stimuli since under normal conditions these cells constitute the bulk of skin cells. Moreover, it has been shown that this enzyme activity is inducible in cultured human skin fibroblasts as well. In these studies, when skin fibroblasts were treated for 24 hr with heme there was a three- to four-fold increase observed in heme oxygenase activity (Kappas, Maines, and Sassa, unpublished observations). However, when skin heme oxygenase activity is increased as a result of stimuli such as tissue injury, the response is undoubtedly a more complex phenomenon because of changes in the cell composition of injured skin through proliferation or migration of macrophages, and so on.

Among other tissues in which induction of heme oxygenase activity by hemoglobin and heme compounds has been noted are cultured rat parenchymal and sinusoidal cells (Bissell *et al.*, 1972) and cultured chick liver embryo cells (Maines and Sinclair, 1977). It is noteworthy that the heme oxygenase activity of spleen is not induced by heme compounds (Maines and Kappas, 1975a). A plausible explanation for the lack of induction of spleen heme oxygenase activity is that spleen heme oxidation activity may have already reached the limit of its capacity to synthesize increased amounts of the enzyme as a response to the high concentrations of hemoglobin in the tissue under normal conditions.

An important consequence of the inducibility of heme oxygenase by heme and hemoglobin is its probable association with the development of hyperbilirubinemia in the newborn. Animal studies show that the rate of hepatic heme oxygenase activity in newborn rats immediately after birth is high, reaching levels three to five times that of the adult values during the first week postpartum (Maines and Kappas, 1975c; Thaler *et al.*, 1972). During the first week postpartum skin heme oxygenase activity is also elevated several-fold over adult levels (Maines and Cohn, 1977). These findings suggest that in the newborn increased rates of heme oxidation activity in different organs could be a significant contributing factor to the development of postpartum jaundice. This factor would operate, in addition to the well-known depressed levels of hepatic UDP glucuronyl transferase activity (Levi *et al.*, 1969b), to exaggerate the degree of jaundice occurring at this stage of development. The high levels of heme oxygenase activity in the newborn could be due to the presence of higher levels of hemoglobin in the circulation at this time of development.

### 1.4.2. Metals

The discovery (Maines and Kappas, 1974b) that trace metals regulate synthesis of heme oxygenase and other enzymes involved in heme metabolism (Maines and Kappas, 1975b–d; Maines *et al.*, 1976; Maines, 1977) provided a major new impetus for studies of the biology of this essential pigment and its relation to a number of critical cellular functions. The first metal which was shown to have an inductive effect on microsomal heme oxygenase was cobalt. Divalent cobalt when administered to rats was found to cause a striking increase in the activity of this hepatic enzyme system. This effect, shown to result from *de novo* enzyme induction, was found not to be limited to the liver, but extended to other organs studied such as kidney, heart, lung, and intestine (Maines and Kappas, 1975d,e). In addition, intact skin (Maines and Cohn, 1977), cultured chick embryo hepatic and renal cells (Maines and Sinclair, 1977), and cultured skin fibroblasts (Kappas, Maines, and Sassa, unpublished observations) were responsive to the heme oxygenase-inducing action of cobalt as well. Cobalt was unable to induce heme oxygenase in the spleen and in brain.

Heme oxygenase-inducing activity was subsequently shown to extend to other metals studied, i.e., $Cr^{2+}$, $Mn^{2+}$, $Fe^{2+,3+}$, $Ni^{2+}$, $Cu^{1+,2+}$, $Zn^{2+}$, $Cd^{2+}$, $Hg^{2+}$, $Pb^{2+}$, $Sn^{2+}$ (Maines and Kappas, 1976a; Kappas and Maines, 1976), and recent data indicate that $Pt^{2+,4+}$ (Maines and Kappas, 1977c) and Se (Maines and Kappas, 1976b) also induce this enzyme. An important observation from these studies was the finding that the potency of metals varied from one tissue to another; for example, whereas cobalt most strongly induced hepatic heme oxygenase activity (7- to 12-fold), nickel, tin, and platinum were considerably more potent inducers of heme oxygenase in the kidney (10- to 30-fold). On the other hand, the ability of mercury to induce heme oxygenase activity in myocardium exceeded that of other metals studied. The effect of metals on cellular heme oxygenase activity gained wide physiological significance when it was demonstrated that as a result of metal induction of this enzyme there was marked depletion of cellular hemoproteins, particularly those of microsomal origin such as cytochrome P-450 and cellular "free heme" (Maines and Kappas, 1975d,e; Maines, 1977). The role of heme oxygenase in the *in vivo* metabolism of cellular hemoproteins is discussed in more detail in a later section of this chapter.

The potent induction effect of metals on heme oxygenase has been confirmed in studies in other laboratories in which the effect of cobalt on hepatic microsomal heme oxygenase was investigated (DeMatteis and Gibbs, 1976; DeMatteis and Unseld, 1976). The induction by cobalt of intestinal mucosal heme oxygenase as well as hepatic heme oxygenase has recently been reported by Correia and Schmid (1975).

The mechanism by which cobalt and other transition elements or heavy metals induce heme oxygenase has been examined in detail in studies from this laboratory. Trace metals having similar physiochemical properties apparently share a common mode of regulatory action on cellular heme degradation. For example, one injection of iron dextran, which by itself caused only a doubling of heme oxygenase activity, when given in combination with a small dose of cobalt (which produced only a threefold increase in enzyme activity) caused a tenfold enhancement in heme oxygenase activity. This finding indicates the existence of a synergistic effect of these closely related metals on the control of heme oxygenase formation (Maines and Kappas, 1977b).

Other studies have shown that none of the metals which cause the induction of heme oxygenase are capable of increasing the rate of enzyme activity when added directly to the incubation medium for the assay of this enzyme activity. At high concentrations some metals are in fact inhibitory to the enzyme activity *in vitro*. Further, it has been established that heme oxygenase-inducing metals do not produce an activator molecule or compound in the cell sap, since the addition of hepatic cell sap from cobalt-treated rats to the enzyme preparation does not increase the rate of enzyme activity (Maines and Kappas, 1974b). Studies with inhibitors of nucleic acid and protein synthesis indicate that the effect of the metal on heme oxygenase is a true induction phenomenon (Maines and Kappas, 1975b; Maines and Sinclair, 1977). Therefore it is apparent that in order for the metal to initiate inductive effects on this enzyme it must react with some physiological component which has a metal binding or complexing site and which is involved in the regulation of heme oxygenase synthesis.

The possibility that metals act indirectly by alteration of endogenous extracellular substances such as hormones, heme (from hemoglobin), or metabolic intermediates present in the plasma has been ruled out by studies in which it has been demonstrated that metals are effective inducers of heme oxygenase in chick liver embryo cells cultured in a synthetic medium (Maines and Sinclair, 1977). Moreover, in these preparations it was shown that the induction of heme oxygenase by metals requires *de novo* synthesis of enzyme protein since cycloheximide was inhibitory to the induction of the enzyme by metal.

One common characteristic which all heme oxygenase-inducing metals studied have in common is their ability to form stable complexes with sulfhydryl (—SH) groups. Therefore, the relationships between cellular content of —SH and the availability of free metal ions to the induction of heme oxygenase have been intensively investigated. Some of these findings are presented in Table II. Studies in whole animals have shown that

**Table II.** Blocking Effect of Cysteine and Glutathione on Induction of Heme Oxygenase and Degradation of Hepatic Hemoprotein Content, and Augmentation of Effects by Diethyl Maleate

| Treatment[a] | Heme oxygenase (nmol bilirubin/mg hr) | Cytochrome P-450 (nmol/mg) |
|---|---|---|
| Control | 1.80 | 0.72 |
| $Co^{2+}$ | 12.59 | 0.43 |
| Co and cysteine complex (1:3 M:M) | 1.52 | 0.61 |
| Co and glutathione complex (1:3 M:M) | 1.49 | 0.65 |
| Cysteine (60 min before cobalt) + $Co^{2+}$ | 1.90 | 0.70 |
| $Co^{2+}$ + cysteine (15 min after cobalt) | 1.95 | 0.69 |
| Diethyl maleate (30 min before cobalt) + $Co^{2+b}$ | 16.70 | 0.30 |

[a]Rats were treated as indicated 24 hr before killing. The dose of $CoCl_2 \cdot 6H_{20}$ was 25 $\mu$ml/100 g, sc; diethyl maleate was 0.5 ml/kg, sc; and cysteine was orally administered.
[b]12.5 $\mu$mol/100 g.

when the cellular content of glutathione (GSH) is reduced by pretreatment with agents such as diethyl maleate (Boyland and Chausseaud, 1970), the inductive effect of cobalt on enzyme activity is greatly increased (Maines and Kappas, 1976b). Also, the effects of iron, when administered in the form of iron dextran, on hepatic heme oxygenase were doubled by prior depletion of cellular GSH content (Maines and Kappas, 1977b). Conversely, when animals were given an oral dose of cysteine (1 hr) before metal ($Co^{2+}$, $Ni^{2+}$) treatment, the effect of the metal was totally blocked; in addition, when rats were orally treated with cysteine shortly after injection with cobalt the effect of the metal on the enzyme was prevented. Cobalt and nickel are totally ineffective in inducing heme oxygenase when injected in the trivalent state (obtained by complexing the metals covalently with GSH or cysteine in a 1:3 molar ratio of metal to the thiol agent), prior to their administration to animals (Maines and Kappas, 1976a, 1977b). The involvement of cellular thiol compounds such as GSH in the regulation of heme oxygenase by metals has been substantiated in cell culture studies in which it has been shown that the presence of diethyl maleate highly intensified the chick embryo liver cell heme oxygenase response to cobalt (Maines and Sinclair, 1977).

These findings make clear that cellular sulfhydryl-containing compounds serve as a protective mechanism against the action of metals by binding the free metal ion; and, on the other hand, suggest that the metal, in order to initiate the induction effect on heme oxygenase, must react directly with some cellular component which has a metal binding or complexing site and which is involved in the regulation of heme oxygenase synthesis. This cellular component (regulator site) which binds ionic metal must either directly complex the metal—in which case the regulator site would reside either on the membranes of the endoplasmic reticulum or at the cell nucleus (or both)—or, alternatively, the possibility must be considered that heme oxygenase-inducing metals may, in the course of forming an intracellular complex of nonspecific type, indirectly induce heme oxygenase by depleting some regulatory system of an essential component involved in repressing synthesis of the enzyme, or synthesis of some substance controlling its activity. In the latter case, the following mechanism may be postulated for the mode of action of metals to induce heme oxygenase. There may exist a repressor component in the regulatory mechanism of heme oxygenase fraction, and this repressor is an —SH active constituent, the oxidation–reduction capacity of which is necessary for controlling heme oxygenase production. If the oxidation–reduction cycle of the —SH groups of this component is blocked, as would occur after treatment with cobalt and related metals, the regulatory function of this cellular constituent on heme oxygenase would be lost. The system would then function without repressive regulation, leading to an exaggerated synthesis of the enzyme. This high level of enzyme production would continue until more repressor is synthesized, the metal is excreted, or its effective concentration is reduced by complexing with nonregulatory —SH-containing cell components.

At this time, it is impossible to define the precise mechanism by which metals induce heme oxygenase in tissues of man. However, at this point it can be inferred that metals are in fact the physiological regulators of heme oxygenase, and therefore, the induction of heme oxygenase by heme results from a regulatory action of the central iron metal of this metalloporphyrin, rather than an action of the intact metalloporphyrin molecule. Other factors such as endotoxins and metabolic agents which alter heme oxygenase activity could obviously act indirectly by altering intracellular flux or concentrations of trace metals as is known to occur, for example, in infectious disease states in man.

### 1.4.3. Hormonal and Metabolic Factors

There has been considerable interest in the effects of steroids on heme metabolism. This interest has been mainly directed toward the effects of steroid hormones on heme synthesis (Granick and Kappas, 1967; Kappas and Granick, 1968) and bile pigment transport and excretion, and there is no current evidence, with the possible exception of De Schepper and Vander Stock's (1971) studies, indicating that steroid sex hormones play a role in cellular heme oxidation and formation of bile pigments. The effects of sex steroids on the drug-metabolizing microsomal enzyme system are well known, and as the glucuronidation pathway is closely related to this enzyme system, the alterations brought about by steroids on conjugation aspects of bile pigments are not surprising. It is reported that steroid levels in newborn blood and urine are very high (Mitchell, 1967) and that steroids inhibit the enzyme bilirubin UDP glucuronyl acid transferase by competing with UDP glucuronic acid (Adlard and Lathe, 1970) which is already low in infants (Dutton, 1959). This may lead to increased plasma concentration of bilirubin. It is known that during pregnancy there are great alterations in maternal plasma levels of steroid hormones and steroid composition, and these may be reflected in the activities of microsomal drug-metabolizing enzymes. However, pregnancy has no significant effect on hepatic microsomal heme oxygenase activity in rats (Maines and Kappas, 1975c). Moreover, when male rats are castrated, there is no alteration observed in hepatic heme oxygenase activity when compared to sham operated rats. This is in contrast to the marked decrease in the activity of the hepatic microsomal drug-metabolizing system and of the content of its terminal oxidase, cytochrome P-450. Also, in castrated rats there is no significant difference in the magnitude of the induction response of hepatic microsomal heme oxygenase (Maines, unpublished observations) to cobalt. Bakken *et al.* (1972) also did not note any effect of ovariectomy on hepatic heme oxygenase activity of rats. In contrast to steroids, adrenal medullary hormones and factors which alter cellular glucose metabolism have been reported to affect microsomal heme oxygenase systems. Bakken *et al.* (1972) studied the effects of a number of such agents on hepatic heme oxygenase activity in rats and they reported that hypoglycemia, induced by injection of insulin or mannose, increased hepatic heme oxygenase activity up to sevenfold. On the other hand, feeding of glucose to animals treated with insulin diminished the magnitude of the increased heme oxygenase response to insulin. Parenteral glucagon and epinephrine treatments caused a five- to sixfold increase in hepatic heme oxygenase when microsomal fractions were assayed 7 hr after injection of the hormones. In this laboratory, when hepatic microsomal heme oxygenase activity of rats treated with epinephrine for 20 hr was measured, only a 10–20% increase in heme oxygenase activity was noted. This difference in response to epinephrine could be due to an activation phenomenon observed by Bakken *et al.* (1972) produced soon after the injection of epinephrine into the rats rather than a true induction effect. The biological half-life of hepatic heme oxygenase has been determined in this laboratory to be about 24 hr (Maines, unpublished observations). Moreover, it has been noted that hepatic heme oxygenase activity following induction with metals (Maines and Kappas, 1975b) does not return to a normal value for 72 hr or longer. Therefore, the idea that the epinephrine-mediated increase in heme oxygenase is a true induction phenomenon remains open to question. Bakken *et al.* (1972) also reported that AMP and cyclic AMP increased hepatic heme oxygenase activity 7 hr after injection by two- to threefold. In contrast hormones such as thyroxine and hydrocortisone, as well as glucose in drinking water, had no effect on hepatic heme oxygenase activity. It is of particular interest that of all the agents tested by a number of investigators, only cyclic nucleotides, AMP and db (dibutyryl) AMP, and glucagon cause increases in splenic heme oxygenase activity (two- to threefold).

Somewhat different results of an apparently contradicting nature were obtained when similar experiments were conducted on the effect of various hormonal factors on induction of heme oxygenase in peritoneal macrophages by engulfed erythrocytes (Gemsa *et al.*, 1974, 1975). In these studies it was noted that although the erythrophagocytic action of the macrophages for antibody-coated erythrocytes was not altered by the addition of the nucleotides AMP, cyclic AMP, db cyclic AMP, or theophylline, the extent of induction of heme oxygenase as a response to engulfed erythrocytes was decreased in a dose-related manner with the nucleotide, with concentrations greater than 1 mM greatly inhibiting the induction response. No inhibition of induction was observed at concentrations of nucleotides in the range 10–100 $\mu$M. Theophylline at concentrations of 100–1000 $\mu$M was inhibitory to the induction response. Epinephrine and isoproterenol (500 $\mu$M) decreased the extent of induction by about 50% Epinephrine was by far a less effective inhibitor of induction of heme oxygenase, and at high concentrations (500 $\mu$M) reduced the induction response by only about 25%. Several prostaglandins were also found inhibitory to the induction of heme oxygenase by engulfed erythrocytes, with prostaglandins $E_1$ (PGE$_1$) being the most effective. The incorporation of [$^{14}$C]leucine into macrophage proteins was decreased by 10–20% in the presence of 1mM concentration of cyclic nucleotides and theophylline, and by 10–15% in the presence of 10 $\mu$M PGE$_1$ and 500 $\mu$M epinephrine. The results reported by Gemsa *et al.* (1975) regarding the suppressive effect of cyclic nucleotides and related agents on induction of heme oxygenase in this system not only contrast with the inductive effects of such agents in liver but must be interpreted cautiously in relation to their significance for the physiological mode of regulation of heme oxygenase since extremely large concentrations of nucleotides and other compounds were used to obtain relatively small variations in the measured parameters.

Although a causal relationship between the rise in cyclic AMP and the suppression of substrate-mediated induction of heme oxygenase was suggested by Gemsa *et al.* (1974, 1975), it has been observed (Maines, unpublished observations) that pretreatment of rats with high concentrations of theophylline before cobalt induction of heme oxygenase does not alter the extent of induction.

An interesting and controversial factor which has been studied by several laboratories relates to the effect on the heme oxygenase system and bile pigment formation of starvation or caloric intake and the ultimate relationship of blood glucose levels and hormonal regulation to heme oxygenase activity. Bakken *et al.* (1971) reported that when newborn or adult rats were fasted for 6 hr and 3 days, respectively, there was a two- to threefold increase in hepatic heme oxygenase activity relative to the controls. Refeeding of these animals returned hepatic heme oxygenase activity to normal in 6 to 24 hr, respectively. This finding suggested to these authors that hormones associated with hypoglycemia may mediate the increase in the level of heme oxidation activity. Accordingly, rats were injected intraperitoneally with glucagon and epinephrine and a twofold increase of heme oxygenase activity was obtained 7 hr after injection. These results were interpreted to indicate that fasting induces heme oxygenase in hepatocytes, and glucagon and epinephrine reproduce and accelerate the effects of fasting. These findings further suggested to

Bakken *et al.* (1971) that increased enzyme activity is due to one or both of these hormones which are released during hypoglycemia or depletion of glucagon. However, Rothwell *et al.* (1973) reported an observation which was quite different from that of the former group in respect to the effect of starvation on heme oxygenase activity. The latter demonstrated that in adult rats starvation for 24 hr causes only a 30–40% increase in hepatic heme oxygenase activity; however, by 48 hr the activity falls below normal, and 3 days of starvation causes a nearly 30–40% reduction in hepatic heme oxygenase activity when compared to the baseline values.

Bensinger *et al.* (1973) studied the effect of a low caloric diet in normal young adults (male and female) and patients with Gilbert's syndrome, on endogenous carbon monoxide production and plasma levels of bilirubin. They found that 48 hr of a low caloric intake (consisting of 400 cal/24 hr, with a composition of 46% carbohydrate and 15% each of protein and fat) did not change the rate of carbon monoxide production in normal subjects or in patients with Gilbert's syndrome. However, there was an 80% increase in the concentration of unconjugated plasma bilirubin in the normals and a 200% increase in the patients with Gilbert's syndrome. These findings indicate that fasting and caloric restriction do not increase the rate of heme turnover but rather that these circumstances (caloric restriction) primarily interfere with the plasma clearance of bilirubin. It should be recalled that the synthesis and activity of UDP glucuronyl transferase is a function of the microsomal enzyme system closely related to the activity of the mixed-function oxidase complex which metabolizes drugs; and the activity of the latter system is known to be susceptible to caloric intake and the composition of diet in man (Kappas *et al.*, 1976; Conney *et al.*, 1976; Alvares *et al.*, 1976). In contrast to the conclusion reached by Bensinger *et al.* as to the lack of an effect of caloric intake restriction on the turnover rate of heme, Lundh *et al.* (1972) reported that consumption of 360 cal/24 hr (evenly distributed) in the form of skimmed milk caused a 68% increase in the endogenous rate of carbon monoxide production in healthy adults. A close examination of these two studies revealed no difference in the technical aspects of CO measurements; however, there was a difference in the composition of the diets. Most importantly, though, in the Lundh *et al.* study, apparently the basal levels of CO production were measured a few weeks earlier than the time the measurement of CO production as a response to caloric intake was done. Since there is a considerable variation for normal males and females in the rates of endogenous carbon monoxide production both between individuals and within each individual (Lynch and Moede, 1972), it is possible that the data obtained by Lundh *et al.* may have been reflective of these factors.

### 1.4.4. Effect of Endotoxins and Drugs on Heme Degradation

Bacterial endotoxins were reported by Edington and Kampschmidt (1968) to increase bilirubin production in rats 24 hr after intraperitoneal administration. In these animals the ability of the liver to conjugate bilirubin was not affected, indicating that the induction of heme degradation activity caused by the endotoxin accounted for the increase in bilirubin production. Gemsa *et al.* (1974) confirmed this effect of endotoxins on heme degradation activity reported by Edington and Kampschmidt and showed that hepatic heme oxygenase activity in the whole liver of endotoxin-treated rats is about fourfold higher than in control animals. Edington and Kampschmidt (1968) also reported an increase in plasma bilirubin concentrations in rats 7 days after intramuscular transplants of Walker carcinoma 256. The mechanism by which endotoxins produce induction of heme oxygenase activity in whole animals is not clear. Endotoxins may induce heme oxygenase indirectly through alterations in a number of physiological parameters, which could be expected since endotoxins are well known to produce widespread physiological changes in animals. Moreover, under diseased states such as infections, there are well-documented changes in plasma and cellular contents of metals, and it would not be unreasonable to suppose that injection of bacterial endotoxins could easily cause changes in the cellular and plasma concentrations of metals, which regulate heme oxygenase.

A number of drugs and chemicals have been studied in regard to their effects on microsomal heme oxygenase activity and bile pigment formation. Drugs produce mainly three types of hepatic disorders which are related to heme catabolism activity. One type of dysfunction would result from alterations in cellular metabolism of heme; another type would result from alterations in cell and plasma clearance of bilirubin; lastly, a drug may produce a mixed type heme–bile pigment aberration comprising both features. Chemicals and drugs which produce the first types of dysfunctions are of main concern in this chapter.

Carbon tetrachloride ($CCl_4$) is a known hepatotoxin which destroys hepatic parenchymal cells and markedly reduces oxidative and other hepatic cell functions such as drug-metabolizing activities (Castro *et al.*, 1968). This hepatotoxin has been studied in this laboratory regarding its effect on hepatic microsomal heme oxygenase activity. Rats were treated with $CCl_4$ (0.1 ml/100 g) for 24 hr. In contrast to the drug-metabolizing activity of liver, which was reduced greatly, hepatic microsomal heme oxidation activity in these animals was somewhat increased (approximately two times) by such treatment, indicating that heme oxygenase enzyme protein is not as susceptible to destruction by free radicals (which are believed to be produced by $CCl_4$ metabolites) as is the microsomal mixed-function oxidase system. The effect of another lipid-soluble compound carbon disulfide ($CS_2$), which decreases drug-metabolizing activity, on hepatic microsomal heme oxygenase was also investigated. Rats were given an oral dose of $CS_2$ (0.1 ml/100 g) or intraperitoneally injected with the compound once. After 24 hr a three- to fivefold increase in microsomal heme oxygenase activity was noted. Carbon disulfide simultaneously decreased other oxidative functions of microsomal fractions of liver such as drug-metabolizing activity by 50–60%. The mechanism by which carbon disulfide increases heme oxygenase activity is not known; but in addition to the possible direct action of compounds on heme oxygenase or on the regulation of its synthesis, it is plausible to believe that $CS_2$ may indirectly bring about alterations in heme oxygenase as a result of direct effects on other physiological parameters, such as cellular levels of heme, rates of heme synthesis, or on other factors such as plasma levels of hemoglobin—as a result, for example, of changes in RBC membrane permeability.

A number of drugs used therapeutically are known to alter cellular heme metabolism. Interestingly, the rate of enzymatic heme degradation is not subject to change by drugs to the same extent as is the activity of the P-450-dependent drug-metabolizing enzyme system. Barbiturates, for example, are one class of drugs whose effects on the mixed-function enzyme system have been used as the prototype for a number of drugs. Polycyclic hydrocarbon carcinogens such as 3-methylcholanthrene (3-MC) represent another type of modifier of microsomal drug-metabolizing activities (Conney, 1967). Accordingly, several laboratories have studied the effects of these classes of compounds, particularly the effects of phenobarbital, on the heme degradation pathway. The general view is that phenobarbital does not induce hepatic heme oxygenase activity. These studies include the original investigations by Tenhunen et al. (1969a) on phenobarbital effects on hepatic heme oxygenase; that of Schacter and Mason (1974) on the effect of phenobarbital, 3-MC, and 3,4-benzo(a)pyrene on splenic heme oxygenase; and that of Blaschke et al. (1974) who studied the influence of phenobarbital on various aspects of heme metabolism in man, including the rate of CO production, bilirubin clearance, and plasma turnover. In none of these studies was any induction in the rate of heme oxidation activity noted. Actually, studies by Maines and Kappas (1975d) have demonstrated that treatment of rats with phenobarbital causes a somewhat decreased rate of hepatic heme oxygenase activity. It should be noted that although phenobarbital does not increase the rate of this microsomal enzyme activity, it does alter heme metabolizing activity, mainly by altering the hepatic clearance of bilirubin and its rate of conjugation with glucuronic acid (Robinson, 1968; Yaffe *et al.*, 1966; Arias *et al.*, 1969) and by increasing the rate of synthesis of hepatic heme (Schmid *et al.*, 1966; Israel *et al.*, 1966; Robinson *et al.*, 1966). The effects of other compounds, which are known to alter microsomal drug-metabolizing enzymes, on the microsomal heme oxygenase system have also been investigated including compounds such as the barbiturate analog allylisopropylacetamide (AIA) and dicarbethoxydihydrocollidine (DDC). Rothwell *et al.* (1973), Maines and Kappas (1975d), and Maines *et al.* (1976) noted that these two potent porphyrinogenic agents do not change the levels of microsomal heme oxygenase activity. DeMatteis and Unseld (1976) utilizing AIA made similar findings. Acute intoxication with α-naphthylisothiol cyanate (ANIT) has been shown to cause hyperbilirubinemia in animals (Eliakim *et al.*, 1959); this compound also causes alterations in the hepatic microsomal drug-metabolizing system (Plaa *et al.*, 1965). Several hypotheses have been offered as to the mechanism by which hyperbilirubinemia is produced by ANIT. The data obtained by Roberts and Plaa (1968) indicate that enhanced excretion of bilirubin, as a result of ANIT treatment, coincided with increased incorporation of hepatic heme precursor (δ-aminolevulinate) into bilirubin, strongly supporting the view that an increase in the rate of hepatic heme oxygenase activity is produced by ANIT.

## 1.5. Catabolism of Heme Compounds *in Vivo*

### 1.5.1. Hemoglobin

Hemoglobin in average humans produces about 200–250 mg of bilirubin a day; of this, 80–85% is derived from the breakdown of hemoglobin heme (London *et al.*, 1950) in senescent erythrocytes. It is well known that aging erythrocytes are destroyed in the reticuloendothelial system, specifically in spleen, bone marrow, lung, liver, and peritoneal macrophages (Rich, 1925). Spleen with its high cellular population of reticulocytes is very active in the degradation of senescent erythrocytes, and this organ is also effective in the removal of intravascular hemoglobin since in the presence of hemolysis there is an extensive splenomegaly observed (Tenhunen *et al.*, 1970). Injected hemoglobin, when administered in small doses, i.e., in doses not exceeding the binding capacity of plasma haptoglobin for hemoglobin, is quantitatively converted to bilirubin. In contrast, when hemoglobin is injected in large doses or when antibody-sensitized red blood cells are administered, only 65–80% of administered heme is recovered as bilirubin (Ostrow *et al.*, 1962). Moreover, it appears that the degradation of heme produces an equimolar ratio of carbon monoxide to bilirubin under normal conditions (Landaw et al., 1970; Coburn et al., 1967); but under certain conditions which were discussed earlier, such as treatment with allylisopropylacetamide and related compounds, this ratio changes such that the value exceeds unity (Landaw et al., 1970).

Recently more detailed aspects of hemoglobin metabolism, such as the role of cells other than reticuloendothelial cells, in the metabolism of hemoglobin and erythrocytes and the influence of a binding protein on the degradation of heme have been investigated. Bissell et al. (1972), utilizing $^{59}$Fe-labeled RBC in a preparation of isolated rat liver parenchymal and sinusoidal cells, studied the cellular site of erythrocyte and hemoglobin metabolism. It was noted that the site of ingestion of intact RBC was a subpopulation of sinusoidal cells—named erythrophagocytes—whereas the dissolved hemoglobin, free or hepatoglobin bound, was mainly detected in parenchymal cells. Heme oxygenase activity was present both in the parenchymal and the sinusoidal cells, although under normal conditions the heme oxygenase activity of sinusoidal cells is apparently 10 to 20 times greater than that of parenchymal cells (Hupka and Karler, 1973). Bissell et al. (1972) also demonstrated, using double-labeled heme and protein, that, whereas the intact hemoglobin molecule is removed by isolated parenchymal cells, when heme–albumin was presented to the cells, heme was detached from albumin before it was taken in by the cells. This was in accordance with the earlier observation made by Muller-Eberhard and co-workers (1969) who observed that when heme bound to human albumin was injected into rabbits, there was transfer of heme from albumin to rabbit hemopexin prior to the removal of the heme–albumin complex from the circulation. The transfer of heme from heme–albumin to hemopexin was detected as early as 3 min after injection of heme–albumin. Moreover, the plasma levels of hemopexin were elevated as a response to the administration of heme to the rabbits, although the most rapid increase was observed when the amount of heme was below the binding capacity of hemopexin for heme.

The ability to remove dissolved hemoglobin and degrade its heme moiety is shared by a number of anatomically distinct types of cells; for example, the epithelial cells of small intestine were shown to be able to remove hemoglobin from dietary sources and to metabolize its heme moiety to release iron (Turnbull et al., 1962). Weintraub et al. in 1968 demonstrated that the epithelial mucosa of small intestine of dog behaves like that of man with respect to the absorption of dietary hemoglobin. They detected the presence of an enzyme which they referred to as "heme splitting" enzyme in the mucosal homogenate. This protein had a molecular weight greater than 64,000 and could degrade the heme of hemoglobin to release iron. The heme-splitting enzyme of Weintraub et al. could well be the same enzyme that is now referred to as "heme oxygenase." Raffin *et al.* (1974) confirmed this finding by demonstrating that heme, in the form of the heme–albumin complex, is metabolized *in vitro* by epithelial cells of rat small intestine to release iron and form bilirubin. Raffin *et al.* also noted that the rate of heme oxygenase activity of microsomal fractions prepared from the intestinal mucosa of iron-deficient rats was increased by two- to threefold in the duodenal and jejunal sections of the small intestine and that the hemoglobin iron absorption from these sections of intestine was increased. It is interesting that there is no evidence that prolonged ingestion of large amounts of hemoglobin or prolonged consumption of high hemoglobin diets induces heme oxygenase or fractional hemoglobin iron absorption in the gut. Therefore, it appears reasonable to speculate that the rate of intestinal heme oxygenase activity, and consequently release of iron from the ingested heme molecules, is principally a function of the physiological need for the metal.

The degradation of RBC by bone marrow in certain pathological disorders becomes a major source of bile pigments. For example, in certain kinds of anemias such as pernicious anemia and primary refractory anemia as well as thalassemia (in which conditions the degradation rate of immature RBC is increased due to ineffective erythropoiesis) there is also a marked increase in bile pigment and carbon monoxide derived from bone marrow (White *et al.,* 1967; London and West, 1950). Moreover, bone marrow appears to be another tissue in which the presence of hemoglobin per se does not appear to regulate the rate of heme degradation; reticulocytes in the peripheral blood also show this property. Again, in these tissues other factors seem to be involved in the regulation of this activity. White (1969) has shown that the heme oxidation activity in aspirated bone marrow cells of patients with sideroblastic anemia is more than seven times greater than the heme oxidizing activity of normal subjects. Moreover, it was established that this increased heme degradation activity reflects the actual cellular heme degradation rate rather than being a manifestation of increased extracellular availability of substrate due to hemolysis. Although the heme degradation activity of the reticulocytes in peripheral blood was considerably lower than that of the bone marrow, in the patients with sideroblastic anemia or thalassemia, heme degradation activity was nearly 11 times higher than that of the controls.

## 1.5.2. Microsomal Cytochromes

As was mentioned earlier approximately 80–85% of the bilirubin produced in a day is derived from the breakdown of RBC hemoglobin. The remaining 15–20% originates from the breakdown of nonerythropoietic heme, such as cytochromes and myoglobin. In 1964 Schwartz *et al.* reported that in bile fistula dogs 20% of an administered dose of [$^{14}$C]aminolevulinic acid (ALA) (a heme precursor which almost exclusively labels nonhemoglobin heme) was excreted in the bile in the form of bilirubin 3–6 hr after injection. Israel *et al.* (1963) studied the incorporation of [$^{14}$C]glycine (a precursor of both hemoglobin and nonerythropoietic heme) into bilirubin in bile fistula dogs and normal humans. They reported the existence of an early labeled bilirubin peak in the bile or plasma which occurred 12–24 hr after injection; this activity clearly could not have had an erythropoietic origin because of the long half-life of RBC. A second and larger peak which occurred in 3–5 days corresponded with the rate of RBC formation. This pattern of bilirubin formation varied significantly from that observed by Yamamoto *et al.* (1965) utilizing [$^{14}$C]ALA as heme precursor, which, as just noted, is preferentially incorporated into nonhemoglobin heme. The latter group observed that when [$^{14}$C]ALA was used as heme precursor instead of glycine, only a single sharp peak of radioactivity was observed in the bile, which reached its maximum in 1 hr, indicating a nonerythroid source of bilirubin in the bile and pointing to the rapid turnover rate of nonhemoglobin heme and its metabolism *in vivo*. Robinson *et al.* (1966) studied the source of this "early labeled" bilirubin further; they indicated that in man this fraction accounts for 13% of the total labeled pigment produced from injected [$^{14}$C]glycine and suggested that the origin of the early labeled peak is liver heme. The work of Schmid *et al.* (1966) refined this point further and indicated microsomal hemoproteins as the source of this peak. Moreover, they demonstrated that in phenobarbital-treated rats, the increase in microsomal cytochromes (cytochromes P-450 and $b_5$) closely paralleled the formation of bilirubin from the heme precursor [$^{14}$C]glycine.

A theoretical formulation of heme transfer and catabolism in liver was proposed in 1973 by Maines and Anders who, on the basis of a series of studies involving the transfer of heme from microsomal hemoproteins to heme binding proteins, proposed that in order for the heme of cytochrome P-450 to be degraded, the cytochrome must first be converted to its nonreactive form, i.e., P-420, the heme of which would then be oxidatively degraded by the microsomal heme oxygenase (Maines and Anders, 1973b, Maines *et al.*, 1974). Cytochrome P-450 constitutes more than two-thirds of the hepatic microsmal hemoproteins and has a half-life of 8–12 hr in comparison to that of cytochrome $b_5$, which has a half-life of 24–36 hr and constitutes the other one-third of microsomal hemoproteins. Of the two hemoproteins, cytochrome P-450 has been more intensively studied and has attracted wide interest, since it is the terminal oxidase of the drug-metabolizing system which biotransforms drugs and steroids. The fact that cytochrome P-450 was initially believed to be essential for the function of heme oxygenase (Schmid, 1972; Tenhunen *et al.*, 1972), but was later shown not to be involved in this enzyme action (Maines and Kappas, 1974b in liver; Yoshida *et al.*, 1974 in spleen) added new dimensions to the study of this hemoprotein. In the course of experiments dissociating the oxidation of heme from cytochrome P-450 in liver (Maines and Kappas, 1975b) it was noted that the induction of heme oxygenase was followed by a reduction in the microsomal content of hemoproteins (P-450 and $b_5$) and the cellular content of heme. Although the original observation was made utilizing cobalt, this observation has been extended to a number of metals which include various divalent or transition elements as well as several heavy metals and trace elements; among these are Cr, Mn, Fe, Co, Ni, Cu, Zn, Cd, Sn, Pt, Hg, Pb, and Se. Moreover, this induction of heme oxygenase and the subsequent decrease in microsomal hemoprotein was observed in other tissues as well (e.g., kidney and heart) (Maines and Kappas, 1975d,e; 1976a,b, 1977b; Kappas and Maines, 1976). The effect of metals on cellular heme metabolism and the relationship between heme synthesis and heme degradation were studied in great detail using the prototype element, cobalt. It was noted that the reduction in the microsomal heme and cytochrome P-450 which occurred following metal administration took place within the framework of normal levels of cellular heme synthesis activity, as indicated by the presence of normal or above-normal activities of $\delta$-aminolevulinic acid synthetase, ALAS (following a transient inhibition of this enzyme), as well as normal ferrochelatase activity and total porphyrin contents (Maines and Kappas, 1975b,e; 1976b, 1977b; Maines *et al.*, 1976). ALAS is the initial and rate-limiting enzyme of the heme biosynthetic sequence and ferrochelatase is the terminal enzyme of the pathway.

These findings clearly demonstrated that an increased rate of heme oxygenase activity is responsible for the increased rate of microsomal heme degradation, rather than the former being due to a decreased rate of heme synthesis. The concept that hepatic microsomal cytochrome P-450 and heme are degraded by microsomal heme oxygenase was further substantiated (Maines and Kappas, 1975e; Maines, 1976, 1977) in studies in which the formation of bilirubin from microsomal heme was measured in bile fistula rats under experimental conditions in which the sequence of induction of heme oxygenase and injection of [14C]ALA was altered. It was noted that in animals in which heme oxygenase was induced prior to the injection of labeled ALA the biliary excretion of bile pigment and 14C activity was immediate, whereas in animals in which the microsomal heme was prelabeled and who then were treated with heme oxygenase inducer ($Co^{2+}$), there was a lag period before the peak of excretion of 14C activity into the bile. The lag period corresponded with the length of time required for the induction of hepatic heme oxygenase (2 hr). These findings indicate that not only is heme from preformed microsomal hemoprotein, including P-450, degraded by heme oxygenase but that "free heme"—that is, heme prior to its binding with various cytochromes—is degraded by microsomal heme oxygenase as well. As was mentioned earlier, apocytochrome P-450 has been shown to have a very high affinity for heme; its heme moiety is not dissociable from the cytochrome unless it is converted to the inactive form, i.e., cytochrome P-420 (Maines and Anders, 1973b; Maines et al., 1974). Accordingly, it was postulated that in order for the heme of cytochrome P-450 to be oxidized the cytochrome must first be converted to cytochrome P-420, the heme of which would be released readily. This hypothesis was tested experimentally (Maines, 1977) and it was found that indeed only the heme of cytochrome P-420 is degraded by microsomal heme oxygenase to produce bilirubin whereas the heme of cytochrome P-450 serves as substrate for heme oxygenase only after transformation of P-450 to P-420. Thus, in order for cytochrome P-450 to be degraded *in vivo* by heme oxygenase, the cytochrome must first be converted to its inactive form in which the heme moiety is more labile; there is, therefore, a necessity for the existence of an intermediary factor in cells involved in the conversion of cytochrome P-450 to P-420. This intermediary factor must be a P-450 denaturing agent or a process which facilitates the conversion of P-450 to its inactive form. The increased rate of microsomal P-450 degradation produced by cobalt and other inducers of heme oxygenase thus not only could be due to an increased rate of heme degradation, but may also involve the additional factor of an increased rate of conversion of P-450 to P-420. The same considerations apply to the oxidation of the heme moiety of cytochrome P-448 (Maines, 1976).

The accelerated rate of conversion of cytochrome P-450 to cytochrome P-420 by metals could be brought about through the following mechanisms: (a) by increasing the concentration of a natural component which is the endogenous "denaturant" of cytochrome P-450. This increase could be brought about by increased synthesis of this "substance" or by the release of the denaturant from a specific cellular compartment (e.g., lysosomes). (b) Metals could directly interfere with proper binding of heme to apo-P-450 which could then result in the formation of an aberrant form of the cytochrome—that is, an apoprotein which binds heme less tightly than the unaltered apo-P-450. This alteration could result from the covalent binding of metal ion at or near the receptor site(s) for the heme, with resultant changes in the protein configuration or the electronic potential of the heme binding site. (c) The last and least likely means by which the conversion of P-450 to P-420 could be accelerated by metals is a direct effect of the metal on the hemoprotein, causing its denaturation. The proposed mechanism for the catabolism of cytochrome P-450 and cytochrome P-448 and the effect of metals on this activity is schematically presented in Fig. 3.

There are some controversial data from other laboratories which indicate the presence of relationships, contrary to those described herein for heme oxygenase activity and microsomal hemoproteins, in primary cultures of rat hepatocytes (Bissell *et al.*, 1974) and in rat intestine (Correia and Schmid, 1975). Bissell *et al.* reported that in primary cultures of adult rat hepatocytes a decrease in cellular cytochrome P-450 takes place *prior* to the occurrence of an increase in heme oxygenase activity, which may be interpreted to indicate that in this system heme of cytochrome P-450 is degraded by means other than through degradation by heme oxygenase. These investigators also reported that in rats treated with [¹⁴C]ALA the

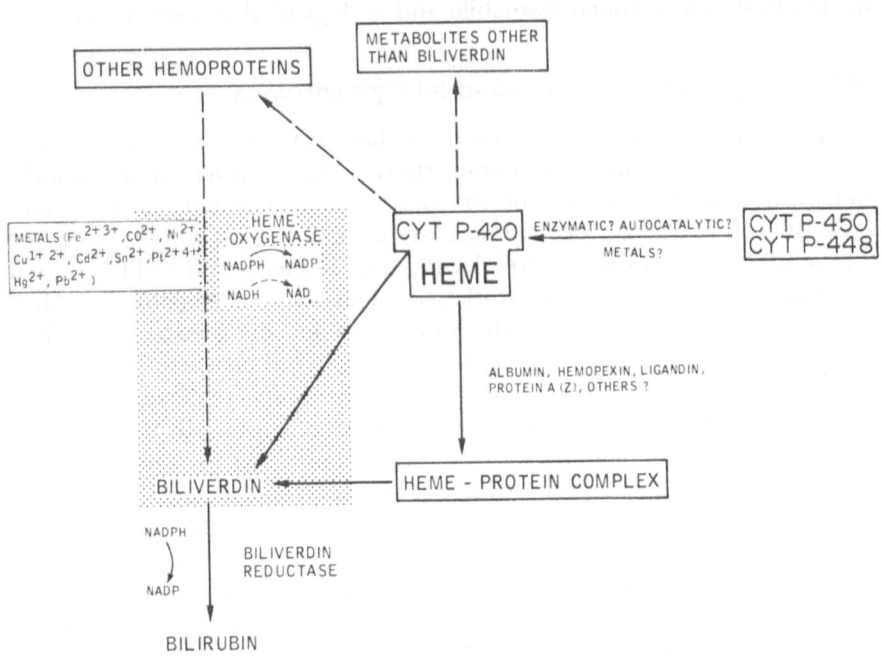

**Fig. 3.** Proposed mechanism of microsomal heme metabolism.

production of $^{14}CO$, presumably derived from degradation of cyto-chrome P-450 heme, preceded the induction of heme oxygenase by endo-toxin and heme.

A third and a totally different relationship between heme oxygenase activity and cytochrome P-450 is the observation of Correia and Schmid (1975) that in the intestinal mucosa of rat the increase in heme oxygenase by cobalt is accompanied by an increase in cytochrome P-450 content. The authors suggest that the mechanism of the cobalt-mediated stimulation of microsomal heme oxygenase in liver and intestinal mucosa either is differ-ent and/or is unrelated to the turnover of cytochrome P-450.

There has been little direct study of the metabolism of the other microsomal hemoprotein, cytochrome $b_5$. This cytochrome has a longer half-life and a lower microsomal concentration in hepatocytes than does cytochrome P-450. It is very likely that this hemoprotein is also degraded by the microsomal heme oxygenase system since it has been noted that induction of heme oxygenase results in decrease of both cytochromes P-450 and $b_5$ (Maines and Kappas, 1975b). However, due to the structural relationship between the heme of cytochrome $b_5$ and the apocytochrome, this hemoprotein is much less labile and is degraded at a slower rate.

### 1.5.3. Myoglobin and Mitochondrial Cytochromes

In contrast to the vast amount of literature documenting various aspects of hemoglobin degradation, there is little information available concerning the degradation of the hemes of myoglobin, catalase, and tryptophan pyrrolase, which contain $b$-type hemes as prosthetic group, or of hemoproteins with non-$b$-type hemes, i.e., hemes $a$ and $c$. There are a few studies concerning the degradative metabolism of cytochrome $c$ but none available concerning the fate of cytochromes of $a$ type ($a$, $a_3$). This is partly because cytochrome oxidase has resisted full characterization and purification. Beinert in 1950 reported the first study concerning the fate of injected cytochrome $c$ in rat. Prior to that time, apparently the injection of cytochrome $c$ had been used to some extent as a therapeutic procedure in man. Beinert injected rats with [$^{55}Fe$]cytochrome $c$ and 24 hr later attempted to isolate intact cytochrome $c$ and $^{55}Fe$ activity in various tissues. No intact cytochrome $c$ was detected thereafter in any organs or other physiological materials, and intact cytochrome $c$ could be detected only in the urine 2 hr after injection of the hemoprotein. On the other hand, after 24 hr a number of tissues exhibited substantial $^{55}Fe$ activity; tissues such as kidney, liver, muscle, bone, skin, blood, and spleen had high activity whereas brain, lung, gonads, heart, and thyroid gland had negligi-ble activity.

Some $^{55}Fe$ activity in part was associated with ferritin, but the bulk of the activity was associated with the residue of cytochrome $c$. This pattern of tissue distribution of [55]Fe activity may be interpreted to indicate the tissue site of cytochrome $c$ degradation; however, it does not provide any information concerning the intracellular site of heme type $c$ degradation. Schwartz *et al.* (1975) also studied the fate of [14]C-labeled cytochrome $c$ in the bile fistula dog. They noted that the total amount of [14]C injected was recovered in urine within 6 days after injection. However, no intact cytochrome was detected in the urine. The urine excreted within the first several hours after injection of cytochrome $c$ contained a green pigment which was not identifiable as biliverdin. Wise (1964), who also injected cytochrome $c$ in bile fistula rats, did not detect any increase in the bilirubin excretion in these rats. Furthermore, liberation of carbon monoxide was not detected in these studies involving cytochrome $c$ degradation in mammals. Therefore, apparently the system which degrades cytochrome $c$ is not identical with the heme oxygenase system for heme of the $b$ type. In contrast to cytochrome $c$, which is degraded to pigments other than biliverdin and bilirubin, myoglobin, which has a $b$-type heme as its prosthetic group, is metabolized in most part to form bile pigments in the same fashion as hemoglobin. Daly *et al.* (1967) administered [3]H-labeled myoglobin intravenously to bile fistula rats and noted that 75% of the injected radioactivity was recovered in bile; of this activity 80–90% was identified as bilirubin. The excretion of activity was detectable in the bile within 1 hr after injection and proceeded to increase linearly in rate up to 7 hr, with the maximum being reached in 24 hr. However, myoglobin isolated from the animals retained significant amounts of [3]H activity up to 6 months. This finding not only reflects the long half-life of myoglobin, but it may be interpreted as indicating that there may be some exchange of heme taking place among myoglobin protein molecules; also, this may be a reflection of the low heme oxygenase activity of muscle tissue. That the degradation of myoglobin is mediated by heme oxygenase is further substantiated by the recent studies of Maines and Cohn (1977) in which myoglobin when injected subcutaneously was found to be an inducer of skin microsomal heme oxygenase activity, indicating the degradation of myoglobin by the skin microsomal heme oxygenase system.

ACKNOWLEDGMENTS

I am grateful to Professor Attallah Kappas for his valuable suggestions, advice, and support of the work reported here.

I am indebted to Mrs. Patricia Macklin and in particular to Miss Ann Quatela for the typing of the manuscript.

# References

Adlard, B. P. F., and Lathe, G. H., 1970, The effect of steroids and nucleotides on solubilized bilirubin uridine diphosphate-glucuronyltransferase, *Biochemistry* **119**:437.

Alvares, A. P., Anderson, K., Cooney, A. H., and Kappas, A., 1976, Interaction of nutritional factors and drug biotransformations in man, *Proc. Nat. Acad. Sci. U.S.A.* **73**:2501–2504.

Arias, I. M., Gartner, L. M., Cohen, M., Ben Ezzer, J., and Levi, A. J., 1969, Chronic nonhemolytic unconjugated hyperbilirubinemia with glucuronyl transferase deficiency. Clinical, biochemical, pharmacologic and genetic evidence of heterogeneity, *Am. J. Med.* **47**:395.

Bakken, A. F., Thaler, M. M., Pimstone, N. R., and Schmid, R., 1971, Stimulation of hepatic heme oxygenase activity by fasting and by hormones, *Gastroenterology* **60**:177 (Abstract #1).

Bakken, A. F., Thaler, M. M., and Schmid, R., 1972, Metabolic regulation of heme catabolism and bilirubin production, *J. Clin. Invest.* **51**:530.

Beinert, H., 1950, Studies on the metabolism of administered cytochrome C by the aid of iron-labelled cytochromes, *Science* **111**:469.

Bensinger, T., Maisels, M. J., Carlson, D. E., and Conrad, M. E., 1973, Effect of low caloric diet on endogenous carbon monoxide production: Normal adults and Gilbert's syndrome, *Proc. Soc. Exp. Biol. Med.* **144**:417–419.

Bissell, D. M., Hammaker, L., and Schmid, R., 1972, Hemoglobin erythrocyte catabolism in rat liver. The separate roles of parenchymal and sinusoidal cells, *Blood* **40**:812.

Bissell, D. M., Guzelian, P. S., Hammaker, L. E., and Schmid, R., 1974, Stimulation of heme oxygenase and turnover of cytochrome P-450 may be related, *Fed. Proc.* **33**:1246 (Abstract).

Blaschke, T. F., Berk, P. D., Rodkey, F. L., Scharschmidt, B. F., Collison, H. A., and Waggoner, J. G., 1974, Drugs and the liver—Effects of glutethimide and phenobarbital on hepatic bilirubin clearance, plasma bilirubin turnover and carbon monoxide production in man. *Biochem. Pharmacol.* **23**:2795.

Boyland, E., and Chausseaud, L. F., 1970, The effect of some carbonyl compounds on rat liver glutathione levels, *Biochem. Pharmacol.* **19**:1526–1529.

Castro, J. A., Sasame, H., and Gillette, J. R., 1968, Diverse effects of SKI 525-A and antioxidants on carbon tetrachloride-induced changes in liver microsomal P-450 content and ethylmorphine metabolism, *Life Sci.* **7**:129.

Coburn, R. F., Williams, W. J., and Forster, R. E., 1964, Effect of erythrocyte destruction on carbon monoxide production in man, *J. Clin. Invest.* **43**:1098.

Coburn, R. F., Williams, W. J., and Kahn, B., 1966, Endogenous carbon monoxide production in patients with hemolytic anemia, *J. Clin. Invest.* **45**:460.

Coburn, R. F., Williams, W. J., White, P., and Kahn, S. B., 1967, Production of carbon monoxide from hemoglobin in vivo, *J. Clin. Invest.* **46**:346–356.

Colleran, E., and O'Carra, P., 1969, Breakdown of pyridine haemichrome by liver extract, *Biochem. J.* **115**:13 (Abstract).

Conney, A. H., 1967, Pharmacological implications of microsomal enzyme induction, *Pharmacol. Rev.* **19**:317.

Conney, A. H., Pantuck, E. J., Hsiao, K.-C., Garland, W. A., Anderson, K. E., Alvares, A. P. and Kappas, A., 1976, Nutrition and chemical biotransformations: Enhanced phenacetin metabolism in humans fed charcoal-broiled beef, *Clin. Pharmacol. Ther.* (in press).

Cooke, J. R., and Roberts, L. B., 1969, The binding of bilirubin to serum proteins, *Clin. Chim. Acta* **26**:425.

Cooper, D. Y., Levin, S., Narasimhulu, S., Rosenthal, O., and Estabrook, R. W., 1965, Photochemical action spectrum of the terminal oxidase of mixed function oxidase systems, *Science* **147**:400–402.

Correia, M. A., and Meyer, V., 1975, *Proc. Nat. Acad. Sci. U.S.A.* **72**:400.

Correia, M. A., and Schmid, R., 1975, Effect of cobalt on microsomal cytochrome P-450: Differences between liver and intestinal mucosa, *Biochem. Biophys. Res. Commun.* **65**:1378.

Daly, J. S. F., Lillte, J. M., Troxler, R. F., and Lester, R., 1967, Metabolism of $^3$H myoglobin, *Nature* **216**:1031.

DeMatteis, F., and Gibbs, A. H., 1976, The effect of cobaltous chloride on liver haem metabolism in the rat, *Ann. Clin. Res.* **8**:193.

DeMatteis, F., and Unseld, A., 1976, Increased liver haem degradation caused by foreign chemicals: A comparison of the effects of 2-allyl-2-iso-propylacetamide and cobaltous chloride, *Biochem. Soc. Trans.* **4**:205–214.

DeSchepper, J., and Vander Stock, J., 1971, Influence of sex on the urinary bilirubin excretion at increased free plasma hemoglobin levels in whole dogs and in isolated normal thermic perfused dog kidneys, *Experientia* **27**:1264.

Dutton, G. J., 1959, Glucuronide synthesis in foetal liver and other tissues, *Biochem. J.* **71**:141.

Edington, C. L., and Kampschmidt, R. P., 1968, Bilirubin production in endotoxin-treated or tumor-bearing rats, *Proc. Soc. Exp. Biol. Med.* **129**:580.

Elder, G., Gray, L. H., and Nicholson, D. C., 1972, Bile pigment fat in gastrointestinal tract, *Semin. Hematol.* **9**:71.

Eliakim, M., Eisner, M., and Unger, H., 1959, Experimental intrahepatic obstructive jaundice following ingestion of α-naphthyl-isothiolcyanate, Bulletin Research Council Israel 8E, pp. 7–17.

Engel, R. R., Matsen, J. M., Chapman, S. S., and Schwartz, S., 1972, Carbon monoxide production from heme compounds by bacteria, *J. Bacteriol.* **112**:1320.

Fischer, H., and Hess, R., 1931, Uber neo-xanthone obilirubins und partialsynthese des mesobilirubins und mesobilirubin organs (urobilinogens, Hoppe-Seyler Z.), *Physiol. Chem.* **194**:193.

Foulkes, E. S., Lemberg, R., and Pardom, P., 1951, Verdohaem and verdoglobins, *Proc. Roy. Soc. Lond. B* **138**:386.

Gemsa, D., Fudenberg, H. H., and Schmid, R., 1974, Erythrocytosis: Regulation of the heme-degrading enzyme system, *in Activation of Macrophages* (W. H. Wagnor, H. Han, and R. Evans, eds.), pp. 40–53, American Elsevier, New York.

Gemsa, D., Woo, C. H., Webb, D., Fudenberg, H. H., and Schmid, R., 1975, Erythrocytosis by macrophages: Suppression of heme oxygenase by cyclic AMP, *Cell. Immunol.* **15**:21–36.

Goldstein, G. W., Hammaker, L., and Schmid, R., 1968, The catabolism of Heinz bodies: An experimental model demonstrating conversion to non-bilirubin metabolites, *Blood* **31**:385.

Granick, S., and Kappas, A., 1967, Steroid induction of porphyrin synthesis in liver cell culture. I. Structural basis and possible physiological role in the control of heme formation, *J. Biol. Chem.* **242**:4587.

Gray, C. H., and Nakajima, O., 1967, Studies on haem $\alpha$-methenyl oxygenase: Isomeric structure of formylbiliverdin, a possible precursor of biliverdin, *Biochem. J.* **104**:20.

Gray, C. H., Nicholson, D. C., and Nicolaus, R. A., 1958, The IX$\alpha$ structure of the common bile pigments, *Nature (London)* 181–183.

Hayaishi, O., Katageri, M., and Rothberg, S., 1955, Mechanism of the pyrocateclase reaction, *J. Am. Chem. Soc.* **77**:2914.

Hupka, R., and Karler, J., 1973, Biotransformation of ethylmorphine and heme by isolated parenchymal and reticuloendothelial cell of rat liver, *Reticuloendothel. Soc.* **14**:225.

Israel, L. G., Skanderberg, J., Guyda, H., Zingg, W., and Zipursky, A., 1963, Study of the early-labelled fraction of bile pigment: Effect of altering erythropoiesis on incorporation of [2-$^{14}$C]glycine into haem and bilirubin, *Br. J. Haematol.* **9**:50–62.

Israel, L. G. Levitt, M., Novak, W., and Zipursky, A., 1966, The early bilirubin, *Medicine* **45**:517.

Kappas, A., and Granick, S., 1968, Steroid induction of porphyrin synthesis in liver cell culture. II. The effects of heme, uridine diphosphate glucuronic acid, and inhibitors of nucleic acid and protein synthesis on the induction process, *J. Biol. Chem.* **243**:346–351.

Kappas, A., and Maines, M. D., 1976, Tin: A potent inducer of heme oxygenase in kidney, *Science* **192**:60–62.

Kappas, A., Anderson, K. E., Conney, A. H., and Alvares, A. P., 1976, Influence of dietary protein and carbohydrate on antipyrine and theophylline metabolism in man, *Clin. Pharmacol. Ther.* **20**:643–653.

Kendrew, J. C., Dickerson, R. E., Standberg, B. D., Hart, R. G., Davis, R., Phillips, O. C., and Shore, V. C., 1960, Structure of myoglobin: A three-dimensional Fourier synthesis, at 2A resolution, *Nature (London)* **185**:422.

Ketterer, B., Ross-Mansell, P., and Whitehead, J. K., 1967, The isolation of carcinogen-binding protein from livers of rats given 4-methyl aminoazobenzene, *Biochem. J.* **103**:316.

Kikuchi, G., and Yoshida, T., 1976, Heme catabolism by the reconstituted heme oxygenase system, *Ann. Clin. Res.* **8** (Suppl. 17):10.

Klatskin, G., and Bungards, L., 1950, Bilirubin in protein linkages in serum and their relationships to Vandernberg reaction, *J. Clin. Invest.* **29**:660.

Kreimer-Birnbaum, M., Pinkerton, P. H., Bannerman, R. M., and Hutchinson, H. E., 1966, Dipyrrole urinary pigments in congenital Heinz-body anemia due to Hb Koeln and in thalassemia, *Br. Med. J.* **2**:396.

Landaw, S., Callahan, E. W., and Schmid, R., 1970, Catabolism of heme *in vivo:* Comparison of the simultaneous production of bilirubin and carbon monoxide, *J. Clin. Invest.* **49**:914.

Levi, A. J., Gatmaitan, Z., and Arias, I. M., 1969a, Two hepatic cytoplasmic protein factors Y and Z and their possible role in the hepatic uptake of bilirubin sulfabromophthalein and other anions, *J. Clin. Invest.* **48**:2156.

Levi, A. J., Gatmaitan, Z., and Arias, I. M., 1969b, Deficiency of hepatic organic anion-binding protein as a possible cause of nonhemolytic conjugated hyperbilirubinemia in the newborn, *Lancet* **19**:139.

London, I. M., and West, R., 1950, Formation of bile pigment in pernicious anemia, *J. Biol. Chem.* **184**:359.

London, I. M., West, K., Schmid, R., and Rittenberg, D., 1950, On the origin of bile pigment in normal man, *J. Biol. Chem.* **184**:351.

Ludwig, G. D., Blakemore, W. S., and Drabkin, D. L., 1957, Production of carbon monoxide by hemin oxidation, *J. Clin. Invest.* **36**:912.

Lundh, B., Johansson, M. B., Mercke, C., and Cavallin-Stahl, E., 1972, Enhancement of heme catabolism by caloric restriction in man, *Scand. J. Clin. Lab. Invest.* **30**:421–427.

Lynch, S. R., and Moede, A. L., 1972, Variation in the rate of endogenous carbon monoxide production in normal human beings, *J. Lab. Clin. Invest.* **79**:85.

Maines, M. D., 1975, Discussion (Results of a conference entitled, The biological role of porphyrins and related studies, held by the N.Y. Acad. of Sciences on Oct. 23–26, 1973), *Ann. N.Y. Acad. Sci.* **244**:552.

Maines, M. D., 1976, Evidence for the catabolism of PCB-induced cytochrome P-448 by microsomal heme oxygenase; and the inhibition of δ-aminolevulinic dehydratase by PCB, *J. Exp. Med.* **144**:1509–1519.

Maines, M. D., 1977, Mechanism of degradation of endogenous heme and cytochrome P-450 by heme oxygenase, *in Proceedings of the Third International Symposium on Microsomes and Drug Oxidations* (A. G. Hildebrandt, V. Ulrich, R. W. Estabrook, and A. H. Conney, eds.), Pergamon, Oxford, in press.

Maines, M. D., and Anders, M. W., 1973a, Reconstitution of CO-binding particles after removal of heme by serum albumin, *Mol. Pharmacol.* **9**:219–228.

Maines, M. D., and Anders, M. W., 1973b, The implication of heme transfer from cytochrome P-420 to albumin in the metabolism of cytochrome P-450, *in Microsomes and Drug Oxidations* (R. W. Estabrook, J. R. Gillette, and R. C. Leibman, eds.), Williams & Wilkins, Baltimore, Maryland.

Maines, M. D., and Cohn, J., 1977, Bile pigment formation by skin heme oxygenase; with studies on the inducibility of the enzymes by heme and related compounds, *J. Exp. Med.* **145**:1054–1059.

Maines, M. D., and Kappas, A., 1974a, Effects of hemoproteins on cytochrome P-450 and microsomal components, *Fed. Proc.* **33**:421 (Abstract).

Maines, M. D., and Kappas, A., 1974b, Cobalt induction of hepatic heme oxygenase; with evidence that cytochrome P-450 is not essential for this enzyme activity. *Proc. Nat. Acad. Sci. U.S.A.* **71**:4293–4297.

Maines, M. D., and Kappas, A., 1975a, The degradative effects of porphyrins and heme compounds on the components of the microsomal mixed function oxidase, *J. Biol. Chem.* **250**:2363–2369.

Maines, M. D., and Kappas, A., 1975b, Cobalt stimulation of heme degradation in the liver: Dissociation of microsomal oxidation of heme from cytochrome P-450, *J. Biol. Chem.* **250**:4171–4177.

Maines, M. D., and Kappas, A., 1975c, Study of the developmental pattern of heme catabolism in liver and the effects of cobalt on cytochrome P-450 and the rate of heme oxidation during the neonatal period, *J. Exp. Med.* **141**:1400–1410.

Maines, M. D., and Kappas, A., 1975d, The induction of heme oxygenase by metals, *in Porphyrins in Human Disease* (M. Doss, ed.), pp. 43–52 (Proceedings 1st Intl. Porphyrin Meeting, Freiburg, May 1975), Karger, Basel.

Maines, M. D., and Kappas, A., 1975e, The induction of heme oxidation in various tissues by trace metals: Evidence for the catabolism of endogenous heme by hepatic heme oxygenase, *Ann. Clin. Res.* **8** (Suppl. 17):39–46 (Proceedings of the Intl. Conference on Porphyrin Metabolism, Sannas, Finland, July, 1975).

Maines, M. D., and Kappas, A., 1976a, Studies on the mechanism of induction of haem oxygenase by cobalt and other metal ions, *Biochem. J.* **154**:125–131.

Maines, M. D., and Kappas, A. 1976b, Selenium regulation of hepatic heme metabolism: Induction of δ-aminolevulinate synthase and heme oxygenase, *Proc. Nat. Acad. Sci. U.S.A.* **73**:4428–4431.

Maines, M. D., and Kappas, A., 1977a, Enzymatic degradation of cobalt-protoporphyrin IX: Observations on the mechanism of heme oxygenase, *Biochemistry* **16**:419–423.

Maines, M. D., and Kappas, A., 1977b, Regulation of cytochrome P-450 dependent drug metabolizing enzymes by the transition metals, nickel, iron and cobalt, *Clin. Pharmacol. Ther.* (in press).

Maines, M. D., and Kappas, A., 1977c, Regualtion of heme pathway enzymes and cellular glutathione content by metals that do not chelate with tetrapyroles: Blockade of metal effects by phiols, *Proc. Nat. Acad. Sci.* **74**:1875–1878.

Maines, M. D., and Sinclair, P., 1977, Cobalt regulation of heme synthesis and degradation in avian liver cell culture, *J. Biol. Chem.* **252**:219–223.

Maines, M. D., Anders, M. W., and Muller-Eberhard, U., 1974, Studies on the possible role of heme transfer from microsomal hemoproteins to heme binding plasma proteins in the metabolism of cytochrome P-450, *Mol. Pharmacol.* **10**:204–213.

Maines, M. D., Janousek, V., Tomio, J. M., and Kappas, A., 1976, Cobalt inhibition of synthesis and induction of δ-aminolevulinate synthase in liver, *Proc. Nat. Acad. Sci. U.S.A.* **73**:1499–1503.

Maines, M. D., Ibrahim, N., and Kappas, A., 1977a. Solubilization and partial purification of heme oxygenase from rat liver, *J. Biol. Chem.* (in press).

Mann, F. C., Sheard, C., Bollman, J. L., and Blades, E. J., 1926, The formation of bile pigment from hemoglobin, *Am. J. Physiol.* **76**:306.

Mason, H. S., Foulkes, W. B., and Peterson, E. W., 1955, Oxygen transfer and electron transport by the phenolase complex, *J. Am. Chem. Soc.* **77**:2914.

Mason, H. S., North, J. C., and Vanneste, M., 1965, Microsomal mixed-function oxidations: The metabolism of xenobiotics, *Fed. Proc.* **24**:1172.

Masters, B. S. S., and Schacter, B. A., 1976, The catalysis of heme degradation by purified NADPH-cytochrome C reductase in the absence of other microsomal proteins, *Ann. Clin. Res.* **8** (Suppl. 17):18.

Mitchell, F. L., 1967, Steroid metabolism in the fetoplacental unit and in early childhood, *Vitam. Horm.* **25**:191.

Muller-Eberhard, U., Liem, H. H., Hanstein, A., and Saarinen, P. A., 1969, Studies on the disposal of intravascular heme in the rabbit, *J. Lab. Clin. Med.* **73**(21):210.

Nakajima, H., Takemura, T., Nakajima, O., and Yamaoka, K., 1963, Studies on heme α-methenyl oxygenase, *J. Biol. Chem.* **238**:3784.

Nichol, A. W., 1970, The formation of biliverdin by chicken macrophages in tissue culture—Observation on the effect of inhibitors, *Biochim. Biophys. Acta* **222**:28.

Nichol, A. W., 1971, The formation of biliverdin from haem in suspensions by chicken macrophages in culture, *Biochim. Biophys. Acta* **244**:595.

Nichol, A. W., and Morell, D. B., 1969, Studies with isomeric composition of biliverdin and bilirubin by mass spectrometry, *Biochim. Biophys. Acta* **184**:173.

O'Carra, P., 1975, Heme cleavage: Biological systems and chemical analogs, *in Porphyrins and Metalloporphyrins* (K. M. Smith, ed.), p. 122, Elsevier, Amsterdam.

O'Carra, P. A., and Colleran, E., 1969, Haem catabolism and coupled oxidation of haemoproteins, *FEBS Lett.* **5**:295.

Odell, G. B., 1959, Studies in kernicterus I. The protein binding of bilirubin, *J. Clin. Invest.* **38**:823.

Ostrow, J. D., and Schmid, R., 1963, The protein-binding of [$^{14}$C]bilirubin in human and murine serum, *J. Clin. Invest.* **42**:1286.

Ostrow, J. D., Jandle, J. H., and Schmid, R., 1962, The formation of bilirubin from hemoglobin *in vivo*, *J. Clin. Invest.* **41**:1628.

Pimstone, N. R., Engel, P., Tenhunen, R., Seitz, P. T., Marver, H. S., and Schmid, R., 1971a, Inducible heme oxygenase in the kidney: A model for the homeostatic control of hemoglobin catabolism, *J. Clin. Invest.* **50**:2042.

Pimstone, N., Tenhunen, R., Seitz, P. T., Marver, H. S., and Schmid, R., 1971b, The enzymatic degradation of hemoglobin to bile pigments by macrophages, *J. Exp. Med.* **133**:1264.

Plaa, G. L., Rogers, L. A., and Fouts, J. R., 1965, Effect of acute α-naphthylisothiocyanate administration on hepatic microsomal drug metabolism in the mouse, *Proc. Soc. Exp. Biol. Med.* **119**:1045–1048.

Raffin, S. B., Woo, C. H., Roost, K. T., Price, D. C,, and Schmid, R., 1974, Intestinal absorption of hemoglobin iron-heme cleavage by mucosal heme oxygenase, *J. Clin. Invest.* **54**:1344.

Rich, A., 1925, The formation of bile pigment, *Physiol. Rev.* **5**:182.

Roberts, R. J., and Plaa, G. L., 1968, Alteration in biliary bilirubin content and non-erythropoietically derived bilirubin synthesis in rats after α-aphthylisothiocyanate administration, *J. Pharmacol. Exp. Ther.* **161**:382–388.

Robinson, S. H., 1968, The origins of bilirubin, *N. Engl. J. Med.* **279**:143.

Robinson, S. H., Tsong, M., Brown, B. W., and Schmid, R., 1966, The sources of bile pigment in the rat: Studies of the "early-labeled" fraction, *J. Clin. Invest.* **45**:1569.

Roost, K. T., Pimstone, N. R., Diamond, I., and Schmid, R., 1972, The formation of cerebrospinal fluid xanthochromia after subarachnoid hemorrhage, *Neurology* **22**:973.

Rothwell, J. D., Lacroix, S., and Sweeney, G. D., 1973, Evidence against regulatory role for heme oxygenase in hepatic heme synthesis, *Biochim. Biophys. Acta* **304**:871–847.

Schacter, B. A., and Mason, J. I., 1974, The effect of phenobarbital 3M-methyl-cholanthrene, 3,4-benzpyrene and pregnanalone-16 carbonitrate on microsomal heme oxygenase and splenic cytochrome P-450, *Arch. Biochem. Biophys.* **166**:274.

Schacter, B. A., and Waterman, M. R., 1974, Activity of various metalloporphyrin protein complexes with microsomal heme oxygenase, *Life Sci.* **14**:47–53.

Schmid, R., 1972, Bilirubin metabolism in man, *Engl. J. Med.* **287**:703.

Schmid, R., Marver, H. S., and Hammaker, L., 1966, Enhanced formation of rapidly labeled bilirubin by phenobarbital: Hepatic microsomal cytochromes as a possible source, *Biochem. Biophys. Res. Commun.* **24**:319.

Schwartz, S., and Ikeda, K., 1955, Studies of porphyrin synthesis and interconversion with special reference to certain green porphyrins in animals with experimental hepatic porphyria, *in Porphyrin Biosynthesis and Metabolism* (G. E. W. Wolstenholme and E. C. P. Miller, eds.), pp. 209–226, Churchill, London.

Schwartz, S., Ibrahim, G., and Watson, C. J., 1964, Contribution of nonhemoglobin hemes to early labeling of bile bilirubin, *J. Lab. Clin. Med.* **64**:1003.

Schwartz, S., Barelkovski, J., Stephenson, B., Edmondson, P., and Johnson, J., 1975, The metabolic fate of [porphyrin-$^{14}$C]cytochrome *c* in dogs, *Life Sci.* **17**:1737–1746.

Sjörstrand, T., 1949, Endogenous formation of carbon monoxide in man under normal and pathological conditions, *Scand. J. Clin. Lab. Invest.* **1**:201.

Sjörstrand, T., 1952, The formation of carbon monoxide by the decomposition of haemoglobin *in vivo*, *Acta Physiol. Scand.* **26**:336.

Tenhunen, R., Marver, H. S., and Schmid, R., 1968, The enzymatic conversion of heme to bilirubin by microsomal heme oxygenase, *Proc. Nat. Acad. Sci. U.S.A.* **61**:748–755.

Tenhunen, R., Marver, H. S., and Schmid, R., 1969a, Microsomal heme oxygenase characterization of the enzyme, *J. Biol. Chem.* **244**:6388.

Tenhunen, R., Marver, H. S., and Schmid, R., 1969b, The enzymatic conversion of hemoglobin to bilirubin, *Trans. Assoc. Am. Physicians* **82**:363.

Tenhunen, R., Marver, H. S., and Schmid, R., 1970, The enzymatic catabolism of hemoglobin: Stimulation of microsomal heme oxygenase by hemin, *J. Lab. Clin. Med.* **75**:410–421.

Tenhunen, R., Marver, H. S., Pimstone, N. R., Trager, W. F., Cooper, D. Y., and Schmid, R., 1972, Enzymatic degradation of heme: Oxysensitive cleavage requiring cytochrome P-450, *Biochemistry* **11**:1716–1720.

Thaler, M. M,, Gemsa, D. L., and Bakken, A. F., 1972, Enzymatic conversion of heme to bilirubin in normal to starved fetuses and newborn rats, *Pediatr. Res.* **6**:1971.

Troxler, R. F., Dawber, N. H., and Lester, R., 1968, Synthesis of urobilinogen by broken cell preparation of intestinal bacteria, *Gastroenterology* **54**:568.

Turnbull, A., Cleton, F., and Finch, C. A., 1962, Iron absorption IV. The absorption of hemoglobin iron in man, *J. Clin. Invest.* **41**:1897.

Virchow, R., 1847, Die pathologischen pigments, *Arch. Pathol. Anat.* **1**:379.

Weintraub, L. R., Weinstein, M. B., Huser, H. J., and Rafal, S., 1968, Absorption of hemoglobin iron: The role of a heme splitting substance in the intestinal mucosa, *J. Clin. Invest.* **47**:531.

White, P., 1969, Carbon monoxide production of heme catabolism, *Ann. N.Y. Acad. Sci.* **1969**:23.

White, P., Coburn, R. F., Williams, W. J., Goldwein, M. I., Rother, M. L., and Shafer, B. C., 1967, Carbon monoxide production associated with ineffective erythropoiesis, *J. Clin. Invest.* **46**:1968.

Wise, C. D., 1964, Studies on the degradation of hemoglobin into bile pigment, Ph.D. Dissertation, University of Pennsylvania Microfilms, Inc., Ann Arbor, Michigan.

Wise, C. D., and Drabkin, D. C., 1964, Degradation of hemoglobin and hemin to bilirubin by a new cell-free system obtained from the organ of dog placenta, *Fed. Proc.* **23**:223.

Yaffe, S. J., Levy, G., Matsuzawa, T., and Beliah, T., 1966, Enhancement of glucuronide-conjugating capacity in a hyperbilirubinemic infant due to apparent enzyme induction by phenobarbital, *Engl. J. Med.* **275**:1461.

Yamamoto, T., Skanderberg, J., Zipursky, Z., and Israel, L. G., 1965, Early appearing bilirubin: Evidence for two components, *J. Clin. Invest.* **44**:31–41.

Yoshida, T., Takahashi, S., and Kikuchi, G., 1974, Partial purification and reconstitution of heme oxygenase system for pig spleen microsomes, *Biochemistry* **75**:1187.

# 2

# Hemoglobin Synthesis in Normal and Abnormal States

## Michael L. Freedman

The study of hemoglobin synthesis has been one of the major areas of biomedical research for the past 20 years. The information obtained has led to a better understanding of genetics, molecular biology, protein chemistry, and mammalian physiology, as well as clinical hematology. It is beyond the scope of any review article to cover this prolific field completely. However, in this chapter an attempt will be made to summarize the major molecular control mechanisms in normal hemoglobin synthesis, as well as the molecular basis of some of the diseases of abnormal hemoglobin synthesis.

## 2.1. Normal Hemoglobin Synthesis

### 2.1.1. Ontogeny of Hemoglobin Synthesis

Human erythropoiesis begins very early in fetal life, probably at 2–3 weeks of gestation in embryonic yolk sac islands containing erythroid cells (Kazazian, 1974). Three embryonic hemoglobins have been described: hemoglobin Gower$_1$ ($\epsilon_4$), hemoglobin Gower$_2$ ($\alpha_2\epsilon_2$) (Huehns *et al.*, 1961,

MICHAEL L. FREEDMAN • Department of Medicine, New York University Medical Center, New York, New York 10016.

1964a,b), and hemoglobin Portland$_1$ ($\zeta_2\gamma_2$) (Capp $et$ $al.$, 1967, 1970). Hemoglobins Gower$_1$ and Gower$_2$ appear to be the earliest hemoglobins synthesized; they are replaced by hemoglobin F (Hb F) by the tenth week of pregnancy (Huehns, 1974). Since Hb Portland$_1$ migrates closely with hemoglobin A, disappearance is not yet well documented, but small amounts have been demonstrated in cord blood samples from normal (Capp $et$ $al.$, 1967) and abnormal (Todd $et$ $al.$, 1970) infants. Hemoglobin F ($\alpha_2\gamma_2$) synthesis in small amounts has been estimated to begin in the fifth fetal week, whereas hemoglobin A ($\alpha_2\beta_2$) synthesis is estimated to begin in the sixth fetal week (Kazazian and Woodhead, 1974).

Kazazian and Woodhead (1974) have recently proposed that the cells of the yolk sac origin are restricted to $\alpha$- and $\epsilon$-chain production (thus, Hb Gower$_1$ and Gower$_2$). The erythroid cells of hepatic origin, which later populate the bone marrow, can synthesize $\alpha$, $\beta$, $\gamma$, $\delta$, and $\zeta$ globin chains (thus, Hb A, F, A$_2$, and Portland$_1$). Consistent with this hypothesis are the observations that $\epsilon$ chains disappear by the tenth week of fetal life and are not found in infants with homozygous $\alpha$-thalassemia (Todd $et$ $al.$, 1970; Weatherall $et al.$, 1970). These infants, on the other hand, do synthesize $\beta$, $\gamma$, $\delta$, and $\zeta$ chains, but not $\epsilon$ chains. The earlier observation of tiny amounts of Hb Gower$_2$ in developmentally retarded infants (Huehns $et$ $al.$, 1964; Wilson $et$ $al.$, 1967), however, would tend to argue against this hypothesis.

By 10 weeks of normal gestation the Gower hemoglobins have disappeared and Hb F has become the predominant hemoglobin, making up over 95% of the total (Kazazian and Woodhead, 1974). By 12–14 weeks, Hb A has become 3–4% of the total hemoglobin. During this period both Hb A and Hb F are made in cells from various fetal erythropoietic sites (liver, spleen, and bone marrow) (Wood and Weatherall, 1973). Between 12 and 32 weeks of gestation, Hb A makes up 4–6% of the total hemoglobin; at that time predominant $\gamma$-chain production gives way to predominant $\beta$-chain production, and at term 10–30% of the hemoglobin is Hb A (Wood and Weatherall, 1973; Hallenberg $et$ $al.$, 1971; Pataryas and Stamatoyannopoulos, 1972).

## 2.1.2. Hemoglobin Synthesis during Erythropoiesis

### 2.1.2.1. Cells Making Hemoglobin

All normal mammalian hemoglobin molecules consist of tetramers of four globin chains with each chain bound to a heme prosthetic group. In the normal adult each hemoglobin molecule contains two $\alpha$ chains and two non-$\alpha$ chains. It is the non-$\alpha$ chain which determines the identity of the hemoglobin. In the normal human, hemoglobin A $(\alpha_2\beta_2)$ is 97% of the hemoglobin present, while hemoglobin $A_2$ $(\alpha_2\delta_2)$ and hemoglobin F $(\alpha_2\gamma_2)$ represent less than 3 and 1 %, respectively (Rhinesmith *et al.*, 1957). Mature red cells contain virtually only complete hemoglobin molecules and do not synthesize hemoglobin. There are only minute amounts of free chains (Baglioni and Campana, 1967; Winterhalter and Glotthaar, 1971; Gill and Schwartz, 1973). Thus, strict control of both polypeptide chain synthesis and heme synthesis must occur throughout erythropoiesis to assure this balanced synthesis of hemoglobin.

It is now generally accepted that erythrocytes are derived from primitive pluripotential stem cells in the bone marrow (Till and McCulloch, 1965). Present evidence points to either a cell resembling a marrow lymphocyte or monocyte as this pluripotential stem cell (Cudkowicz *et al.*, 1964; Barnes and Oxon, 1967).

Hemoglobin is produced primarily in the bone marrow in differentiating erythroblasts and continues for a short time in the circulating reticulocyte. Synthesis and accumulation of hemoglobin continue during the 6–8 days of erythroid differentiation. The details of erythroid development are given elsewhere (Wintrobe *et al.*, 1974).

The least mature recognizable erythrocyte precursor is known as the pronormoblast. This is a round or oval cell, 14–19 $\mu$m in diameter, with a large nucleus and a rim of basophilic cytoplasm. Nucleoli are present and may be very prominent. At this stage no hemoglobin is present in the cytoplasm, which makes differentiation from myeloblasts and lymphoblasts very difficult. Features that tend to differentiate this cell from other blast cells are a prominent small pale area in the cytoplasm (possibly corresponding to the Golgi apparatus), and a tendency for the chromatin to be more homogeneous and condensed. At this stage, the cells already contain small amounts of cytoplasmic globin messenger RNA (Marks and Rifkind, 1972; Terada *et al.*, 1972; Krantz, 1973).

The basophilic normoblast is smaller (12–17 $\mu$m in diameter) and the nucleoli are no longer visible. The chromatin is coarse and granular and may appear in a wheel–spoke arrangement *(Radkern)*. The cytoplasm is even more darkly basophilic than the pronormoblast because of the presence of ribonucleic acid.

As hemoglobin synthesis increases, acidophilic pink areas appear in the normoblast and the cell is termed the polychromatophilic normoblast. The nuclear chromatin becomes increasingly clumped and the nucleus becomes smaller. This cell is 12–15 $\mu$m in diameter.

When nearly the full amount of hemoglobin is present, the cell is termed an orthochromic normoblast. The cytoplasm is distinctly acidophilic due to hemoglobin. The nucleus is small and appears almost homogeneous as it undergoes pyknotic degeneration. This cell is 8–12 $\mu$m in diameter. During this stage the cell loses its nucleus and nuclear remnants may assume bizarre shapes.

After the nucleus is lost, certain cytoplasmic organelles such as ribosomes, mitochondria, and the Golgi apparatus are maintained for a short time. Hemoglobin synthesis still continues in these cells, the reticulocytes. Because of the presence of ribosomal RNA the cell will still have a faint basophilic staining superimposed on the acidophilic hemoglobin to give a polychromatophilic hue. Reticulocytes can be differentiated on routine staining of peripheral blood by their polychromatophilia and sometimes basophilic stippling. Basophilic stippling also results from ribosomal RNA and is probably no different from diffuse basophilia but just represents prolonged staining. The "reticulum" of reticulocytes can only be seen by supravital staining, and the staining with new methylene blue or crystal blue precipitates ribosomes which produce the reticular network. Reticulocytes are approximately 20% larger in volume than mature erythrocytes.

### 2.1.2.2. Hormonal Control of Erythropoiesis

Erythropoiesis is maintained by a hormonal mechanism. The hormone erythropoietin is a glycoprotein which is thought to be formed in response to reduced oxygen tension, principally in the kidney. Evidence has been presented that erythropoietin itself does not form in the kidney, rather an enzyme is produced (renal erythropoietic factor, REF, or erythrogenin) that reacts with a plasma substance produced in the liver (erythropoietinogen) (Gordon *et al.*, 1967; Camiscoli and Gordon, 1970; Gordon and Zanjani, 1970; Hodgson, 1970) to form erythropoietin. There are other sources of erythropoietin since removal of the kidney does not abolish erythropoiesis or cause complete disappearance of erythropoietin activity (Gordon *et al.*, 1967; Mirand and Murphy, 1970).

It appears that the main site of action of erythropoietin is on committed erythroid precursors to differentiate into pronormoblasts and thereby expand the erythroid marrow (Gordon and Zanjani, 1970; Hodgson, 1970). Erythropoietin also causes the red cell marrow generation time to be shortened, premature denucleation to occur, and reticulocytes to be released into the circulation at an earlier stage of maturity ("shift reticulocytes"). These prematurely released reticulocytes are macrocytic, hypochromic, and polychromatophilic and have a shorter than normal life span (Papayannopoulous and Finch, 1972).

Erythropoietin increases the synthesis of heme, protein, DNA, and RNA in bone marrow cells. The earliest effect of adding erythropoietin to marrow cultures is an increase in RNA, which occurs within minutes (Gross and Goldwasser, 1971). This RNA is short-lived and has a sedimentation coefficient of 150S (Gross and Goldwasser, 1969). As the amount of RNA decreases, various smaller RNAs with sedimentation coefficients consistent with those of messenger RNA, ribosomal RNA, and transfer RNA appear. In addition, a substance appears that permits iron delivered to the cells as transferrin to affect cell functions (iron effector) (Gross and Goldwasser, 1969). The hypothesis proposed to explain this phenomenon states that the 150S RNA is a "translational unit" which subsequently gives rise to the various RNAs responsible for translation of globin or for some enzyme essential for hemoglobin synthesis (Gross and Goldwasser, 1969; Bottomley and Smithee, 1969; Terada *et al.*, 1972). After these events and probably as a result of them, there is an increase in the rate of DNA synthesis and cell division (Powsner and Berman, 1968). Chang and Goldwasser (1973) have extracted a protein from the cytoplasm of marrow cells incubated for a short time with erythropoietin, which increases the rate of RNA synthesis by marrow cell nuclei (marrow cytoplasmic factor). The following hypothesis has been proposed by Goldwasser (1975) to explain these phenomena: Erythroid cell differentiation is the sum of three interrelated processes, termed (a) sensitization, (b) induction, and (c) specialization.

Sensitization is the process by which erythropoietin-responsive cells become competent to be acted upon by erythropoietin. Goldwasser (1975) has proposed a tentative, probably overly simplified, model in which stem cells, erythropoietin-responsive cells, granulopoietin-responsive cells, and thrombopoietin-responsive cells are the same cells in different phases of the cell cycle. These cells are defined by the presence of specific receptors for erythropoietin, granulopoietin, and thrombopoietin, with each class of receptor having a short life span on the surface of the cell.

Induction is defined as the primary biochemical step that occurs as the result of the specific interaction with erythropoietin. After erythropoietin interacts with cell surface receptors marrow cytoplasmic factor appears. This protein acts nonspecifically on nuclei to increase the rate of RNA synthesis. The first RNA to be synthesized in erythropoietin-exposed cells is the 150S nuclear RNA just discussed.

Specialization is defined as the complex series of molecular changes which occur in the induced cells to acquire those new functions that distinguish them as being differentiated. An early event in specialization is the synthesis of ribosomal RNA precursor which begins at about 15 min. This is followed by the synthesis of processed ribosomal RNA, followed by transfer RNA, iron effector, and 9S RNA (messenger RNA, possibly globin mRNA). These substances are formed at about 45 min.

Hemoglobin synthesis does not start until approximately 10 hr after erythropoietin addition. Glass *et al.* (1975) have shown in murine bone marrow cultures that erythropoietin first stimulates δ-aminolevulinic acid synthetase activity and heme synthesis prior to its effect on globin synthesis. These investigators also showed that heme synthesis is maximal in the earliest precursor cells and decreases with cell maturity, whereas globin synthesis increases with cell maturity. These findings suggest that sufficient heme must be present in the cell before globin synthesis may proceed.

Recently Piantadosi *et al.* (1976) have shown that erythropoietin sequentially activates multiple forms of nuclear RNA polymerase. As a result of this the RNA synthesis seen in induction and specialization occurs. Furthermore, Spivak (1976) has presented data indicating that erythropoietin stimulates the synthesis of both histone and nonhistone chromosomal proteins, and the synthesis of these proteins is maximal before appearance of morphologically identifiable erythroblasts. Other events which must take place during specialization include DNA synthesis, membrane synthesis, and the synthesis of the various other proteins of the erythroid cell (Goldwasser, 1975).

The role of cyclic AMP in the mechanism of action of erythropoietin is still controversial. Dukes (1971) found that erythropoietin stimulation of heme synthesis in marrow cultures was enhanced by dibutyryl cAMP. Bottomley *et al.* (1971) showed that δ-aminolevulinic acid synthetase was increased in the presence of dibutyryl cAMP in marrow cultures. In her *in vivo* studies she showed enhancement of erythropoietin stimulation of erythropoiesis by cAMP and theophylline. Gorshein *et al.* (1975) have also shown in marrow culture *in vitro* that dibutyryl cAMP stimulated heme synthesis and that the effect was enhanced by theophylline. Still other investigators have reported that dibutyryl cAMP enhanced heme synthesis and/or erythropoiesis *in vivo* (Gidari *et al.*, 1971; Schooley and Mahlmann, 1971; Brown and Adamson, 1974, 1976; Freedman *et al.*, 1976a). George *et al.* (1975) have presented evidence that cyclic AMP is involved in the renal production and/or release of erythropoietin.

On the other hand, Graber *et al.* (1972) and Goldwasser (1975) were unable to demonstrate any effect of dibutyryl cAMP on heme synthesis in their *in vitro* marrow culture systems. It is possible that differences in methodology might explain their results, which are in contrast to those described *in vitro*. Another possible explanation is that erythropoietin and cAMP work upon different cells or different portions of cells and that the differences in techniques used in various laboratories are selecting out certain cells and/or interactions. In any event, the majority of the evidence now seems to indicate that cAMP does play some role in erythropoiesis, perhaps via an effect on heme synthesis (Freedman *et al.*, 1976a).

### 2.1.2.3. Erythropoiesis with "Friend Leukemia Virus"

Considerable insight into mechanisms controlling hemoglobin synthesis during erythropoiesis might also be gained by studies of murine erythroleukemia cells transformed by "Friend leukemia virus" in tissue culture (Friend *et al.*, 1971). In the presence of dimethyl sulfoxide (DMSO) these cells begin to differentiate into early erythroid cells with an increase in globin mRNA and hemoglobin, and are recognizable as erythroblasts (Friend *et al.*, 1971; Sherton and Kabat, 1976; Peterson and McConkey, 1976). Thus, they may be used as models for the initial steps of erythropoiesis. It is also possible to introduce globin genes from differentiated cells into spontaneously proliferating erythroleukemia cells, which then may be expressed after exposure to DMSO (Deisseroth *et al.*, 1976). Studies of these hybrids should be useful in gaining information of the chromosomal locations of structural and regulatory loci involved in the regulation of human globin genes. In addition, hybrid cells of this type offer an opportunity to study control of expression of the three linked globin structural genes ($\gamma$, $\delta$, $\beta$) in man.

## 2.1.3. Transcription, Processing, and Translation of Globin Messenger RNA

See reviews by Benz and Forget (1974), Clegg (1974), and Lehninger (1975).

### 2.1.3.1. Nuclear Synthesis and Processing of mRNA

The genetic information for the amount and structure of a protein, in this case globin, is present in the nucleotide sequence of DNA. The DNA makes up the gene, located on the chromosome within the cell nucleus. At the present time the best evidence seems to indicate that $\alpha$ and $\beta$ genes are located on different chromosomes (Price *et al.*, 1972; Deisseroth *et al.*, 1976). Price *et al.* (1972) have presented evidence that the $\alpha$ gene is on chromosome 2, whereas $\beta$, $\delta$, and $\gamma$ genes appear to be closely linked on a B-group chromosome (either 4 or 5).

The genetic information is transferred from the DNA of the gene to a strand of messenger RNA (mRNA). The nucleotide sequence of the mRNA is complementary (mirror image) to the DNA according to Watson–Crick base pairing (dC in DNA gives G in mRNA; dA gives U; dG gives C; and dT gives A). This process of synthesis of mRNA from DNA is termed transcription.

In both DNA and RNA, the nucleotides are linked by phosphodiester bonds which join the 5′-hydroxyl groups on the deoxyribose (DNA) or ribose (RNA) moiety of one nucleotide with the 3' group, whereas the other end has a free 5' group. This asymmetry confers a beginning and an end to each nucleotide sequence during the process of decoding the genetic information in both DNA and RNA. Transcription of DNA into mRNA proceeds from the 3' end of mRNA. Translation of mRNA into protein proceeds from the 5' end of the mRNA to the 3' end. The mRNA for globin is larger than if it only contained the minimum information required for the translation of the amino acid sequences of globin chains. Globin mRNA has a sedimentation coefficient of 9–10S and a molecular weight of 200,000–220,000. Thus, the globin mRNA must contain about 650–670 nucleotides, including initiation and termination codons, instead of the 429 and 444 residues necessary for the 141 amino acids in $\alpha$ chains and 146 amino acids in $\beta$ chains. The mRNA therefore contains untranslated nucleotide sequences.

A portion of the untranslated sequences of globin mRNA may be accounted for by a poly A sequence located at the 3' end of globin mRNA (Lim and Canellakis, 1970; Burr and Lingrel, 1971). In addition, at least five abnormal hemoglobins which contain abnormally long $\alpha$ globin chains (Milner et al., 1971; Seid-Akhavan et al., 1972; Clegg et al., 1974; DeJong et al., 1975; Bradley et al., 1975) and two abnormally long $\beta$-chain variants have been described (Flatz et al., 1971; Bunn et al., 1975). Nucleotide sequence analysis of normal and abnormal hemoglobin mRNA has now shown what the usual untranslated sequences are in both $\alpha$ (Marotta et al., 1974; Forget et al., 1974) and $\beta$ chains (Forget et al., 1975; Lehmann et al., 1975) beyond the normal termination codon and before the poly A sequence at the 3' end. In addition, there has to be a nontranslated portion of mRNA at the 5' end of globin mRNA to account for the remainder of the untranslated residues.

Like other eukaryotic mRNAs globin mRNA does not appear to be synthesized initially in its final form in cells. Most eukaryotic mRNAs are initially synthesized as heterogeneous nuclear RNA (HnRNA) which is a very high molecular weight RNA, up to 10 times the final size of translatable mRNA (Darnell et al., 1973). The poly A sequence found in mature mRNAs is added to HnRNA as a posttranscriptional event, presumably one base residue at a time (Darnell et al., 1973). The poly A in HnRNA is located at the very 3' end of the HnRNA, just as in mRNA, and is approximately the same size. After the addition of the poly A segment the HnRNA is processed to produce mRNA. It appears that poly A plays an important role in this step, since if poly A addition to HnRNA is inhibited, newly synthesized mRNA does not appear in cytoplasmic polyribosomes, although HnRNA synthesis continues (Darnell et al., 1973). The processing of HnRNA to mRNA in the nucleus involves cleavage of the HnRNA through intermediates (pre-mRNA). Most of the HnRNA is turned over in the nucleus. Subsequent processing of nuclear mRNA involves association with protein to form messenger ribonucleoprotein (mRNP) particles (Scherrer, 1973). Some of the proteins appear to be specifically bound to the poly A of the mRNA (Kwan and Braverman, 1972; Blobel, 1973). This association with proteins appears to represent intermediate steps in the transport process and thus the poly A is probably required for transport to the cytoplasm.

The specific mechanisms controlling the transcription of globin genes into globin mRNAs are not yet known. It is not known how transcription is initiated and in response to what stimuli. Furthermore, it is possible to imagine that considerable control of genetic expression occurs at a post-transcriptional but pretranslational level. For example, differences in the amount of a specific gene product might be regulated by differences in processing of HnRNA, instead of, or in addition to, transcription. It is imaginable, for example, that the closely linked $\gamma$, $\delta$, and $\beta$ chains are transcribed as a polycistronic mRNA from which processing in the nucleus allows only large amounts of $\beta$ mRNA to be released to the cytoplasm.

### 2.1.3.2. Cytoplasmic Processing of mRNA

Globin mRNA appears first as free cytoplasmic mRNA and is not delivered directly from nucleus to ribosomes (Scherrer, 1973). The free cytoplasmic mRNA is complexed with proteins to form messenger ribonucleoprotein (mRNP) particles with a sedimentation coefficient of 15S (Jacobs-Lorena and Baglioni, 1972, 1973; Olson et al., 1972). This intact mRNP cannot serve as a template for protein synthesis. However, the 9–10S mRNA is quite active if it is released from the protein. The mammalian free globin mRNP is almost entirely $\alpha$-chain-specific mRNA (Jacobs-Lorena and Baglioni, 1972, 1973).

The 9–10S mRNA associated with polyribosomes appears also to be associated with protein. The 14–15S "polysomal mRNP" particles contain 10S globin mRNA bound to two proteins of different molecular weight. These proteins are different from that of free cytoplasmic mRNP, and therefore it would seem that mRNA exchanges proteins before or during its association with ribosomes (Scherrer, 1973). These mRNP particles, therefore, appear to be involved in the handling of cytoplasmic mRNA, in the protection against degradation of ribonucleases and proteases, and perhaps in the selection of specific mRNA for translation. Therefore, control of globin synthesis also seems to involve cytoplasmic pretranslational events.

### 2.1.3.3. Translation of Globin mRNA in the Cytoplasm

*2.1.3.3a. Polyribosomes.* Hemoglobin synthesis occurs on ribosome–messenger RNA complexes, the polyribosomes. This process, translation, may be subdivided into three stages: initiation, elongation, and release. Initiation is the association of a ribosome with the 5'-nucleotide end of mRNA. Elongation is the process of ribosomal movement along mRNA translating the nucleotide triplet code into an amino acid sequence. At the 3'-nucleotide end of mRNA, the completed globin chain is released and the ribosome separates from mRNA. The ribosome is then reutilized and will reinitiate.

Optimal hemoglobin synthesis occurs when approximately five to six ribosomes are attached simultaneously to a single mRNA at different sites of the mRNA. Each ribosome is involved in translating a different portion of the mRNA sequence. The number of ribosomes on an mRNA strand is directly proportional to the rate of initiation, and inversely proportional to the rate of release (Waxman *et al.*, 1967; Freedman *et al.*, 1967; Rabinovitz *et al.*, 1969). Therefore, when initiation is selectively inhibited but elongation and release occur normally, the polyribosomes disaggregate to single ribosomes not attached to mRNA (Velez *et al.*, 1971; Freedman *et al.*, 1972). When elongation is inhibited at codons uniformly distributed throughout the mRNA, the polyribosomes are "frozen" at five or six ribosomes on an mRNA. On the other hand, if elongation is selectively inhibited at the 5'-nucleotide end of mRNA of both globin chains, the polyribosomes disaggregate to predominantly single ribosomes. Since the critical inhibition is close to the 5'-nucleotide end, very few ribosomes can attach to mRNA due to the impaired secondary initiation delay. Thus, if the rate of movement beyond the critical codon is normal and ribosomes are released at a faster rate than they may be initiated, the end result is a failure to maintain the steady state of ribosomes on mRNA (Freedman *et al.*, 1968a,b; Freedman and Rabinovitz, 1970). In contrast, selective inhibition at release or at or near the 3'-nucleotide ends of both mRNAs results in larger than normal polyribosomes due to maximal packing of ribosomes proximal to the critical codon (Freedman *et al.*, 1968b).

An interesting and useful phenomenon was noted when rabbit reticulocytes were incubated with L-*O*-methylthreonine to induce an isoleucine deficiency which is coded for only at the 5'-nucleotide end of mRNA for α chains, and only at the 3'-nucleotide end of the mRNA for β chains (Rabinovitz *et al.*, 1969; Kazazian and Freedman, 1968; Freedman and Rabinovitz, 1971). These isoleucine-deficient cells contained new large polyribosomes consisting of approximately 12 ribosomes, and there was an increase in polyribosomes consisting of two and three ribosomes. At the same time, there was a decrease in the normal aggregates of four to six ribosomes. Peptide analysis of tryptic digests of these fractions demonstrates that the new peak of large polyribosomes contained mainly β-chain peptides, and the small peaks contained mainly α-chain peptides blocked at the isoleucine codons near the 5'-nucleotide end (Kazazian and Freedman, 1968). Further studies showed that the large polyribosomes formed by maximal packing on a β-chain mRNA inhibited at the isoleucine codon at the 3'-nucleotide end (Freedman and Rabinovitz, 1971). This technique of separating α- and β-chain polyribosomes has proved useful as a means of separating and purifying α- and β-chain mRNA (Temple and Housman, 1972).

*2.1.3.3b. Initiation.* Initiation may be defined as the process in which the first amino acid of the protein attaches to the ribosome–messenger RNA complex. The N-terminal amino acid is the first amino acid added whereas the C-terminal amino acid is the last (5'-nucleotide end to 3'-nucleotide end of the mRNA). In mammalian cells the triplet codon AUG, which codes for methionine, is the start or initiator codon for normal protein synthesis. This codon calls for a specific methionine-transfer RNA (tRNA$_f^{Met}$) which is the first amino acid of every mammalian protein beginning to be synthesized (Chattergee *et al.*, 1971; Culp *et al.*, 1970; Housman *et al.*, 1970; Hunter and Jackson, 1971; Jackson and Hunter, 1970; Shafritz and Anderson, 1970). The N-terminal methionine, however, is cleaved off during elongation on the ribosomes. The first permanent amino acid (valine) of both α and β chains is added to the methionine in the initial dipeptide formation (which is usually considered part of the initiation process).

All steps in protein synthesis, including initiation, require the properly charged tRNA species. For example, only methionyl-tRNA$_f^{Met}$ can participate in initiation; deacylated tRNA$_f^{Met}$ is inactive (Chen *et al.*, 1972; Culp *et al.*, 1970; Gupta and Aerni, 1973). A number of "charging enzymes" (aminoacyl-tRNA synthetases) have been described (Pain and Clemens, 1973). These enzymes recognize the three-dimensional structure of each tRNA species so that only the amino acid that is called for by the anticodon is linked.

Initiation appears to occur as follows. The ribosome (80S) completing translation is dissociated by a "dissociation factor" to a 40S and 60S subunit (Kaempfer and Kaufman, 1972a; Lubsen and Davis, 1972; Merrick *et al.*, 1973; Mizuno and Rabinovitz, 1973). The 40S subunit interacts with GTP, Met-tRNA$_f^{Met}$, and an initiation factor, IF-MP, to form the 40S initiation complex, which then combines with the codon AUG on mRNA (Nombela *et al.*, 1976). The next step is interaction of the 40S initiation complex with the 60S subunit. This step requires initiation factors IF-

M2A and IF-M2B. At this stage there is GTP hydrolysis, which is probably accompanied by release of IF-MP (Nombela *et al.*, 1976). No IF-M3, ATP, or other factors seem to be required to form an 80S complex when AUG is the template (Nombela *et al.*, 1976). GTP hydrolysis is probably catalyzed by IF-M2A, which has ribosome-dependent GTPase activity (Merrick *et al.*, 1973). There are at least several other factors that have been described (e.g., IF-M1 and IF-M3), but their mode of action is still not completely known. (This subject has been reviewed by Benz and Forget, 1974.) It appears that the initiation factors as well as the ribosomes are recycled, but this has not yet been definitively shown. It should be emphasized that initiation, as well as all steps in protein synthesis, requires the correct concentration of $Mg^{2+}$ and $K^+$, proper pH, and favorable oxidation–reduction conditions within the cell. The role of hemin and the hemin-controlled repressor is considered in a later section.

*2.1.3.3c. Initial Dipeptide Formation.* The formation of the first N-terminal dipeptide is often considered as part of the initiation process since this reaction does not occur in the absence of initiation factors (Crystal *et al.*, 1971; Shafritz *et al.*, 1971a,b, 1972). However, this initial methionine–valine formation is also very similar to elongation. It is probably then best described as a transitional step between initiation and elongation.

Two specific aminoacyl-tRNA binding sites exist on ribosomes: the "A" (aminoacyl) site and the "P" (peptidyl) site. Activated or charged tRNAs are first bound onto the A site, while the partially completed polypeptide is on the P site awaiting entry of the next aminoacyl-tRNA into the A site (Crystal *et al.*, 1971; Baglioni *et al.*, 1972; Busiello and DiGirolamo, 1973). The initiator Met-tRNA$_f^{Met}$ appears to be on the P site (Crystal *et al.*, 1971; Shafritz *et al.*, 1971a,b, 1972). Valyl-tRNA$^{Val}$ enters the A site. Elongation factor EF$_1$ and GTP are required (Arlinghaus *et al.*, 1968; Collins *et al.*, 1972; Culp *et al.*, 1969; Lin *et al.*, 1969; McKeehan and Hardesty, 1969a; Shafritz *et al.*, 1971a). Then in a reaction cooperatively catalyzed by EF$_1$ (a structural ribosomal protein having "transpeptidase" activity) and perhaps other proteins, the carboxyl group of methionine is linked to the amino group of valine by peptide bond formation (Arlinghaus *et al.*, 1968). During this "transpeptidation reaction" the bond between the carboxyl group of methionine and the initiator tRNA$_f^{Met}$ is broken. Methionine is therefore transferred to the valyl-tRNA$^{Val}$ creating dipeptidyl-methionyl-valyl-tRNA$^{Val}$. The P site now contains deacylated tRNA$_f^{Met}$ while the A site is occupied by dipeptidyl-Met-Val-tRNA$^{Val}$. At this point the requirement for initiation factors seems ended, and elongation, or addition of more amino acids and movement of the ribosome from the 5' end to the 3' end of mRNA, proceeds.

*2.1.3.3d. Elongation.* Immediately after initial dipeptide formation deacylated $tRNA_f^{Met}$ is released from the P site, while $Met\text{-}Val\text{-}tRNA^{Val}$ is on the A site. $Met\text{-}Val\text{-}tRNA^{Val}$ is shifted from the A site to the P site, leaving the A site vacant. The ribosome simultaneously advances one codon toward the 3' end of the mRNA, maintaining the dipeptidyl-$tRNA^{Val}$ in the P site with its valine codon. The next codon is now aligned with the vacant A site. The shifts of the dipeptidyl-$tRNA^{Val}$ and the movement of the ribosome require elongation factor $EF_2$ (or translocase) and GTP hydrolysis. These simultaneous processes are termed "translocation" (Arlinghaus *et al.*, 1968; Brot *et al.*, 1969; Culp *et al.*, 1969; McKeehan and Hardesty, 1969b; Shafritz *et al.*, 1971a,b).

Following translocation, the A site is vacant and the next aminoacyl-tRNA can bind the ribosome by entering the A site. This tRNA is charged with the proper amino acid called for by the next codon. The P site is occupied by $Met\text{-}Val\text{-}tRNA^{Val}$. Transpeptidation then occurs in a reaction analogous to initial dipeptide formation. $EF_1$, GTP, and GTP hydrolysis are required. Thus, a tripeptide has formed; the dipeptide has transferred to the new aminoacyl-tRNA at the A site. The P site contains deacylated $tRNA^{Val}$, which will be released. Translocation again occurs with the tripeptidyl-tRNA shifting to the P site, and the ribosome moving one codon. Elongation of the entire mRNA continues in this fashion. Fairly early in elongation methionine is cleaved off, leaving valine as the first amino acid (Suzuki and Itano, 1972a,b; Yoshida *et al.*, 1970; Yoshida and Lin, 1972). The entire assembly of a globin chain takes approximately 60–80 sec (Clegg *et al.*, 1968; Dintzis, 1961; Hunt *et al.*, 1969; Lodish and Jacobsen, 1972; Rieder, 1972).

*2.1.3.3e. Termination and Release.* At the 3' end of mRNA the ribosome comes to a termination codon either UAA or UAG. These codons are called nonsense codons as they do not direct the incorporation of any amino acid. At this point elongation stops, the completed globin chain is released, and the ribosome falls off mRNA. This step requires a protein termination or release (R) factor and GTP (Beaudet and Caskey, 1971; Goldstein *et al.*, 1970; Tate *et al.*, 1973). The ribosome seems to fall off as an 80S ribosome, which is then dissociated by "dissociation factor" (DF) into the 40S and 60S subunits for reinitiation. However, DF might also be working by preventing the reassociation of the subunits. It is possible that the ribosome spontaneously dissociates into subunits as it falls off the mRNA and DF prevents it from reassociating to form inactive 80S ribosomes (Kaempfer and Kaufman, 1972a).

Efficient protein synthesis requires the recycling of all the initiation, elongation, and release factors, as well as ribosomal subunits. tRNA is also recycled. After it is released from the ribosome, aminoacyl-tRNA synthetase recharges it with its amino acid.

## 2.1.4. Assembly of Hemoglobin

### 2.1.4.1. Tetramer Formation

After release of the globin chain from the ribosome it is rapidly incorporated into complete hemoglobin molecules (Rossi-Fanelli et al., 1958; Winterhalter et al., 1969). This reaction is spontaneous, extremely rapid, and seems to require only heme. It is not yet known whether heme combines with globin in its physiologically active divalent form, or whether heme first binds in its trivalent form, forming methemoglobin which is then enzymatically reduced to functional hemoglobin. However, it is known that heme is not added to globin until after release from the polyribosome (Felicetti et al., 1966; Rabinovitz et al., 1969). Complete functional hemoglobin contains four heme groups, each of which is bound to a separate globin chain. Minor hemoglobin components containing only one, two, or three heme groups per tetramer have been identified (Winterhalter, 1966; Winterhalter and Glotthaar, 1971). Evidence has been presented that heme has a higher affinity for $\alpha$ chains than for $\beta$ chains in these partially heme-saturated tetramers. Thus, it is possible that partially heme-saturated tetramers, with heme attached to the $\alpha$ chains, are intermediates in normal hemoglobin assembly, but this still has not been conclusively proven.

However, heme-depleted globin chains can form dimers and tetramers with other heme-depleted or heme-saturated globin chains. Small pools of heme-depleted free $\alpha$ chains, heme-containing free $\alpha$ chains, and $\alpha$–non-$\alpha$ dimers have been found (Baglioni and Campana, 1967; Gill and Schwartz, 1973; Shaeffer, 1967; Tavill et al., 1968, 1972; Winterhalter et al., 1969; Zucker and Schulman, 1968). Newly labeled $\alpha$ chains are first found in the free $\alpha$-chain pool; later in the pool of $\alpha\beta$ dimers; and finally in complete hemoglobin molecules. Newly labeled $\beta$ chains are rapidly detected in small $\alpha\beta$ dimer pools and then in complete hemoglobin molecules. In heme deficiency states, discussed in greater detail later, newly synthesized globin chains accumulate in free $\alpha$-chain pools and $\alpha\beta$ dimers. When these systems are repleted with heme the globin chains are chased into complete hemoglobin tetramers (Felicetti et al., 1966; Tavill et al., 1968, 1972; Winterhalter et al., 1969). Thus, it seems that the combination of globin chains to form tetramers and the combination of heme with each globin chain are interdependent processes. Furthermore, it appears that $\alpha\beta$ dimers are physiologic intermediates in hemoglobin assembly.

## 2.1.4.2. Coordination of $\alpha$-Chain and Non-$\alpha$-Chain Synthesis

The synthesis of $\alpha$ chains and non-$\alpha$ chains is strictly regulated so that essentially equimolar amounts of each are produced. The question that has been raised is whether or not the synthesis of one chain controls the synthesis of the other. In the past, studies in cell-free systems suggested a theory whereby $\alpha$-chain synthesis is partially regulated through feedback inhibition of $\alpha$-chain synthesis by free $\alpha$ chains (Shaeffer *et al.*, 1969; Blum *et al.*, 1970). $\beta$-Chain synthesis, according to this view, is also subject to feedback inhibition, but the inhibition is indirect via depletion of the free $\alpha$-chain pool which in turn is required for maximal rates of $\beta$-chain release from polyribosomes. According to this view, $\alpha$-chain synthesis controls $\beta$-chain synthesis, but $\beta$-chain synthesis has essentially no effect on $\alpha$-chain synthesis.

Evidence against this theory, however, has come from several sources. Intact reticulocytes were obtained from rabbits with a variant hemoglobin containing less than one isoleucine residue per $\beta$ chain. It was assumed that the $\beta$ chain isolated from these rabbits was a mixture of two different $\beta$ chains, one containing one isoleucine residue and the other, none. When these reticulocytes were incubated with L-$O$-methylthreonine to induce an isoleucine deficiency, it was found that the synthesis of the isoleucine-containing $\beta$ chain, as well as the $\alpha$ chain, was inhibited. However, the synthesis of the isoleucine-deficient $\beta$ chain was stimulated. These studies suggest that at least in the intact reticulocyte neither chain is required for or aids the synthesis of the other (Rabinovitz *et al.*, 1969). They also suggest that neither chain regulates its own synthesis via feedback inhibition, since this would require its removal and combination with the other chain to prevent such inhibition. These conclusions have been confirmed in human cord blood reticulocytes where $O$-methylthreonine (OMT) inhibited the synthesis of the isoleucine-containing $\gamma$ chains, but the synthesis of the non-isoleucine-containing $\alpha$ chains continued and free $\alpha$ chains accumulated (Honig, 1967; Honig *et al.*, 1969). Wolf *et al.* (1973) and Garrick *et al.* (1975) confirmed the findings of Rabinovitz *et al.* (1969) using rabbit reticulocytes with variant hemoglobins (non-isoleucine-containing $\beta$ chains). $O$-Methylthreonine inhibited the isoleucine-containing $\alpha$-chain synthesis while $\beta$-chain synthesis continued normally. However, in bone marrow cells from these variant rabbits, inhibition of $\alpha$-chain synthesis was followed by a delayed but appreciable reduction in $\beta$-chain synthesis (Wolf *et al.*, 1973). This finding, together with the work of

Shaeffer *et al.* (1969) and Blum *et al.* (1970), suggests that there might be coarse but imperfect control of synthesis by one chain in order to make the other. However, as is demonstrated in thalassemic cells as well as in the studies with O-methylthreonine in reticulocytes, there is no absolute requirement for the synthesis of one chain in order to make the other.

There are two important differences, however, between the synthesis of $\alpha$ and $\beta$ chains. The first is that $\alpha$ chains are made on smaller polyribosomes than are $\beta$ chains (Hunt *et al.*, 1968a,b, 1969). This difference is accounted for by the fact that ribosomes initiate synthesis more frequently on $\beta$-chain mRNA than on $\alpha$-chain mRNA, whereas elongation and termination are the same (Lodish and Jacobsen, 1972). Studies by Lodish (1974) have shown that $\alpha$-mRNA has a lower affinity for ribosomes than $\beta$-mRNA; thus each $\beta$-mRNA directs the synthesis of more globin chains than each $\alpha$-mRNA. The second difference between the synthesis of $\alpha$ and $\beta$ chains is that there seems to be an excess of $\alpha$-chain mRNA (Lodish, 1971; Boyer *et al.*, 1974), perhaps corresponding to the duplicated genes for $\alpha$ chains (Lehmann and Carrell, 1968). It appears that the lower affinity of $\alpha$-chain mRNA has been selected for in order to compensate for the increase in $\alpha$-gene dosage.

### 2.1.4.3. Coordination of Heme and Globin Synthesis

There is excellent evidence that heme and globin synthesis are closely coordinated. Heme synthesis is at least partially controlled by end product inhibition (by heme) of the rate-limiting enzyme, ALA synthetase (Granick and Kappas, 1967; Kappas and Granick, 1968; Karibian and London, 1965; Freedman *et al.*, 1977). Thus, if intracellular heme levels are high, heme synthesis is inhibited. Similarly, if heme concentration is low, globin synthesis will be diminished. There is also evidence that heme synthesis is controlled by globin synthesis; when protein synthesis is inhibited, heme synthesis is also reduced (Grayzel *et al.*, 1967). In the absence of globin synthesis heme would accumulate, and it is probably this excessive heme which in turn then inhibits ALA synthetase. Thus, there is a control mechanism to coordinate closely the synthesis of heme and globin during erythropoiesis, which is discussed in a subsequent section.

### 2.1.5. Molecular Control Mechanisms in Normal Hemoglobin Synthesis

There are at least six points of potential molecular control of the synthesis of globin chains (Fig. 1). Some of these have been less well studied than others (e.g., nuclear processing or posttranscription). However, this does not necessarily imply that these are any less important. In this section the current understanding of these control mechanisms will be summarized.

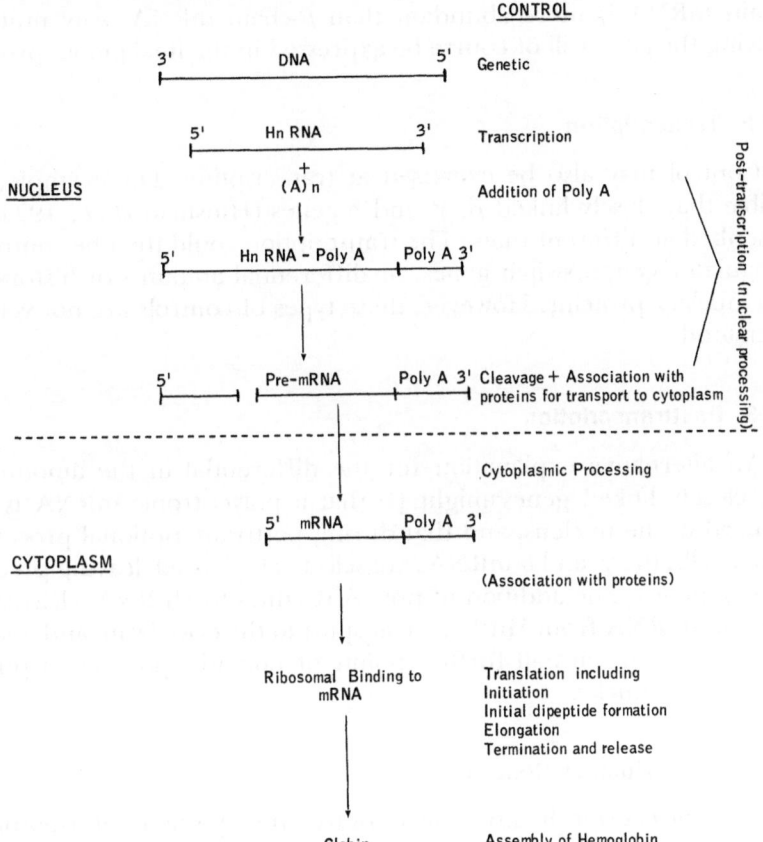

**Fig. 1.** Schematic representation of the control mechanisms involved in synthesis, processing, transport, and translation of mRNA into globin. Globin mRNA is first transcribed from DNA in the form of heterogeneous RNA (HnRNA). Poly A is added to the 3'-terminal end. Most of the HnRNA is turned over in the nucleus. The pre-mRNA becomes associated with proteins, and is transported to the cytoplasm. In the cytoplasm mRNA becomes associated with ribosomes, translation occurs, and globin is released for assembly into hemoglobin. Details of the control mechanisms are given in the text.

### 2.1.5.1. Gene Dosage

The first point of control is at the level of the gene, or DNA. It is now clear that the γ-chain and the α-chain loci are duplicated genes in humans, whereas β- and δ-chain genes are single copies (Weatherall and Clegg, 1972; Weatherall *et al.*, 1974; Schroeder and Huisman, 1974; Gambino *et al.*, 1974; Ottolenghi *et al.*, 1974, 1975; Taylor *et al.*, 1974; Kan *et al.*, 1975b; Lanyon *et al.*, 1975; Old *et al.*, 1976; Tolstoshev *et al.*, 1976). "Gene dosage" may play some role in the control of globin synthesis since

$\alpha$-chain mRNA is more abundant than $\beta$-chain mRNA. Any mutation involving the gene will of course be expressed in the final globin product.

### 2.1.5.2. Transcription

Control may also be exercised at transcription. For example, it is possible that closely linked $\beta$, $\gamma$, and $\delta$ genes (Huisman *et al.*, 1974) are transcribed at different rates. The transcription could then be controlled by regulator genes, switch genes, or differential amounts of histones or acidic nuclear proteins. However, these types of controls are not yet well understood.

### 2.1.5.3. Posttranscription

An alternative explanation for the differential in the amounts of these closely linked genes might be that a polycistronic mRNA is first produced in the nucleus, and that during posttranscriptional processing in adult cells, the $\gamma$- and $\delta$-mRNAs are selectively cleaved, leaving predominantly $\beta$ genes. The addition of poly A residues to HnRNA, cleavage of globin pre-mRNA from HnRNA, transport to the cytoplasm, and association with proteins are all further points of potential posttranscriptional control in the nucleus.

### 2.1.5.4. Other Nuclear Controls

Intranuclear mechanisms also control the synthesis of ribosomes: tRNA, transcriptional processing and translational factors, amino acid availability, and other requirements for globin synthesis. All of these nuclear requirements appear to be extremely complex and at this time poorly understood.

### 2.1.5.5. Cytoplasmic Pretranslation

As discussed in a preceding section, the cytoplasmic pretranslational control mechanisms are not yet well understood. However, the association with the correct proteins are potentially an important site of cytoplasmic control.

### 2.1.5.6. Translation

Most of the current knowledge of regulation of hemoglobin synthesis is on mechanisms of translational control.

*2.1.5.6a. mRNA and Ribosomes.* Globin mRNA is of course necessary for any translation to occur. In the reticulocyte globin mRNA seems to be quite stable since globin synthesis continues for 24–48 hr in the absence of a nucleus. Globin mRNA is quite susceptible to ribonuclease, and ribonuclease is present in erythroid cells (Burka, 1968, 1969, 1971; Farkas and Marks, 1968; Rowley and Morris, 1967; Rowley *et al.*, 1971). Furthermore, it has been demonstrated that mRNA is more resistant to ribonuclease when ribosomes are attached to them (as polyribosomes) than when it is free (DelMonte and Kazazian, 1971; Velez *et al.*, 1971; Freedman *et al.*, 1972). Thus, it is possible that in normal maturation and loss of mRNA, heme synthesis ceases, ribosomes are thus unable to initiate protein synthesis (see below), and mRNA is free and degraded by ribonuclease.

*2.1.5.6b. Heme Control of Globin Synthesis.* One of the most important controls of translation appears to be the interdependence of heme and globin synthesis. Heme (as hemin) has been shown to be necessary for maximal globin synthesis both in intact rabbit reticulocytes (Kruh and Borsook, 1956; Bruns and London, 1965; Waxman and Rabinovitz, 1965, 1966; Grayzel *et al.*, 1966; Waxman *et al.*, 1967; Rabinovitz *et al.*, 1969) and their cell-free preparations (Adamson *et al.*, 1968; Zucker and Schulman, 1968; Maxwell and Rabinovitz, 1969; Rabinovitz *et al.*, 1969; Howard *et al.*, 1970; Maxwell *et al.*, 1971; Hunt *et al.*, 1972). When intact cells are incubated in the absence of hemin and are rendered iron deficient by an iron chelating agent, the polyribosomes are converted to single ribosomes not attached to mRNA. Furthermore, globin synthesis is markedly inhibited. These results suggest that inhibition of heme synthesis results in an inhibition of initiation of globin synthesis. Both hemin and a ferrous iron–transferrin mixture prevent and reverse this effect on initiation in intact cells. Studies utilizing rabbit reticulocyte cell-free lysate preparations have shown that in the absence of hemin, a hemin-controlled translational repressor of initiation (HCR) forms in the postribosomal supernatant at the same time globin synthesis stops (Rabinovitz *et al.*, 1969; Maxwell and Rabinovitz, 1969; Mizuno *et al.*, 1972; Gross and Rabinovitz, 1972a,b; Adamson *et al.*, 1972; Legon *et al.*, 1973; Darnborough *et al.*, 1973; Balkow *et al.*, 1973a,b; Clemens *et al.*, 1974; Freedman *et al.*, 1974). Hemin markedly retards the formation of this repressor. A similar HCR may be isolated from human or rabbit mature erythrocytes, but not from reticulocytes (Freedman *et al.*, 1974). This is evidence that HCR indeed plays a physiological role in maturation and cessation of protein synthesis.

HCR has now been shown to reduce the level of Met-tRNA$_f^{Met}$ associated with ribosomal subunits (Darnborough *et al.*, 1973; Balkow *et al.*, 1973a; Clemens *et al.*, 1974; London *et al.*, 1976; Hunt, 1976). This inhibition may be overcome by a ribosomal preparation which has been subfractionated to yield an initiation factor "IF-MP" which mediates binding of Met-tRNA$_f^{Met}$ to the 40S ribosomal subunit. Clemens *et al.* (1974) have proposed that HCR directly inhibits IF-MP-dependent binding of Met-tRNA$_f^{Met}$ to the 40S ribosomal subunit. Balkow *et al.* (1973a), however, suggested that the impaired binding is a secondary phenomenon with the primary effect of HCR being deacylation of the Met-tRNA$_f^{Met}$ on the 40S subunit (initial dipeptide formation). To add to this complexity, Raffel *et al.* (1974) presented evidence that hemin promotes protein synthesis by mediating the formation of an active initiation factor complex (stimulator) from inactive lower molecular weight components. It is certainly possible that the "inactive" component (minus hemin) is a repressor whereas the "active" component (plus hemin) is a stimulator (perhaps even IF-MP). However, there is no evidence yet to support this view.

HCR has been partially purified and shown to be a protein which acts catalytically, since one molecule can inactivate up to 1000 ribosomes (Gross and Rabinovitz, 1972a). It forms from a "proinhibitor" which is normally present in the cytoplasm and does not inhibit protein synthesis. Incubation of a postribosomal supernatant or the partially purified proin-hibitor results in the formation of the inhibitor. This incubation does not require added energy or factors, only temperature elevation (Maxwell and Rabinovitz, 1969; Rabinovitz *et al.*, 1969; Freedman *et al.*, 1974). Formation of this repressor occurs rapidly (within 2–10 min) at 34–37°C but much slower at 25°C (Gross and Rabinovitz, 1972a,b). It has been suggested on the basis of incubation of reticulocyte postribosomal super-nates without hemin, that a "hemin reversible" repressor first forms from the proinhibitor state. According to this view, with prolonged incubations minus hemin the repressor converts to a "hemin irreversible" state (Gross, 1974). Recently we diluted samples of "irreversible repressor" and observed kinetics identical to that of "reversible repressor" (Freedman and Rosman, 1976). These results suggest that the differences in kinetics observed between so-called reversible and irreversible forms of HCR reflect differences in the quantity of the same protein. Since high concen-trations of hemin also inhibit reticulocyte–lysate cell-free systems (Kaplan *et al.*, 1974), it might be that in these test systems insufficient hemin is added to reverse large quantities of HCR, and thus we see "irreversible" kinetics.

HCR formation is accelerated by the presence of ATP and largely prevented by high levels of GTP (Balkow *et al.*, 1975). Thiol-reactive agents such as *N*-ethylmaleimide also accelerate the formation of this inhibitor. There is always a lag period of normal protein synthesis before

HCR-induced inhibition is apparent; in cell-free systems this is of the order of 5–15 min. Of interest is that similar inhibitory kinetics is found in the presence of oxidized glutathione (Zehavi-Willner et al., 1971; Kosower et al., 1972) or with the addition of double-stranded RNA (dsRNA) (Ehrenfeld and Hunt, 1971).

Recently, several groups have shown that very high concentrations (nonphysiological) of cyclic AMP are capable of reversing the inhibitory properties of HCR in cell-free systems (Legon et al., 1974; Levin et al., 1975). In addition other purines such as adenine, 2-aminopurine, caffeine, and theophylline could reverse HCR inhibition. Hunt (1976) has postulated the following mechanisms to explain the action of HCR in cell-free systems. He states that HCR has an absolute requirement for ATP in order to prevent the binding of Met-tRNA$_f^{Met}$ to 40S ribosomal subunits, and that IF-MP becomes phosphorylated and inactive during incubation of ribosomes with HCR and ATP. According to this theory, cyclic AMP prevents this phosphorylation. He has evidence that HCR fractions, which are not yet completely purified, contain a protein kinase which is rather specific for IF-MP, and which can catalytically prevent the binding of Met-tRNA$_f^{Met}$ to 40S ribosomal subunits in an ATP-dependent reaction. Furthermore, he has found similar results with dsRNA, but the inhibitor which phosphorylates IF-MP appears to be different from HCR and seems to require phosphorylation itself in order to be activated. It is not yet clear how the effects of oxidized glutathione are mediated.

If inhibition of globin synthesis is the result of the action of this protein kinase, presumably a protein phosphatase is also involved in reversing its activity. Thus, Hunt has suggested that the role of hemin might be regulation of this protein phosphatase (Hunt, 1976). Hirsch and Martelo (1976), however, have recently isolated a specific cytoplasmic cyclic AMP-dependent protein kinase from rabbit reticulocytes which was inhibited by hemin. These investigators suggested that this protein kinase might be HCR and that hemin could reverse it directly.

Recently in our laboratory we have looked at the control of HCR activity in intact reticulocytes (Freedman et al., 1976a). We have used the intact cell rather than the cell-free system since the latter lacks membrane sites for adenyl cyclase and heme synthesis. We were able to demonstrate that agents which are known to stimulate adenyl cyclase (epinephrine and isoproterenol) or inhibit phosphodiesterase (theophylline), or enter the cell as cyclic AMP (dibutyryl cAMP) protected against inhibitors of heme synthesis. In addition, these compounds elevated cAMP concentrations in the intact reticulocyte, prevented HCR activation, and prevented inhibition of reticulocyte protein synthesis. The cAMP reversal of inhibition of heme synthesis occurred prior to the reversal of protein synthesis, suggesting that the physiological control in the intact cell is hemin concentration. Thus we have postulated that the primary effect of cAMP in hemin control of protein synthesis is maintenance of a maximal rate of heme synthesis. Our data, however, do not contradict the observations in cell-free systems discussed previously. It is possible that there are several control points for hemin control. A tentative model for hemin control is shown in Fig. 2.

This model of hemin control is consistent with the large amount of work discussed previously, showing that cAMP can stimulate *in vitro* erythropoiesis and heme synthesis. Recently, Glass *et al.* (1975), using bone marrow precursors in tissue culture, showed that erythropoietin first stimulates δ-ALA synthetase and heme synthesis prior to its effect on globin synthesis. In this system, heme synthesis is maximal in the earliest precursor cells and decreases with cell maturity, whereas globin synthesis increases with cell maturity. These findings are compatible with the postulate that there must first be sufficient intracellular hemin to convert HCR from its inhibitory to its noninhibitory state before protein synthesis may proceed. Even though it is possible that the effects of cAMP are independent of erythropoietin and/or of different cells, it appears that cAMP can stimulate heme synthesis in at least some erythroid precursors.

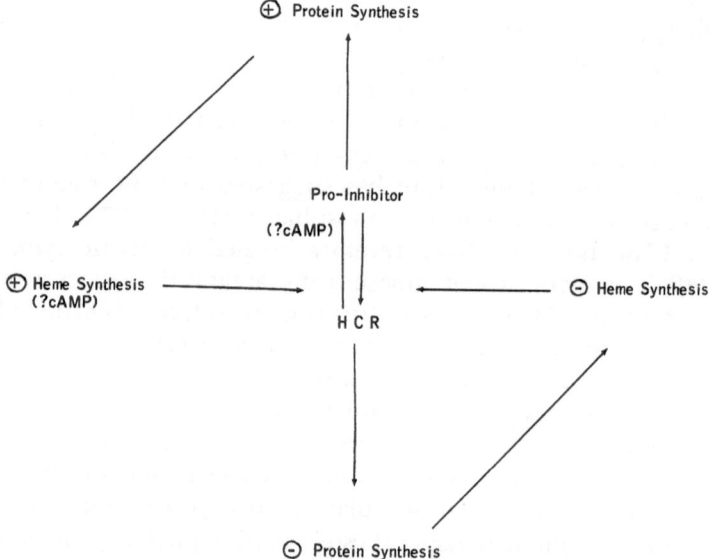

**Fig. 2.**  Relationship between heme synthesis, HCR formation from the proinhibitor, and protein synthesis. In the presence of heme synthesis ⊕ , the noninhibitory proinhibitor allows protein synthesis ⊕ . In the absence of heme synthesis ⊖ , HCR forms to inhibit initiation of protein synthesis ⊖ . Cyclic AMP (cAMP) has been postulated to be required for stabilization of the proinhibitor and/or for maintenance of heme synthesis. When protein synthesis is inhibited at a nonheme-requiring step, the excess heme inhibits heme synthesis by feedback inhibition at ALA synthetase. See the text for details.

In our studies we found that the effect of cAMP was to maintain maximal heme synthesis in the presence of inhibitors of heme synthesis. The inhibitors of heme synthesis used were ethanol, $\alpha,\alpha$-dipyridyl, and benzene. Ethanol has been reported to inhibit pyridoxal phosphokinase (Hines and Grasso, 1970) and uroporphyrinogen cosynthetase (Chu and Chu, 1970) whereas benzene exerts its effect at or before $\delta$-aminolevulinic acid synthetase (Freedman et al., 1977). $\alpha,\alpha$-Dipyridyl is a ferrous iron chelating agent. Of note is that $Fe^{2+}$ has been reported to be necessary for the enzyme function of many of the heme synthetic enzymes, including $\delta$-aminolevulinic acid synthetase, aminolevulinic acid dehydratase, copro-porphyrinogen oxidase, and ferrochelatase (Moore and Goldberg, 1974). The mechanism by which iron combines with protoporphyrin and globin to form heme is not yet completely understood. It has been proposed that there are intracellular iron compounds of small molecular weight to which iron attaches as it passes from transferrin to hemoglobin (Mazur and Carleton, 1963; Zail et al., 1964; Primosigh and Thomas, 1968). Chelates of iron with ATP or ADP have been proposed as being candidates for this role, but other soluble chelates are also possible. The iron deficiency induced by $\alpha,\alpha$-dipyridyl is a deficiency of ionic iron and does not neces-sarily have to result in an inability of other forms of iron to combine with protoporphyrin to form heme. This view is supported by the observation that heme synthesis continues normally in the presence of elevated cAMP and dipyridyl. These results suggest that iron is still available for combin-ing with protoporphyrin even when ionic iron is unavailable. In support of this explanation is our inability to find elevated levels of free erythro-cyte protoporphyrin in these cells treated with dipyridyl.

In order to best explain the observations that elevation of cAMP concentration resulted in continued heme synthesis in the presence of these three different-acting inhibitors of heme synthesis, a common point of toxicity requiring cAMP has to be demonstrated. One possibility not yet demonstrated might be iron release from transferrin which has been reported by Ponka and Neuwirt (1975) to require cAMP.

Furthermore, the hemin effect does not seem specific to the synthesis of globin. Recently, it has been shown that hemin is necessary for maximal protein synthesis of the nonglobin proteins of the reticulocyte (Mizuno et al., 1972; Lodish and Desalu, 1973; Lodish, 1974; Beuzard et al., 1973), as well as for Krebs II ascites tumor cells (Beuzard et al., 1973), platelets (Freedman and Karpatkin, 1973; Karpatkin et al., 1974), brain and liver cells (Raffel et al., 1974), as well as mRNAs for nonmammalian proteins (Rhoads et al., 1973; Matthews et al., 1973). Although it still remains to be shown if the hemin control in all these systems is via the hemin-controlled repressor, it appears that hemin control might be a major universal point of control of initiation.

*2.1.5.6c. Specificity of Ribosomes and Initiation Factors.* There are other possible control points of initiation. Postulated mechanisms include specificity of reticulocyte ribosomes for $\alpha$- and $\beta$-mRNA as well as messenger RNA-specific initiation factors (Hall and Arnstein, 1973; Nudel *et al.,* 1973). The evidence with O-methylthreonine, however, tends to argue against absolute specificity of ribosomes for a particular mRNA (Kazazian and Freedman, 1968). When reticulocytes were made isoleucine deficient with this amino acid analog, 70% of the total quality of $\alpha$ and $\beta$ ribosomes were found participating in $\beta$-chain synthesis Thus, a large part of the ribosomes that normally would have been involved in $\alpha$-chain synthesis were capable of being initiated on $\beta$-chain mRNA. Further evidence has been presented that ribosomes from many different species and tissues are nonspecific in their ability to translate mammalian globin mRNA (Benz and Forget, 1974). Similarly, initiation factors from many different species and tissues seem to be interchangeable with reticulocyte initiation factors in translating globin mRNA (Benz and Forget, 1974). Thus, it appears that there are no absolute mRNA-specific initiation factors required for globin mRNA translation. It is still possible, however, that there are "fine" control mechanisms involving either specificity of ribosomes or specific initiation factors.

*2.1.5.6d. Elongation and Release.* Modulation is a term that has been given to a control mechanism when the addition of some amino acids to the nascent chain on the ribosome occurs more slowly than the addition of other amino acids (Itano, 1966). According to this theory, translation will be slower at the 5'-nucleotide end of mRNA or proximal to the rate-limiting codon, whereas distally (3'-nucleotide end) it will be normal. Thus, ribosomes will accumulate proximal to the rate-limiting step. Modulation can occur from deficiencies of amino acids, as we have demonstrated experimentally (Freedman *et al.,* 1968a,b; Kazazian and Freedman, 1968; Rabinovitz *et al.,* 1969; Freedman and Rabinovitz, 1970, 1971). In addition, since the genetic code is degenerate, there are several codons coding for the same amino acid. Thus, different codons could exist within an mRNA calling for the same amino acid but a different tRNA. Some tRNAs could be scarce and thus translation would be retarded at this step (Anderson, 1969; Anderson and Gilbert, 1969a,b).

If modulation occurred in normal elongation, then there would have to be an asymmetrical distribution of ribosomes on mRNA and an asymmetrical rate of synthesis of the nascent chain. If modulation occurred toward the 3'-nucleotide end of mRNA or at release, there would be maximal packing of ribosomes as seen with cysteine deficiency (Freedman *et al.,* 1968b) or isoleucine deficiency (Kazazian and Freedman, 1968; Rabinovitz *et al.,* 1969; Freedman and Rabinovitz, 1971) in rabbit reticulocytes. Studies investigating this possibility in normal cells have shown that there is no retardation of either ribosomes or chain synthesis along globin mRNA (Hunt *et al.*, 1968b; Luppis *et al.*, 1970; Rieder, 1972). Thus, it is now accepted that modulation does not occur in normal globin synthesis. Similarly there is no retardation at release. It is now well accepted that initiation is the major site of control of normal translation.

## 2.2. Abnormal Globin Synthesis

This section reviews the molecular abnormalities that have been shown or postulated to exist in a wide variety of red cell disorders. No attempt is made to discuss all the pathophysiology of these illnesses or the clinical, diagnostic, and therapeutic problems. Rather, the focus is on mechanisms of abnormal globin synthesis and how they relate to disease.

### 2.2.1. Synthesis of Globin in Thalassemia and Related States

Thalassemia is a term used to describe a heterogeneous group of diseases characterized by the following three common features: (a) they are all hereditary disorders; (b) there is a decrease (or absence) of synthesis of one of the normal globin chains, with (c) a normal rate of synthesis of the other normal chains resulting in a relative overproduction of these chains. This imbalance in globin chain synthesis leads to precipitation of the chain produced in excess which results in ineffective erythropoiesis and hemolysis of the erythrocyte (Weatherall and Clegg, 1972; Freedman, 1974).

The thalassemias are broadly classified as $\alpha$- or $\beta$-thalassemia. Thus, in $\alpha$-thalassemia there is a decrease in $\alpha$-chain synthesis (Clegg and Weatherall, 1976) and a relative overproduction of $\beta$ chains. Since $\alpha$ chains are also part of Hb F, there is also an excess of $\gamma$ chains. In $\beta$-thalassemia it is the $\beta$-chain synthesis which is depressed, and there is a relative overproduction of $\alpha$ chains (Weatherall *et al.*, 1965; Heywood *et al.*, 1965; Bank and Marks, 1966; Bargellesi *et al.*, 1967; Modell *et al.*, 1969).

#### 2.2.1.1. $\beta$-Thalassemia

*2.2.1.1a. Definition.* Most evidence now indicates that there is a single $\beta$-gene locus on a chromosome (Rucknagel and Winter, 1974). The homozygote for $\beta$-thalassemia has both chromosomes affected, whereas the heterozygote has only one chromosome affected. The deficiency in adequate amounts of $\beta$ chains results in a decreased amount of Hb A and total hemoglobin in the red cells. $\alpha$-Chain synthesis is not impeded, which results in a large relative excess of $\alpha$ chains (Bank, 1968; Huehns and Modell, 1967) that precipitate in the cells (Fessas *et al.*, 1966; Weatherall *et al.*, 1969). In $\beta$-thalassemia the precipitated $\alpha$ chains form inclusion bodies (Heinz bodies) which are present both in the soluble and stromal fractions of the cells. Thus, the membranes of these cells are damaged. The inclusions form rigid areas of the cells which are removed by the spleen and other reticuloendothelial organs (Nathan and Gunn, 1966; Nathan *et al.*, 1969), resulting in deformation of cell shape. The membrane damage induced by the $\alpha$-chain inclusion bodies leads to marked premature destruction in the bone marrow (ineffective erythropoiesis). This ineffective erythropoiesis is responsible for the iron overload seen in patients with $\beta$-thalassemia.

In $\beta$-thalassemia there is an attempt to compensate for the diminished $\beta$-chain synthesis by increasing the production of either $\gamma$ chains (Hb F) or $\delta$ chains (Hb A$_2$), or both. However, the compensation is never complete. Furthermore, the increase in Hb F is heterogeneous; some cells have a great increase in Hb F, others no increase (Shepard *et al.*, 1962). If it were possible to have a homogeneous distribution of Hb F as well as balanced $\alpha$- and $\gamma$-chain synthesis, it would be possible to restore normal functional hemoglobin levels. In the rare homozygous condition of hereditary persistence of Hb F, there is no $\beta$- or $\delta$-chain production (see later) and yet the markedly increased $\gamma$-chain production which is homogeneously distributed in all erythrocytes is sufficient to prevent anemia or other symptomatology of thalassemia. The recent demonstration that marrow cells placed into an *in vitro* culture system synthesize increased amounts of Hb F indicates that it might be possible either to induce hemoglobin synthesis or at least select out clones of cells that are more capable of producing Hb F (Papayannopoulous *et al.*, 1976). If it were possible to accomplish this *in vivo*, thalassemia could be cured.

*2.2.1.1b. Molecular Mechanisms.* The $\beta$-thalassemias may be subdivided into those that produce some $\beta$ chains ($\beta^+$-thalassemia); those that do not ($\beta^0$); and those that produce neither $\beta$ or $\delta$ chains ($\delta\beta^0$). It has been shown by many investigators that the defect in thalassemia is not in the ribosomes (Bank and Marks, 1966), the rate of translation (Clegg *et al.*, 1968; Rieder, 1972), or in the factors needed for initiation (Nathan *et al.*, 1971; Gilbert *et al.*, 1970; Nienhius *et al.*, 1971). The defect is now accepted to be in the amount of functional ability of the mRNA specific for the affected chain (see reviews by Forget, 1974; Nienhuis and Anderson, 1974; Benz and Forget, 1975; Clegg and Weatherall, 1976).

The type of experiments to show this depended on several findings in molecular biology research. First, these experiments utilized the enzyme RNA-dependent DNA polymerase ("reverse transcriptase") which could synthesize a DNA copy of globin mRNA (Verma *et al.*, 1972; Ross *et al.*,

1972; Kacian *et al.*, 1972). Secondly, these experiments used a method of isolation of chain-specific mRNAs (Temple and Housman, 1972; Jacobs-Lorena and Baglioni, 1972) from L-$O$-methylthreonine-separated rabbit $\alpha$- and $\beta$-chain polyribosomes (Kazazian and Freedman, 1968).

Using these chain-specific mRNAs and the RNA-dependent DNA polymerase of avian myeloblastosis virus, a radioactive DNA copy was made of specific rabbit $\alpha$- and $\beta$-mRNA. Then with hybridization techniques it was possible to show that in $\beta$-thalassemia there was decreased or absent $\beta$-mRNA, and in $\alpha$-thalassemia a similar deficiency in $\alpha$-mRNA. This technique showed that in the thalassemic patients studied there was a deficiency of mRNA. It also made it possible to isolate chain-specific human mRNA. For example, in a $\beta$-thalassemia without detectable $\beta$-mRNA, there is a large amount of $\alpha$-chain mRNA. Similarly, in the $\alpha$-thalassemias (see below) there is a great amount of $\beta$-chain mRNA. Specific DNA copies could now be made of these mRNAs and used as probes in hybridization studies to determine in other patients if there was a deficiency of mRNA. Similarly, these probes could be used to quantitate the number of genes (Forget, 1974; Nienhuis and Anderson, 1974; Benz and Forget, 1975; Clegg and Weatherall, 1976).

Using these techniques it has been possible to show that $\beta^+$-thalassemia results from a reduced production of $\beta$-chain mRNA (Housman *et al.*, 1973; Kacian *et al.*, 1973). Since there is some $\beta$-chain synthesis (and $\beta$-mRNA) this condition could not be the result of gene deletion. Thus, it must result from either abnormal transcription or processing of mRNA (Table I).

**Table I.** Reported Molecular Abnormalities in the $\beta$-Thalassemias and $\beta$-Thalassemia-like States

| Disease | Molecular abnormality | Postulated primary defect |
|---------|----------------------|---------------------------|
| $\beta^+$-Thal | ↓ $\beta$-mRNA | Transcription or processing |
| $\beta^0$-Thal | $\beta$-mRNA absent, $\beta$ genes present | Transcription or processing |
| $\beta^0$-Thal | $\beta$-mRNA present but nonfunctional | Abnormal mRNA |
| $\beta^0$-Thal | $\beta$-mRNA present, $\beta$-chain synthesis inducible | $\beta$-mRNA requires additional translational factors |
| $\delta\beta^0$-Thal | $\beta$-mRNA absent, $\delta\beta$ genes absent | $\delta\beta$ gene deletion |
| HPHF (Negro type) | $\beta$-mRNA absent, $\delta\beta$ genes absent | $\delta\beta$ gene deletion (? also deletion of additional DNA regulating switch to $\beta$-gene production) |
| Hb Lepore | $\delta\beta$-mRNA | $\delta\beta$ fusion gene |

At least three types of $\beta^0$-thalassemia exist (Table I). The most common type is where there is absent $\beta$-mRNA (Dow et al., 1973; Pritchard et al., 1976), but $\beta$ genes are present (Tolstoshev et al., 1976). This then would result from a defect in transcription or nuclear processing. The second type is where there is $\beta$-mRNA demonstrable by hybridization techniques, but which cannot be induced to synthesize $\beta$ chains (Kan et al., 1975a). Thus, this $\beta$-mRNA is nonfunctional, presumably due to an alteration in some critical portion of the molecule. The third type would be where $\beta$-mRNA is present and functional but cannot be utilized until a soluble cell fraction, presumably containing translational requirements, is added (Conconi et al., 1972) (Table I). It is also easy to imagine a type of $\beta^0$-thalassemia existing which would result from $\beta$-gene deletion, even though this has not yet been described and is not shown in Table I.

However, in $\delta\beta^0$-thalassemia (Table I) absence of both $\beta$-mRNA and $\delta$ and $\beta$ genes has been demonstrated. This type then seems to occur as a result of a deletion of the closely linked $\delta$- and $\beta$-gene loci (Clegg and Weatherall, 1976). One could also imagine similar heterogeneity in the $\delta\beta^0$-thalassemias as is seen in the $\beta^0$-thalassemias.

Studies of the heterozygous form of $\beta$-thalassemia have shown that in bone marrow cells of these patients surprisingly there is a balanced $\beta/\alpha$ synthetic ratio of 1.0, whereas the peripheral blood ratio is 0.5 (Schwartz, 1970; Kan et al., 1972; Clegg and Weatherall, 1972). Wood and Stamatoyannopoulos (1975) have recently shown evidence that in $\beta$-thalassemia heterozygotes a large $\alpha$-chain pool is present throughout erythroid cell maturation and that the observed balance in chain synthesis is a function of the ability of the early marrow cells to degrade the excess $\alpha$ chains. This finding then points to a potentially important control point in globin synthesis.

### 2.2.1.2. Hereditary Persistence of Hb F

*2.2.1.2a. Definition.* Hereditary persistence of Hb F is a term which is used to describe the persistent production of Hb F beyond the neonatal period. There appears to be several varieties of this condition, all of which are unassociated with any major hematological abnormalities (Edington and Lehmann, 1955; Conley et al., 1963). There is increasing evidence that many of these disorders are extremely mild forms of $\beta$-thalassemia with minimal chain imbalance due to the almost complete compensation for defective $\beta$-chain synthesis by the production of $\gamma$ chains (Weatherall and Clegg, 1974; Clegg and Weatherall, 1976).

*2.2.1.2b. Molecular Mechanisms.* Hemoglobin F is a mixture of two molecules which are identical except for one amino acid at position 136.

The chains containing glycine and alanine at position 136 are designated $^G\gamma$ and $^A\gamma$, respectively (Huisman *et al.*, 1974). The $\gamma$ gene is duplicated and there are at least four genes for $\gamma$ chains; furthermore, each chain is the product of a separate gene. The postulated order of genes on the chromosome for the non-$\alpha$ chains is $^G\gamma$, $^A\gamma$, $\delta$, $\beta$ (Huisman *et al.*, 1974). At least one type of hereditary persistence of Hb F (Negro type) has been shown to result from a gene deletion of the $\delta\beta$ locus (Kan *et al.*, 1975c). Thus it appears that there is at least some area of DNA that suppresses neonatal $\gamma$-chain production (Table I).

$\delta\beta^0$-Thalassemia also results from a gene deletion, but in thalassemia the hemoglobin F is distributed heterogeneously and does not make up for the lack of $\beta$-chain production. In contrast, in the Negro type of HPHF, the Hb F is homogeneously distributed and almost completely compensates for the lack of $\beta$ chains, even though there is slight imbalance in globin chain production (Charache *et al.*, 1975). The reason for these differences between $\delta\beta^0$-thalassemia and this type of HPHF is not yet well understood but might involve the areas of DNA that suppress $\gamma$-chain production.

Finally, a form of hereditary persistence of Hb F with heterogeneous distribution of Hb F has been studied in which there was no evidence of thalassemia (Clegg and Weatherall, 1976). In this family the homozygote made both $\gamma$ and $\beta$ chains on each chromosome with no chain imbalance detectable. The heterogeneous distribution of Hb F, however, suggests that there are genetic loci controlling the selection of cell populations during fetal maturation. Thus, the change from Hb F to Hb A production during development appears to depend both on genetic control areas on the chromosome containing $\gamma$ and $\beta$ chains, as well as on genetic controls selecting clones of cells.

### 2.2.1.3. Hemoglobins Lepore

*2.2.1.3a. Definition.* The hemoglobins Lepore are often classified with the $\beta$-thalassemias. These are a group of hemoglobins that consist of normal $\alpha$ chains combined with non-$\alpha$ chains which have the N-terminal end of the $\delta$ chain fused to the C-terminal end of the $\beta$ chain.

*2.2.1.3b. Molecular Mechanisms.* It is believed that the hemoglobins Lepore have arisen by chromosomal misalignment with unequal crossover between the $\delta$- and $\beta$-chain genes (Baglioni, 1962). This results in a $\delta\beta$ fusion gene which directs the synthesis of the non-$\alpha$ chains (Table I). The kinetics of $\beta$-chain synthesis are the same as those of $\delta$-chain synthesis (Rieder and Weatherall, 1965), resulting in a marked reduction in the amount of this non-$\alpha$ chain. In addition, the anti-Lepore hemoglobin (Hb

Miyada) which is a $\beta\delta$ fusion product has been described, and it also has kinetics of $\delta$-chain synthesis. This is in contrast with a $\gamma\beta$ fusion product, Hb Kenya (Huisman *et al.*, 1972), which is synthesized normally. Clegg and Weatherall (1974, 1976) have suggested that the instability of $\delta$-, $\beta$-, and $\delta\beta$-mRNAs results from the lack of sequences at the 5' and 3' ends of their mRNAs, which are present in $\alpha$-, $\beta$-, and $\gamma$-chain mRNAs and act as stabilizing regions. Degradation of such susceptible mRNA molecules soon after synthesis would lead to low levels in affected cells.

#### 2.2.1.4. $\alpha$-Thalassemias

*2.2.1.4a. Definition.* In the $\alpha$-thalassemias there is normal $\beta$-chain and $\gamma$-chain synthesis. The $\beta_4$ tetramers (Hemoglobin H) and the $\gamma$-chain tetramers (hemoglobin Bart's) are more soluble and stable than excessive $\alpha$ chains. As a result the cells in $\alpha$-thalassemia are more likely to be delivered to the peripheral circulation, and there is less ineffective erythropoiesis and iron overload than in the $\beta$-thalassemias. Both Hb H and Hb Bart's have extremely high oxygen affinity and are thus useless as oxygen carriers (Clegg and Weatherall, 1976).

*2.2.1.4b. Molecular Mechanisms.* In recent years it has become easier to understand the $\alpha$-thalassemia syndromes. The $\alpha$ genes in many, if not all, humans are duplicated (Rucknagel and Winter, 1974). Thus, there are two $\alpha$ genes on each chromosome and each of the four genes perhaps produces 25% of the total $\alpha$ chains. The types of $\alpha$-thalassemia found support this view. It is now believed that the silent carrier state represents a deletion of one gene; $\alpha$-thalassemia minor is a deletion of two genes; Hb H disease, a deletion of three genes; and the $\alpha$-thalassemia hydrops fetalis is the total deletion of four genes (Kan *et al.*, 1975b) (Table II).

#### 2.2.1.5. Chain Termination Mutants: Hb Constant Spring

*2.2.1.5a. Definition.* An interesting variant of Hb H disease has been found and is being described with increasing frequency. In these cases a small quantity of an $\alpha$-chain hemoglobin variant is found, which has been called hemoglobin Constant Spring. There is now good genetic evidence that patients who received the Hb Constant Spring gene from one parent and a deleted pair of $\alpha$ genes from the other have this type of Hb H disease (Clegg and Weatherall, 1976) (Table II).

*2.2.1.5b. Molecular Mechanisms.* Hb Constant Spring has an elongated $\alpha$ chain in which there are 31 extra residues at the C-terminal end. The best evidence is that there was a single base change in the termination

**Table II.** Probable Genetic Defects in the α-Thalassemias and α-Thalassemia-like States

| Clinical | Postulated genetic defect |
|---|---|
| Silent carrier | One α gene deleted |
| α-Thalassemia minor | Two α genes deleted |
| Hb H disease | Three α genes deleted |
| Hydrops fetalis | Four α genes deleted |
| Hb Constant Spring | Mutation in termination codon resulting in abnormally long α chain |
| Hb Constant Spring: Hb H disease | Two deleted genes (α-thal minor) together with Hb Constant Spring gene |

codon UAA to CAA which codes for glutamine. Thus, the mRNA is read through at the 3' end of α-chain mRNA until it reaches another termination codon at position 173 (Milner *et al.*, 1971; Forget *et al.*, 1974) (Fig. 3). Single base changes in the termination codon could result in other amino acid substitutions. Indeed, additional hemoglobins with elongated chains (both α and β chains) have recently been described (see Sections 2.1.3 and 2.2.2.1b). The reason these chain-termination mutant hemoglobins are synthesized only in small amounts is not yet completely understood. However, it appears that as the Hb Lepore, the mRNA is unstable. This might be because areas at the 3' end are translated, and this somehow alters the stability of the mRNA (Clegg and Weatherall, 1976).

Position

| α chain | | 137 | 138 | 139 | 140 | 141 | Term |
|---|---|---|---|---|---|---|---|
| NORMAL | mRNA codon | (ACC) | (UCC) | (AAA) | (UAC) | GCU | UAA |
| | Amino acid | Threo | Ser | Lys | Tyr | (Arg) | |

| CONSTANT SPRING | | | | | | | mutation U → C |
|---|---|---|---|---|---|---|---|
| | mRNA codon | (ACC) | (UCC) | (AAA) | (UAC) | (GCU) | (CAA) --------- 172 |
| | Amino acid | Threo | Ser | Lys | Tyr | Arg | Gln |

| WAYNE | | | | ↓Deletion & Frameshift | | | |
|---|---|---|---|---|---|---|---|
| | mRNA codon | (ACC) | (UCC) | (AAU) ACG | CUU | AAX --------- 146 |
| | Amino acid | Threo | Ser | Asn | Threo | Leu | Lys |

**Fig. 3.** Postulated lesions in α-chain termination mutants, Hbs Constant Spring and Wayne.

## 2.2.2. Synthesis of Structurally Abnormal Hemoglobins

### 2.2.2.1. Genetic Mechanisms

Hundreds of structurally abnormal hemoglobins have been described. They arise from mutations in a globin chain gene which cause the addition, deletion, or substitution of amino acids in the amino acid sequence.

*2.2.2.1a. Point Mutations.* By far the most common genetic alteration resulting in an abnormal hemoglobin is a point mutation, or the substitution of a single DNA nucleotide base for another (Lehmann and Carrell, 1969). This change in the genetic code can result in the substitution of one amino acid for another in the globin chain. For example, Hb S contains normal $\alpha$ chains and altered $\beta$ chains with a valine replacing the glutamic acid in the $\beta6$ position (Pauling *et al.,* 1949). This change can be explained by a single mutational event in which a single base in the $\beta$-chain gene is altered. For example, Hb S could arise by mutation of the GAA mRNA codon for glutamic acid to GAU which codes for valine. The mutation in the corresponding DNA would of course be CTT→CTA (Benz and Forget, 1974).

Two types of point mutations have been described. A transition is a substitution of a pyrimidine for another pyrimidine or a purine for another purine. A transversion is a substitution of a purine for a pyrimidine or vice versa. Transversions tend to result in more radical alterations in protein structure than transitions. If mutations occurred at random, twice as many transversions as transitions should be observed. However, transitions and transversions are found about equally (Lehmann and Carrell, 1969). If only substitutions affecting the molecular surface of hemoglobin are investigated, twice as many transversions are found. However, changes in the molecular core are usually produced by transitions. Purine transitions are more common than pyrimidine and the most common of all is adenine→guanine in DNA (Bunn *et al.,* 1972). The reason for these findings is not yet well understood.

The only exception to the one base change appears to be Hb Bristol where at $\beta67$ aspartic acid replaces valine (Lehmann and Carrell, 1969). None of the valine codons differ from any of the aspartic acid codons by only one base. Thus, either there has been a change of two bases, or a mutation has occurred in a previously mutated gene, or some other mechanism must be invoked.

*2.2.2.1b. Abnormally Long Hemoglobins.* The second type of mutation is the abnormally long hemoglobins, such as hemoglobin Constant Spring or hemoglobin Wayne (Fig. 3). Hemoglobin Constant Spring can be explained by a single base substitution in the normal termination codon (Milner *et al.*, 1971; Forget *et al.*, 1974). Hb Wayne can be explained by a single base deletion in the termination codon of α-mRNA with a shift in mRNA reading phase (frameshift mutation). As a result, a portion of the 3'-terminal end of α-mRNA is translated (Seid-Akhavan *et al.*, 1972). In the past few years increasing numbers of these abnormally long hemoglobins have been described, involving both the α and β chains. Different genetic mechanisms involving either mutations affecting the termination codon or unequal crossover between chromosomes may explain them (Marotta *et al.*, 1974; Forget *et al.*, 1974, 1975; Bunn *et al.*, 1975; Lehmann *et al.*, 1975).

*2.2.2.1c. Abnormally Short Hemoglobins.* The third type of mutant hemoblobin is the abnormally short globin chains. In those, one or a few amino acids are missing, and the remainder of the sequences are normal. These variants appear to arise by deletion of one or more intact codons which code for the missing amino acids (Stamatoyannopoulos, 1972). Therefore, no frameshift occurs.

*2.2.2.1d. Chain Fusions.* The fourth type of mutation is the hemoglobins with fused chains, such as Hb Lepore (Baglioni, 1962) or Hb Kenya (Huisman *et al.*, 1972). These have been considered previously and appear to arise by unequal crossing over between complementary chromosomes during meiosis.

### 2.2.2.2. Mechanisms of Reduced Synthesis of Abnormal Globins

*2.2.2.2a. β-Chain Mutants.* Most of the mutant hemoglobins are found in somewhat reduced amounts. This could result from many different causes. In the β-chain mutants, the abnormal hemoglobin is usually about 40% of the total hemoglobin in the heterozygote. Transcription, processing, or transport of these mutated mRNAs might be inefficient; the abnormal mRNA might be unstable and degraded rapidly; or translation might be slow due to the mutant codon acting as a modulation codon. The reduced amount of abnormal globin could also be explained by abnormal elongation of the globin chain on mRNA due to a configurational change in the nascent chain. Finally, the synthesis of the mutant chain could be normal, but due to instability and/or inability to form tetramers normally, there is preferential loss due to precipitation or catabolism. This last mechanism appears to be quite common and has been reviewed (White, 1971).

*2.2.2.2b.  α-Chain Mutants.* Hemoglobins with abnormal α chains are present usually at only 10–25% of the total hemoglobin in heterozygotes. This is best explained by the duplication of the α-chain loci, with each locus producing about 25% of the total hemoglobin (gene dosage) (Lehmann and Carrell, 1968).

In Hb Constant Spring (as with Hb Lepore, Hb A₂) and other abnormal hemoglobins, synthesis occurs only in bone marrow cells and not in reticulocytes. It has been suggested that this results from instability of the mRNA (Clegg and Weatherall, 1974, 1976).

### 2.2.2.3. Structure : Function Relationships in the Abnormal Hemoglobins

The Perutz (1976) model of the hemoglobin molecule demonstrates that the water-free molecular care is stabilized by nonpolar van der Waals interactions. Amino acids with polar side chains are completely excluded from the interior and are found only on the molecular surface, where they interact with water to solubilize the hemoglobin molecule. Heme is covalently bound to histidine residues but also forms about 60 contacts with nonpolar amino acids, thereby contributing to the stability of the tertiary structure. Because of this environment heme iron ($Fe^{2+}$)can associate with oxygen without being converted to $Fe^{3+}$ (methemoglobin). There are two kinds of contacts between the four polypeptide chains in each molecule. The larger contact, $\alpha_1\beta_1$, is a result of nonpolar interactions among 34 amino acids; the smaller contact, $\alpha_1\beta_2$, involves 19 amino acids. With oxygenation, the $\alpha_1\beta_2$ contact moves 7 Å, producing the subunit ("heme–heme") interaction. Using this model it has been possible to understand the effect of amino acid substitutions on the function of hemoglobin (Heller, 1966; Perutz and Lehmann, 1968) (Table III).

*2.2.2.3a.  Polymerization of Hemoglobin Molecules.* Most substitutions at the molecular surface are innocuous and do not affect tertiary structure, heme function, or subunit interaction. However, some surface substitutions can result in hemoglobin molecules that tend to polymerize. For example, Hb S is this type of mutant and results in an altered molecular surface that interacts with a complementary site on an adjacent molecule. The pathophysiology of the illness, sickle cell anemia, is a consequence of this polymerization of hemoglobin molecules and the relative insolubility of these aggregates. A recent review of this subject has been written by May and Huehns (1976).

**Table III.** Classification of Abnormal Hemoglobins by Functional Abnormality

| Functional abnormality of Hb | Location of amino acid substitution | Clinical presentation | Example |
|---|---|---|---|
| None | Surface | Normal | Hb G Philadelphia |
| Aggregation and ↓ solubility | Surface | Hemolytic anemia; abnormal rheology (homozygote) | Sickle cell anemia |
| Unstable | Internal, non-polar residues | Hemolytic anemia (heterozygote) | Hb Köln |
| ↑ $O_2$ affinity | $\alpha_1\beta_2$ contact or $\beta$ C terminus | Erythrocytosis | Hb Chesapeake |
| ↓ $O_2$ affinity | Near heme and $\alpha_1\beta_2$ contact | Cyanosis | Hb Kansas |
| Methemoglobin formation | Proximal F8 or distal E7 histidine | Cyanosis | Hb M |

*2.2.2.3b. The Unstable Hemoglobins.* Hemoglobin variants arising from neutral substitutions involving internal, nonpolar residues will result in hemoglobins with reduced stability. These hemoglobins tend to precipitate. Many of these substitutions affect residues that contact the heme groups, thus reducing heme–globin bonding. It is therefore possible for water to gain access to the heme pocket and heme may drop out of the molecule. Both heme-free normal globin and partially heme-free hemoglobin are unstable. This area has recently been reviewed by White (1976).

*2.2.2.3c. Increased Oxygen Affinity of Hemoglobin.* When an abnormality is in an $\alpha_1\beta_2$ contact point, subunit interaction is impaired and the hemoglobin has increased oxygen affinity, often leading to erythrocytosis. A few similar hemoglobins have been described where the substitution is at the C-terminal end of the $\beta$ chain. These substitutions can interfere with the Bohr effect, 2,3-DPG binding, or with the formation of salt bridges needed to stabilize hemoglobin in the deoxy, low-oxygen-affinity state.

*2.2.2.3d. Decreased Oxygen Affinity of Hemoglobin.* Hemoglobins have been described for which oxygen affinity is reduced. The substitution in at least some of these is at a residue-forming part of the $\alpha_1\beta_2$ contact which also contacts the heme group.

*2.2.2.3e. Methemoglobin Formation.* Five abnormal hemoglobins form methemoglobin (Hb M). Of these, three have reduced and two have normal oxygen affinity. These Hb Ms usually arise when a tyrosine substitutes for either the proximal (F8:$\alpha$87, $\beta$92) or distal (E7:$\alpha$58, $\beta$63) histidine. These substitutions allow an ionic bond to form between heme iron and the phenolic oxygen of tyrosine, thereby stabilizing iron in the nonfunctional, ferric state. In Hb M Milwaukee [$\beta$67 (E11) Val→Glu] a similar ionic bond forms with the glutamic carboxyl group. Such heme groups cannot bind oxygen, and patients have methemoglobinemia and cyanosis.

This subject of hemoglobins with altered oxygen affinity and methemoglobin formation has been reviewed recently by Bellingham (1976).

## 2.2.3. Synthesis of Hemoglobin in Heme-Deficient States

In both experimental and clinical heme deficiency, globin synthesis is severely impaired, with $\alpha$-chain synthesis being impaired more than $\beta$-chain synthesis (White *et al.*, 1971; White and Harvey, 1972; White and Ali, 1973; White and Hoffbrand, 1974). These findings may possibly be explained by considering the role of hemin in control of globin synthesis as discussed in Section 2.1.5.6b. IF-MP promotes the formation of active initiation complexes, but the $\beta$-chain mRNA has a greater affinity for these complexes than does $\alpha$-mRNA. In heme deficiency, the rate of formation of the initiation complex is diminished due to the action of the hemin-controlled repressor (HCR). It is possible that the synthesis of both $\alpha$ and $\beta$ chains declines, but since $\alpha$-mRNA has a lesser affinity for the 40S Met-tRNA$_f^{Met}$ complex than $\beta$-mRNA, the decline in $\alpha$-chain synthesis is more marked and the $\alpha/\beta$ ratio falls.

### 2.2.3.1. Models for Iron Deficiency Anemia, the Anemia of Chronic Disease, and the Sideroblastic Anemias

Recent work in this laboratory (Freedman and Rosman, 1976) has shown that when intact rabbit reticulocytes are incubated in the presence of a ferrous iron chelating agent ($\alpha,\alpha$-dipyridyl) or an inhibitor of the enzymes of heme synthesis (ethanol) (Ali and Brain, 1974; Freedman *et al.*, 1975), heme synthesis is inhibited, HCR is activated prematurely, and protein synthesis is thus inhibited. On the basis of this evidence we have postulated that the dipyridyl experiments are models of iron deficiency anemia. Furthermore, these experiments serve as a model for the anemia of chronic disease, where iron is not available to the developing red cell (Douglas and Adamson, 1975). In these conditions there would be prema-

**Table IV.** Postulated Role of the Hemin-Controlled Repressor (HCR) in Various Anemias

| Disease | HCR | Protein synthesis | Postulated primary lesion |
|---|---|---|---|
| Iron deficiency | ↑ | ↓ | Lack of body iron |
| Chronic disease | ↑ | ↓ | Lack of iron for normoblasts, total body iron normal |
| Sideroblastic anemia | ↑ | ↓ | Decreased heme synthetic enzymes |
| Benzene-induced aplastic anemia | ↑ | ↓ | Decreased heme synthesis in stem cells due to inhibition at δ-ALA synthetase |

ture appearance of HCR to inhibit protein synthesis due to lack of intracellular iron for heme synthesis. When the heme synthetic enzymes are inhibited in the presence of adequate iron, as with ethanol, HCR also appears prematurely and protein synthesis is also inhibited. However, iron would continue to accumulate in these conditions, overload the ferritin system, and appear as mitochondrial iron. The end result of this type of inhibition then would be a sideroblastic anemia (Ali and Brain, 1974; Freedman et al., 1975; Freedman and Rosman, 1976). Ferritin itself appears to be nontoxic to protein synthesis (Freedman et al., 1976b), whereas mitochondrial nonferritin iron appears to damage the mitochondria further by peroxidation of the mitochondrial lipids (Hunter et al., 1963). The postulated role of HCR in these three anemias is shown in Table IV.

Sideroblastic anemias result when there is inadequate protoporphyrin synthesis (Goodman and Hall, 1967; Aoki et al., 1974; Cartwright and Deiss, 1975); a deficiency of the iron-inserting enzyme, ferrochelatase (Lee et al., 1966; Rothstein et al., 1969; Vogler and Mingioli, 1968); or impaired globin chain synthesis (thalassemia) (Bessis and Breton-Gorius, 1962; Heller et al., 1965; Kramer et al., 1969). The end result of these states is an iron-overloaded but heme-deficient cell. We have postulated that the deficiency of heme will lead to a premature activation of HCR which in turn will lead to a deficiency of protein and polyribosomes. Grasso and Hines (1969) have shown that the normoblasts in sideroblastic anemias have few ribosomes, inconspicuous polyribosomes, and decreased hemoglobin.

### 2.2.3.2. Speculations on Hemin and Aplastic Anemia

Recently, we have presented evidence that benzene also inhibits reticulocyte heme and globin synthesis and prematurely activates HCR (Forte et al., 1976). The major effect of benzene in this *in vitro* system was at or before δ-aminolevulinic acid synthetase (Freedman *et al.*, 1977). Benzene has long been implicated as a cause of aplastic anemia in man. On the basis of this work performed in our laboratory it is possible to speculate that the primary toxic effect of benzene on bone marrow cells also might be inhibition of heme synthesis at or before δ-ALA synthetase. Considerable evidence has been presented in the past few years that ALA synthetase plays a central role in erythropoiesi. Levere and Gidari (1974) recently summarized the data showing that erythropoietin as well as the 5-β-H steroids stimulate erythropoiesis, heme, and globin synthesis in marrow cultures. These hormones appear to exert a major part of their action by first inducing the synthesis of ALA synthetase. Glass *et al.,* (1975) showed that heme synthesis is maximal in the earliest marrow precursor cells and decreases with cell maturity, whereas globin synthesis increases with cell maturity. These results are compatible with the postulate that there must first be sufficient intracellular hemin to reverse HCR, and thus allow globin synthesis to proceed. It is interesting to postulate that benzene, by its action at or before δ-ALA synthetase, thereby prevents hormonal activation of heme synthesis and derepression of HCR, which in turn is necessary for globin synthesis and erythropoiesis. The hemin requirement in other cell types might explain why there is involvement of the entire marrow.

This speculative theory also implies that to develop aplastic anemia with an inhibitor of heme synthesis, it is necessary to affect very early marrow precursor cells (Table IV). Since ALA synthetase is the rate-limiting enzyme (Moore and Goldberg, 1974), an inhibitor would either have to affect this enzyme or decrease one of the other enzymes in the pathway below the activity of ALA synthetase. The highly lipid-soluble benzene with a pronounced affinity for bone marrow is such an agent (Schrenk *et al.*, 1941). Furthermore, the interaction of benzene with other inhibitors of heme synthesis in the environment might accelerate the development of benzene toxicity. In this regard, we have shown additive *in vitro* toxicity with lead (Wildman *et al.*, 1976) and ethanol (Greenblatt *et al.*, 1977), two other inhibitors of heme synthesis.

Finally, the role of cyclic AMP in protecting and reversing heme deficiency must be considered. It is still not clear if cyclic AMP works directly to reverse a protein kinase (which could be HCR itself); or works on a phosphatase which in turn reverses the activity of HCR; or finally, if cAMP works to prevent inhibition of heme synthesis, and it is the hemin itself which is the only physiological regulator of HCR activity. There are still many questions to be answered in this scheme. It is clear, though, that hemin control is one of the central control points in translational regulation of both normal and abnormal hemoglobin synthesis.

# References

Adamson, S. D., Herbert, E., and Godchaux, W., III, 1968, Factors affecting the rate of protein synthesis in lysate systems from reticulocytes, *Arch. Biochem. Biophys.* **125**:671.

Adamson, S. D., Yan, R. M. P., Herbert, E., and Zucker, W. V., 1972, Involvement of hemin, a stimulatory function from ribosomes and a protein synthesis inhibitor in the regulation of hemoglobin synthesis, *J. Mol. Biol.* **63**:247.

Ali, M. A. M., and Brain, M. C., 1974, Ethanol inhibition of haemoglobin synthesis: In vitro evidence for a haem correctable defect in normal subjects and in alcoholic patients, *Br. J. Haematol.* **28**:311.

Anderson, W. F., 1969, The effect of tRNA concentration on the rate of protein synthesis, *Proc. Nat. Acad. Sci. U.S.A.* **62**:566.

Anderson, W. F., and Gilbert, J., 1969a, Translational Control of *in vitro* hemoglobin synthesis, *Cold Spring Harbor Symp. Quant. Biol.* **34**:585.

Anderson, W. F., and Gilbert, J., 1969b, tRNA dependent translational control of *in vitro* hemoglobin synthesis, *Biochem. Biophys. Res. Commun.* **36**:456.

Aoki, Y., Urata, G., Wada, O., and Takaku, F., 1974, Measurement of δ-aminolevulinic acid synthetase activity in human erythroblasts, *J. Clin. Invest.* **53**:1326.

Arlinghaus, R., Shaeffer, J., Bishop, J., and Schweet, R., 1968, Purification of the transfer enzymes from reticulocytes and properties of the transfer reaction, *Arch. Biochem. Biophys.* **125**:604.

Baglioni, C., 1962, The fusion of two peptide chains in hemoglobin Lepore and its interpretation as a genetic deletion, *Proc. Nat. Acad. Sci. U.S.A.* **48**:1880.

Baglioni, C., and Campana, T., 1967, Alpha chain and globin intermediates in the formation of rabbit hemoglobin, *Eur. J. Biochem.* **2**:480.

Baglioni, C., Jacobs-Lorena, M., and Meade, H., 1972, The site of action of inhibitors of initiation of protein synthesis in reticulocytes, *Biochim. Biophys. Acta* **271**:188.

Balkow, K., Mizuno, S., Fisher, J. M., and Rabinovitz, M., 1973a, Hemin control of globin synthesis: Effect of a translational repressor on met-tRNA$_f$ binding to the small ribosomal subunit and its relation to the activity and availability of an initiation factor, *Biochim. Biophys. Acta* **324**:397.

Balkow, K., Mizuno, S., and Rabinovitz, M., 1973b, Inhibition of an initiation codon function by hemin deficiency and the hemin-controlled translational repressor in the reticulocyte cell-free system, *Biochem. Biophys. Res. Commun.* **54**:315.

Balkow, K., Hunt, T., and Jackson, R. J., 1975, Control of protein synthesis in reticulocyte lysates: The effect of nucleotide triphosphates on formation of the translational repressor, *Biochem. Biophys. Res. Commun.* **67**:366.

Bank, A., 1968, Hemoglobin synthesis in β-thalassemia: The properties of the free α chains, *J. Clin. Invest.* **47**:860.

Bank, A., and Marks, P. A., 1966, Excess alpha-chain synthesis relative to beta-chain synthesis in thalassemia major and minor, *Nature (London)* **212**:1198.

Bargellesi, A., Pontremoli, S., and Conconi, F., 1967, Absence of beta-globin synthesis and excess of alpha-globin synthesis in homozygous β-thalassemia and its removal from the red blood cell cytoplasm, *Eur. J. Biochem.* **3**:364.

Barnes, D. W. H., and Oxon, B. M., 1967, Haemopoietic stem cells in the peripheral blood, *Lancet* **2**:1138.

Beaudet, A. L., and Caskey, C. T., 1971, Mammalian peptide chain termination. II Codon specificity and GTPase activity of release factor, *Proc. Nat. Acad. Sci. U.S.A.* **68**:619.

Bellingham, A. J., 1976, Haemoglobins with altered oxygen affinity, *Br. Med. Bull.* **32**:234.

Benz, E. J., Jr., and Forget, B. G., 1974, The biosynthesis of hemoglobin, *Semin. Hematol.* **11**:463.

Benz, E. J., Jr., and Forget, B. G., 1975, The molecular genetics of the thalassemia syndromes, *Prog. Hematol.* **9**:107.

Bessis, M. C., and Breton-Gorius, J., 1962, Iron metabolism in the bone marrow as seen by electron microscopy: A critical review, *Blood* **19**:635.

Beuzard, Y., Rodvien, R., and London, I. M., 1973, Effect of hemin in the synthesis of hemoglobin and other proteins in mammalian cells, *Proc. Nat. Acad. Sci. U.S.A.* **70**:1022.

Blobel, G., 1973, A protein of molecular weight 78,000 bound to the polyadenylate region of eukaryotic messenger RNA's, *Proc. Nat. Acad. Sci. U.S.A.* **70**:924.

Blum, N., Maleknia, M., and Schapira, G., 1970, α- et β-globines lebres et biosynthese de l'hemoglobine, *Biochim. Biophys. Acta* **199**:236.

Bottomley, S. S., and Smithee, A. G., 1969, Effect of erythropoietin on Δ-aminolevulinic acid synthetase and heme synthetase, *J. Lab. Clin. Med.* **74**:445.

Bottomley, S. S., Whitcomb, W. H., and Smithee, G. A., 1971, Effect of cyclic adenosine 3′,5′-monophosphate on bone marrow δ-aminolevulinic acid synthetase and erythrocyte iron uptake, *J. Lab. Clin. Med.* **77**:793.

Boyer, S. H., Smith, K. D., Noyes, A. N., and Mullen, M. A., 1974, Immunological characterization of rabbit hemoglobin α and β-chain synthesizing polysomes: Estimation of relative numbers of active α and β-messenger ribonucleic acid, *J. Biol. Chem.* **249**:7210.

Bradley, T. B., Wonl, R. C., and Smith, G. J., 1975, Elongation of the α globin chain in a black family: Interaction with Hb G Philadelphia, *Clin. Res.* **23**:131A.

Brot, H., Spears, C., and Weissbach, H., 1969, The formation of a complex containing ribosomes, transfer factor G and a guanosine dinucleotide, *Biochem. Biophys. Res. Commun.* **34**:843.

Brown, J. E., and Adamson, J. W., 1974, Cyclic nucleotide influence on *in vitro* heme synthesis, *Blood* **44**:913(a).

Brown, J. E., and Adamson, J. W., 1976, Beta (β) adrenergic modulation of *in vitro* erythropoiesis, *Clin. Res.* **24**:304(a).

Bruns, G. P., and London, I. M., 1965, The effect of hemin on the synthesis of globin, *Biochem. Biophys. Res. Commun.* **18**:236.

Bunn, H. F., Bradley, T. B., Davis, W. E., Drysdale, J. W., Burke, J. F., Beck, W. S., and Laver, M. B., 1972, Structural and functional studies on hemoglobin

Bethesda, $\alpha_2\beta_2^{145His}$, a variant associated with compensatory erythrocytosis, *J. Clin. Invest.* **51**:2299.

Bunn, H. F., Schmidt, G. J., Haney, D. N., and Dluhy, R. G., 1975, Hemoglobin Cranston, an unstable variant having an elongated $\beta$ chain due to nonhomologous crossover between two normal $\beta$ chain genes, *Proc. Nat. Acad. Sci. U.S.A.* **72**:3609.

Burka, E. R., 1968, Hemin, an inhibitor of erythroid cell ribonuclease, *Science* **162**:1287.

Burka, E. R., 1969, RNAase activity in erythroid cell lysates, *J. Clin. Invest.* **48**:1724.

Burka, E. R., 1971, Erythroid cell RNAase: Activation by urea and localization to the cell membrane, *J. Clin. Invest.* **50**:60.

Burr, H., and Lingrel, J. B., 1971, Poly A sequences at the 3' termini of rabbit globin mRNAs, *Nature (London) New Biol.* **233**:41.

Busiello, E., and DiGirolamo, M., 1973, Aminoacyl tRNA binding sites in *E. coli* and reticulocyte ribosomes, *FEBS Lett.* **35**:341.

Camiscoli, J. F., and Gordon, A. S., 1970, Bioassay and standardization of erythropoietin, *in Regulation of Hematopoiesis*, Vol. I (A. S. Gordon, ed.), p. 369, Appleton, New York.

Capp, G. L., Rigas, D. A., and Jones, R. T., 1967, Hemoglobin Portland₁: A new human hemoglobin unique in structure, *Science* **157**:65.

Capp, G. L., Rigas, D. A., and Jones, R. T., 1970, Evidence for a new haemoglobin chain ($\varphi$-chain), *Nature (London)* **228**:278.

Cartwright, G. E., and Deiss, A., 1975, Sideroblasts, siderocytes and sideroblastic anemia, *N. Engl. J. Med.* **29**:185.

Chang, S. S., and Goldwasser, E., 1973, On the mechanism of erythropoietin-induced differentiation XII: A cytoplasmic protein mediating induced nuclear RNA synthesis, *Dev. Biol.* **34**:246.

Charache, S., Clegg, J. B., Weatherall, D. J., and Conley, C. L., 1975, Unbalanced globin synthesis in hereditary persistence of fetal hemoglobin (HPFH), *Clin. Res.* **23**:397A.

Chattergee, N. K., Bose, K. K., Woodley, C. L., and Gupta, N. K., 1971, Protein synthesis in rabbit reticulocytes: Factors controlling terminal and internal methionine codon (AUG) recognition by methionyl tRNA species, *Biochem. Biophys. Res. Commun.* **43**:771.

Chu, T. C., and Chu, E. J. H., 1970, Effects of various additives on porphyrin biosynthesis, *Biochim. Biophys. Acta* **215**:377.

Clegg, J. B., 1974, Haemoglobin synthesis, *Clin. Haematol.* **3**:225.

Clegg, J. B., and Weatherall, D. J., 1972, Haemoglobin synthesis during erythroid maturation in $\beta$-thalassemia, *Nature New Biol.* **240**:190.

Clegg, J. B., and Weatherall, D. J., 1974, $\beta^0$-Thalassemia—Time for a reappraisal? *Lancet* **2**:133.

Clegg, J. B., and Weatherall, D. J., 1976, Molecular basis of thalassemia, *Br. Med. Bull.* **32**:262.

Clegg, J. B., Weatherall, D. J., Na-Nakorn, S., and Wasi, P., 1968, Hemoglobin synthesis in $\beta$-thalassemia, *Nature (London)* **220**:664.

Clegg, J. B., Weatherall, D. J., Contopolou-Griva, I., Caroutsos, K., Poungouras,

P., and Tsevrenis, H., 1974, Haemoglobin Icaria, a new chain termination mutant which causes α-thalassemia, *Nature (London)* **251**:245.

Clemens, M. J., Henshaw, E. C., Rahaminoff, H., and London, I. M., 1974, Met-tRNA$_f^{met}$ binding to 40S ribosomal units. A site for the regulation of protein synthesis by hemin, *Proc. Nat. Acad. Sci. U.S.A.* **71**:2946.

Collins, J., Moon, H., and Maxwell, G., 1972, Multiple forms and some properties of amino acyl transferase 1 (EF$_1$) from rat liver, *Biochemistry* **11**:4187.

Conconi, F., Rowley, P. T., Del Senno, L., and Pontremoli, S., 1972, Induction of β-globin synthesis in the β-thalassemia of Ferrara, *Nature (London) New Biol.* **238**:83.

Conley, C. L., Weatherall, D. J., Richardson, S. N., Shepard, M. K., and Charache, S., 1963, Hereditary persistence of fetal hemoglobin: A study of 79 affected persons in 15 Negro families in Baltimore, *Blood* **21**:261.

Crystal, R., Shafritz, D., Prichard, P., and Anderson, W. F., 1971, Initial dipeptide formation in hemoglobin biosynthesis, *Proc. Nat. Acad. Sci. U.S.A.* **68**:1810.

Cudkowicz, G., Upton, A. C., Smith, L. H., Goslee, D. G., and Hughes, W. L., 1964, Characterization of stem cells in mouse bone marrow, *Ann. N.Y. Acad. Sci.* **114**:571.

Culp, W., McKeehan, W., and Hardesty, B., 1969, The mechanism of mRNA translocation through ribosomes, *Proc. Nat. Acad. Sci. U.S.A.* **64**:388.

Culp, W., McKeehan, W., and Hardesty, B., 1970, Initiation tRNA for the synthesis of globin peptides, *Biochem. Biophys. Res. Commun.* **40**:777.

Darnborough, C., Legon, S., Hunt, T., and Jackson, R. J., 1973, Initiation of protein synthesis: Evidence for messenger RNA-independent binding of methionyl-transfer RNA to the 40S ribosomal subunit, *J. Mol. Biol.* **76**:379.

Darnell, J. E., Jelinek, W. R., and Molloy, G. R., 1973, Biogenesis of mRNA: Genetic regulation in mammalian cells, *Science* **181**:1215.

Deisseroth, A., Velez, R., and Nienhuis, A. W., 1976, Hemoglobin synthesis in somatic cell hybrids: Independent segregation of the human alpha and beta-globin genes, *Science* **191**:1262.

DeJong, W. W., Meerakhan, P., and Bernini, L. F., 1975, Hemoglobin Koya Dora: High frequency of α-chain termination mutant. *Am. J. Hum. Genet.* **27**:81.

DelMonte, M., and Kazazian, H. H., Jr., 1971, Unequal synthesis of globin chains after extended incubation of rabbit reticulocytes with L-O-methylthreonine, *J. Mol. Biol.* **56**:429.

Dintzis, H., 1961, Assembly of the peptide chains of hemoglobin, *Proc. Nat. Acad. Sci. U.S.A.* **47**:247.

Douglas, S. W., and Adamson, J. W., 1975, The anemia of chronic disorders: Studies of marrow regulation and iron metabolism, *Blood* **45**:55.

Dow, L. W., Terada, M., Natta, C., Metafora, S., Grassbard, E., Marks, P. A., and Bank, A., 1973, Globin synthesis of intact cells and activity of isolated mRNA in β-thalassemia, *Nature New Biol* **243**:114.

Dukes, P. P., 1971, Potentiation of erythropoietin effects of marrow cell cultures by prostaglandin E$_1$ or cyclic 3′,5′-AMP, *Blood* **38**:822.

Edington, G. M., and Lehmann, H., 1955, Expression of the sickle cell gene in Africa, *Br. Med. J.* **1**:1308.

Ehrenfeld, E., and Hunt, R. T., 1971, Double-stranded poliovirus RNA inhibits initiation of protein synthesis by reticulocyte lysates, *Proc. Nat. Acad. Sci. U.S.A.* **68**:1075.

Farkas, W., and Marks, P. A., 1968, Partial purification and properties of a ribonuclease from rabbit reticulocytes, *J. Biol. Chem.* **243**:6464.

Felicetti, L., Columbo, B., and Baglioni, C., 1966, Assembly of hemoglobin, *Biochim. Biophys. Acta* **129**:380.

Fessas, P., Loukopoulos, D., and Kaltsoy, A., 1966, Peptide analysis of the inclusions of erythroid cells in β-thalassemia, *Biochim. Biophys. Acta* **124**:430.

Flatz, G., Kinterlerer, J. C., Kilmartin, J. V., and Lehmann, H., 1971, Hemoglobin Tak: A variant with additional residues at the end of the β chains, *Lancet* **1**:732.

Forget, B. G., 1974, The molecular basis of thalassemia, *CRC Crit. Rev. Biochem.* **2**:311.

Forget, B. G., Marotta, C. A., Weissman, S. M., Verma, I. M., McCaffrey, R. P., and Baltimore, D., 1974, Nucleotide sequences of human globin messenger RNA, *Ann. N.Y. Acad. Sci.* **241**:290.

Forget, B. G., Marotta, C. A., Weissman, S. M., and Cohen-Solal, M., 1975, Nucleotide sequences of the 3'-terminal untranslated region of messenger RNA for human beta globin chains, *Proc. Nat. Acad. Sci. U.S.A.* **72**:3614.

Forte, F. J., Cohen, H. S., Rosman, J., and Freedman, M. L., 1976, Hemin reversal of benzene-induced inhibiton of reticulocyte protein synthesis, *Blood* **47**:145.

Freedman, M. L., 1974, Thalassemia: An abnormality in globin chain synthesis, *Am. J. Med. Sci.* **267**:256.

Freedman, M. L., and Karpatkin, S., 1973, Requirement of iron for platelet protein synthesis, *Biochem. Biophys. Res. Commun.* **54**:475.

Freedman, M. L., and Rabinovitz, M., 1970, Ribosomal subunits in rabbit reticulocytes under different conditions of polyribosome disaggregation, *Exp. Cell Res.* **60**:480.

Freedman, M. L., and Rabinovitz, M., 1971, Structure of the large β-chain polyribosome from O-methylthreonine-induced isoleucine deficient rabbit reticulocytes, *Mol. Pharmacol.* **7**:317.

Freedman, M. L., and Rosman, J., 1976, A rabbit reticulocyte model for the role of hemin-controlled repressor in hypochromic anemias, *J. Clin. Invest.* **57**:594.

Freedman, M. L., Hori, M., and Rabinovitz, M., 1967, Membranes in polyribosome formation by rabbit reticulocytes, *Science* **157**:323.

Freedman, M. L., Fisher, J. M., and Rabinovitz, M., 1968a, Puromycin interference of reticulocyte polyribosome disaggregation caused by tryptophan deficiency, *J. Mol. Biol.* **33**:315.

Freedman, M. L., Hori, M., and Rabinovitz, M., 1968b, Polyribosome structure: Relationship to codon location in amino acid deficiencies of rabbit reticulocytes, *Fed. Proc.* **27**:397a.

Freedman, M. L., Velez, R., and Mucha, J., 1972, Resistance of messenger RNA-bound ribosomes to proteolytic dissociation, *Exp. Cell Res.* **72**:431.

Freedman, M. L., Geraghty, M., and Rosman, J., 1974, Hemin control of globin synthesis: Isolation of a hemin-reversible translational repressor from human mature erythrocytes, *J. Biol. Chem.* **249**:7290.

Freedman, M. L., Cohen, H. S., Rosman, J., and Forte, F., 1975, Ethanol inhibition of reticulocyte protein synthesis: The role of haem, *Br. J. Haematol.* **30**:351.

Freedman, M. L., Wildman, J. M., and Rosman, J., 1976a, The role of cyclic AMP in regulating hemin-controlled repressor activity in intact rabbit reticulocytes, *Clin. Res.* **24**:308(a).

Freedman, M. L., Cohen, H. S., Rosman, J., and Forte, F. J., 1976b, Ferritin and sideroblastic anaemias: Inhibition of protein synthesis by protease contaminants in commercial preparations of ferritin, *Br. J. Haematol.* **32**:579.

Freedman, M. L., Wildman, J. M., Rosman, J., Eisen, J., and Greenblatt, D. R., 1977, Benzene inhibition of *in vitro* rabbit reticulocyte haem synthesis at δ-aminolaevulinic acid synthetase: Reversal of benzene toxicity by pyridoxine, *Br. J. Haematol.* **35**:43.

Friend, C., Scher, W., Holland, J. G., and Sato, T., 1971, Hemoglobin synthesis in murine virus-induced leukemia cells *in vitro*. Stimulation of erythroid differentiation by dimethyl sulfoxide, *Proc. Nat. Acad. Sci. U.S.A.* **68**:378.

Gambino, R., Kacian, D., O'Donnell, J., Ramirez, F., Marks, P. A., and Bank, A., 1974, A limited number of globin genes in human DNA, *Proc. Nat. Acad. Sci. U.S.A.* **71**:3966.

Garrick, L. M., Dembure, P. P., and Garrick, M. D., 1975, Interaction between the synthesis of α and β globin, *Eur. J. Biochem.* **58**:339.

George, W. J., Rodgers, G. M., Briggs, D. W., and Fisher, J. W., 1975, Role of cyclic AMP in the regulation of erythropoietin production, *in Erythropoiesis: Proceedings of the 4th International Conference on Erythropoiesis* (K. Nakao, J. W. Fisher, and F. Tokaku, eds.), p. 277, University Park Press, Baltimore, Maryland.

Gidari, A. S., Zanjani, E. D., Gizzi, C. A., Gordon, A. S., and Rappaport, I. A., 1971, Stimulation of erythropoiesis by adenine nucleotides, 14th Annual Meeting, American Society of Hematology, San Francisco, California, p. 144.

Gilbert, J. M., Thornton, A. G., Nienhaus, A. W., and Anderson, W. F., 1970, Cell-free hemoglobin synthesis in beta-thalassemia, *Proc. Nat. Acad. Sci. U.S.A.* **67**:1854.

Gill, F., and Schwartz, E., 1973, Free α globin pool in human bone marrow, *J. Clin. Invest.* **52**:3057.

Glass, J., Lavidor, L. M., and Robinson, S. H., 1975, Studies of murine erythroid cell development, *J. Cell Biol.* **65**:298.

Goldstein, J., Beaudet, A., and Caskey, C., 1970, Peptide chain termination with mammalian release factor, *Proc. Nat. Acad. Sci. U.S.A.* **67**:99.

Goldwasser, E., 1975, Erythropoietin and the differentiation of red blood cells, *Fed. Proc.* **34**:2285.

Goodman, J. R., and Hall, S. G., 1967, Accumulation of iron in mitochondria of erythroblasts, *Br. J. Haematol.* **13**:335.

Gordon, A. S., and Zanjani, E. D., 1970, Some aspects of erythropoietin physiology, *in Regulation of Hematopoiesis*, Vol. 1 (A. S. Gordon, ed.), p. 413, Appleton, New York.

Gordon, A. S., Cooper, G. W., and Zanjani, E. D., 1967, The kidney and erythropoiesis, *Semin. Hematol.* **4**:337.

Gorshein, D., Reisner, E. H., Jr., and Gardner, F. H., 1975, Tissue culture of bone marrow. V. Effect of 5β(H) steroids and cyclic AMP on heme synthesis, *Am. J. Physiol.* **228**:1024.

Graber, S. E., Carrillo, M., and Krantz, S. B., 1972, The effect of cyclic AMP on heme synthesis by rat bone marrow cells *in vitro, Proc. Soc. Expt. Biol. Med.* **141**:206.

Granick, S., and Kappas, A., 1967, Steroid induction of porphyrin synthesis in liver cell culture. I. Structural basis and possible physiological role in the control of heme formation, *J. Biol. Chem.* **24**:4587.

Grasso, J. A., and Hines, J. D., 1969, A comparative electron microscopic study of refractory and alcoholic sideroblastic anaemia, *Br. J. Haematol.* **17**:35.

Grayzel, A. I., Horchner, P., and London, I. M., 1966, The stimulation of globin synthesis by heme, *Proc. Nat. Acad. Sci. U.S.A.* **55**:650.

Grayzel, A., Fuhr, J., and London, I. M., 1967, The effects of inhibitors of protein synthesis on the synthesis of heme in rabbit reticulocytes, *Biochem. Biophys. Res. Commun.* **28**:705.

Greenblatt, D. R., Rosman, J., and Freedman, M. L., 1977, Benzene and ethanol additive inhibition of rabbit reticulocyte heme and protein synthesis, *Environ. Res.* (in press).

Gross, M., 1974, Control of globin synthesis by hemin: An intermediate form of the translational repressor in rabbit reticulocyte lysates, *Biochim. Biophys. Acta* **366**:319.

Gross, M., and Goldwasser, E., 1969, On the mechanism of erythropoietin-induced differentiation. V. Characterization of the ribonucleic acid formed as a result of erythropoietin action, *Biochemistry* **8**:1795.

Gross, M., and Goldwasser, E., 1971, On the mechanism of erythropoietin-induced differentiation. IX. Induced synthesis of 9S ribonucleic acid and hemoglobin, *J. Biol. Chem.* **246**:2480.

Gross, M., and Rabinovitz, M., 1972a, Control of globin synthesis by hemin: Factors influencing formation of an inhibitor of globin chain initiation in reticulocyte lysates, *Biochim. Biophys. Acta* **287**:340.

Gross, M., and Rabinovitz, M., 1972b, Control of globin synthesis in cell-free preparations of reticulocytes by formation of a translational repressor that is inactivated by hemin, *Proc. Nat. Acad. Sci. U.S.A.* **69**:1565.

Hall, N. D., and Arnstein, H. R. V., 1973, Differential translation of α- and α-globin messenger RNA in a cell-free system, *FEBS Lett* **35**:45.

Hallenberg, M. D., Kaback, M. M., and Kazazian, H. H., Jr., 1971, Adult hemoglobin synthesis by reticulocytes from the human fetus at midtrimester, *Science* **174**:698.

Heller, P., 1966, Hemoglobinopathic dysfunction of the red cell, *Am. J. Med.* **41**:799.

Heller, P., VanStone, J., Apple, D., and Coleman, R. D., 1965, Defective globin synthesis in hypochromic hypersideremic anemia (α-thalassemia?), *Blood* **25**:635.

Heywood, J. D., Karon, M., and Weissman, S., 1965, Asymmetrical incorporation of amino acids into the alpha and beta chains of hemoglobin synthesized in thalassemic reticulocytes, *J. Lab. Clin. Med.* **66**:476.

Hines, J. D., and Grasso, J. A., 1970, The sideroblastic anemias, *Semin. Hematol.* **7**:86.

Hirsch, J. D., and Martelo, O. J., 1976, Inhibition of rabbit reticulocyte protein kinases by hemin, *Biochem. Biophys. Res. Commun.* **71**:926.

Hodgson, G., 1970, Mechanism of action of erythropoietin, *in Regulation of Hematopoiesis*, Vol. I (A. S. Gordon, ed.), p. 459, Appleton, New York.

Honig, G. R., 1967, Inhibition of synthesis of fetal hemoglobin by an isoleucine analogue, *J. Clin. Invest.* **46**:1778.

Honig, G. R., Rowan, B., and Mason, R., 1969, Unequal synthesis of complementary globin chains of human fetal hemoglobin by the effect of L-O-methyl-threonine, *J. Biol. Chem.* **244**:2027.

Housman, D., Jacobs-Lorena, M., Ragbhandary, U. L., and Lodish, H. F., 1970, Initiation of hemoglobin synthesis by methionyl tRNA, *Nature (London)* **227**:913.

Housman, D., Forget, B. G., Skoultchi, A., and Benz, E. J., Jr., 1973, Quantitative deficiency of chain-specific globin messenger ribonucleic acid in the thalassemia syndromes, *Proc. Nat. Acad. Sci. U.S.A.* **70**:1809.

Howard, G. A., Adamson, S. D., and Herbert, E., 1970, Studies on the cessation of protein synthesis in a reticulocyte lysate cell-free system, *Biochim. Biophys. Acta* **213**:237.

Huehns, D. R., and Modell, C. B., 1967, Hemoglobin synthesis in thalassemia, *Trans. Roy. Soc. Trop. Med. Hyg.* **61**:157.

Huehns, D. R., Hecht, F., Keil, J. V., and Motulsky, A. G., 1964, Developmental hemoglobin anomalies in a chromosomal triplication: $D_1$ trisomy syndrome, *Proc. Nat. Acad. Sci. U.S.A.* **51**:89.

Huehns, E. R., 1974, Haemoglobin: The haemoglobinopathies, *in Blood and Its Disorders* (R. M. Hardesty and D. J. Weatherall, eds.), p. 526, Blackwell, Oxford.

Huehns, E. R., Flynn, F. V., Butler, E. A., and Beaven, G. H., 1961, Two new hemoglobin variants in a very young human embryo, *Nature (London)* **189**:496.

Huehns, E. R., Dance, N., Beaven, G. H., Hecht, F., and Motulsky, A. G., 1964a, Human embryonic hemoglobins, *Cold Spring Harbor Symp. Quant. Biol.* **29**:327.

Huehns, E. R., Dance, N., Beaven, G. H., Keil, J. V., Hecht, F., and Motulsky, A. G., 1964b, Human embryonic hemoglobins, *Nature (London)* **201**:1095.

Huisman, T. H. J., Wrightstone, R. N., Wilson, J. B., and Schroeder, W. A., 1972, Hemoglobin Kenya, the product of fusion of $\gamma$ and $\beta$ polypeptide chains, *Arch. Biochem. Biophys.* **153**:850.

Huisman, T. H. J., Schroeder, W. A., Efremov, G. D., Duma, H., Mladenovski, B., Hyman, C. B., Rachmilewitz, E. A., Bouver, N., Miller, A., Brodie, A., Shelton, J. R., Shelton, J. B., and Apell, G., 1974, The present status of the heterogeneity of fetal hemoglobin in $\beta$-thalassemia: An attempt to unify some observations in thalassemia and related conditions, *Ann. N.Y. Acad. Sci.* **232**:107.

Hunt, R. T., Munro, A. J., and Hunter, A. R., 1968a, Control of hemoglobin synthesis: A difference in the size of polysomes making $\alpha$ and $\beta$ chains, *Nature (London)* **220**:481.

Hunt, R. T., Hunter, A. J., and Munro, A., 1968b, Control of hemoglibin synthesis: Distribution of ribosomes on the mRNA for α and β chains, *J. Mol. Biol.* **36**:31.

Hunt, R. T., Hunter, A. J., and Munro, A., 1969, Control of hemoglobin synthesis: Rate of translation of the messenger RNA for the α and β chains, *J. Mol. Biol.* **43**:123.

Hunt, T., 1976, Control of globin synthesis, *Br. Med. Bull.* **32**:257.

Hunt, T., Vanderhoff, G., and London, I. M., 1972, Control of globin synthesis: The role of heme, *J. Mol. Biol.* **66**:471.

Hunter, A., and Jackson, R., 1971, The origin and nature of the methionine residue initiation the synthesis of hemoglobin *in vivo* and *in vitro*, *Eur. J. Biochem.* **19**:316.

Hunter, F. E., Jr., Gebicki, J. M., Hoffsten, P. E., Weinstein, J., and Scott, A., 1963, Swelling and lysis of rat liver mitochondria induced by ferrous ions, *J. Biol. Chem.* **238**:828.

Itano, H. A., 1966, Genetic regulation of peptide synthesis in hemoglobins, *J. Cell. Physiol.* **67** (Suppl. 1):65.

Jackson, R., and Hunter, T., 1970, Role of methionine in the initiation of haemoglobin synthesis, *Nature (London)* **227**:672.

Jacobs-Lorena, M., and Baglioni, C., 1972, Messenger RNA for globin in the postribosomal supernatant of rabbit reticulocytes, *Proc. Nat. Acad. Sci. U.S.A.* **69**:1425.

Jacobs-Lorena, M., and Baglioni, C., 1973, Synthesis of rabbit globin by reticulocyte postribosomal supernatants and heterologous ribosmes, *Eur. J. Biochem.* **35**:559.

Kacian, D. L., Spiegelman, S., Bank, A., Terada, M., Metafora, S., Dow, L., and Marks, P. A., 1972, *In vitro* synthesis of DNA components of human genes for globins, *Nature New Biol.* **235**:167.

Kacian, D. L., Gambino, R., Dow, L. W., Crossbard, E., Natta, C., Ramirez, F., Spiegelman, S., Marks, P. A., and Bank, A., 1973, Decreased globin messenger RNA in thalassemia detected by molecular hybridization, *Proc. Nat. Acad. Sci. U.S.A.* **70**:1886.

Kaempfer, R., and Kaufman, J., 1972a, Translational control of synthesis by an initiation factor required for recycling of ribosomes and their binding to messenger RNA, *Proc. Nat. Acad. Sci. U.S.A.* **69**:3317.

Kaempfer, R., and Kaufman, J., 1972b, Inhibition of cellular protein synthesis by double-stranded RNA. Inactivation of an initiation factor, *Proc. Nat. Acad. Sci. U.S.A.* **70**:1222.

Kan, Y. W., Nathan, D. G., and Lodish, H. F., 1972, Equal synthesis of α and β globin chains in erythroid precursors in heterozygous β-thalassemia, *J. Clin. Invest.* **51**:1906.

Kan, Y. W., Holland, J. P., Dozy, A. M., and Varmus, H. E., 1975a, Demonstration of nonfunctional β-globin mRNA in homozygous β⁰-thalassemia, *Proc. Nat. Acad. Sci. U.S.A.* **72**:5140.

Kan, Y. W., Dozy, A. M., Varmus, H. E., Taylor, J. M., Holland, J. P., Lie-Ingo, L. E., Ganesan, J., and Todd, D., 1975b, Deletion of α-globin genes in haemoglobin H disease demonstrates multiple 2-globin structural loci, *Nature (London)* **255**:255.

Kan, Y. W., Holland, J. P., Dozy, A. M., Charache, S., and Kazazian, H. H., 1975c, Deletion of the β-globin structure gene in hereditary persistence of fetal hemoglobin, *Nature (London)* **258**:162.

Kaplan, B. H., Tricoche, M., and Vanderhoff, G., 1974, Regulatory role of heme, *Ann. N.Y. Acad. Sci.* **241**:334.

Kappas, A., and Granick, S., 1968, Steroid induction of porphyrin synthesis in liver cell culture: II. The effects of heme, uridine diphosphate, glucuronic acid and inhibition of protein synthesis in the process, *J. Biol. Chem.* **243**:346.

Karibian, D., and London, I. M., 1965, Control of heme synthesis by feedback inhibition, *Biochem. Biophys. Res. Commun.* **18**:293.

Karpatkin, S., Garg, S. K., and Freedman, M. L., 1974, The role of iron in thrombopoiesis, *Am. J. Med.* **57**:521.

Kazazian, H. H., Jr., 1974, Regulation of fetal hemoglobin production, *Semin. Hematol.* **11**:525.

Kazazian, H. H., Jr., and Freedman, M. L., 1968, The characterization of separate alpha- and beta-chain polyribosomes in rabbit reticulocytes, *J. Biol. Chem.* **243**:6446.

Kazazian, H. H., Jr., and Woodhead, A. P., 1974, Adult hemoglobin synthesis in the human fetus, *Ann. N.Y. Acad. Sci.* **241**:691.

Kosower, N. S., Vanderhoff, G. A., and Kosower, E. M., 1972, Glutathione. VIII. The effects of glutathione disulfide on initiation of protein synthesis, *Biochim. Biophys. Acta* **272**:623.

Kramer, S., Vilgoen, E., Becker, D., Zail, S. S., and Metz, J., 1969, The relationship between haem and globin synthesis by erythroid precursors in refractory normoblastic anaemia, *Scand. J. Haematol.* **6**:293.

Krantz, S. B., 1973, Recent contributions to the mechanism of action and clinical relevance of erythropoietin, *J. Lab. Clin. Med.* **82**:897.

Kruh, J., and Borsook, H., 1956, Hemoglobin synthesis in rabbit reticulocytes *in vitro*, *J. Biol. Chem.* **220**:905.

Kwan, S. W., and Braverman, G., 1972, A particle associated with the polyadenylate segment in mammalian messenger RNA, *Proc. Nat. Acad. Sci. U.S.A.* **69**:3247.

Lanyon, W. G., Ottolenghi, S., and Williamson, R., 1975, Human globin gene expression and linkage in bone marrow and fetal liver, *Proc. Nat. Acad. Sci. U.S.A.* **72**:258.

Lee, G. R., Cartwright, G. E., and Wintrobe, M. M., 1966, The response of free erythrocyte protoporphvrin to pyridoxine therapy in a patient with sideroachrestic (sideroblastic) anemia, *Blood* **27**:557.

Legon, S., Jackson, R. J., and Hunt, T., 1973, Control of protein synthesis in reticulocyte lysates by haemin, *Nature New Biol.* **241**:150.

Legon, S., Brayley, A., Hunt, T., and Jackson, R. J., 1974, The effect of cyclic AMP and related compounds on the control of protein synthesis in reticulocyte lysates, *Biochem. Biophys. Res. Commun.* **56**:745.

Lehmann, H., and Carrell, R. W., 1968, Differences between α- and β-chain mutants of human haemoglobin and between α- and β-thalassemia. Possible duplication of the α-chain gene, *Br. Med. J.* **4**:748.

Lehmann, H., and Carrell, R. W., 1969, Variations in the structure of human haemoglobin with particular reference to the unstable haemoglobins, *Br. Med. Bull.* **25**:14.

Lehmann, H., Casey, R., Lang, A., Stathopoulou, R., Imai, K., Tuchinda, S., Vinai, P., and Flatz, G., 1975, Haemoglobin Tak: A β chain elongation, *Br. J. Haematol.* **31** (Suppl.):19.

Lehninger, A. L., 1975, *Biochemistry,* Worth, New York.

Levere, R. D., and Gidari, A. S., 1974, Steroid metabolites and the control of hemoglobin synthesis, *Bull. N.Y. Acad. Med.* **50**:563.

Levin, D. H., Ranu, R. S., Vivian, E., Fifer, M. A., and London, I. M., 1975, Association of cyclic AMP-dependent protein kinase with a purified translational inhibitor isolated from hemin-deficient rabbit reticulocyte lysates, *Proc. Nat. Acad. Sci. U.S.A.* **72**:4849.

Lim, L., and Cannellakis, E. S., 1970, Adenine rich polymer associated with rabbit reticulocyte messenger RNA, *Nature (London)* **227**:710.

Lin, S. Y., McKeehan, W. L., Culp, W., and Hardesty, B., 1969, Partial characterization of the enzymatic properties of the amino acyl transfer ribonucleic acid binding enzyme, *J. Biol. Chem.* **244**:4340.

Lodish, H. F., 1971, Alpha and beta globin messenger ribonucleic acid: Different amounts and rate of initiation of translation, *J. Biol. Chem.* **246**:7131.

Lodish, H. F., 1974, Model for the regulation of mRNA translation applied to haemoglobin synthesis, *Nature (London)* **251**:385.

Lodish, H. F., and Desalu, O., 1973, Regulation of synthesis of nonglobin proteins in cell-free extracts of rabbit reticulocytes, *J. Biol. Chem.* **248**:3520.

Lodish, H. F., and Jacobsen, M., 1972, Regulation of hemoglobin synthesis: Equal rates of translation and termination of α and β chains, *J. Biol. Chem.* **247**:3622.

London, I. M., Clemens, M. J., Ranu, R. S., Levin, D. H., Cherbas, L. F., and Ernst, V., 1976, The role of hemin in the regulation of protein synthesis in erythroid cells, *Fed. Proc.* **35**:2218.

Lubsen, N. W., and Davis, B. D., 1972, A ribosome dissociation factor from rabbit reticulocytes, *Proc. Nat. Acad. Sci. U.S.A.* **69**:353.

Luppis, B., Bargellesi, A., and Conconi, F., 1970, Control of hemoglobin synthesis at the translational level: Nascent polypeptide chain distribution on rabbit reticulocyte ribosomes, *Biochemistry* **9**:4175.

Marks, P. A., and Rifkind, R. A., 1972, Protein synthesis: Its control in erythropoiesis, *Science* **175**:955.

Marotta, C. A., Forget, B. G., Weissman, S. M., Verma, I. M., McCaffrey, R. P., and Baltimore, D., 1974, Nucleotide sequences of human globin messenger RNA, *Proc. Nat. Acad. Sci. U.S.A.* **71**:2300.

Matthews, M. B., Hunt, T., and Brayley, A., 1973, Specificity of the control of protein synthesis by haemin, *Nature New Biol.* **243**:230.

Maxwell, C. R., and Rabinovitz, M., 1969, Evidence for an inhibitor in the control of globin synthesis by hemin in a reticulocyte lysate, *Biochem. Biophys. Res. Commun.* **35**:79.

Maxwell, C. R., Kamper, C. S., and Rabinovitz, M., 1971, Hemin control of globin synthesis: An assay for the inhibitor formed in the absence of hemin and some characteristics of its formation, *J. Mol. Biol.* **58**:317.

May, A., and Huehns, E. R., 1976, Mechanism and prevention of sickling, *Br. Med. Bull.* **32**:223.

Mazur, A., and Carleton, A., 1963, Relation of ferritin iron to heme synthesis in marrow and reticulocytes, *J. Biol. Chem.* **238**:1817.

McKeehan, W., and Hardesty, B., 1969a, Purification and partial characterization of the amino acyl tRNA binding enzyme from rabbit reticulocytes, *J. Biol. Chem.* **244**:4330.

McKeehan, W., and Hardesty, B., 1969b, The mechanism of cycloheximide inhibition of protein synthesis in rabbit reticulocytes, *Biochem. Biophys. Res. Commun.* **36**:625.

Merrick, W. C., Lubsen, H. H., and Anderson, W. F., 1973, A ribosome dissociation factor from rabbit reticulocytes distinct from initiation factor M3, *Proc. Nat. Acad. Sci. U.S.A.* **70**:2220.

Milner, P. F., Clegg, J. B., and Weatherall, D. J., 1971, Haemoglobin H disease due to a unique haemoglobin variant with an elongated $\alpha$ chain, *Lancet* **1**:729.

Mirand, E. A., and Murphy, G. P., 1970, Extrarenal erythropoietin activity in man and experimental animals, *in Regulation of Hematopoiesis,* Vol. I (A. S. Gordon, ed.), p. 495, Appleton, New York.

Mizuno, S., and Rabinovitz, M., 1973, Factor-promoted dissociation of free ribosomes in a rabbit reticulocyte lysate system. Inhibition and requirement for an energy source, *Proc. Nat. Acad. Sci. U.S.A.* **70**:787.

Mizuno, S., Fisher, J. M., and Rabinovitz, M., 1972, Hemin control of globin synthesis: Action of an inhibitor formed in the absence of hemin in the reticulocyte cell-free system and its reversal by a ribosomal factor, *Biochim. Biophys. Acta* **272**:638.

Modell, C. B., Latter, A., Steadman, J. H., and Huehns, E. R., 1969, Hemoglobin synthesis in $\beta$-thalassemia, *Br. J. Haematol.* **17**:485.

Moore, M. R., and Goldberg, A., 1974, Normal and abnormal haem synthesis, *in Iron in Biochemistry and Medicine* (A. Jacobs and M. Warwood, eds.), p. 115, Academic Press, New York.

Nathan, D. G., and Gunn, R. B., 1966, Thalassemia: The consequences of unbalanced hemoglobin synthesis, *Am. J. Med.* **41**:815.

Nathan, D. G., Stossel, T. B., Gunn, R. B., Zarkowsky, H. S., and Laforet, M. T., 1969, Influence of hemoglobin precipitation of erythrocyte metabolism in alpha and beta thalassemia, *J. Clin. Invest.* **48**:33.

Nathan, D. G., Lodish, H. F., Kan, J. W., and Housman, D., 1971, Beta-thalassemia and translation of globin messenger RNA, *Proc. Nat. Acad. Sci. U.S.A.* **68**:2514.

Nienhuis, A. W., and Anderson, W. F., 1974, The molecular defect in thalassemia, *Clin. Haematol.* **3**:437.

Nienhuis, A. W., Laycock, D. G., and Anderson, W. F., 1971, Translation of rabbit hemoglobin messenger RNA by thalassemic and non-thalassemic ribosomes, *Nature (London) New Biol.* **231**:205.

Nombela, C., Nombela, N. A., Ochoa, S., Safer, B., Anderson, W. F., and Merrick, W. C., 1976, Polypeptide chain initiation in eukaryotes: Mechanism of formation of initiation complex, *Proc. Nat. Acad. Sci. U.S.A.* **73**:298.

Nudel, U., Lebleu, B., and Revel, M., 1973, Discrimination between messenger ribonucleic acids by a mammalian translation initiation factor, *Proc. Nat. Acad. Sci. U.S.A.* **70**:2139.

Old, J., Clegg, J. B., Weatherall, D. H., Ottolenghi, S., Comi, P., Giglioni, B., Mitchell, J., Toltoshev, P., and Williamson, R., 1976, A direct estimate of the number of human γ-globin genes, *Cell* **8**:13.

Olson, G., Gaskill, G., and Kabat, D., 1972. Presence of hemoglobin messenger RNA in a reticulocyte supernatant fraction, *Biochim. Biophys. Acta* **272**:297.

Ottolenghi, S., Lanyon, W. G., Paul, J., Williamson, R., Weatherall, D. J., Clegg, J. B., Pritchard, J., Pootrakul, S., and Wong, H. B., 1974, Gene deletion as the cause of α-thalassemia, *Nature (London)* **251**:389.

Ottolenghi, S., Lanyon, W. G., Williamson, R., Weatherall, D. J., Clegg, J. B., and Pitcher, C. S., 1975, Human globin gene analysis for a patient with beta⁰/delta-beta thalassemia, *Proc. Nat. Acad. Sci. U.S.A.* **72**:2294.

Pain, W. M., and Clemens, M. J., 1973, The role of soluble protein factors in the translational control of protein synthesis in eukaryotic cells, *FEBS Lett.* **32**:205.

Papayannopóulous, T., and Finch, C. H., 1972, On the *in vivo* action of erythropoietin, *J. Clin. Invest.* **51**:1179.

Papayannopoulous, T., Brice, M., and Stamatoyannopoulos, G., 1976, Stimulation of fetal hemoglobin synthesis in bone marrow cultures from adult individuals, *Proc. Nat. Acad. Sci. U.S.A.* **73**:2033.

Pataryas, H. A., and Stamatoyannopoulos, G., 1972, Hemoglobins in human fetuses: Evidence for adult hemoglobin production after the 11th gestational week, *Blood* **39**:688.

Pauling, L., Itano, H. A., Singer, S. J., and Wells, I. C., 1949, Sickle cell anemia, a molecular disease, *Science* **110**:543.

Perutz, M. F., 1976, Structure and mechanism of haemoglobin, *Br. Med. Bull.* **32**:195.

Perutz, M. F., and Lehmann, H., 1968, Molecular pathology of human haemoglobin, *Nature (London)* **219**:902.

Peterson, J. C., and McConkey, E. H., 1976, Proteins of Friend leukemia virus, *J. Biol. Chem.* **251**:555.

Piantadosi, C. A., Dickerman, H. W., and Spivak, J. L., 1976, Sequential activation of splenic nuclear RNA polymerases by erythropoietin, *J. Clin. Invest.* **57**:20.

Ponka, P., and Neuwirt, J., 1975, Regulation of iron delivery from transferrin to reticulocytes, in *Proteins of Iron Storage and Transport in Biochemistry and Medicine* (R. R. Crighton, ed.), p. 147, North-Holland, Publ., Amsterdam.

Powsner, E. R., and Berman, L., 1968, Effect of erythropoietin on DNA synthesis by erythroblasts *in vivo*, *Blood* **30**:189.

Price, P. M., Conover, J. H., and Hirschhorn, K., 1972, Chromosomal localization of human haemoglobin structural genes, *Nature (London)* **237**:340.

Primosigh, J. V., and Thomas, E. D., 1968, Studies in the partition of iron in the bone marrow, *J. Clin. Invest.* **47**:1473.

Pritchard, J., Longley, J., Clegg, J. B., and Weatherall, D. J., 1976, Assay of thalassemic messenger RNA in the wheat germ system, *Br. J. Haematol.* **32**:473.

Rabinovitz, M., Freedman, M. L., Fisher, J. M., and Maxwell, C. R., 1969,

Translational control in hemoglobin synthesis, *Cold Spring Harbor Symp. Quant. Biol.* **34**:567.

Raffel, C., Stein, S., and Kaempfer, R., 1974, Role for heme in mammalian protein synthesis: Activation of an initiation factor, *Proc. Nat. Acad. Sci. U.S.A.* **71**:4020.

Rhinesmith, H., Schroeder, W., and Pauling, L., 1957, A qualitative study of the hydrolysis of human dinitrophenyl globin: The number and kinds of polypeptides in normal adult hemoglobin, *J. Am. Chem. Soc.* **79**:4682.

Rhoads, R. E., McKnight, G. S., and Schimke, R. T., 1973, Quantitative measurement of ovalbumin messenger ribonucleic acid activity, *J. Biol. Chem.* **248**:2031.

Rieder, R. F., 1972, Translation of $\beta$-globin mRNA in $\beta$-thalassemia and the S and C hemoglobinopathies, *J. Clin. Invest.* **51**:364.

Rieder, R. F., and Weatherall, D. J., 1965, Studies on hemoglobin biosynthesis: Asyndhronous synthesis of hemoglobin A and hemoglobin $A_2$ by erythrocyte precursors, *J. Clin. Invest.* **44**:42.

Ross, J., Aviv, H., Scolnick, E., and Leder, P., 1972, *In vitro* synthesis of DNA complementary to purified rabbit globin mRNA, *Proc. Nat. Acad. Sci. U.S.A.* **69**:264.

Rossi-Fanelli, A., Antonio, G., and Caputo, A., 1958, Studies on the structure of hemoglobin, *Biochim. Biophys. Acta* **30**:608.

Rothstein, G., Lee, G. R., and Cartwright, G. E., 1969, Sideroblastic anemia with dermal photosensitivity and greatly increased erythrocyte protoporphyrin, *N. Engl. J. Med.* **280**:587.

Rowley, P. T., and Morris, J., 1967, Protein synthesis in the maturing reticulocyte, *J. Biol. Chem.* **242**:1533.

Rowley, P. T., Midthun, R. A., and Adams, M. A., 1971, Solubilization of a reticulocyte ribosomal fraction responsible for the decline in ribosomal activity with cell maturation, *Arch. Biochem. Biophys.* **145**:6.

Rucknagel, D. L., and Winter, W. P., 1974, Duplication of structural genes for hemoglobin $\alpha$ and $\beta$ chains in man, *Ann. N.Y. Acad. Sci.* **241**:80.

Scherrer, K., 1973, Messenger RNA in eukaryotic cells. The life history of duck globin messenger RNA, *Acta Endocrinol.* **74** (Suppl. 80):95.

Schooley, J. C., and Mahlmann, L. J., 1971, Stimulation of erythropoiesis in the plethoric mouse by cyclic AMP and its inhibition by anti-erythropoietin, *Proc. Soc. Exp. Biol. Med.* **137**:1289.

Schrenk, H. H., Yant, W. P., Pearce, S. J., Patty, F. A., and Sayers, R. R., 1941, Absorption, distribution and elimination of benzene by body tissues and fluids of dogs exposed to benzene vapor, *J. Ind. Hyg. Toxicol.* **23**:20.

Schroeder, W. A., and Huisman, T. H. J., 1974, Multiple cistrons for fetal hemoglobins in man, *Ann. N.Y. Acad. Sci.* **241**:70.

Schwartz, E., 1970, Heterozygous beta thalassemia: Balanced globin synthesis in bone marrow cells, *Science* **167**:1513.

Seid-Akhavan, M., Winter, W. P., Abramson, R. K., and Rucknagel, D. L., 1972, Hemoglobin Wayne: A frameshift variant occurring in two distinct forms, *Blood* **40**:927a.

Shaeffer, J. R., 1967, Evidence for soluble $\alpha$ chains as intermediates in hemoglobin synthesis in the rabbit reticulocyte, *Biochem. Biophys. Res. Commun.* **28**:647.

Shaeffer, J. R., Trostle, P. K., and Evans, R. F., 1969, Inhibition of the biosynthetic completion of rabbit hemoglobin by isolated human hemoglobin chains, *J. Biol. Chem.* **244**:4284.

Shafritz, D., and Anderson, W. F., 1970, Factor dependent-binding of methionyl tRNA to reticulocyte ribosomes, *Nature (London)* **227**:918.

Shafritz, D., Laycock, D., and Anderson, W. F., 1971a, Puromycin–peptide bond formation with reticulocyte initiation factors M1 and M2, *Proc. Nat. Acad. Sci. U.S.A.* **68**:496.

Shafritz, D., Laycock, D., Crystal, R., and Anderson, W. F., 1971b, Requirement for GTP in the initiation process on reticulocyte ribosomes and ribosomal subunits, *Proc. Nat. Acad. Sci. U.S.A.* **68**:2246.

Shafritz, D. A., Prichard, P. M., Gilbert, J. M., Merrick, W. C., and Anderson, W. F., 1972, Separation of reticulocyte initiation factor M2 into two components, *Proc. Nat. Acad. Sci. U.S.A.* **69**:983.

Shepard, M. K., Weatherall, D. J., and Conley, C. L., 1962, Semi-quantitative estimation of the distribution of fetal hemoglobin in red cell populations, *Bull. Johns Hopkins Hosp.* **110**:293.

Sherton, C. C., and Kabat, D., 1976, Changes in RNA and protein metabolism proceeding onset of hemoglobin synthesis in cultured Friend leukemia cells, *Dev. Biol.* **48**:118.

Spivak, J. L., 1976, Effect of erythropoietin on chromosomal protein synthesis, *Blood* **47**:581.

Stamatoyannopoulos, C., 1972, The molecular basis of hemoglobin disease, *Annu. Rev. Genet.* **6**:47.

Suzuki, H., and Itano, H. A., 1973a, Removal of N-terminal methionine from nascent globin chains in sickle cell anemia reticulocytes, *Proc. Nat. Acad. Sci. U.S.A.* **70**:2059.

Suzuki, H., and Itano, H. A., 1973b, Quantitative differences between N-terminal methionyl nascent globin chains of human and rabbit reticulocytes, *Nature New Biol.* **246**:107.

Tate, W. P., Beaudet, A. L., and Caskey, C. T., 1973, Influence of guanine nucleotides and elongation factors on interaction of release factors with the ribosome, *Proc. Nat. Acad. Sci. U.S.A.* **70**:2350.

Tavill, A. S., Grayzel, A. I., London, I. M., Williams, M. K., and Vanderhoff, G. A., 1968, The role of heme in the synthesis and assembly of hemoglobin, *J. Biol. Chem.* **243**:4987.

Tavill, A. S., Vanderhoff, G., and London, I. M., 1972, The control of hemoglobin synthesis: A comparison of the role of heme in rabbit bone marrow and reticulocytes, *J. Biol. Chem.* **247**:366.

Taylor, J. M., Dozy, A., Kan, Y. W., Varmus, H. E., Lie-Ingo, L. E., Ganesan, J., and Todd, D., 1974, Genetic lesion in homozygous α-thalassemia (hydrops fetalis), *Nature (London)* **251**:392.

Temple, G., and Housman, D., 1972, Separation and translation of the messenger RNA's coding for α and β chains of rabbit globin, *Proc. Nat. Acad. Sci. U.S.A.* **69**:1574.

Terada, M., Cantor, L., Metafora, S., Rifkind, R. A., Bank, A., and Marks, P. A., 1972, Globin messenger RNA activity in erythroid precursor cells and the effect of erythropoietin, *Proc. Nat. Acad. Sci. U.S.A.* **69**:3575.

Till, J. E., and McCulloch, E. A., 1965, A direct measurement of the radiation sensitivity of normal mouse bone marrow cells, *Radiat. Res.* **74**:213.

Todd, D., Lai, M. C. S., Beaven, G. H., and Huehns, E. R., 1970, The abnormal haemoglobins in homozygous α-thalassemia, *Br. J. Haematol.* **19**:27.

Tolstoshev, P., Mitchell, J., Lanyon, G., Williamson, R., Ottolenghi, S., Comi, P., Giglioni, B., Masera, G., Modell, B., Weatherall, D. J., and Clegg, J. B., 1976, Presence of gene for β globin in homozygous $β^0$-thalassemia, *Nature (London)* **259**:95.

Velez, R., Farrell, N. L., and Freedman, M. L., 1971, Selective proteolytic dissociation of rabbit reticulocyte single ribosomes not attached to messenger RNA, *Biochim. Biophys. Acta* **228**:719.

Verma, I. M., Temple, G. F., Fan, H., and Baltimore, D., 1972, *In vitro* synthesis of RNA complementary to rabbit reticulocyte 10S RNA, *Nature New Biol.* **235**:163.

Vogler, W. R., and Mingioli, E. S., 1968, Porphyrin synthesis and heme synthetase activity in pyridoxine-responsive anemia, *Blood* **32**:979.

Waxman, H. S., and Rabinovitz, M., 1965, Iron supplementation *in vitro* and the state of aggregation and function of reticulocyte ribosomes in hemoglobin synthesis, *Biochem. Biophys. Res. Commun.* **19**:538.

Waxman, H. S., and Rabinovitz, M., 1966, Control of reticulocyte polyribosome content and hemoglobin synthesis by heme, *Biochim. Biophys. Acta* **129**:369.

Waxman, H. S., Freedman, M. L., and Rabinovitz, M., 1967, Studies with [59]Fe-labeled hemin on the control of polyribosome formation in rabbit reticulocytes, *Biochim. Biophys. Acta* **145**:353.

Weatherall, D. J., and Clegg, J. B., 1972, *The Thalassemia Syndromes*, 2nd ed., Blackwell, Oxford.

Weatherall, D. J., and Clegg, J. B., 1975, Hereditary persistence of fetal hemoglobin, *Br. J. Haematol.* **29**:191.

Weatherall, D. J., Clegg, J. B., and Naughton, M. A., 1965, Globin synthesis in thalassemia: An *in vitro* study, *Nature (London)* **208**:1061.

Weatherall, D. J., Clegg, J. B., Na-Nakorn, S., and Wasi, P., 1969, The pattern of disordered haemoglobin synthesis in homozygous and heterozygous β-thalassemia, *Br. J. Haematol.* **16**:251.

Weatherall, D. J., Clegg, J. B., and Boon, W. H., 1970, The haemoglobin constitution of infants with the haemoglobin Bart's hydrops fetalis syndrome, *Br. J. Haematol.* **18**:357.

Weatherall, D. J., Pembrey, M. E., and Pritchard, J., 1974, Fetal haemoglobin, *Clin. Hematol.* **3**:467.

White, J. M., 1971, The synthesis of abnormal hemoglobins, *Ser. Hematol.* **4**:116.

White, J. M., 1976, The unstable haemoglobins, *Br. Med. Bull.* **32**:219.

White, J. M., and Harvey, D. R., 1972, Defective synthesis of α and β globin chains in lead poisoning, *Nature (London)* **236**:71.

White, J. M., and Ali, M., 1973, Globin synthesis in sideroblastic anemia. II. Effect of pyridoxine, δ-aminolevulinic acid and haem *in vitro*, *Br. J. Haematol.* **29**:481.

White, J. M., and Hoffrand, A. U., 1974, Haem deficiency and chain synthesis, *Nature (London)* **248**:88.

White, J. M., Brain, M. C., and Ali, M., 1971, Globin synthesis in sideroblastic anemia. I. α and β peptide chain synthesis, *Br. J. Haematol.* **20**:263.

Wildman, J. M., Freedman, M. L., Rosman, J., and Goldstein, B., 1976, Benzene and lead inhibition of rabbit reticulocyte heme and protein synthesis: Evidence for additive toxicity of these two components of commercial gasoline, *Res. Commun. Chem. Pathol. Pharmacol.* **13**:473.

Wilson, M. G., Schroeder, W. A., Graves, D. A., and Kach, V. D., 1967, Hemoglobin variations in D-trisomy syndrome, *N. Engl. J. Med.* **277**:953.

Winterhalter, K. H., 1966, The sequence of linkage between the prosthetic groups and the polypeptide chains of hemoglobin, *Nature (London)* **211**:932.

Winterhalter, K. H., and Glotthaar, B., 1971, Intermediates of hemoglobin and their relation to biosynthesis, *Ser. Haematol.* **4**:84.

Winterhalter, K. H., Heywood, J., Huehns, E. R., and Finch, C. A., 1969, The free globin in human erythrocytes, *Br. J. Haematol.* **16**:523.

Wintrobe, M. M., Lee, G. R., Boggs, D. R., Bithell, T. C., Athens, J. W., and Foerster, J., 1974, Morphology, intrinsic metabolism, function, laboratory evaluation, *in Clinical Hematology* (M. M. Wintrobe, ed.), Chap. 3, Lea & Febiger, Philadelphia.

Wolf, J. R., Mason, G., and Honig, G., 1973, Regulation of hemoglobin β chain synthesis in bone marrow by α chains, *Proc. Nat. Acad. Sci. U.S.A.* **70**:3405.

Wood, W. G., and Weatherall, D. J., 1973, Haemoglobin synthesis during foetal development, *Nature New Biol.* **244**:162.

Wood, W. G., and Stamatoyannopoulos, C., 1975, Globin synthesis in fractionated normoblasts of β-thalassemia heterozygote, *J. Clin. Invest.* **55**:567.

Yoshida, A., and Lin, W., 1972, Amino terminal formylmethionine and amino terminal methionine cleaving enzymes in rabbit reticulocytes, *J. Biol. Chem.* **247**:952.

Yoshida, A., Watanabe, S., and Morris, J., 1970, Initiation of rabbit hemoglobin synthesis: Methionine and formylmethionine at the N-terminus, *Proc. Nat. Acad. Sci. U.S.A.* **67**:1600.

Zail, S. S., Charlton, R. W., Torrance, J. D., and Bothwell, T. H., 1964, Studies on the formation of ferritin in red cell precursors, *J. Clin. Invest.* **43**:670.

Zehavi-Willner, T., Kosower, E. M., Hunt, R. T., and Kosower, N. S., 1971, Glutathione V. The effects of the thiol-oxidizing agent diamide on initiation and translation in rabbit reticulocytes, *Biochim. Biophys. Acta* **228**:245.

Zucker, W., and Schulman, H., 1968, Stimulation of globin chain initiation by hemin in the reticulocyte cell-free system, *Proc. Nat. Acad. Sci. U.S.A.* **59**:582.

**3**

# Clinical Significance of 2,3-Diphosphoglycerate in Hematology

## Frank A. Oski and Julia A. McMillan

A decade has now elapsed since the observations of Chanutin and Curnish (1967) and Benesch and Benesch (1967) that intraerythrocytic organic phosphates play a central role in modulating hemoglobin's affinity for oxygen. In the ensuing years many clinical conditions have been identified in which the position of the oxygen–hemoglobin equilibrium curve has deviated from normal as a result of variations in the concentration of red cell organic phosphates. Numerous studies have been performed in both animals and man in an attempt to elucidate the significance of these deviations in terms of oxygen delivery. Much of the data are highly suggestive but as yet it remains unclear just how important a shift in the oxygen–hemoglobin equilibrium curve is in the adaptation of man to both physiologic and pathologic processes.

This chapter will focus on the information that has accumulated in the study of humans that bears on the clinical significance of alterations in the position of the curve that are produced by changes in red cell organic phosphates.

FRANK A. OSKI and JULIA A. McMILLAN • Department of Pediatrics, State University of New York, Upstate Medical Center, Syracuse, New York.

## 3.1. Oxygen Transport and Delivery

The oxygen transport system in man is the erythrocyte. The erythrocyte serves this role because it contains the iron protein conjugate, hemoglobin. The red cell's primary function is to bring oxygen to the tissues in adequate quantities, at a sufficient partial pressure, to permit its rapid diffusion from the blood. The ultimate supply of oxygen to the cell is determined by a number of factors, including the content of oxygen in the inspired air; the partial pressure of oxygen in the inspired air; the pulmonary and alveolar ventilation; the diffusion of oxygen from the alveolar air to the capillary bed; the cardiac output; the blood volume; the hemoglobin concentration; and the passive diffusion of oxygen from the capillaries to the cells.

*In vivo*, the total amount of oxygen made available to the tissues per minute can be calculated from the relationship

$$O_2 \text{ transport} = Q \times CaO_2$$

in which $Q$ is the blood flow in liters per minute, and $CaO_2$ is the arterial oxygen content in milliliters per liter of blood.

The consumption of oxygen by any given tissue or by the whole organism can be expressed by the equation

$$V_{O_2} = 1.39 \times Hb \times Q(Sat_A - Sat_V)$$

where 1.39 represents the amount of oxygen in milliliters that can be bound to 1 g of hemoglobin; Hb the hemoglobin concentration in grams per 100 ml of blood; $Q$ the blood flow in liters per minute; and $Sat_A$ and $Sat_V$ the oxygen saturation of arterial and venous blood, respectively.

Simple calculations reveal that under most circumstances the quantity of oxygen transported to the tissues exceeds the amount delivered to them. The amount delivered to the tissues is determined not only by the tissue requirements but also by the rate of diffusion of oxygen from the blood to the tissues. The position of the oxygen–hemoglobin equilibrium curve plays a major role in the final process of diffusion of oxygen from the capillary to the tissues. This principle is illustrated by the equation

$$dV_{O_2}/dt = D \times (P_{O_2} \text{ capillary} - P_{O_2} \text{ cell interior})$$

where $dV_{O_2}/dt$ represents the volume of oxygen that has diffused over a period of time, and $D$ represents a diffusion coefficient for a given tissue. This diffusion coefficient is dependent on the oxygen solubility in a given tissue, and the surface area and thickness of the tissue involved. From this equation it follows that the higher the partial pressure of oxygen in the capillary at which oxygen can be released, the greater is the amount of oxygen that may diffuse over any period in time.

The oxygen–hemoglobin equilibrium curve (Fig. 1) reflects the affinity of hemoglobin for oxygen and is thus a measure of the partial pressure of oxygen at which hemoglobin may be released for tissue diffusion. As blood circulates in the normal lung, the arterial oxygen tension rises from 40 mm Hg and reaches approximately 110 mm Hg, sufficient to ensure at least 95% saturation of the arterial blood. The shape of the curve is such that a further increase in the oxygen tension in the lung results in only a very small increase in the degree of saturation of the blood. As blood travels from the lung, the oxygen tension falls as it is released to the tissues from hemoglobin. In the normal adult when the oxygen tension has fallen to approximately 27 mm Hg, at a pH of 7.4 and a temperature of 37°C, 50% of the oxygen bound to hemoglobin has been released. The $P_{50}$, the whole blood oxygen tension at 50% oxygen saturation, is thus stated to be 27 mm Hg. When the affinity of hemoglobin for oxygen is reduced, more oxygen is released to the tissues at a given oxygen tension. In such situations the oxygen–hemoglobin equilibrium curve is shifted to the right of normal. When the affinity of hemoglobin for oxygen is increased, the equilibrium curve appears shifted to the left and the tension must drop lower than normal before the hemoglobin releases an equivalent amount of oxygen.

If the arteriovenous oxygen saturation difference remains constant, a decrease in affinity of hemoglobin for oxygen, a rightward shift in the position of the curve, would be accompanied by an increase in mixed venous oxygen tension and a leftward shift by a decrease. If the mixed

Fig. 1. The oxygen dissociation curve of normal adult blood. The $P_{50}$, the oxygen tension at 50% oxygen saturation, is approximately 27 mm Hg. As the curve shifts to the right the oxygen affinity of hemoglobin decreases and more oxygen is released at a given oxygen tension. With a shift to the left the opposite effects are observed. A decrease in pH or an increase in temperature decreases the affinity of hemoglobin for oxygen.

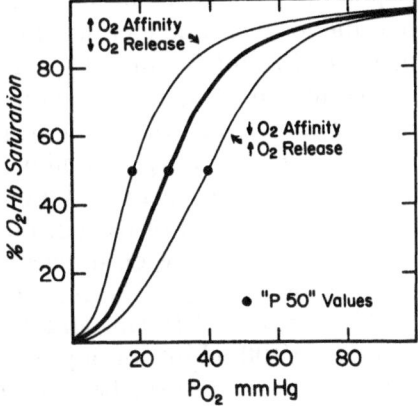

venous oxygen tension remains constant, then the arteriovenous oxygen saturation difference increases with a shift in the curve to the right and decreases with a shift to the left. Since the rate of oxygen diffusion from blood to cell interior is related to the oxygen pressure differential, it may be assumed that a shift to the right facilitates oxygen diffusion and a shift to the left limits it.

From the initial equations it is also apparent that compensations may occur which would keep the oxygen consumption constant despite alterations in hemoglobin's affinity for oxygen. These compensations may include an increase in flow (cardiac output), or an increase in the oxygen-carrying capacity of the blood (erythrocytosis). If compensation is unsatisfactory, then the physiological consequences of impaired tissue oxygenation may be evident. These manifestations include elevations in plasma or urinary erythropoietin, alterations in the plasma lactate-to-pyruvate ratio, or alterations in organ function. Organ dysfunction is most apparent in the heart and brain, the two major oxygen-consuming tissues of the body.

A certain partial pressure gradient is needed for the transfer of oxygen from capillary to tissue. Below this critical capillary oxygen tension, diffusion is impaired and tissue hypoxia results. Kety (1957) and Landis and Pappenheimer (1973) have stated that the end-capillary oxygen tension necessary for adequate tissue oxygenation is at least 20 mm Hg. In support of this figure is the observation of Opitz and Schneider (1950) that brain oxygen uptake decreased when the venous oxygen tension fell into the 20- and 25-mm Hg range. Similarly, Berne *et al.* (1957) found that coronary vasodilatation occurred when the arterial oxygen pressure was 22–24 mm Hg and that loss of myocardial function was severe at an oxygen tension of 10–12 mm Hg.

A critical capillary oxygen tension cannot be defined precisely for all tissues under all metabolic conditions because of the inherent variability in requirements from tissue to tissue. Bendixen and Laver (1965) suggest that the term "average critical range" be employed, and place this value between 20 and 30 mm Hg. At a normal pH and temperature this represents an oxygen saturation in the range of 35 to 55%. Thus, a normal individual with a hemoglobin concentration of 16 g/100 ml, having an arterial oxygen content of 22.2 vol/100 ml (16.0 × 1.39 ml, the oxygen-carrying capacity of 1 g of hemoglobin), would have between 7.7 and 12.1 vol/100 ml of oxygen unavailable to the tissues.

The average oxygen uptake is approximately 5 vol/100 ml. Contributing to this average is the very small arteriovenous oxygen difference in the kidneys, 1.5 vol/100 ml, and the large arteriovenous oxygen difference of 11.5 vol/100 ml in working muscle and the heart. These latter organs have no oxygen reserve because they are extracting as much oxygen as possible from the blood at the optimal partial pressure for diffusion.

## 3.2. Factors Modifying Hemoglobin's Affinity for Oxygen

Numerous factors influence the affinity of hemoglobin for oxygen. In addition to the structure of the hemoglobin itself, they include the intraerythrocytic pH, temperature, $P_{CO_2}$, and the red cell concentration of organic phosphate. Although these factors, working in concert, are the major determinants of the position of the oxygen–hemoglobin equilibrium curve, it is apparent from a variety of studies that other factors, some as yet unidentified, also play a role in regulating the $P_{50}$ (Shappell and Lenfant, 1972). These factors are summarized in Table I.

Over a pH range of 6.0 to 8.5 oxygen affinity varies directly with pH (Bohr effect). The rise in $P_{50}$ that accompanies a fall in pH appears to offer a physiological advantage in facilitating oxygen unloading. At the tissue level, the drop in pH caused by $CO_2$ production lowers oxygen–hemoglobin affinity, thus enhancing oxygen release. At the pulmonary level, the efflux of $CO_2$ leads to a rise in pH and thus increases hemoglobin's affinity for oxygen and oxygen uptake. At a constant $P_{CO_2}$, the magnitude of this effect is given by the relation $\Delta \log P_{50}/\Delta pH = -0.40$

**Table I.** Causes of Alterations in Hemoglobin–Oxygen Affinity[a]

| Factors that increase $P_{50}$ | Factors that decrease $P_{50}$ |
|---|---|
| By direct or unknown action | By direct action |
| Increased temperature | Decreased temperature |
| Increased {$H^+$} | Decreased {$H^+$} |
| Increased DPG (and ATP) | Decreased $P_{CO_2}$ |
| Increased Hb concentration | Decreased DPG (and ATP) |
| Increased ionic strength | Decreased Hb concentration |
| Abnormal hemoglobin | Decreased ionic strength |
| Cortisol | Abnormal hemoglobin |
| Aldosterone | Carboxyhemoglobin |
| Pyridoxol phosphate (in Hb solution) | Methemoglobin |
| Cell age? | Cell age? |
| By increasing DPG in cells | By decreasing DPG in cells |
| Decreased {$H^+$} | Increased {$H^+$} |
| Thyroid hormone | Decreased thyroid hormone |
| Erythrocytic enzyme deficiency | Erythrocytic enzyme deficiency |
| Cell age | Cell age |
| Increased inorganic phosphate | Decreased inorganic phosphate |
| Inosine | |
| Increased sulfate | |

[a]Taken from Shappell and Lenfant (1972).

(Naeraa *et al.*, 1966). Although it has long been assumed that the value of the Bohr effect was the same at all degrees of oxygen saturation, recent evidence suggests that the numerical value of the Bohr effect may be smaller at the extremes of the oxygen–hemoglobin dissociation curve (Siggaard-Anderson *et al.*, 1972).

Carbon dioxide affects hemoglobin function in two ways. It readily diffuses into red cells where, in the presence of carbonic anhydrase, carbonic acid is formed. This fall in pH, as previously mentioned, reduced hemoglobin's affinity for oxygen. In addition, $CO_2$ can bind free amino groups on hemoglobin to form carbamino compounds by the reaction

$$RNH_2 + CO_2 \rightleftharpoons RNHCOO^- + H^+$$

Only nonprotonated amino groups can react with $CO_2$. The only amino groups in globin whose p$K$ values are low enough to be partially nonprotonated at physiological pH are the N termini. Deoxyhemoglobin forms carbamino compounds more readily than oxyhemoglobin, and this is why $CO_2$ tends to reduce the affinity of hemoglobin for oxygen. It is likely that at the usual pH of the red cell of approximately 7.20, only 10% of the $CO_2$ produced by tissue metabolism is transported to the lungs in the form of carbamino compounds.

The Bohr effect measured by changing the pH by varying the $P_{CO_2}$ is larger (−0.48) than the Bohr effect measured by changing the pH by adding other acids or bases (−0.40). In addition, the concentration of 2,3-diphosphoglycerate within the red cell also alters the Bohr effect (Wranne *et al.*, 1972). All of these interacting effects have made calculations of the $P_{50}$ utilizing the Bohr factor extremely complex. *In vivo* determinations of the $P_{50}$ employing a single venous sample (Lichtman *et al.*, 1976) may provide a more reliable and more convenient measure of the position of the oxygen–hemoglobin dissociation curve.

Temperature changes also produce an immediate influence on the affinity of hemoglobin for oxygen. An increase in temperature produces a rightward shift in the position of the curve. The magnitude of this effect can be expressed by the equation $\Delta \log P_{50}/T = -0.024$.

The effects of pH, temperature, and $P_{CO_2}$ on hemoglobin–oxygen affinity attracted little clinical attention until 1967 when Benesch and Benesch (1967) and Chanutin and Curnish (1967) demonstrated that the affinity of a hemoglobin solution for oxygen could be decreased by an interaction with a number of organic phosphates. Of the organic phosphates tested, 2,3-diphosphoglycerate (2,3-DPG) and adenosine triphosphate were most effective in lowering oxygen affinity, whereas adenosine diphosphate, adenosine monophosphate, pyrophosphate, and inorganic phosphate had progressively decreasing degrees of effectiveness. The highly charged anion 2,3-DPG was demonstrated by Benesch and co-workers (1967) to bind to deoxyhemoglobin but not to the oxygenated form of the molecule. They found that 1 mole of 2,3-DPG bound reversibly to 1 mole of deoxyhemoglobin tetramer under physiological conditions of intraerythrocytic solute concentration and pH.

Of the organic phosphates normally found in the human erythrocyte, 2,3-DPG is the one found in largest concentration and thus is quantitatively the most important with respect to modulation of hemoglobin–oxygen affinity. The content of 2,3-DPG in the red cell averages 5.1 $\mu$mol/ml of red blood cells (range 3.4–6.2 $\mu$mol/ml of red blood cells) and adenosine triphosphate 1.0 $\mu$mol/ml of red blood cells (range 0.8–1.4 $\mu$mol/ml of red blood cells), whereas the remainder of the organic phosphates generally total less than 0.4 $\mu$mol/ml.

A comparison of the reactivities of a number of animal and human hemoglobins of known structure with 2,3-DPG has suggested that the N-terminal amino acids of the $\beta$ chains and the imidazoles of $\beta$143 histidine are specific residues responsible for 2,3-DPG binding (Bunn and Briehl, 1970).

Model fitting and X-ray diffraction studies have confirmed these as the likely binding sites and indicate that 2,3-DPG is situated in the central cavity between the two chains (Arnone, 1972). Its negative charges are neutralized by the positively charged groups just cited. In addition, the $\beta$82 lysine and $\beta$2 histidine are also thought to be involved in 2,3-DPG binding. Bunn (1974) has proposed the following equation to reflect this interaction:

$$HbDPG + O_2 \rightleftharpoons Hb(O_2) + DPG$$

This equilibrium demonstrates both the preferential binding of 2,3-DPG for deoxyhemoglobin and the 1:1 stoichiometry involved.

The regulation of the red cell concentration of 2,3-DPG is not completely understood, although it appears that most clinical conditions associated with hypoxia are accompanied by a rise in the concentration of red cell 2,3-DPG.

Although it has been recognized since 1925 (Greenwold, 1925) that the human erythrocyte, unlike most other cells of the body, contains large quantities of 2,3-DPG, its role within the red cell and the factors regulating its metabolism have remained a puzzle. The red cell synthesizes 2,3-DPG from 1,3-DPG in the presence of the enzyme 2,3-diphosphoglycerate mutase. The 2,3-DPG formed is then eventually hydrolyzed to 3-phosphoglycerate and inorganic phosphate by the enzyme 2,3-diphosphoglycerate phosphatase. The conversion of glyceraldehyde-3-phosphate to 1,3-DPG is controlled by the ratio of nicotinamide adenine dinucleotide/nicotinamide adenine dinucleotide, reduced, within the cell. The conversion of 1,3-DPG to either 2,3-DPG or 3-PGA is governed in part by the concentration of unbound 2,3-DPG within the cell, the level of 3-PGA, and the ratio of adenosine diphosphate–adenosine triphosphate. Increased concentrations of adenosine diphosphate facilitate conversion of 1,3-DPG to 3-PGA. High levels of 3-PGA appear to inhibit the phosphoglycerate kinase reaction and direct synthesis of 1,3-DPG to 2,3-DPG.

Studies of 2,3-diphosphoglycerate mutase have indicated that it is inhibited by very low concentrations of its product 2,3-DPG (Rose, 1970). The observation that deoxygenated hemoglobin binds 2,3-DPG has provided one explanation for the ability of the cell to synthesize this compound. When 2,3-DPG is bound to deoxyhemoglobin, the inhibition of 2,3-diphosphoglycerate mutase by its product 2,3-DPG is removed, and thus further production of this compound is facilitated. This binding of 2,3-DPG by deoxyhemoglobin appears to be a partial explanation for the increased levels of 2,3-DPG observed in situations of hypoxemia. Deoxygenation also produces a rise in intraerythrocytic pH. This would result in an increase in red cell glycolysis and an increase in 2,3-DPG synthesis. Additionally, patients with hypoxia commonly exhibit respiratory alkalosis which then may also contribute to an acceleration of 2,3-DPG synthesis.

The studies of Keitt and co-workers (1974) have helped to clarify the relative importance of arterial pH and oxygen saturation in patients with stable chronic obstructive pulmonary disease and in the same patients during episodes of acutely induced hypoxemia. In the stable state, red cell 2,3-DPG correlated with arterial $P_{O_2}$. It would thus appear that chronic hypoxemia and reduced oxygen saturation stimulate 2,3-DPG synthesis by the binding of 2,3-DPG to deoxyhemoglobin, whereas in acute situations accompanied by alterations in pH, the effects of alkalosis or acidosis predominate in regulating red cell 2,3-DPG. Alkalosis stimulates glycolysis via relief of phosphofructokinase inhibition whereas acidosis has an inhibitory effect on red cell glucose metabolism.

## 3.3. Clinical Conditions Associated with Alterations in Red Cell 2,3-DPG

In a wide variety of clinical conditions, the position of the oxygen–hemoglobin equilibrium curve, as reflected by the $P_{50}$, bears a striking relationship to the red cell 2,3-DPG content (Oski et al., 1970). Throughout the physiological range (2–10 $\mu$mol DPG/ml RBC), the relationship between $P_{50}$ and 2,3-DPG has been found to be linear, a change of 0.43 $\mu$mol of DPG/ml RBC producing a change of 1 mm Hg in the $P_{50}$. Exceptions to this relationship have been observed in patients with hepatic encephalopathy (Zimmon, 1973), and in the coronary sinus blood of patients with angina during atrial pacing (Shappell *et al.*, 1970). These exceptions indicate that other factors also play a role in modulating hemoglobin's affinity for oxygen. Drugs or humoral agents may act to affect the distribution of 2,3-DPG within the cell or alter the hydrogen ion gradient between the inside and outside of the erythrocyte.

Many clinical conditions associated with alterations in hemoglobin's affinity for oxygen have now been described (Table II). In many these effects are mediated by changes in red cell 2,3-DPG; others are a consequence of intrinsic abnormalities of hemoglobin structure.

### 3.3.1. Cardiac Disease

#### 3.3.1.1. Cyanotic Heart Disease

In infants and children with congenital heart disease associated with cyanosis an increase in red cell concentrations of 2,3-DPG and a right shift in the position of the oxygen–hemoglobin equilibrium curve have been

**Table II.** Clinical Conditions Associated with Changes in the Oxygen Affinity of Blood

| |
|---|
| I. Increased red blood cell 2,3-DPG, increased $P_{50}$ |
|     Adaptation to high altitude |
|     Hypoxemia associated with chronic pulmonary disease |
|     Hypoxemia associated with cyanotic heart disease |
|     Anemia |
|         Secondary to iron deficiency |
|         Secondary to chronic renal disease |
|         Caused by sickle cell anemia |
|     Decreased red cell mass |
|     Chronic liver disease |
|     Hyperthyroidism |
|     Red cell pyruvate kinase deficiency, phosphoglycerate deficiency |
|     Hyperphosphatemia |
|     Myocardial infarction |
| II. Decreased red blood cell 2,3-DPG, decreased $P_{50}$ |
|     Septic shock |
|     Severe acidosis |
|     Following massive transfusions of stored blood |
|     Neonatal respiratory distress syndrome |
|     Hypophosphatemia |
| III. Increased $P_{50}$, no consistent alteration in red blood cell DPG |
|     Abnormal hemoglobins (Kansas, Seattle, Hammersmith, Tacoma, E) |
|     Vigorous exercise |
| IV. Decreased $P_{50}$, no consistent alteration in red blood cell DPG |
|     Abnormal hemoglobins (Kempsey, Philly, Chesapeake, J, Capetown, Yakima, Ranier) |

observed. In general this right shift in the curve is evident when the arterial oxygen saturation falls below 85% or when the cardiac output falls below 70% of normal.

Miller (1972) has described two infants in whom the quantitative significance of this type of red cell adaption to hypoxemia could be demonstrated. Measurements of arteriovenous oxygen difference were made in a 6-month-old infant with intractable cardiac failure secondary to large shunts through a ventricular septal defect and a patent ductus arteriosus. Before surgical correction the patient's $P_{50}$ was 33.2 mm Hg, the red cell DPG 6.6 $\mu$mol/ml RBC, and the cardiac output 60% of normal. The AV oxygen content difference was 6.0 ml 02/100 ml blood and the central venous oxygen tension was 42 mm Hg. Following surgical correction the $P_{50}$ fell to 25.8 mm Hg, the red cell 2,3-DPG was 4.9 $\mu$mol/ml RBC, and the cardiac output had normalized. The AV oxygen content difference was 3.5 ml $O_2$ and the central venous oxygen tension was 43 mm Hg. Miller (1972) concluded that:

> during the period of severe heart failure that the rightward-shifted curve provided for significant amounts of systemic oxygen transport and that without such a change in oxygen unloading capacity that a large, and probably intolerable demand for additional cardiac output of blood would have been required to meet the same tissue oxygen flow.

In a second infant with significant hypoxemia from pulmonary atresia and a ventricular septal defect the $P_{50}$ was 37.6 mm Hg, the red cell 2,3-DPG 7.9 $\mu$mol/ml RBC, and the cardiac output 70% of normal. The infant had a huge AV $O_2$ difference of 6.2 ml $O_2$ as a result of the rightward shifted curve and an accompanying polycythemia. Six months after palliative surgery the $P_{50}$ measured 26.3 mm Hg, the 2,3-DPG 5.2 $\mu$mol/ml RBC, the cardiac output was normal, and the AV oxygen content difference was 4.0 ml. This patient again illustrates the protective role of a rightward shift in the curve in providing for sufficient oxygen unloading in the presence of significant hypoxemia.

Rosenthal *et al.* (1971) examined the relationships between red cell 2,3-DPG, $P_{50}$, arterial oxygen tension, and systemic oxygen transport (systemic blood flow times arterial oxygen content) in 73 children with congenital heart disease who were catheterized as part of their diagnostic evaluation. Although a decrease in arterial oxygen tension was found to be associated with an increase in $P_{50}$ and red cell 2,3-DPG, there was great variability at any given arterial oxygen tension. The red cell response appeared to be more directly related to systemic oxygen transport. The reversibility of this adaptive mechanism was demonstrated following surgical correction of the cardiac defect.

### 3.3.1.2. Noncyanotic Heart Disease

Woodson *et al.* (1970) studied 39 patients with a variety of noncyanotic cardiac defects. These authors also observed a progressive rise in red cell 2,3-DPG and $P_{50}$ as cardiac disease increased in severity. The severity of the cardiac disease was determined by the measurement of cardiac index and the cardiac symptoms. The $P_{50}$ rose as the cardiac index fell, and was also found to be related to the degree of anemia present in the patients. Both $P_{50}$ and the red cell 2,3-DPG were highest in those with the greatest AV oxygen content difference. When analyzing these results the authors pointed out that in the six patients with the lowest cardiac outputs (cardiac index 1.39 liters/min m$^2$) the arteriovenous oxygen difference was 9.4 vol % (normal 4.5–5.0 vol %) and their oxygen consumption was normal. In these patients the mixed venous oxygen tension was 30 mm Hg (normal 40 mm Hg). If no shift in the curve had occurred, the same oxygen extraction would have resulted in a central mixed venous oxygen tension of 25 mm Hg.

These studies performed in both children and adults, with and without cyanotic heart disease, all appear to indicate that impaired cardiac function is accompanied by a decrease in the affinity of hemoglobin for oxygen. This adaptation appears to be beneficial to the patient in enabling a greater oxygen unloading than would otherwise be possible at reasonable oxygen tensions. As yet a comparison between patients with and without this compensatory mechanism has not been reported in an attempt to determine if the patient without compensation is significantly worse with an equivalent degree of heart disease.

### 3.3.1.3. Ischemic Heart Disease

Attention has focused on patients, generally young, with normal coronary arteries and objective signs of myocardial ischemia and/or infarction. Vokonas *et al.* (1970) studied 13 such patients and found each to have normal oxygen–hemoglobin equilibrium curves and normal red cell concentrations of 2,3-DPG. Guy *et al.* (1971) have observed that in some patients with this form of nonobstructive coronary artery angina the release of oxygen from hemoglobin is delayed although the $P_{50}$ and 2,3-DPG are normal. Studies of purified hemolysates from these patients have suggested that the decrease in the rate of oxygen unloading is a consequence of an intrinsic abnormality of the hemoglobin.

Shappell *et al.* (1970) measured the $P_{50}$ of coronary sinus blood in patients with angina during atrial pacing that produced pain. They found that the $P_{50}$ of blood obtained from the coronary sinus rose whereas blood obtained simultaneously from the radial artery did not. The rise in $P_{50}$

was not accompanied by any change in red cell 2,3-DPG, ATP, or pH. The mechanism by which this apparent adaptive response to myocardial ischemia was produced remains unknown.

Kostuk *et al.* (1973) observed similar increases in $P_{50}$ unaccompanied by elevations in the concentration of red cell organic phosphates in patients with acute myocardial infarctions. These changes, however, were observed in both venous and arterial blood and were manifest as early as 2 h after the infarction. The increase in $P_{50}$ appeared to be proportional to the degree of myocardial injury. Again the stimulus to this abrupt change in hemoglobin–oxygen affinity remains unexplained.

### 3.3.1.4. Cardiac Surgery

Rosenthal *et al.* (1971) observed postoperative rises in red cell 2,3-DPG and $P_{50}$ in patients with congenital heart disease undergoing corrective cardiac surgery. This response, although short-lived, appeared paradoxical in view of the fact that the surgical procedure corrected the preexisting hypoxemia. Similar transient rises in red cell 2,3-DPG and $P_{50}$ have been reported in patients following noncardiac surgery (Proctor *et al.*, 1971).

In contrast, Bordiuk *et al.* (1971) and Young *et al.* (1973) have observed transient decreases in $P_{50}$ and red cell 2,3-DPG during the first 24 h following cardiac surgery. In the patients studied by Young and co-workers (1973) the fall in 2,3-DPG was accompanied by a fall in red cell ATP, and both could be related to the development of postoperative hypophosphatemia. Neither the transfusion of stored blood nor the effect of cardiopulmonary bypass explained this transient decrease in 2,3-DPG and $P_{50}$.

Giannelli and co-workers (1976) have observed that red cell 2,3-DPG declines progressively in patients undergoing open heart surgery while on cardiac bypass with a bubble oxygenator. This fall in red cell 2,3-DPG could be prevented by the administration of solutions of inosine, pyruvate, and phosphate during the course of surgery. No attempt was made to evaluate the protective effect of this procedure against ischemic myocardial damage in patients who were being operated on for aortic valve replacement or myocardial revascularization.

The infusion of red cells with 150% of normal 2,3-DPG content was found to increase postoperative myocardial function in patients undergoing coronary bypass surgery (Dennis *et al.*, 1975). These patients received 2,3-DPG-enriched, previously frozen, washed red cells and were contrasted with patients receiving CPD-stored or fresh blood containing approximately 70% of the normal 2,3-DPG content. When patients were removed from cardiopulmonary bypass and given a volume load, the group that had received the high 2,3-DPG blood had a significant increase in cardiac index at similar filling pressures. At this time, body oxygen consumption, *in vivo* $P_{50}$, and arteriovenous oxygen content difference were all increased while the $P_{V_{O_2}}$ remained normal. In these patients improved oxygen delivery occurred without decreasing the mixed venous oxygen tension. The authors concluded that, with volume loading, the function of the heart with coronary artery disease is limited, in part, by available oxygen. In this study the shift in the oxygen–hemoglobin dissociation curve produced all the expected physiologic phenomena. In the setting where flow was limiting, because of disease, the improved oxygen delivery appeared to have produced a demonstrable beneficial effect.

### 3.3.2. Hypoxemia of Altitude or Pulmonary Disease

It has been known for some time that when residents of low altitudes are exposed to higher altitudes, they experience shortness of breath and decreased exercise tolerance. In 1936 Keys and co-workers first demonstrated a shift of the oxyhemoglobin dissociation curve to the right in long-time residents of high-altitude areas. This shift represents only a small part of the compensation that prevents tissue hypoxia at very high altitudes. Torrance and associates (1970b) found that people living up to 10,000 ft above sea level had increasing red cell 2,3-DPG and $P_{50}$ which corresponded with increases in altitude. The calculations of these investigators, however, indicate that the 2 mm Hg increase in $P_{50}$ found in residents of 12,000 ft accounted for only a slight portion of the total compensation for decreased oxygen saturation. Hyperventilation and erythrocytosis accounted for the remainder of the compensation seen. When subjects who lived at 14,000 ft were studied, the effect of the shifted oxygen–hemoglobin dissociation curve was even less significant. The pH of the arterial blood was normal in all these subjects.

Lenfant and co-workers (1969) found an increase of 4.2 mm Hg in the $P_{50}$ of residents at high altitudes when compared to controls. Dempsey and collaborators (1975) found no change in 2,3-DPG and no increase in $P_{50}$ that could not be accounted for by decreased pH and increased temperature in subjects after prolonged work at high altitudes. These subjects were not permanent residents of the high altitude but had experienced the high-altitude conditions for 2–3 weeks before being tested.

Acute exposure to high-altitude conditions has also been associated with an increase in red cell 2,3-DPG and $P_{50}$, but the rise does not seem to be mediated by a decreased oxygen saturation. Prevention of the respiratory alkalosis that accompanies this acute change has been found to eliminate the 2,3-DPG and $P_{50}$ rises (Lenfant et al., 1971), and, if the subjects are kept at rest, there is no significant increase in 2,3-DPG or $P_{50}$ even though respiratory alkalosis develops (Rørth et al., 1973).

Subjects exposed to a low-pressure chamber environment for 24 h and allowed to pursue a normal amount of exercise exhibited a significant rise in hemoglobin, hematocrit, and white blood cell count. There was a 30% rise in 2,3-DPG and a decrease in $P_{CO_2}$ (Rørth et al., 1973). The respiratory alkalosis resulting from a decrease in $P_{CO_2}$ tends to cause a shift in the $P_{50}$ opposing that of the increased red cell 2,3-DPG. The hemoglobin–oxygen affinity is thus changed very little by these counteracting forces.

The relationship of various stimuli to increased levels of 2,3-DPG upon exposure to altitude is thus unclear. It is felt that in the steady state conditions of chronic high-altitude exposure, increased 2,3-DPG is the result of decreased arterial oxygen saturation and is not due to alkalosis. The rise in 2,3-DPG that is seen in acute exposure to high-altitude conditions is attributed to respiratory alkalosis in some studies and in other cases is unexplained.

Increased levels of red cell 2,3-DPG have also been found in patients with chronic obstructive pulmonary disease (COPD). Orzalesi and Motoyama (1973) found significantly higher 2,3-DPG and right-shifted oxygen–hemoglobin dissociation curves in hypoxic patients with cystic fibrosis. Block and co-workers (1974) found that the increased 2,3-DPG they detected in COPD patients returned to normal levels when oxygen treatment was instituted. Their testing showed a significant correlation between 2,3-DPG levels and arterial oxygen tension and arterial oxygen saturation. However, there was no correlation between 2,3-DPG and pH. These investigators suggested that in the steady state 2,3-DPG is regulated by arterial oxygen saturation, whereas acute changes are mediated by hydrogen ion concentration. These findings and conclusions were shared by Keitt and associates (1974). As previously discussed, they found increased 2,3-DPG concentrations in the red cells of COPD patients on oxygen therapy. The 2,3-DPG levels were not significantly related to arterial pH, but did correlate significantly with arterial oxygen saturation. Abrupt withdrawal of oxygen in these patients produced changes in pH and related changes in red cell 2,3-DPG.

All investigators do not agree with these findings. Lenfant et al. (1969) found that not all their patients with COPD exhibited an increased $P_{50}$. They found that patients whose hematocrit was increased did have a right-shifted oxygen–hemoglobin dissociation curve, whereas those with lower hematocrit values had curves which were shifted to the left. They postulated that this leftward shift allowed for more efficient oxygenation of blood in the lungs.

In five patients with COPD and severe arterial hypoxemia and respiratory acidosis, Edwards and Cannon (1972) found no increase in 2,3-DPG or $P_{50}$. Weiss and Desforges (1972) studied patients with asthma and found that in the steady state their patients showed no shift in their ODC. The pH was elevated (7.44), and hypoxia was noted. During acute asthmatic attack these investigators noted no change in these parameters except that pH fell to a mean of 7.39. The $P_{50}$ in the asthmatic patients who were judged to be hypoventilating was significantly lower than that in the other asthmatic patients, and the red cell 2,3-DPG in these patients was reduced.

Attempts to compensate for hypoxia appear to involve complex and interlocking phenomena which operate differently in individual patients and in particular phases of disease states. 2,3-DPG is but one variable, and its increase or decrease depends on the net effect of the many other variables, including arterial and venous oxygen saturation, tissue oxygen levels, hemoglobin, pH, cardiac output, and probably others. Complete understanding of the interaction of these mechanisms will require technologic advances that allow rapid and accurate *in vivo* measurement of all parameters involved.

### 3.3.3. Anemia

Early studies measuring levels of red cell 2,3-DPG in anemic subjects described an inverse correlation between 2,3-DPG and hemoglobin (Eaton and Brewer, 1968; Hjelm, 1969). Torrance et al. (1970a) were able to show a predictable relationship between the degree of anemia and the red cell 2,3-DPG. They found that a decrease of 1 g of hemoglobin was accompanied by an increase in red cell 2,3-DPG of 0.23 mmol/ml RBC and an increase in $P_{50}$ of 0.30 mm Hg. These investigators proposed a correlation between levels of mixed venous $O_2$ saturation and red cell 2,3-DPG that was later confirmed by Thomas et al. (1974).

Slawsky and Desforges (1972) were unable to find a direct correlation between hemoglobin levels and red cell 2,3-DPG, though they too demonstrated increased 2,3-DPG in iron-deficient subjects. It seems likely that the etiology of the anemia may have some effect on the response of erythrocyte 2,3-DPG. Opalinski and Beutler (1971) found that 2,3-DPG was higher in younger red cells and demonstrated smaller rises in 2,3-DPG in the anemia resulting from an aplastic phenomenon than from other causes.

Fernandez and Erslev (1972) attempted to explain the stimulus for increased erythropoiesis that occurs as a compensation for the hemolysis of hereditary spherocytosis (HS). They found that the $P_{50}$ of presplenectomy patients with HS was the same as that of a control group. The level of 2,3-DPG in the red cells of the presplenectomy HS patients was one-half that of the normal group and of the postsplenectomy patients with HS. They felt that change in oxygen affinity of HS patients was not the basis on which to explain the compensation for hemolysis that occurs. They postulated that the increased MCHC which occurs in HS is responsible for the normal position of the oxygen–hemoglobin dissociation curve despite lowered levels of red cell 2,3-DPG. The decrease in 2,3-DPG in HS patients is probably due to the drop in intracellular pH that occurs during splenic erythrostasis (Palek *et al.*, 1969).

Valeri and Fortier (1969) have shown that there is a significant relationship between red cell mass deficit and 2,3-DPG response.

Subjects phlebotomized over a period of 1 to 3 weeks' time (250–750 ml of blood removed) had an increase in $P_{50}$ which showed significant correlation to the number of young cells produced (Edwards and Cannon, 1972). Increased erythropoiesis and a right shift in the oxygen–hemoglobin dissociation curve seemed more than adequate compensation for the loss of blood that occurred, since the cardiac output actually decreased during the time under study. This finding may be the basis for the "blood doping" that was alleged to have occurred during the 1976 summer Olympics. This practice involves bleeding an athlete 2 to 3 weeks prior to competition and then returning the blood shortly before the competition. This would produce both a right-shifted curve and an increased red cell mass.

### 3.3.4. Abnormalities of Serum Inorganic Phosphate

Serum levels of inorganic phosphate serve to influence the red cell concentration of 2,3-diphosphoglycerate. Hyperphosphatemia is generally accompanied by an increase in red cell 2,3-DPG whereas hypophosphatemia results in a decrease in 2,3-DPG. Relationships between plasma levels of inorganic phosphate and red cell 2,3-DPG have been described in uremia (Lichtman *et al.*, 1969; Lichtman and Miller, 1970; Ninness *et al.*, 1974), in diabetic ketoacidosis (Ditzel and Standl, 1975), and in prolonged intravenous alimentation (Travis *et al.*, 1971). Card and Brain (1973) have proposed that the normal changes of 2,3-DPG that occur with age are a result of the gradual decline in the serum inorganic phosphate level.

In uremic patients the presence of acidosis, hyperphosphatemia, and the increased red cell 2,3-DPG levels serve to shift the oxygen–hemoglobin equilibrium curve to the right and thus partially or totally compensate for the anemia that invariably accompanies chronic renal failure. The role of dialysis on influencing oxygen transport and delivery in this condition is far from clear (Szwed *et al.*, 1974; Hirszel *et al.*, 1975). With the presence of multiple variables that influence hemoglobin's affinity for oxygen in such situations it is not surprising that conclusions of clinical relevance are difficult to obtain.

In patients in diabetic ketoacidosis the initial decrease in pH serves to compensate for the lowered red cell 2,3-DPG levels and $P_{50}$ values are often normal (Ditzel and Standl, 1975). With correction of the acid–base disturbance the red cell 2,3-DPG remains reduced as a result of the accompanying hypophosphatemia, and $P_{50}$ values may be reduced by as much as 5 mm Hg. It has been proposed that oxygen unloading may be reduced by as much as one-third of normal under such circumstances. Rehydration fluids in such patients should always include inorganic phosphorus. Hypophosphatemia of a profound degree, serum phosphorus levels of less than 1.0 mg/dl, may also produce a lowering of red cell adenosine triphosphate levels in addition to the decline in 2,3-diphosphoglycerate. In such situations a hemolytic anemia has been observed (Klock *et al.*, 1974; Jacobs and Amsden, 1971).

The relationship of red cell 2,3-DPG to $P_{50}$ in diabetes may be altered by virture of the presence of variable quantities of hemoglobin $A_{1C}$ (Trivelli *et al.*, 1971; Koenig *et al.*, 1976). This altered hemoglobin, which is produced as a result of persistent hyperglycemia, has an increased affinity for oxygen and does not bind 2,3-DPG.

### 3.3.5. Liver Disease

Cirrhosis of the liver is associated with both an increased level of red cell 2,3-DPG and an increased $P_{50}$ (Mulhausen *et al.*, 1967; Astrup and Rörth, 1973; Thomas *et al.*, 1974). Patients with cirrhosis frequently have anemia and acid–base disturbances, and occasionally demonstrate modest degrees of arterial hypoxemia. Thomas *et al.* (1970) examined the relationship of anemia and pH to 2,3-DPG and $P_{50}$ in a group of 41 patients with alcohol-induced liver disease. The mean $P_{50}$ was increased by 2.8 mm Hg. The mean oxygen-carrying capacity was reduced by 5.8 vol %. This would be equivalent to a reduction in hemoglobin of approximately 4 g/dl, a degree of anemia that usually produces a rise in red cell 2,3-DPG concentration. In this group of patients, however, the degree of anemia did not correlate with the $P_{50}$, suggesting that other factors were operative. In another study by these same workers (Thomas *et al.*, 1974), the changes in 2,3-DPG and $P_{50}$ appeared most closely related to the arterial pH. The authors concluded that both anemia and blood pH were factors in regulating the $P_{50}$ in patients with liver disease but, like Astrup and Rörth (1973), they proposed that in liver disease and certain other disorders, currently unrecognized factors were also responsible for producing alterations in the affinity of hemoglobin for oxygen.

One possible solution to this problem has been proposed by Zimmon (1973) who measured increased amounts of unbound red cell 2,3-DPG in patients with hepatic coma. He proposed that a false neurotransmitter, such as octopamine, could act to displace 2,3-DPG from the red cell membrane, thus increasing the intracellular pool interacting with hemoglobin. The net effect of such a displacement would be to increase the $P_{50}$ without increasing the total 2,3-DPG. Further evidence for such a regulatory mechanism awaits confirmation.

As yet no studies have been reported that demonstrate that this observed shift to the right of the oxygen–hemoglobin dissociation curve in patients with liver disease actually provides compensation for the anemia or is required to maintain adequate oxygen consumption.

### 3.3.6. Endocrine Disorders

Increases in both red cell 2,3-DPG and $P_{50}$ have been observed in patients with hyperthyroidism (L. R. Miller *et al.*, 1970; W. W. Miller *et al.*, 1970; Monti, 1974). Triiodothyronine has been reported to raise red cell 2,3-DPG *in vitro* (Snyder and Reddy, 1970) although other investigators have not confirmed this observation (Gerlach and Duhm, 1972). Hypothyroidism produces a shift to the left in the position of the oxyhemoglobin dissociation curve (Schussler and Ranney, 1971). In panhypopituitarism 2,3-DPG levels are normal or low; treatment with thyroid produces an increase in red cell 2,3-DPG until the red cell mass deficit is corrected (Rodriguez and Shahidi, 1971).

Androgen therapy appears to produce an increase in red cell 2,3-DPG levels (Parker *et al.*, 1972; Gorshein *et al.*, 1974).

### 3.3.7. Blood Storage and Transfusion

Valtis and Kennedy (1954) were the first to observe that the $P_{50}$ of blood stored in the anticoagulant, acid citrate dextrose (ACD), decreased markedly over the first week of storage, and that transfusion of such blood could lower the $P_{50}$ of the recipient. This fall in $P_{50}$ was subsequently demonstrated to be the result of the decline in red cell 2,3-DPG (Bunn *et al.*, 1969).

Massive transfusions of stored blood with a reduced 2,3-DPG content can reduce the level of 2,3-DPG in the recipient to one-third of normal and lower the $P_{50}$ to approximately 19 mm Hg (McConn and Derrick, 1972). Transfused cells regain normal levels of 2,3-DPG over several days in healthy recipients (Valeri and Hirsch, 1969; Beutler and Wood, 1969).

The decline in red cell 2,3-DPG is slower in blood stored in the anticoagulant, citrate phosphate dextrose, and can be prevented by prompt freezing of blood after collection (Valeri, 1973). The decline in red cell 2,3-diphosphoglycerate can be retarded by a variety of chemical modifications of the storage conditions, and red cell 2,3-diphosphoglycerate can be restored to normal, and even supranormal levels, by the addition of phosphate, pyruvate, and inosine (Valeri, 1973).

The clinical consequences of producing an acute increase in the affinity of hemoglobin by massive transfusions of 2,3-DPG-poor blood remain a subject of speculation. In combat injured, otherwise previously healthy subjects, the transfusions of 2,3-DPG-poor blood produced no alterations in oxygen consumption (Bowen and Fleming, 1974). In this circumstance it appeared that circulatory compensations were adequate to correct for the increase in hemoglobin's affinity for oxygen.

It is probable that only in clinical situations in which flow is limited, as a result of cardiac disease or vascular disease, can abrupt decreases in $P_{50}$ be shown to have undesirable effects. The previously cited studies of Dennis and associates (1975) in patients undergoing coronary artery surgery are a specific instance of this clinical setting.

Employing isolated canine hindlimbs, Harken and Woods (1976) were able to demonstrate clearly physiological alterations produced by shifts in the curve mediated by 2,3-DPG. In this experimental situation blood flow, temperature, arterial oxygen and carbon dioxide content, and pH were kept constant while the limbs were perfused alternatively with blood high or low in 2,3-DPG. When blood with a $P_{50}$ that was only 70% of normal was perfused the oxygen uptake of the limb dropped to 65% of the control value.

### 3.3.8. The Newborn Infant

Anselmino and Hoffman (1930) first observed that the oxygen affinity of human fetal blood was greater than that of maternal blood. Fetal blood had a $P_{50}$ value some 6–8 mm Hg lower than that of the normal adult. Allen *et al.* (1953) demonstrated that although intact fetal cells possess a higher affinity for oxygen than do the red cells of adults, when adult and fetal hemoglobin solutions were dialyzed against the same buffer, the resulting oxygen affinities were identical.

This puzzling observation was resolved by the finding that the affinity of fetal hemoglobin for 2,3-DPG is far less than that of adult hemoglobin (Bauer *et al.*, 1968). When 2,3-DPG is added to solutions of fetal hemoglobin the decrease in oxygen affinity produced by this compound is much less than that observed with adult hemoglobin. The fetal hemoglobin obtained from the red cells of patients with β-thalassemia behaves in a manner identical to that of fetal hemoglobin obtained from the erythrocytes of the newborn infant (Maurer *et al.*, 1970).

From these studies it appears that the major reason the blood of the newborn infant possesses an oxygen–hemoglobin equilibrium curve that is shifted to the left of that of the normal adult is due to the failure of fetal hemoglobin to bind 2,3-DPG to the same degree as does adult hemoglobin.

The position of the oxygen–hemoglobin equilibrium curve in the neonate is determined by the relative proportions of adult and fetal hemoglobin present and the red cell 2,3-DPG concentration. Infants with similar fetal hemoglobin concentrations can have different $P_{50}$ values if they differ significantly in their red cell 2,3-DPG concentrations; alternatively, infants with similar 2,3-DPG concentrations may have dissimilar $P_{50}$ values if they differ in their percent fetal hemoglobin. The need to consider both the proportion of adult and fetal hemoglobin, as well as the 2,3-DPG content of the cells explains why previous investigators failed to find a direct relationship between fetal hemoglobin values alone and the position of the curve. Employing all three variables Orzalesi and Hay (1971) developed the term "the effective DPG fraction." "The effective DPG fraction" bears a precise relationship to the $P_{50}$ value and is similar to the "functioning DPG fraction" of Delivoria-Papadopoulos et al. (1971b).

In the term infant the oxygen–hemoglobin equilibrium curve gradually shifts to the right and the $P_{50}$ value approximates that of the normal adult by approximately 4 to 6 months of age. A significant increase in $P_{50}$ can be observed during the first week of life (Delivoria-Papadopoulos et al., 1971b). This increase is a result of the rise in the red cell 2,3-DPG level. It is tempting to speculate that it is caused by the transient rise in the serum inorganic phosphate level which so commonly occurs during this period.

In the premature infant, born with lower 2,3-DPG levels and higher fetal hemoglobin values, the shift in the position of the curve is far more gradual. In all infants the position of the curve appears to be directly correlated with the "effective" (Orzalesi and Hay, 1971) or "functioning" DPG fraction (Delivoria-Papadopoulos et al., 1971b).

Red cell 2,3-DPG levels are profoundly decreased in infants with severe respiratory distress. This decrease, with its associated lowering of the $P_{50}$ value, is most marked in infants with profound acidosis.

When adult erythrocytes are transfused into the fetus or newborn infant they retain their characteristic oxygen–hemoglobin equilibrium curve. Novy and associates (1971) and Mathers et al. (1970) have shown that following intrauterine transfusions the adult cells retain their normal properties for periods of as long as 8 weeks. In these instances in which the fetal oxygen–hemoglobin equilibrium approximates that of the maternal blood, no deleterious effects have been observed (Novy et al., 1971). This observation has resulted in a reexamination of the belief that a difference in hemoglobin–oxygen affinity between mother and infant is required for adequate oxygen delivery to the fetus *in utero*. These findings, in association with observations in situations in which mothers with hemoglobin variants with very high affinities for oxygen have given birth to apparently normal infants (Parer, 1970), suggest that a higher level than maternal blood affinity for oxygen is not an absolute necessity for intrauterine existence. Before this concept is totally accepted it should be recognized that the intrauterine transfusion of lambs appears to produce subtle evidence of hypoxic stress (Battaglia *et al.*, 1969).

MacLennan and co-workers (1976) observed that red cell 2,3-DPG levels were significantly lower in mothers whose fetus was stillborn or growth retarded.

Exchange transfusion following birth produces rapid alterations in the infant's oxygen–hemoglobin equilibrium curve (Delivoria-Papadopoulos *et al.*, 1971a). The early changes are produced as a function of the storage characteristics of the blood employed.

Because exchange transfusions in newborn infants can promptly produce an acute shift to the right in the position of the oxygen–hemoglobin dissociation curve when relatively fresh blood anticoagulated with citrate phosphate dextrose is employed, this procedure has been examined as an adjunct to conventional therapy in children with severe respiratory distress and tissue hypoxemia (Delivoria-Papadopoulos *et al.*, 1976; Gottuso *et al.*, 1976). In both studies infants with severe respiratory distress who received exchange transfusions early in the course of their illness were found to have significantly lower mortality.

Exchange transfusion was demonstrated to produce the expected increase in $P_{50}$. This was accompanied by a rise in central venous oxygen tension (Delivoria-Papadopoulos *et al.*, 1976). In the study of Gottuso and associates (1976), a study of both alterations in coagulation factors and red cell concentrations of fetal hemoglobin and 2,3-DPG failed to demonstrate any significant relationship between these variables and the improved survival of infants receiving exchange transfusions. Following exchange transfusion there was a significant decrease in the concentrations of inspired oxygen required to maintain arterial oxygen tension, suggesting that pulmonary perfusion and/or ventilation was improved by the procedure.

When premature infants who have received either exchange transfusions or multiple small transfusions with adult blood are studied hematologically during the first 12 weeks of life, it has been observed that their hemoglobin values fall lower than do the hemoglobin values of infants who are permitted to maintain normally high concentrations of fetal hemoglobin (Stockman *et al.*, 1976). This right shift in the position of the oxygen–hemoglobin equilibrium curve produced by the replacement of adult for fetal hemoglobin appears to facilitate oxygen unloading as reflected by the fact that such infants, with less than 30% fetal hemoglobin, can tolerate hemoglobin levels 3–4 g/dl less than infants with fetal hemoglobin concentrations of greater than 60% before they begin to elaborate increased amounts of erythropoietin (Stockman *et al.*, 1976).

## 3.4. Physiologic Significance of Shifts in the Oxygen–Hemoglobin Dissociation Curve

The studies of hemoglobin mutants with increased and decreased affinities for oxygen, discussed elsewhere in this volume, and the studies performed in premature infants indicate that the position of the oxygen–hemoglobin equilibrium curve does influence tissue oxygenation and the regulation of erythropoiesis.

It is of interest to note that $P_{50}$, as regulated by the red cell concentration of 2,3-DPG, produces a constancy in oxygen delivery, despite changes in hemoglobin concentration that normally accompany maturation. In Table III we have placed the values which represent the mean $P_{50}$, and the mean hemoglobin concentration from birth to adolescence. An arbitrarily selected central venous oxygen tension of 40 mm Hg was selected for purposes of calculating the amount of oxygen unloaded from 100 ml of blood if the cardiac output per meter squared remained constant. The table illustrates that from the time of 8 months of age and on into adult life the amount of oxygen unloaded remains virtually constant despite the progressive rise in hemoglobin. This constancy is a consequence of the

**Table III.** Oxygen Unloading Changes with Age

| Age | $P_{50}$ (mm Hg) | % saturation of venous oxygen (tension of 40 mm Hg) | Hemoglobin (g %) | Oxygen unloaded[b] (ml/100 ml) |
|---|---|---|---|---|
| 1 day | 19.4 | 87 | 17.2 | 1.84 |
| 3 weeks | 22.7 | 80 | 13.0 | 2.61 |
| 6–9 weeks | 24.4 | 77 | 11.0 | 2.65 |
| 3–4 months | 26.5 | 73 | 10.5 | 3.10 |
| 6 months | 27.8 | 69 | 11.3 | 3.94 |
| 8–11 months | 30.0 | 65 | 11.8 | 4.74 |
| 5–8 years | 29.0[a] | 67 | 12.6 | 4.73 |
| 9–12 years | 27.9[a] | 69 | 13.4 | 4.67 |
| Adult | 27.0 | 71 | 15.0 | 4.92 |

[a]Derived from data of Card and Brain (1973); remainder of $P_{50}$'s as previously reported (Delivoria-Papadopoulos *et al.*, 1971b).
[b]Assumes arterial oxygen saturation of 95%.

progressive rise in oxygen's affinity for hemoglobin that accompanies the increase in hemoglobin concentration. What still remains unexplained are the factors responsible for the stimulus to reach the oxygen unloading value of 4.75–5.00 ml of oxygen which must operate during the first 8 months of life.

Although the regulation of erythropoiesis appears related to the $P_{50}$ it still remains unclear how important shifts in the $P_{50}$ may be in the adaptation to pathologic processes. Because of the many compensatory mechanisms that exist, critical clinical experiments are difficult to design. Studies of organs with the greatest oxygen extraction and the least reserve for augmenting flow, such as the myocardium, will be required before the clinical relevance of red cell alterations in 2,3-DPG can be placed in proper perspective.

# References

Allen, D. W., Wyman, T., and Smith, C. A., 1953, The oxygen equilibrium of fetal and adult human hemoglobin, *J. Biol. Chem.* **203**:84.

Anselmino, K. T., and Hoffman, F., 1930, Die Ursachen des Icterus neonatorum, *Arch. Gynaekol.* **143**:477.

Arnone, A., 1972, X-ray diffraction study of binding of 2,3-diphosphoglycerate to human deoxyhemoglobin, *Nature (London)* **235**:146.

Astrup, J., and Rörth, M., 1973, Oxygen affinity of hemoglobin and red cell 2,3-diphosphoglycerate in hepatic cirrhosis, *Scand. J. Clin. Lab. Invest.* **31**:311.

Battaglia, F. C., Bowes, W., McGaughey, H. R., Makouski, E. L., and Meschia, G., 1969, The effect of fetal exchange transfusion with adult blood upon fetal oxygenation, *Pediatr. Res.* **3**:60.

Bauer, C., Ludwig, I., and Ludwig, M., 1968. Different effects of 2,3-diphosphoglycerate and adenosine triphosphate on the oxygen affinity of adult and foetal human hemoglobin, *Life Sci.* **7**:1339.

Bendixen, H. H., and Laver, M. B., 1965, Hypoxia in anesthesia: A review, *Clin. Pharmacol. Ther.* **6**:510.

Benesch, R., and Benesch, R. E., 1967, The effect of organic phosphates from the human erythrocyte on the allosteric properties of hemoglobin, *Biochem. Biophys. Res. Commun.* **26**:162.

Benesch, R. E., Benesch, R., and Yu, C. I., 1967, The oxygenation of hemoglobin in the presence of 2,3-diphosphoglycerate. Effect of temperature, pH, ionic strength and hemoglobin concentration, *Biochemistry* **8**:2567.

Berne, R. M., Blackman, J. R., and Gardner, T. H., 1957, Hypoxemia and coronary blood flow, *J. Clin. Invest.* **36**:1101.

Beutler, E., and Wood, L., 1969, The *in vivo* regeneration of red cell 2,3-diphosphoglyceric acid (DPG) after transfusion of stored blood, *J. Lab. Clin. Med.* **74**:300.

Block, A. J., Castle, J. R., and Keitt, A. S., 1974, Chronic oxygen therapy:

Treatment of chronic obstructive pulmonary disease at sea level, *Chest* **65**:279.

Bordiuk, J. M., McKenna, P. J., Gianelli, S., Jr., and Ayers, S. M., 1971, Alterations on 2,3-diphosphoglycerate and $O_2$ hemoglobin affinity in patients undergoing open-heart surgery, *Circulation* **43**:141.

Bowen, J. C., and Fleming, W. H., 1974, Increased oxyhemoglobin affinity after transfusion of stored blood, *Ann. Surg.* **180**:760.

Bunn, H. F., 1974, The structure and function of normal and abnormal human hemoglobins, *in Hematology of Infancy and Childhood* (D. G. Nathan and F. A. Oski, eds.), Saunders, Philadelphia.

Bunn, H. F., and Briehl, R. W., 1970, The interaction of 2,3-diphosphoglycerate with various human hemoglobins, *J. Clin. Invest.* **49**:1088.

Bunn, H. F., May, M. H., Kochalaty, W. F., and Shields, C. E., 1969, Hemoglobin function in stored blood, *J. Clin. Invest.* **48**:311.

Card, R. T., and Brain, M. C., 1973, The "anemia" of childhood: Physiologic response to hyperphosphatemia, *N. Engl. J. Med.* **288**:388.

Chanutin, A., and Curnish, R. R., 1967, Effect of inorganic and organic phosphates with hemoglobin, *Arch. Biochem.* **131**:180.

Delivoria-Papadopoulos, M., Morrow, G., III, and Oski, F. A., 1971a, Exchange transfusion in the newborn infant with "fresh" and "old" blood. The role of storage on 2,3-diphosphoglycerate hemoglobin-oxygen affinity, and oxygen release, *J. Pediatr.* **79**:898.

Delivoria-Papadopoulos, M., Roncevic, N. P., and Oski, F. A., 1971b, Postnatal changes in oxygen transport of term, premature and sick infants. The role of adult hemoglobin and red cell 2,3-diphosphoglycerate, *Pediatr. Res.* **5**:235.

Delivoria-Papadopoulos, M., Miller, L. D., Forster, R., and Oski, F. A., 1976, The role of exchange transfusion in the management of low-birth-weight infants with and without severe respiratory distress syndrome. I. Initial observations, *J. Pediatr.* **89**:273.

Dempsey, J. A., Thomson, J. M., and Forster, H. V., 1975, $HbO_2$ dissociation in man during prolonged work in chronic hypoxia, *J. Appl. Physiol.* **38**:1022.

Dennis, R. C., Vito, L., Weisel, R. D., Valeri, C. R., Berger, R. L., and Hechtman, H. B., 1975, Improved myocardial performance following high 2,3-diphosphoglycerate red cell transfusions, *Surgery* **77**:741.

Ditzel, J., and Standl, E., 1975, The oxygen transport system of red blood cells during diabetic ketoacidosis and recovery, *Diabetologia* **11**:255.

Eaton, J. W., and Brewer, G. J., 1968, The relationship between red cell 2,3-diphosphoglycerate and levels of hemoglobin in the human, *Proc. Nat. Acad. Sci. U.S.A.* **61**:756.

Edwards, M. J., and Cannon, B., 1972, Normal levels of 2,3-diphosphoglycerate in red cells despite severe hypoxemia of chronic lung disease, *Chest* **61**:258.

Fernandez, L. A., and Erslev, A. J., 1972, Oxygen affinity and compensated hemolysis in hereditary spherocytosis, *J. Lab. Clin. Med.* **80**:780.

Gerlach, E., and Duhm, J., 1972, 2,3-DPG metabolism of red cells: Regulation and adaptive changes during hypoxia, *in Oxygen Affinity of Hemoglobin and Red Cell Acid–Base Status* (M. Rørth and P. Astrup, eds.), p. 552, Munksgaard, Copenhagen.

Giannelli, S., Jr., McKenna, J. P., Bordiuk, J. M., Miller, L. D., and Jerome, C. R., 1976, Prevention of increased hemoglobin-oxygen affinity in open-heart operations with inosine-phosphate-pyruvate solution, *Ann. Thor. Surg.* **21**:386.

Gorshein, D., Oski, F. A., and Delivoria-Papadopoulos, M., 1974, Effect of androgens on the red cell 2,3-diphosphoglycerate, hemoglobin oxygen affinity and red cell mass in mammals, *Proc. Soc. Exp. Biol. Med.* **147**:616.

Gottuso, M. A., Williams, M. L., and Oski, F. A., 1976, The role of exchange transfusions in the management of low-birth-weight infants with and without severe respiratory distress syndrome, *J. Pediatr.* **89**:279.

Greenwold, I., 1925, A new type of phosphoric acid compound isolated from blood, with some remarks on the effect of substitution on the rotation of *l*-glyceric acid, *J. Biol. Chem.* **63**:339.

Guy, C. R., Salhany, J. M., and Eliot, R. S., 1971, Disorders of hemoglobin-oxygen release in ischemic heart disease, *Am. Heart J.* **82**:824.

Harken, A. H., and Woods, M., 1976, The influence of oxyhemoglobin affinity on tissue oxygen consumption, *Ann. Surg.* **183**:130.

Hirszel, P., Maher, J. F., Tempel, G. E., and Mengel, C. E., 1975, Influence of peritoneal dialysis on factors affecting oxygen transport, *Nephron* **15**:438.

Hjelm, M., 1969, The content of 2,3-diphosphoglycerate and some other phospho compounds in human erythrocytes from healthy adults and subjects with different kinds of anemia, *Forsvorsmedicin* **5**:219.

Jacobs, H. S., and Amsden, T., 1971, Acute hemolytic anemia with rigid red cells in hypophosphatemia, *N. Engl. J. Med.* **285**:1446.

Keitt, A. S., Hinkes, C., and Block, A. J., 1974, Comparison of factors regulating red cell 2,3-diphosphoglycerate in acute and chronic hypoxemia, *J. Lab. Clin. Med.* **84**:275.

Kety, S. S., 1957, Determinants of tissue oxygen tension, *Fed. Proc.* **16**:666.

Keys, A., Hall, F. G., and Barron, E. S., 1936, The position of the oxygen dissociation curve of human blood at high altitude, *Am. J. Physiol.* **115**:292.

Klock, J. C., Williams, H. E., and Mentzer, W. C., 1974, Hemolytic anemia and somatic cell dysfunction in severe hypophosphatemia, *Arch. Intern. Med.* **134**:360.

Koenig, R. J., Peterson, C. M., Jones, R. L., Saudek, C., Lehrman, M., and Cerami, A., 1976, Correlation of glucose regulation and hemoglobin $A_{Ic}$ in diabetes mellitus, *N. Engl. J. Med.* **295**:417.

Kostuk, W. J., Suwa, K., Bernstein, E. F., and Sobel, B. E., 1973, Altered hemoglobin oxygen affinity in patients with acute myocardial infarction, *Am. J. Cardiol.* **31**:295.

Landis, E. M., and Pappenheimer, J. R., 1973, Exchange of substances through the capillary walls, *in Handbook of Physiology, Circulation*, 2nd ed., Chap. 29, The American Physiological Society, Washington, D.C.

Lenfant, C. J. M., Ways, D., Aucutt, C., and Cruz, J., 1969, Effect of chronic hypoxia on the $O_2$–Hb dissociation curve and respiratory gas transport in man, *Respir. Physiol.* **7**:7.

Lenfant, C. J. M., Torrance, J. D., and Reynafarje, C., 1971, Shift of the $O_2$–Hb dissociation curve at altitude: Mechanism and effect, *J. Appl. Physiol.* **30**:625.

Lichtman, M. A., and Miller, D. R., 1970, Erythrocyte glycolysis, 2,3-dipho-sphoglycerate and adenosine triphosphate concentration in uremic subjects. Relationship to extracellular phosphate concentration, *J. Lab. Clin. Med.* **76**:267.

Lichtman, M. A., Miller, D. R., and Freeman, R. B., 1969, Erythrocyte adenosine triphosphate depletion during hypophosphatemia in a uremic subject, *N. Engl. J. Med.* **280**:240.

Lichtman, M. A., Murphy, M. S., and Adamson, J. W., 1976, Detection of mutant hemoglobins with altered affinity for oxygen, *Ann. Intern. Med.* **84**:517.

MacLennan, A. H., Hunter, D. J. S., and Darley, J. H., 1976, Tissue oxygenation and red cell 2,3-diphosphoglycerate in normal and abnormal pregnancy, *Br. J. Obstet. Gynaecol.* **83**:378.

Mathers, N. P., James, G. B., and Walker, J., 1970, The oxygen affinity of the blood of infants treated by intrauterine transfusions, *J. Obstet. Gynaecol. Br. Commonw.* **77**:648.

Maurer, H. S., Behrman, R. E., and Honig, F. R., 1970, Dependence of the oxygen affinity of blood on the presence of foetal or adult hemoglobin, *Nature (London)* **227**:388.

McConn, R., and Derrick, J. B., 1972, The respiratory function of blood; transfusion and blood storage, *Anesthesiology* **36**:119.

Miller, L. R., Sugarman, H. J., Miller, W. W., Delivoria-Papadopoulos, M., and Oski, F. A., 1970, Increased peripheral oxygen delivery in thyrotoxicosis, *Ann. Surg.* **172**:1051.

Miller, W. W., 1972, Erythrocyte oxygen transport in normal infants and in infants with cardiovascular disease, *in Neonatal Heart Disease* (W. F. Friedman, M. Lesch, and E. H. Sonnenbleck, eds.), p. 263, Grune & Stratton, New York.

Miller, W. W., Delivoria-Papadopoulos, M., Miller, L., and Oski, F. A., 1970, Oxygen releasing factor in hyperthyroidism, *JAMA* **211**:1824.

Monti, M., 1974, Red cell 2,3-diphosphoglycerate in patients with hyperthyroidism before and after treatment, *Acta Med. Scand.* **196**:263.

Mulhausen, R., Astrup, P., and Kjeldsen, K., 1967, Oxygen affinity of hemoglobin in patients with cardiovascular diseases, anemia, and cirrhosis of the liver, *Scand. J. Clin. Lab. Invest.* **19**:291.

Naeraa, N., Petersen, E. S., Boye, E., and Severinghaus, J. W., 1966, pH and molecular $CO_2$ components of the Bohr effect in human blood, *Scand. J. Clin. Lab. Invest.* **18**:96.

Ninness, J. R., Kimber, R. W., and McDonald, J. W. D., 1974, Erythrocyte 2,3-DPG, ATP, and oxygen affinity in hemodialysis patients, *Can. Med. Assoc. J.* **111**:661.

Novy, M. J., Frigoletto, F. D., Easterday, C. L., Umansky, I., and Nelson, N. M., 1971, Changes in cord blood oxygen affinity after intrauterine transfusions for erythroblastosis, *N. Engl. J. Med.* **285**:857.

Opalinski, A., and Beutler, E., 1971, Creatinine, 2,3-diphosphoglycerate and anemia, *N. Engl. J. Med.* **285**:483.

Opitz, E., and Schneider, M., 1950, Über die Sauerstoffversorgung des Gehirns und den mechanismus von Mangelwirkungen, *Ergeb. Physiol.* **46**:126.

Orzalesi, M. M., and Hay, W. W., 1971, The regulation of oxygen affinity of fetal blood. I. *In vitro* experiments and results in normal infants, *Pediatrics* **48**:857.

Orzalesi, M. M., and Motoyama, E. K., 1973, Blood oxygen affinity in children with cystic fibrosis, *Am. Rev. Respir. Dis.* **107**:928.

Oski, F. A., Gottlieb, A. J., Miller, W. W., and Delivoria-Papadopoulos, M., 1970, The effects of deoxygenation of adult and fetal hemoglobin on the synthesis of red cell 2,3-diphosphoglycerate and its *in vivo* consequences, *J. Clin. Invest.* **49**:400.

Palek, J., Mircevova, L., and Brabec, V., 1969, 2,3-Diphosphoglycerate metabolism in hereditary spherocytosis, *Br. J. Haematol.* **17**:59.

Parer, J. T., 1970, Reversed relationship of oxygen affinity in maternal and fetal blood, *Am. J. Obstet. Gynecol.* **108**:323.

Parker, J. P., Beirne, G. J., Desai, J. N., Raich, P. C., and Shahidi, N. T., 1972, Androgen-induced increase in red cell 2,3-diphosphoglycerate, *N. Engl. J. Med.* **287**:381.

Proctor, H. J., Parker, J. C., and Johnson, G., Jr., 1971, Alterations in erythrocyte 2,3-diphosphoglycerate in postoperative patients, *Ann. Surg.* **173**:357.

Rodriguez, J. M., and Shahidi, N. T., 1971, Erythrocyte 2,3-diphosphoglycerate in adaptive red-cell-volume deficiency, *N. Engl. J. Med.* **285**:479.

Rørth, M., Nygaard, S. F., Parving, H. H., Hansen, V., and Kalsig, T., 1973, Human red cell metabolism and *in vivo* oxygen affinity of red cells during 24 hours exposure to simulated high altitude (4500 m), *Scand. J. Clin. Lab. Invest.* **31**:447.

Rose, Z. B., 1970, The enzymes of 2,3-diphosphoglycerate metabolism in the human red cell. Red cell metabolism and function, *Adv. Exp. Med. Biol.* **6**:137.

Rosenthal, A., Mentzer, W. C., Eisenstein, E. B., Nathan, D. G., Nelson, N. M., and Madas, A. S., 1971, The role of red blood cell organic phosphates in adaptation to congenital heart disease, *Pediatrics* **47**:537.

Schussler, G. C., and Ranney, H. M., 1971, Thyroid hormones and oxygen affinity of hemoglobin, *Ann. Intern. Med.* **74**:632.

Shappell, S. D., and Lenfant, C. J. M., 1972, Physiological role of the oxyhemoglobin dissociation curve, *in The Red Blood Cell*, 2nd ed. (D. M. Surgenor, ed.), p. 842, Academic Press, New York.

Shappell, S. D., Murray, J. A., Nasser, M. G., Wells, R. E., Torrance, J. D., and Lenfant, C. J. M., 1970, Acute changes in hemoglobin affinity for oxygen during angina pectoris, *N. Engl. J. Med.* **282**:1218.

Siggaard-Anderson, O., Salling, N., Nörgaard-Pedersen, B., and Rørth, M., 1972, Oxygen-linked hydrogen ion binding of human hemoglobin. Effects of carbon dioxide and 2,3-diphosphoglycerate. III. Comparison of the Bohr effect and the Holdane effect, *Scand. J. Clin. Lab. Invest.* **29**:185.

Slawsky, P., and Desforges, J., 1972, Erythrocyte 2,3-diphosphoglycerate in iron deficiency, *Arch. Intern. Med.* **129**:914.

Snyder, L. M., and Reddy, W. J., 1970, Mechanism of action of thyroid hormones on erythrocyte 2,3-diphosphoglyceric acid synthesis, *J. Clin. Invest.* **49**:1993.

Stockman, J. A., III, Garcia, J. F., and Oski, F. A., 1976, The anemia of prematurity. Factors governing the erythropoietin response, *Pediatr. Res.* **10**:382.

Szwed, J. J., Luft, F. C., and Boyken, J. R., 1974, Effect of hemodialysis on oxygen–hemoglobin affinity in chronic uremics, *Chest* **66**:278.

Thomas, H. M., III, Lefrak, S. S., and Fritts, H. W., Jr., 1970, Blood oxygen affinity and acid-base state in patients with alcoholic liver disease and in normals, *Fed. Proc.* **29**:329.

Thomas, H. M., Lefrak, S. S., Irwin, R. S., Fritts, H. W., Jr., and Caldwell, P. R. B., 1974, The oxyhemoglobin dissociation curve in health and disease, *Am. J. Med.* **57**:331.

Torrance, J., Jacobs, P., Restrepo, A., Eschbach, J., Lenfant, C., and Finch, C. A., 1970a, Intraerythrocytic adaption to anemia, *N. Engl. J. Med.* **283**:165.

Torrance, J. D., Lenfant, C. J. M., Cruz, J., and Marticorena, E., 1970b, Oxygen transport mechanisms in residents at high altitudes, *Respir. Physiol.* **11**:1.

Travis, S. F., Sugerman, H. J., Ruberg, R. L., Dudrick, S. J., Delivoria-Papadopoulos, M., Miller, L. D., and Oski, F. A., 1971, Alterations of red cell glycolytic intermediates and oxygen transport as a consequence of hypophosphatemia in patients receiving intravenous hyperalimentation, *N. Engl. J. Med.* **285**:763.

Trivelli, L. A., Ranney, H. M., and Lai, H.-T., 1971, Hemoglobin components in patients with diabetes mellitus, *N. Engl. J. Med.* **284**:353.

Valeri, R., 1973, Metabolic regeneration of depleted erythrocytes and their frozen storage, *in The Human Red Cell in Vitro* (T. J. Greenwalt and G. A. Jamieson, eds.), p. 281, Grune & Stratton, New York.

Valeri, C. R., and Fortier, N. L., 1969, Red cell 2,3-diphosphoglycerate and creatinine levels in patients with red-cell mass deficits or with cardiopulmonary insufficiency, *N. Engl. J. Med.* **281**:1452.

Valeri, C. R., and Hirsch, N. M., 1969, Restoration *in vivo* of erythrocyte adenosine triphosphate, 2,3-diphosphoglycerate, potassium ion, and sodium ion concentrations following the transfusion of acid-citrate-dextrose-stored human red cells, *J. Lab. Clin. Med.* **73**:822.

Valtis, D. J., and Kennedy, A. D., 1954, Effective gas transport of stored red blood cells, *Lancet* **2**:119.

Vokonas, P. S., Cohn, P. F., Klein, M. D., Laver, M. B., and Gorlin, R., 1970, Hemoglobin affinity for oxygen in the original syndrome with normal coronary arteriograms, *Circulation* **42**:204.

Weiss, E. B., and Desforges, J. F., 1972, Oxyhemoglobin affinity in bronchial asthma: Chronic stable state, acute, and status asthmaticus, *Chest* **62**:709.

Woodson, R. D., Torrance, J. D., Shappell, S. F., and Lenfant, C., 1970, The effect of cardiac disease on hemoglobin–oxygen binding, *J. Clin. Invest.* **49**:1349.

Wranne, B., Woodson, R. D., and Detter, J. C., 1972, Bohr effect: Interaction between $H^+$, $CO_2$, and 2,3-DPG in fresh and stored blood, *J. Appl. Physiol.* **32**:749.

Young, J. A., Lichtman, M. A., and Cohen, J., 1973, Reduced red cell 2,3-diphosphoglycerate and adenosine triphosphate, hypophosphatemia, and increased hemoglobin–oxygen affinity after cardiac surgery, *Circulation* **47**:1313.

Zimmon, D. S., 1973, Membrane mediated reduced red cell oxygen affinity on hepatic coma, *Clin. Res.* **21**:965.

**4**

# The Interaction of Folate Ligands with Macromolecules

## Maria da Costa and Sheldon P. Rothenberg

## 4.1. Introduction

Folic acid was obtained in pure form in 1944 and identified as a water-soluble vitamin essential for normal hematopoiesis in man and animals in 1948. Since then, the biochemical function of folic acid and its active coenzymes as carriers of carbon units for biosynthetic reactions has been well defined (Blakely, 1969). The physiology of folate transport, cellular uptake, and intracellular storage has been less clearly appreciated. Unlike vitamin $B_{12}$ and iron, a carrier protein which is required for transport and cellular uptake of folate* has not been identified. The major fraction of plasma folate circulates free or loosely bound to a variety of proteins; a storage protein for folates in tissues has not been definitely established.

In 1967, Ghitis identified a folate binding protein in milk and when, a few years later, a folate binder was found in chronic myelogenous leukemia cells (Rothenberg, 1970), a new interest in the biochemical and physiologic role of folate binding proteins was stimulated. The purpose of

*The term folic acid refers specifically to pteroylglutamic acid (PGA). The term folate is less specific and refers to any biologically active form of this vitamin.

---

MARIA DA COSTA and SHELDON P. ROTHENBERG • Division of Hematology/Oncology, Department of Medicine, New York Medical College, New York, New York 10029.

this chapter is to present an overall evaluation of the recent studies on these binding macromolecules, and to summarize the current status of the identification, purification, properties, function, and possible clinical implications of these newly defined proteins.

## 4.2. Methods of Identification of Folate Binding Macromolecules

The folate binder could only be identified by indirect methods until an isotopically labeled form of folate with sufficiently high specific activity to detect low concentrations of the unsaturated binder became available. Furthermore, the binding of exogenous folate would be of no value if the binding protein were already saturated by endogenous folate. These problems have been overcome in some measure by the availability in recent years of high specific activity [³H]folic acid (PGA) and by the application of radioimmunoassay techniques which could detect saturated forms of the binding protein.

In general, the methodology for studying folate binders is fairly simple and involves the addition of a tracer quantity of [³H]PGA to the test sample and, following a period of incubation, measuring the bound radioactivity after separation of the free (unbound) [³H]PGA by adsorption to dextran-coated charcoal, dialysis, or gel filtration.

Earlier studies to determine the association of folate with plasma proteins utilized microbiological assay of fractions of plasma separated by column chromatography through Sephadex gels. The association of folate activity with plasma protein fractions was considered sufficient evidence for folate binding. However, these studies did not indicate the type of kinetic reaction between folate and the protein, and such information is necessary to determine whether binding is specific or nonspecific.

Partial purification of the folate binding protein from chronic myelogenous leukemia cells (Fischer *et al.*, 1975) has facilitated the development of a radioimmunoassay which has been used to detect protein(s) with similar immunochemical properties in other tissues or biological fluids. The value of this radioimmunoassay is that it can identify the binder even when it is saturated with endogenous folate.

The principle of this radioimmunoassay is summarized in the following equations:

$$[\text{B-}(^{3}\text{H})\text{PGA}] + [\text{Ab}] \rightleftarrows \quad [\overline{\text{Ab-B-}(^{3}\text{H})\text{PGA}}] \qquad (1)$$

$$[\text{B-}(^{3}\text{H})\text{PGA}] + [\text{B}_s] + [\text{Ab}] \rightleftarrows [\overline{\text{Ab-B-}(^{3}\text{H})\text{PGA}}] + [\overline{\text{Ab-B}_s}] \qquad (2)$$

where B-(³H)PGA is the binder saturated with [³H]PGA and is, therefore, the tracer, and $B_s$ is the binder protein molecule which may be present in other tissues or fluids. Antiserum (Ab) containing antibodies to the partially purified folate binder was obtained by immunization of rabbits. When the antiserum is diluted to bind approximately 50% of the B-($^3$H)PGA, the addition of the test sample containing a similar immunoreactive folate binding protein ($B_s$) will decrease the antibody binding of B-($^3$H)PGA by competitive inhibition.

Because the binder is labeled with [$^3$H]PGA rather than directly by a $\gamma$-emitting isotope such as $^{125}$I, this radioimmunoassay lacks sufficient sensitivity to measure picogram quantities of the protein. However, for preliminary studies, the method was used as a simple screening test to detect the presence of a folate binder in biologic fluids and tissue extracts. Inhibition of the antibody binding of B-($^3$H)PGA by the test sample indicates that it contains an immunochemical determinant similar to the folate binder obtained from CML cells. Table I lists the biological fluids and samples of tissue and cell homogenates tested for the binder protein by radioimmunoassay and for the unsaturated binder by binding of [$^3$H]PGA. It is evident that a protein immunochemically similar to this folate binder is ubiquitous and is not species specific.

A more sensitive radioimmunoassay using $^{125}$I-labeled binder has now been developed in our laboratory (manuscript in preparation) by which picogram quantities of the binder protein can be quantified. We can measure this protein in virtually all normal sera (or plasma), suggesting that it is a constituent of normal blood in the category of trace proteins (i.e., $10^{-9}$M or less).

## 4.3. Definition of Terminology

Because of the earlier notion that there are no specific binders of folate, the subsequent identification of a macromolecule in some tissues and fluids with binding determinants for PGA has not been accepted without some skepticism. Much of this confusion, in fact, has been due to the lack of a precise definition of the types of folate–macromolecular complexes.

The interaction between the folate molecule and its macromolecular binder may exhibit the properties of nonspecific or specific binding. Nonspecific binding is characteristically a weak interaction with a low affinity constant, usually less than $10^4$ or $10^3$ liters/mole. The complexes can be dissociated by adsorption of the small folate ligand to another nonspecific but higher affinity attracting surface such as charcoal, even though gel filtration chromatography or short periods of dialysis may not result in similar dissociation. This type of binding does not exhibit saturation kinetics so that in the presence of a wide range of supersaturating concentrations of folate, the ratio of bound to free folate remains fairly

**Table I.** Tissues Containing Saturated and Unsaturated Folate Binders

| Source | Saturated binder[a] | Unsaturated binder[b] |
|---|:---:|:---:|
| Human serum | | |
|   Normal | + | ± |
|   Folate deficiency | + | + |
|   $B_{12}$ deficiency | + | ± |
|   Pregnancy | + | + |
|   Oral contraceptive administration | + | + |
|   Liver disease | + | + |
|   Myeloproliferative disease | + | + |
|   Chronic myelogenous leukemia | + | + |
|   Malignancy (pancreas, lung) | + | + |
| Biologic fluids | | |
|   Urine | + | ± |
|   Bile | + | + |
|   Malignant peritoneal effusion | + | 0 |
|   Malignant pleural effusion | + | 0 |
| Human tissues | | |
|   Normal leukocytes | + | − |
|   Chronic myelogenous leukemia cells | + | + |
|   Acute myeloblastic leukemia cells | + | − |
|   Acute lymphoblastic leukemia cells | + | − |
|   Chronic lymphocytic leukemia cells | + | − |
|   Normal liver homogenate | + | 0 |
|   Normal skin | + | + |
|   Normal breast | + | 0 |
|   Normal thyroid | + | + |
|   Chronic myelogenous leukemia liver and spleen | + | + |
|   Bronchogenic carcinoma | + | − |
|   Carcinoma of breast | + | ± |
|   Ovarian carcinoma | + | + |
|   Pancreatic carcinoma | + | 0 |
|   Renal carcinoma | + | ± |
|   Lymph node (anaplastic carcinoma, Hodgkin's, sarcoidosis) | + | 0 |
| Animal sources | | |
|   Pig serum | + | + |
|   Cows' milk | + | + |
|   L-1210 leukemia | + | − |
|   Guinea pig intestine | + | 0 |

[a]Tested by radioimmunoassay.
[b]Tested by determination of binding of [$^3$H]PGA.
Symbols: positive, +; negative, −; not tested, 0; positive and negative, ±.

constant. Nonspecific binding of folate to macromolecules is probably mediated by the carboxyl groups of the glutamate moiety of the molecule which are ionized at physiologic pH and interact by weak electrostatic attractions with positive ions on the proteins.

    Specific binders of folate, on the other hand, interact with the pteridine moiety of the folate molecule with equilibrium constants greater than $10^5$–$10^6$ liters/mole. The folate cannot be dissociated by adsorption with charcoal. The reaction demonstrates saturation kinetics and, when all binding sites are saturated, the ratio of bound to free folate decreases as the total folate concentration increases.

## 4.4. Nonspecific Folate Binder Complexes in Serum

The folate binding to proteins in serum may be specific or nonspecific, and recognition of these differences will resolve the conflicting data concerning the nature, significance, and even the existence of a folate binding macromolecule(s).

Earlier investigations provided evidence to support the notion that there were no plasma folate binders. Condit and Grob (1958) showed that endogenous serum folate was freely diffusible, and they could not demonstrate significant protein-bound folate in serum by equilibrium dialysis, paper chromatography, or starch gel electrophoresis. Herbert *et al.* (1962) also showed that serum folate activity could be adsorbed by charcoal, and this was later demonstrated again by Metz *et al.* (1968). Hampers *et al.* (1967) reported that plasma folate could be rapidly dialyzed across Visking cellophane membranes, and the observation that plasma folate decreased during hemodialysis (Mowbray *et al.*, 1965; Whitehead *et al.*, 1968) and during peritoneal dialysis (Sevitt and Hoffbrand, 1969) suggested that there was weak, if any, protein binding of serum folates.

On the other hand, Johns *et al.* (1961) stated that there was little or no free folic acid, and showed that 64% of [$^3$H]PGA added to serum remained protein bound after equilibrium dialysis. Elsborg (1972), using ultrafiltration techniques, reported that approximately 50% of [$^3$H]PGA added to plasma at pH 7.4 is bound to albumin; this ratio of bound to free folate was constant at all concentrations tested, indicating that this was nonspecific binding. Spector *et al.* (1975) also showed that the binding of [$^{14}$C]methyltetrahydrofolate by serum did not demonstrate saturation kinetics; a similar binding pattern could be obtained with albumin. Markkanen (1968), using Sephadex gel filtration, demonstrated that 50–87% of endogenous folate activity was not protein bound, 13–50% was associated with the albumin fraction, and less than 10% filtered with a high molecular weight globulin. In this last fraction, the *L. casei* activity was very firmly bound to protein and could not be separated by $(NH_4)_2SO_4$ precipitation of the protein or by dialysis (Markkanen and Peltola, 1971).

These seeming inconsistencies do not really represent conflicting data, but rather confirm the notion that the major portion of endogenous plasma folate is unbound or weakly and nonspecifically bound to a variety of proteins and, therefore, can be dissociated by charcoal adsorption or prolonged dialysis. The data of Johns et al. (1961), Elsborg (1972), and Spector et al. (1975) demonstrate that such binding is nonspecific by the definition previously described, and the albumin-associated fraction of folate observed by Markkanen et al. (1973a) also represents nonspecific binding of folate by plasma proteins.

Further evidence that the major fraction of endogenous folate in serum is unbound or only weakly associated with proteins is the fact that most folates in serum can be assayed microbiologically (Herbert, 1966) or by radioassay without prior extraction procedures (Rothenberg et al., 1972). This would not be feasible if the serum folates were not readily available for uptake by assay microorganisms or for binding by the macromolecular binding determinants in the radioassays.

## 4.5. Specific Folate Binder Complexes in Serum

In spite of these observations that most of endogenous serum folate is not specifically bound to a protein, paradoxically, there is also recent evidence for a protein in some serums which appears to satisfy the criteria of a specific folate binder. Rothenberg and da Costa (1971) reported the presence of a binder in the sera of some CML patients which bound [$^3$H]PGA and could not be dissociated by even 5% albumin-coated charcoal, or by the anion exchange resin, Dowex 2-X8. A macromolecular factor with specific binding determinants for PGA was subsequently identified in folate-deficient serums, the serum of two subjects with alcoholic folate deficiency (Waxman and Schreiber, 1973), and in women who were pregnant or taking oral contraceptives (da Costa and Rothenberg, 1974; Markkanen et al., 1973b). Additional reports have provided evidence that a similar folate binder may be found in fetal cord blood (Kamen and Caston, 1975b), sera from some uremic patients (Hines et al., 1973), and serum from patients with liver disease (Rothenberg, 1973), on Dilantin therapy (Markkanen et al., 1973c), and with acute myelogenous leukemia (Gorst et al., 1976).

To complicate this subject even further, Zettner and Duly (1974) examined serum from 99 normal volunteers and 916 hospitalized patients and showed that human serum normally contains a macromolecule which can bind picogram quantities of [$^3$H]PGA; that the binding is specific for folates; and that binding is reversible and saturable. Gorst et al. (1976) also found a binding capacity of 20–120 pg/ml in 85% of 94 normal serums. Although a recent study by Retief et al. (1976) failed to demonstrate the binding of exogenous [$^{14}$C]PGA and [$^{14}$C]methyltetrahydrofolate (methyl FH$_4$) by normal serum, the specific activity of their labeled folates was really insufficient to detect the binding of picogram amounts of folate. Nevertheless, they did observe some binding of PGA and methyl $FH_4$ by folate-deficient sera.

It can now be concluded with a fair degree of certainty that there is a macromolecule in the blood of most subjects which has the properties of a specific binder of folate. In some illnesses, such as liver disease, folate deficiency, and leukemia, the serum binds more exogenous [3H]PGA, indicating that the unsaturated binding capacity of the macromolecule has increased. There is as yet no clear correlation between the unsaturated folate binding capacity and the severity of a particular disease process, nor is there a constant relationship between the concentration of total serum folate and the unsaturated [3H]PGA binding capacity (Zettner and Duly, 1974).

It should be appreciated that, heretofore, the quantification of the binding of exogenous [3H]PGA indicated only the degree of unsaturation of the binder in serum and not the *total* concentration of the binder protein. The total concentration of the binding protein may, theoretically, vary directly, inversely, or independently of the unsaturated binding capacity. These theoretical considerations are depicted graphically in Fig. 1, where the unsaturated binding capacity may be normal, high, or low, with a normal, high, or low concentration of the binding protein. The direct measurement of this binding protein by radioimmunoassay will help to correlate its concentration in serum with the unsaturated folate binding capacity. This study is now in progress with normal subjects and

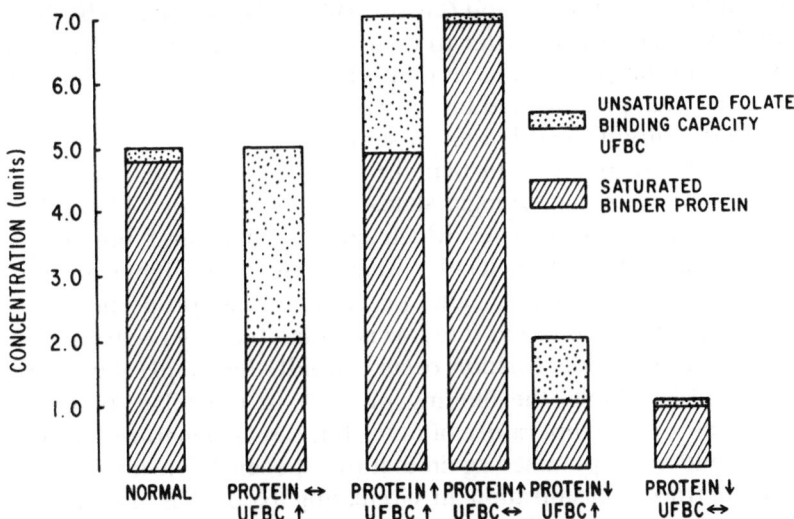

**Fig. 1.** Hypothetical examples of combinations of total binding protein concentration and unsaturated folate binding capacities (UFBC) (normal = ↔; increased ↑ ; decreased ↓ ). (Reprinted with the permission of *Clinics in Haematology.*)

patients with various diseases, and may help to determine whether there is any physiologic or pathologic significance to these variations.

## 4.6. Properties of the Specific Folate Binder in Serum

The specific folate binding protein in adult human serum has not been purified, possibly because of its low concentration. However, by studying the unsaturated folate binder found in some sera from patients with CML (Rothenberg and da Costa, 1971) and folate deficiency (Waxman and Schreiber, 1973), from women who are pregnant or taking oral contraceptives (da Costa and Rothenberg, 1974), and normal subjects (Zettner and Duly, 1975), some properties of the binder have been defined. An important finding is that the folate binder has a much higher affinity for oxidized folate (PGA) than for methyl $FH_4$, and it has an even lower affinity for formyltetrahydrofolate (formyl $FH_4$) and methotrexate. The polyglutamates of PGA as well as pteroic acid are also bound by this protein with somewhat less avidity than the monoglutamate.

Gel filtration and gradient centrifugation indicated that most of the unsaturated binder has a molecular weight in the range of 25,000 to 40,000. The sera from two patients with alcoholic folate deficiency also contained a small fraction of unsaturated binder with a molecular weight approximating 200,000 (Waxman and Schreiber, 1973).

A similar folate binding protein has been demonstrated in serum from cord blood by Kamen and Caston (1975b). Serum had to be dialyzed against 1 M citric acid in order to dissociate endogenous folate. Further purification of this protein was accomplished using a methotrexate affinity column; the final product had binding properties and a molecular weight similar to the unsaturated binder in some sera described previously.

These folate binders, present in the sera of normal subjects and subjects with various pathologic states and in fetal cord blood, have a number of similar properties which suggest structural homology. In addition to their similar molecular weight and their higher affinity for oxidized folate, their kinetic and physicochemical properties are also similar. The forward reaction rate is very rapid, binding occurs over a pH range from 5 to 10, dissociation occurs rapidly below pH 4.0, and 6 M urea reversibly inhibits the binding of PGA to the folate binder. The binder is stable to a temperature of 56°C, but can be denatured by boiling.

It should be emphasized again that this specific folate binder which is present in trace concentration in circulating blood has no role in the binding and transport of the physiologic methyl $FH_4$ which constitutes 80–90% of the circulating folate (Herbert et al., 1962). In fact, picograms of [$^3$H]PGA can be bound by some sera which contain 100-fold greater concentration of methyl $FH_4$. This can be explained by the higher affinity of the binder for PGA which will displace loosely associated methyl $FH_4$. Since all sera do not have an unsaturated PGA binding capacity, yet they do contain folate binding protein by competitive radioimmunoassay, it must be concluded that the folate binder in serum is saturated by a form of oxidized folate. This is the only folate which would not be displaced by the tracer [$^3$H]PGA.

The source of the specific folate binding protein in serum is open to speculation. Markkanen *et al.* (1972) suggested that the folate is bound to transferrin; however, antibodies against transferrin do not block the binding of [$^3$H]PGA to the folate binding protein in serum (Waxman, 1975). There is evidence that it may be the granulocyte since the folate binder in the serum from patients with CML and from pregnant women (and women taking oral contraceptives) cross-reacts immunologically with antibodies obtained against the folate binder from CML cells (da Costa and Rothenberg, 1974). It also appears that normal granulocytes contain a protein with similar immunochemical properties (Rothenberg *et al.*, 1977). In addition, lithium, which causes the *in vitro* release of $B_{12}$ binder(s) from granulocytes, can also cause the release of folate binder when added to whole blood (Colman and Herbert, 1974). Nevertheless, since other tissues also contain an immunochemically similar protein (Rothenberg *et al.*, 1977), more studies will be required to determine the source of this specific folate binder in blood.

Folate binders have also been identified in the serum of several animal species. Pig plasma (Mantzos *et al.*, 1974; Mantzos, 1975) contains the unsaturated folate binder in a concentration high enough to be used as the binding ligand in a radioassay for serum folate. The pig plasma binder has determinants for PGA, $FH_4$, and methyl $FH_4$. Its affinity for the reduced folate analogs is, however, greater than that of human serum folate binder. A folate binder from serum of cattle, sheep, and geldings has been separated by DEAE Sephadex chromatography (Markkanen *et al.*, 1974b), and has a pattern of folate binding similar to that of the human serum binder.

## 4.7. Significance of the Serum Folate Binder

A biologic function cannot as yet be ascribed to the specific folate binder in serum. It is present in extremely low concentration, it has little affinity for methyl $FH_4$, and its affinity for oxidized folate is so high that it virtually prevents the uptake of PGA by cells (Waxman and Schreiber, 1974).

However, there may be a value to measuring the concentration of this protein by competitive radioimmunoassay and its unsaturated folate binding capacity (using exogenous [³H]PGA) because alteration of these values from normal may occur in certain clinical situations or disease processes and these could have diagnostic value. For example, an increase in the unsaturated folate binding capacity has been observed in folate deficiency (Waxman and Schreiber, 1973), liver disease (Rothenberg, 1973), pregnancy (da Costa and Rothenberg, 1974), and some leukemias (Rothenberg and da Costa, 1971; Gorst et al., 1976). Using a radioimmunoassay (which measures the binder molecule directly), we have also observed a high concentration of this protein in many of these clinical disorders. Moreover, in some cases, the binder protein concentration is high and correlates neither with the unsaturated folate binding capacity nor the serum folate concentration.

One can speculate that there must be some pathophysiologic effect of this binder if it is increased in the blood, even though it represents a circulating compartment of oxidized folate which has no apparent metabolic function. Since it is elevated in many clinical conditions where there is frequently a perturbation of folate metabolism (e.g., folate deficiency, liver disease, pregnancy, administration of oral contraceptives and Dilantin), it would seem logical to consider some relationship between this protein and these disorders of folate metabolism. For example, Hines et al. (1973) reported that some uremic patients had high concentrations of bound folate in their serum associated with megaloblastic changes in the bone marrow, which corrected somewhat after the administration of folic acid. Experimental studies have also demonstrated that [³H]PGA and [³H]methyl $FH_4$ bound to the folate binding protein from normal plasma were not available for uptake by HeLa cells, human lymphocytes, Friend and L-1210 leukemia cells, and human lymphocytes in culture (Waxman and Schreiber, 1973).

The nonspecific binding of folate to a variety of plasma proteins (i.e., weak binding, nonsaturable, adsorbable by charcoal) may also serve a physiologic function. Such binding may retard the transfer of methyl $FH_4$ into the glomerular ultrafiltrate and prevent urinary loss of folate (Johns et al., 1961). This nonspecific binding might also play a role in intestinal folate absorption if transport across the intestinal epithelial cell follows a gradient requiring free folate in portal blood.

## 4.8. Serum Folate Binders and Radioassay for Folate

Finally, the effect of the folate binder on the radioassays now used for measuring folate in serum must be mentioned, particularly since much of the interest in folate binders has evolved during the development of these assay procedures. The presence of an unsaturated folate binder in the test sample to be assayed will, understandably, disturb the assay conditions since it will bind the isotopically labeled folic acid ([³H]- or [¹²⁵I]PGA). The competitive binding radioassay for folate (as with all quantitative radioimmunoassays) depends on inhibiting the binding of the tracer folate to a single binding determinant by standard folate or by folate in the test sample. If the test sample also binds the tracer folate, there will be a spuriously high percentage of bound tracer and this will falsely lower the value for the folate concentration in the sample (Rothenberg and da Costa, 1974). This problem can be avoided by extracting the sample by boiling to denature the binding protein (Dunn and Foster, 1973; Eichner et al., 1975). This problem can also be minimized by using a very sensitive sequential radioassay procedure which will permit testing as little as 10 to 20 µl sample volumes (Rothenberg et al., 1972).

## 4.9. Folate Binder in Erythrocytes

A specific binder for folate has not been identified in human erythrocytes. Iwai et al. (1964) reported that erythrocyte folate was bound to a macromolecule because it precipitated at 60% $(NH_4)_2SO_4$ saturation and filtered with hemoglobin through Sephadex gel. This is most likely nonspecific binding because most of the folate is dialyzable and can be measured by radioassay without heat extraction. Unsaturated folate binder in red blood cells has not been reported.

## 4.10. Folate Binder in Granulocytes

A folate binder with the properties defined for specificity was first identified in the granulocytes from some patients with chronic myelogenous leukemia (Rothenberg, 1970). The identification of this folate binder in the CML cells results from the observation that as little as $5 \times 10^{-9}$ M [³H]PGA could not be reduced to tetrahydrofolate (FH₄) by lysates of some of these cells, which generally contain a high concentration of the enzyme dihydrofolate reductase (DHFR). However, when the folate concentration in the reaction mixture was increased by the addition of unlabeled PGA, catalytic reduction of the tracer to tetrahydrofolate occurred. Investigation of this apparent paradox revealed that the tracer folate was actually bound to an unsaturated macromolecule and, therefore, could not react with DHFR. When unlabeled PGA was added to the reaction mixture, it saturated the folate binder and the [³H]PGA could then be enzymatically reduced to [³H]FH₄ by the enzyme.

Further study of this macromolecule demonstrated that it was a specific binder for folate and some of its oxidized analogs, and could be separated from DHFR (Rothenberg and da Costa, 1971). The binder was excluded from G-75 and G-100 Sephadex gels, folate was bound over a pH range from 5 to 9.0, and the binder was resistant to temperatures up to 56°C. It bound [³H]PGA rapidly with a forward velocity rate of 1.0%/sec. There was virtually no dissociation at 25 or 37°C in the first 30 min, and only 14% of the bound [³H]PGA was dissociated after 24 hr. This macromolecule had a significantly greater affinity for PGA, its oxidized analogs, and dihydrofolate, than for the reduced folates.

Partial purification of the folate binder from lysates of CML cells has separated two binding fractions by DEAE anion exchange chromatography (Fischer *et al.*, 1975). One binding fraction (A) eluted from the column with 0.001 M sodium phosphate, pH 6, and a second (B), which in some lysates constituted a larger fraction, eluted from DEAE column with 0.1 M sodium phosphate buffer, pH 7.4, indicating that it is a more acidic protein. Although by gel filtration binder A has a molecular weight of 34,000–35,000, and binder B, 44,000, the specificity of each binder for the folate analogs is similar. They are susceptible to digestion by proteolytic enzymes but not by DNAse or RNAse. The greatest affinity is for dihydrofolate ($FH_2$) followed in decreasing order by PGA, the polyglutamates of PGA, and [¹⁰N]methyl PGA. These partially purified binders did have some reactivity with methyl $FH_4$, but very little for formyl $FH_4$ and methotrexate. The fully oxidized folates and $FH_2$ appeared to be irreversibly bound by both binder A and binder B, whereas methyl $FH_4$ was reversibly bound to binder A. Binder A and binder B are immunochemically identical because antibodies against each binding protein react equally well with the other (Rothenberg *et al.*, 1977).

The binders appear to be under continual synthesis by the granulocytes because the concentration of binding protein increases in cultured cells and this increase is inhibited by puromycin and cycloheximide (da Costa and Rothenberg, 1976). Of particular significance is the observation that the B binder which is secreted into the culture medium has the same chromatographic characteristics as the unsaturated folate binder found in some sera from normal subjects and patients with CML. Since these binders are immunochemically similar to the binder in the CML lysates, it is strong evidence that one source of the specific binder in blood may be the maturing granulocyte precursors in the bone marrow. Gorst *et al.* (1976), who found higher levels of the folate binder in the serum of AML patients than in CML patients, have suggested that the mature granulocyte may not be the source of this binding protein. They found some correlation between the folate binder and lysozyme in serum, suggesting that binding protein may, in part, be derived from the monocyte.

The unsaturated folate binder has been identified in the liver of a CML patient postmortem, but since these tissues were infiltrated with the leukemic cells, the source of the binder cannot be definitely ascribed to the liver cell. However, studies using a qualitative radioimmunoassay have identified the binding protein saturated by folate even in normal leukocytes, lymphocytes from patients with chronic lymphocytic leukemia, granulocytes from women who are pregnant or taking oral contraceptives, and a variety of normal and malignant tissues (Rothenberg et al., 1975).

## 4.11. Significance of Intracellular Folate Binder

The presence of an intracellular folate binder has raised considerable speculation as to its function in the cell, particularly since the binder has the highest affinity for the less physiologic folate, PGA. Because it binds dihydrofolate, a coenzyme in de novo DNA synthesis, it has been postulated that the binder might have some function in the regulation of thymine-DNA synthesis (da Costa et al., 1972). De novo DNA synthesis was studied in vitro using cultures of CML cells containing a high and a low concentration of the unsaturated binder by determining the effect of PGA and $FH_2$ on [$^3$H]deoxyuridine (dU) incorporation by these cells. Cells with the high concentration of the unsaturated binder appeared to have a lower capacity for de novo DNA synthesis when compared to CML cells with a low concentration of the unsaturated binder. $FH_2$, which stimulates the de novo pathway, also had a lesser effect in cells with the high concentration of unsaturated binder.

More recent studies in our laboratory (manuscript in preparation) have demonstrated that the partially purified folate binder from CML cells has binding determinants for enzymatically generated [$^5$N,$^{10}$N]methylene-[$^3$H]tetrahydrofolate, the folate coenzyme which donates the $CH_3$ group to dU for the generation of thymidylate. Moreover, the folate binder can inhibit the reaction of this coenzyme with thymidylate synthetase. These studies support the notion that there is some relationship between de novo thymidylate synthesis and the intracellular folate binder, perhaps by regulating the concentration of free coenzymes.

Another possible function of the binder in the intracellular compartment is for storage. On the basis of the kinetic studies, it would seem that the binder with the lower anionic charge (A binder) would be more suited for this purpose because it binds reduced folate reversibly as compared to the more acidic binder (type B).

The intracellular folate binder(s) may also serve as a structural "anchor" for folate to permit polyglutamate synthesis, since binding to the protein occurs by way of the pteridine moiety of the molecule. There is now evidence that mammalian cells rapidly take up folate monogluta-mates and not the polyglutamates, though the intracellular folates are largely in the polyglutamate form. Polyglutamate synthesis from injected PGA has been demonstrated in liver, kidney, and intestine of rats (Brown *et al.*, 1974), all tissues in which the folate binders are known to be present.

## 4.12. Folate Binders in Other Tissues

There has been previous evidence, albeit indirect, that intracellular folate is complexed with a macromolecule. Magnus *et al.* (1969) have shown that liver slices incubated with plasma released folate from a bound state, and it was estimated that approximately half the hepatic folate was bound to intracellular macromolecules.

Correcher *et al.* (1974) have shown that [³H]PGA administered to rats can be recovered in the X and Z cytoplasmic proteins of the liver. Over a period of 24–48 hr, radioactivity appeared to transfer from the X to the Y protein, suggesting a dynamic process of transference from intracellular stores to the plasma.

Both saturated and unsaturated folate binding porteins have also been identified in rat liver, mitochondria, and cytosol by Zamierowski and Wagner (1976). These appeared to have molecular weights of 25,000, 150,000, and greater than 350,000. The endogenous folates which satu-rated some of these macromolecules were polyglutamates. In folate defi-ciency, there was an increase in the binding of exogenous folate by the 150,000 molecular weight macromolecule with a concomitant decrease in the binding by the other two binding fractions.

Extracts of acetone powder of hog kidney were found to contain a folate binder only after dialysis against an acid buffer to dissociate the endogenous folate. Unlike the folate binder from the CML cells, this binder has a high affinity for both methyl FH₄ and PGA (Kamen and Caston, 1975a).

Leslie and Rowe (1972) have identified a folate binding protein from the brush borders of intestinal epithelial cells of the rat. Shelub and Rosenberg (1976) isolated and purified a folate binding protein from the hog small intestine by using affinity chromatography after removal of the endogenous folate from the extract by acid dissociation and charcoal adsorption. The folate binding protein in the intestinal mucosa may be the mechanism involved in the saturable component of the transport of folates by the intestine. It is of particular interest in this regard that drugs such as Dilantin and oral contraceptives, which may cause malabsorption for folate, are also known to increase the concentration of the unsaturated binding capacity of the specific folate binder in serum. Also consonant with this hypothesis that a specific protein may be necessary for transmembrane transport of folate are the rare cases of congenitally defective absorption of folate (Lanzkowsky *et al.*, 1965). If this is due to the absence of the folate binder, it would suggest the absence of a gene required for the synthesis of this specific protein. The presence of the folate binder in the cell membrane of human lymphocytes (Waxman, 1975) also supports the hypothesis that it may function as a carrier protein for folate transport into the cell.

## 4.13. Folate Binder in Milk

It was the initial identification of a high affinity folate binder in cows' milk (Ghitis, 1967) that stimulated the search for other folate binders. Since the folate binder from this source is readily available in large quantities, it has been purified from the milk of several species of animals and its properties studied by several investigators. The folate binding protein is present in the milk of cows (Ghitis, 1967; Ford *et al.*, 1969), humans (Metz *et al.*, 1968; Waxman and Schreiber, 1975a; Markkanen *et al.*, 1974a), and goats (Rubinoff *et al.*, 1975).

The folate binder in cows' milk is a minor whey protein that migrates with, but is distinct from, $\beta$-lactoglobulin (Waxman and Schreiber, 1975a). The folate binder in cows' milk was partially purified from acid whey by $(NH_4)_2SO_4$ precipitation, DEAE-cellulose, and Sephadex G-150 gel filtration (Ford *et al.*, 1969). Further purification was accomplished by affinity chromatography using an agarose-PGA column (Salter *et al.*, 1972). The purified binder was eluted from the column with 8 M urea. A 600-fold purification was thus achieved and, by thin-layer starch gel electrophoresis, the protein appeared as a homogeneous band. By Sephadex gel filtration, the binder had a molecular weight which was estimated to be 38,000, quite similar to the folate binder in CML cells.

Waxman and Schreiber (1975a) separated the folate binding protein by DEAE-cellulose chromatography from commercially prepared bovine $\beta$-lactoglobulin. By Sephadex gel filtration, the isolated folate binder had an estimated molecular weight of 36,000, and by isoelectric focusing demonstrated isoproteins at pH 7.2, 7.8, and 8.6, each binding [³H]PGA.

Like the binder from CML cells and serum, the binder from cows' milk satisfies the properties of a specific binder. It has a much higher affinity for oxidized folate than for reduced folates at physiologic pH (Rothenberg *et al.*, 1972), but at pH 9.3, it binds PGA and methyl $FH_4$ with equal avidity (Givas and Gutcho, 1975). Bound folate cannot be dissociated by charcoal or dialysis and will not support the growth of microorganisms (Rothenberg *et al.*, 1977). The binding is via hydrogen bonding since the folate–protein complex will dissociate at pH below 4 and by urea or guanidine (Salter *et al.*, 1972).

Human milk contains a folate binding protein similar to that in cows' milk, and Waxman and Schreiber (1975b) obtained a 10,000-fold purification using a combination of charcoal treatment of acidified milk, affinity chromatography through a PGA-Sepharose column, and finally, DEAE-cellulose chromatography. The molecular weight of this protein was 26,500 and appeared as two bands on SDS polyacrylamide electrophoresis. Isoproteins were also demonstrated by isolectric focusing, and affinity for concavalin A indicated that these macromolecules are glycoproteins. During the purification, a small quantity of a folate binding protein with a high molecular weight (greater than 200,000) was separated from this major low molecular weight folate binder and was considered to be particulate membrane material secreted into the milk from apocrine glands.

Goats' milk folate binder was purified and studied by Rubinoff *et al.* (1975), and has similar properties.

The physiologic role of the folate binder in milk may be twofold. First, it could be a means by which folate is concentrated from the maternal circulation into the apocrine mammary glands in order to provide the infant with the high levels of folate required during the period of rapid neonatal growth. It is not likely that the folate binder in milk alters the intestinal absorption of folate since the low gastric pH would dissociate the folate and the binding protein would then be digested by pepsin in the stomach, or by trypsin in the small intestine. In fact, Izak *et al.* (1972) have shown only 20% decrease in absorption of folate even when folate bound to cows' or goats' milk was introduced directly into the jejunum.

A second function of the folate binder in milk, as suggested by Ford (1974), may be to control the ecology of the gut microflora. Since bound folate cannot be utilized by bacteria (Rothenberg *et al.*, 1977), it is possible that the unsaturated binder in milk would suppress growth of folate-dependent bacteria by decreasing the amount of free folate, and thus encourage proliferation of bacteria that provide folate to the host. The evidence to support this hypothesis is very indirect. Cows' milk and goats' milk are very low in folate and high in the unsaturated binder. However, piglets show a rapid increase in liver folate despite the low folate concentration in their milk diet, suggesting folate absorption from bacterial synthesis (Ford, 1974; Ford *et al.*, 1975). Even with a low folate diet, both in pigs and mice, synthesis of folate by intestinal bacteria increases (Klipstein and Lipton, 1970). This speculation as to the role of milk binder, however, is very tenuous, since it is also possible that the binder undergoes peptic digestion in the stomach (as suggested earlier) and has no physiologic role in folate absorption.

## 4.14. Summary

Folate binding proteins have now been identified in a variety of biological fluids and tissues. The binder from milk has been purified from a number of sources, and it appears to be a glycoprotein with a molecular weight ranging from 26,000 to 38,000.

Tissues such as liver, kidney, intestinal epithelium, and blood cells such as leukemic granulocytes also contain a folate binder. Where these macromolecules have been isolated, they appear in some instances to have similar properties with respect to the binding of folate analogs.

Serum from many normal subjects contains a very small amount of an unsaturated folate binder which increases in some cases of leukemia, folate deficiency, liver disease, uremia, and in women who are pregnant or taking oral contraceptives.

The functions of the folate in milk, blood, and cells can only be speculated on at this time. Areas which are under investigation include the role of the intracellular folate binder in the storage of folate, transmembrane transport, polyglutamate synthesis, and *de novo* thymidylate synthesis.

ACKNOWLEDGMENT

This work has been supported by research grants AM 16220 and CA 08976 from the National Institutes of Health.

## References

Blakely, R. L., 1969, *The Biochemistry of Folic Acid and Related Pteridines,* North Holland Pub., Amsterdam; Wiley-InterScience, New York.

Brown, J. P., Davidson, G. E., and Scott, J. M., 1974, The identification of the forms of folate bound in the liver, kidney, and intestine of the monkey and their biosynthesis from exogenous pteroylglutamate (folic acid), *Biochim. Biophys. Acta* **343**:78.

Colman, N., and Herbert, V., 1974, Release of folate binding protein FBP from granulocytes. Enhancement by lithium and elimination by fluoride. Studies with normal pregnant, cirrhotic and uremic persons, Proceedings of the 17th Annual Meeting of the American Society of Hematology, p. 155.

Condit, P. T., and Grob, D., 1958, Studies on the folic acid vitamins. I. Observations on the metabolism of folic acid in man and on the effect of aminopterin, *Cancer* **11**:525.

Correcher, R., De Sandre, G., Pacor, M. L., and Hoffbrand, A. V., 1974, Hepatic protein binding of folate, *Clin Sci. Mol. Med.* **46**:551.

da Costa, M., and Rothenberg, S. P., 1974, Appearance of a folate binder in leukocytes and serum of women who are pregnant or taking oral contraceptives, *J. Lab. Clin. Med.* **83**:207.

da Costa, M., and Rothenberg, S, P., 1976, Studies of the folate binding protein in granulocyte leukemia cells. I: Synthesis and release of binder by cells in short term culture, *Bri. J. Haematol.* **34**:581.

da Costa, M., Rothenberg, S. P., and Kamen, B., 1972, DNA synthesis in chronic myelogenous leukemia cells: Comparison of results in cells containing folate binding factor to replicating cells without binder, *Blood* **34**:621.

Dunn, R. T., and Foster, L. B., 1973, Radioassay of serum folate, *Clin. Chem.* **19**:1101.

Eichner, E. R., Paine, C. J., Dickson, V. L., and Hargrove, M. D., 1975, Clinical and laboratory observations on serum folate-binding protein, *Blood* **46**:599.

Elsborg, L., 1972, Binding of folic acid to human plasma proteins, *Acta Haematol.* **48**:207.

Fischer, C., da Costa, M., and Rothenberg, S. P., 1975, Heterogeneity and properties of folate binding protein from chronic myelogenous leukemia cells, *Blood* **46**:855.

Ford, J. E., 1974, Some observations on the possible nutritional significance of vitamin $B_{12}$ and folate binding proteins in milk, *Br. J. Nutr.* **31**:243.

Ford, J. E., Salter, D. N., and Scott, K. J., 1969, The folate-binding protein in milk, *J. Dairy Res.* **36**:435.

Ford, J. E., Scott, K. S., Sansom, B. F., and Taylor, P. J., 1975, Some observations on the possible nutritional significance of vitamin $B_{12}$ and folate binding proteins in milk. Absorption of [58Co]cyanocobalamin by suckling piglets, *Br. J. Nutr.* **34**:469.

Ghitis, J., 1967, The folate binding in milk, *Am. J. Clin. Nutr.* **20**:1.

Givas, J. K., and Gutcho, S., 1975, pH dependence of the binding of folates to milk binder in radioassay of folates, *Clin. Chem.* **21**:427.

Gorst, D. W., Courtis, M., and Delamore, I. W., 1976, Folic acid binding protein in acute myeloid leukemia, *J. Clin. Pathol.* **29**:60.

Hampers, C. L., Streiff, R., Nathan, D. C., Snyder, D., and Merrill, J. P., 1967, Megaloblastic hematopoiesis in uremia and in patients on long term hemodialysis, *N. Engl. J. Med.* **276**:551.

Herbert, V., 1966, Aseptic addition method for *Lactobacillus casei* assay of folate activity in human serum, *Pathology* **19**:12.

Herbert, V., Larrabee, A. R., and Buchanan, J. N., 1962, Studies on the identification of a folate compound of human serum, *J. Clin. Invest.* **41**:1134.

Hines, J. D., Kamen, B., and Caston, D., 1973, Abnormal folate binding proteins in azotemic patients, *Blood* **42**:997.

Iwai, I., Luttner, P. M., and Toennies, G., 1964, Blood folic acid precursors of human erythrocytes, *J. Biol. Chem.* **239**:2365.

Izak, G., Galewski, M., Rachmilewitz, E., and Grossowicz, N., 1972, The absorption of milk-bound pteroylglutamic acid from small intestine segments, *Proc. Soc. Exp. Biol. Med.* **140**:248.

Johns, D. G., Sperti, S., and Gurgen, A. S. V., 1961, The metabolism of tritiated folic acid in man, *J. Clin. Invest.* **40**:1684.

Kamen, B. A., and Caston, J. D., 1975a, Identification of a folate binder in hog kidney, *J. Biol. Chem.* **250**:2203.

Kamen, B. A., and Caston, J. D., 1975b, Purification of folate binding factor in normal umbilical cord serum, *Proc. Nat. Acad. Sci. U.S.A.* **72**:4261.

Klipstein, F. A., and Lipton, S. D., 1970, Intestinal flora in folate-deficient mice, *Am. J. Clin. Nutr.* **23**:132.

Lanzkowsky, P., Erlandson, M. E., and Bezan, A. I., 1965, Isolated defect of folic acid absorption associated with mental retardation and cerebral calcification, *Blood* **34**:452.

Leslie, G. I., and Rowe, P. B., 1972, Folate binding by the brush border membrane proteins of small intestinal epithelial cells, *Biochemistry* **9**:1696.

Magnus, E. M., Dempsey, H., and Butterworth, C. E., 1969, Release of folate by rat liver and spleen slices, *Blood* **33**:400.

Mantzos, J. D., 1975, Radioassay of serum folate with use of pig plasma folate binders, *Acta Haematol.* **54**:289.

Mantzos, J. D., Terzaki, A., and Gyftaki, E., 1974, Folate binding in animal plasma, *Acta Haematol.* **51**:204.

Markkanen, T., 1968, Pteroylglutamic acid (PGA) activity of serum in gel filtration, *Life Sci.* **7**:887.

Markkanen, T., and Peltola, O., 1971, Carrier proteins of folic acid activity in human serum, *Acta Haematol.* **45**:176.

Markkanen, T., Virtanen, S., Himanen, P., and Pajula, R. L., 1972, Transferrin, the third carrier protein of folic acid activity in human serum, *Acta Haematol.* **48**:213.

Markkanen, T., Pajula, R. L., Himanen, P., and Virtanen, S., 1973a, Serum folic acid activity *(L. casei)* in Sephadex gel chromatography, *J. Clin. Pathol.* **26**:486.

Markkanen, T., Himanen, P., Pajula, R. L., Ruponen, S., and Castren, O., 1973b, Binding of folic acid to serum proteins. Effect of pregnancy, *Acta Haematol.* **50**:85.

Markkanen, T., Himanen, P., Pajula, R. L., and Molnar, G., 1973c, Binding of folic acid to serum proteins. The effect of diphenylhydantoin treatment and various diseases, *Acta Haematol.* **50**:284.

Markkanen, T., Pajula, R. L., Virtanen, S., and Himanen, P., 1974a, Binding of folic acid activity (FAA) to proteins in mother's milk, *Int. J. Vitam. Nutr. Res.* **44**:195.

Markkanen, T., Pajula, R. L., Himanen, P., and Virtanen, S., 1974b, Binding of folic acid to serum proteins. IV. In some animal species, *Int. J. Vitam. Nutr. Res.* **44**:347.

Metz, R., Zalusky, R., and Herbert, V., 1968, Folic acid binding by serum and milk, *Am. J. Clin. Nutr.* **21**:289.

Mowbray, J. F., Cohen, S. L., Coak, P. B., Kenyon, J. R., Owen, K., Percival, A., Porter, K. A., and Peart, W. S., 1965, Human cadaveric renal transplantation. Report of 920 cases, *Br. J. Haematol.* **1**:1387.

Retief, F. P., Heyns, A. du P., Oosthuizen, M., Van Reenen, O. R., and Baden-horst, C. J., 1976, *In vitro* binding of folates by body fluids, *Br. J. Haematol.* **32**:113.

Rothenberg, S. P., 1970, A macromolecular factor in some leukemic cells which binds folic acid, *Proc. Soc. Exp. Biol. Med.* **133**:428.

Rothenberg, S. P., 1973, Application of competitive ligand binding for the radioassay of vitamin $B_{12}$ and folic acid, *Metabolism* **22**:1075.

Rothenberg, S. P., and da Costa, M., 1971, Further observations on the folate-binding factor in some leukemic cells, *J. Clin. Invest.* **50**:719.

Rothenberg, S. P., and da Costa, M., 1974, Letter to the editor, *Blood* **43**:312.

Rothenberg, S. P., da Costa, M., and Rosenberg, Z., 1972, Radioassay for serum folate: Use of sequential-incubation, ligand-binding system, *N. Engl. J. Med.* **286**:1335.

Rothenberg, S. P., da Costa, M., and Fischer, C., 1977, Use and significance of folate binders, *Proceedings of a Workshop on Human Folate Requirements* (H. Broquist, C. Butterworth, and C. Wagner, eds.), National Academy of Science, Washington, D.C., in press.

Rubinoff, M., Schreiber, C., and Waxman, S., 1975, Isolation and characterization of folate binding protein (FBP) from goat milk by affinity chromatography, *Fed. Proc.* **34**:904.

Salter, D. N., Ford, J. E., Scott, K. J., and Anderson, P., 1972, Isolation of the folate binding protein from cows milk by the use of affinity chromatography, *Fed. Eur. Biochem. Soc. Lett.* **20**:302.

Sevitt, L. H., and Hoffbrand, A. V., 1969, Serum folate and vitamin $B_{12}$ levels in acute and chronic renal disease. Effect of peritoneal dialysis, *Br. Med. J.* **2**:18.

Shelub, J., and Rosenberg, I. H., 1976, Isolation of folate binding protein from the intestine with the aid of affinity chromatography, *Clin. Res.* **24**:504A.

Spector, R., Lorenzo, A. V., and Drum, D. E., 1975, Serum binding of methylte-trahydrofolic acid, *Biochem. Pharmacol.* **24**:542.

Waxman, S., 1975, Folate binding proteins, *Br. J. Haematol.* **29**:23.

Waxman, S., and Schreiber, C., 1973, Characteristics of folic acid-binding protein in folate-deficient serum, *Blood* **42**:291.

Waxman, S., and Schreiber, C., 1974, The role of folic acid binding protein (FABP) in the cellular uptake of folates, *Proc. Soc. Exp. Biol. Med.* **147**:760.

Waxman, S., and Schreiber, C., 1975a, The isolation of the folate binding protein from commercially purified bovine β-lactoglobulin, *FEBS Lett.* **55**:128.

Waxman, S., and Schreiber, C., 1975b, The purification and characterization of the low molecular weight human folate binding protein using affinity chromatography, *Biochemistry* **14**:5422.

Whitehead, V. M., Comty, C. H., Posen, G. A., and Kaye, M., 1968, Homeostasis of folic acid in patients undergoing maintenance hemodialysis, *N. Engl. J. Med.* **279**:970.

Zamierowski, M., and Wagner, C., 1976, The characterization of high molecular weight complexes of folic acid in mammalian tissues, *in The Chemistry and Biology of Pteridines*, pp. 209–217, de Gruyter, Berlin.

Zettner, A., and Duly, P. E., 1974, New evidence for a binding principle specific for folates as a normal constituent of human serum, *Clin. Chem.* **20**:1313.

5

# Pure Red Cell Aplasia
## Sanford B. Krantz and S. Donald Zaentz

## 5.1. Definition

Pure red cell aplasia (PRCA) was first described by Kaznelson (1922) as an anemia due to an almost complete cessation of erythropoiesis, but without leukopenia or thrombocytopenia. This condition usually can be clearly distinguished from aplastic anemia in which low blood white cell and platelet concentrations accompany the anemia (Van Der Weyden and Firkin, 1972). In PRCA the bone marrow has an isolated absence of erythroblasts with normal granulocytopoiesis and megakaryocytopoiesis (DiGiacomo et al., 1966; Jacobs et al., 1959), whereas in aplastic anemia all three hematopoietic lineages are markedly reduced (Van Der Weyden and Firkin, 1972). In children PRCA has been called "chronic (congenital) hypoplastic anemia," the Diamond–Blackfan anemia, or erythrogenesis imperfecta (Diamond and Blackfan, 1938; Gasser, 1957; Tsai and Levin, 1957). In adults it has been termed isolated aplastic anemia, aplastic crisis, erythroblastopenia, erythrophthisis, chronic erythrocytic hypoplasia, red cell aplastic anemia, or red cell agenesis (Gasser, 1957; Tsai and Levin, 1957). Although these cases could represent a variety of pathogenetic mechanisms they all have in common an isolated absence of marrow erythroblasts and are now considered together as cases of PRCA.

SANFORD B. KRANTZ and S. DONALD ZAENTZ • Division of Hematology, Departments of Medicine, Vanderbilt University School of Medicine and Veterans Administration Hospital, Nashville, Tennessee 37203.

## 5.2. Classification

### 5.2.1. Congenital PRCA

Although PRCA can be classified in a variety of ways (DiGiacomo *et al.*, 1966; Gasser, 1957), the classification we have found most useful is the one shown in Table I, modified from DiGiacomo *et al.* (1966). Both congenital and acquired cases of PRCA have been recognized, and the acquired form has been further divided into primary and secondary categories. The congenital disease manifests itself before 18 months of age (Hughes, 1961), but there are only a small number of cases in which the disease appears to have been inherited (Gasser, 1957). Twelve well-defined familial occurrences have been reported (Hunter and Hakami, 1972; Hamilton *et al.*, 1974; Lawton *et al.*, 1974). A common incidence in siblings has suggested an autosomal recessive mode of inheritance in some of these cases (Hunter and Hakami, 1972; Lawton *et al.*, 1974). In others, however, the disease appears to have been transmitted as an autosomal dominant trait (Hunter and Hakami, 1972; Hamilton *et al.*, 1974; Lawton *et al.*, 1974). Approximately 25% of patients with congenital PRCA have had a wide variety of associated congenital abnormalities including bilateral double ureters and hydronephrosis, exophthalmos, webbed neck, abnormal osseous development, a presumed congenital heart lesion, strabismus, pterygium colli, extra phalanx or thumb, and 11 pairs of ribs (Diamond *et al.*, 1961; Hughes, 1961). Most had decreased growth and several had a retardation of bone age.

**Table I.**   Classification of Pure Red Cell Aplasia

---

I.   Congenital (Diamond–Blackfan)
II.  Acquired
   A.   Primary
      1.   Immunoglobulin inhibitors
         a.   Inhibitors of marrow erythroid cells
            i.   Immunoglobulins cytotoxic for marrow erythroblasts
            ii.  Immunoglobulins that inhibit erythropoietin-responsive cells (ERC)
         b.   Inhibitors of erythropoietin
      2.   Unknown origin and pathogenesis
   B.   Secondary
      1.   Thymoma
      2.   Infections
      3.   Drugs or chemicals
      4.   Hemolytic anemia (aplastic crisis)
      5.   Systemic lupus erythematosus and rheumatoid arthritis
      6.   Severe renal failure
      7.   Severe nutritional deficiency
      8.   Neoplasms (other than thymoma)

---

### 5.2.2. Acquired Primary PRCA

Primary PRCA occurs in adults and children without a known etiology. It has been thought of as a rare condition since only 43 cases were reported by 1964 (Rosner and Hausser, 1964). However, in the last 5 years we have learned of 80 new cases that we were able to document by review of the bone marrow slides. This disease is probably much more frequent than the literature indicates and many cases may exist that have been overlooked or not reported. In some of these cases the disease has been associated with the presence of immunoglobulins that inhibit marrow erythroid cells (Krantz and Kao, 1967, 1969; Krantz et al., 1973). In other cases the disease was associated with immunoglobulins that inhibit erythropoietin (Jepson and Lowenstein, 1966; Peschle et al., 1975). In the remaining group of these patients, the PRCA had no associated pathogenetic factors and the mechanism for the disease in these patients has remained unknown.

### 5.2.3. Acquired Secondary PRCA

Secondary PRCA has been frequently associated with thymomas (Jacobs et al., 1959; Roland, 1964; Schmid et al., 1965; DiGiacomo et al., 1966; Hirst and Robertson, 1967). PRCA with thymoma has been reported as often as primary acquired PRCA (Jacobs et al., 1959; Hirst and Robertson, 1967), and like the latter it represents a chronic state of markedly reduced erythropoiesis. However, in 29% of these cases removal of the thymoma is followed by remission of the anemia (Jacobs et al., 1959). Thus, all patients with chronic PRCA should be investigated for a thymoma. Lateral tomography should be performed when a thymic tumor is not evident on a routine chest roentgenogram since this has revealed a thymoma not seen by other procedures (Hirst and Robertson, 1967). A few cases of PRCA have appeared following a thymectomy, but the reason for this sequence of events is unknown (Hirst and Robertson, 1967; Safdar et al., 1970).

A chronic form of secondary acquired PRCA has been noted with systemic lupus erythematosus (Doughaday, 1968; Cassileth and Myers, 1973; MacKechnie et al., 1973), rheumatoid arthritis (Krantz, unpublished observations), severe renal failure (Gasser, 1957; Pasternack and Wahlberg, 1967), and severe nutritional deficiency such as that seen with marasmus and kwashiorkor (Foy and Kondi, 1961; Kho et al., 1962). Such cases have also been described with a wide variety of hematologic and nonhematologic neoplasms as indicated in Table II. An etiologic relation between many of these neoplasms and PRCA has not been established since the patients were often elderly and would be expected to have an

**Table II.**   Malignant Neoplasms Associated with Development of PRCA

| Type of malignancy | Number of patients | Reference | Comments |
|---|---|---|---|
| Hodgkin's disease | 2 | Bove, 1956; Field et al., 1968 | One PRCA responded to corticosteroids and nitrogen mustard, and another responded to irradiation of thymoma |
| Multiple myeloma | 1 | Gilbert et al., 1968 | No PRCA remission with thymectomy but response to prednisone and phenylalanine mustard |
| Lymphosarcoma | 4 | Jacobs et al., 1959; Jepson and Vas, 1974; Hunt and Lander, 1975 | Two patients' plasmas inhibited mouse erythropoiesis; in one case PRCA and histiocytic lymphoma responded to prednisone and cyclophosphamide |
| Chronic lymphocytic leukemia | 11 | Battle et al., 1963; Stohlman et al., 1971; Tatarsky, 1972; Abeloff and Waterbury, 1974 | PRCA generally responded to corticosteroids, androgens, or cyclophosphamide |

| | | | |
|---|---|---|---|
| Oat-cell carcinoma of the lung | 1 | Entwistle et al., 1964 | Serum inhibitor of rabbit erythropoiesis disappeared after irradiation of tumor but PRCA persisted |
| Squamous cell carcinoma of the lung | 2 | Brafield and Verbov, 1966; Tsai and Levin, 1957 | One PRCA responded to corticosteroids, and another did not |
| Adenocarcinoma of stomach | 1 | Kark, 1937 | Relation to PRCA unknown |
| Adenocarcinoma of unknown primary site | 1 | Mitchell et al., 1971 | PRCA responded to corticosteroids |
| Carcinoma of the breast | 2 | Green, 1958; Clarkson and Prokop, 1958 | One low-grade carcinoma found at postmortem. Second PRCA developed after thymoma removed and unresponsive to complete removal of breast tumor |
| Kaposi's sarcoma | 2 | Hirst and Robertson, 1967; Marmont et al., 1975 | No evidence of relation between tumor and PRCA |

increased incidence of neoplasms. In most cases the PRCA responded to corticosteroids while the tumor still persisted. Only in the lymphoproliferative conditions has there been a high enough frequency of the association to suggest a real relationship. In two cases of lymphosarcoma the plasma γ-globulins inhibited erythropoietin-induced erythropoiesis of polycythemic mice (Jepson and Vas, 1974) and in one case of oat-cell carcinoma of the lung the patient's serum inhibited rabbit erythropoiesis before the tumor was irradiated, but not afterward, although the anemia was unchanged (Entwistle *et al.*, 1964).

In contrast to the chronic state of PRCA that may occur in the primary disease or in the secondary cases just described, an acute and self-limited cessation of red cell production can arise during the course of such infections as atypical pneumonia, mumps, viral hepatitis, meningococcemia, staphylococcemia, and infectious mononucleosis (Chernoff and Josephson, 1951; Gasser, 1957; Sears *et al.*, 1975). It has also been reported with insect bites (Gasser, 1957). Rapid recovery generally occurs in these cases. A similar disappearance of marrow erythroblasts has been reported after exposure to a wide variety of drugs which are listed in Table III. Most of the patients receiving these drugs recovered quickly when they were discontinued (Gasser, 1957; Recker and Hynes, 1969). In one case the PRCA recurred when the drug was administered again (Yunis *et al.*, 1967). In some cases, however, recovery was incomplete or was delayed and associated with androgen (Stephens, 1974) or corticosteroid treatment (Swineford *et al.*, 1958). PRCA has also occurred in patients

**Table III.** Drugs Associated with Development of PRCA

| Agent | Reference |
|---|---|
| Aminopyrine | Gasser, 1957 |
| Arsphenamine | Sharff and Neumann, 1944 |
| Azathioprine | McGrath *et al.*, 1975 |
| Calomel | Gasser, 1957 |
| Chenopodium | Gasser, 1949 |
| Chloramphenicol | Hirst and Robertson, 1967; Vilan *et al.*, 1973 |
| Chlorpropamide | Recker and Hynes, 1969 |
| Co-trimoxazole | Stephens, 1974 |
| Diphenylhydantoin | Brittingham *et al.*, 1964 |
| Halothane | Jurgensen *et al.*, 1970 |
| Isoniazid | Mielke, 1958; Goodman and Block, 1964 |
| Penicillin | Gasser, 1949 |
| Phenobarbital | Gasser, 1949 |
| Phenylbutazone | Swineford *et al.*, 1958; Ibrahim *et al.*, 1966 |
| Santonin | Gasser, 1957 |
| Sulfathiazole | Strauss, 1943; Tsai and Levin, 1957 |
| Thiamphenicol | Cornet *et al.*, 1974 |
| Tolbutamide | Schmid *et al.*, 1963 |

previously exposed to herbicides or insecticides, but an etiologic relationship has never been demonstrated (Krantz and Kao, 1967, 1969; Zaentz *et al.*, 1976). Recently, three patients with acute lymphocytic leukemia acquired PRCA while under treatment with combination chemotherapy (Sallan and Buchanan, 1977; Lukens and McKenzie, unpublished observations). The drugs involved were 6-mercaptopurine, cyclophosphamide, methotrexate, vincristine, cytosine arabinoside, adriamycin, and prednisone. In two cases when the chemotherapy was stopped the PRCA remitted, whereas in the third case it has persisted.

An acute self-limited PRCA can also occur during the course of a variety of chronic hemolytic anemias such as congenital spherocytosis (Gasser, 1957; Bouroncle, 1964), sickle cell disease (Singer *et al.*, 1950; Gasser, 1957; MacIver, 1961), autoimmune hemolytic anemia (Davis *et al.*, 1952; Eisemann and Dameshek, 1954; Gasser, 1957; Meyer and Bertcher, 1960), and other acquired hemolytic anemias (Gasser, 1957). This is commonly referred to as an "aplastic crisis" but is generally an acute self-limited PRCA. The onset of PRCA in these cases is often associated with an infection and it is possible that the infection is the precipitating factor for the anemia (Chernoff and Josephson, 1951). The short life span of the red cells in these hemolytic anemias coupled with the lack of red cell production would quickly produce a severe anemia and bring these cases to the attention of a physician, whereas many similar self-limited cases of PRCA in patients with a normal red cell life span might go unrecognized.

## 5.3. Laboratory Manifestations

### 5.3.1. Blood and Bone Marrow Morphology

Patients with PRCA are usually very anemic at the time of examination. The red cells are normochromic and normocytic and there is virtually no polychromasia (Gasser, 1957). The reticulocyte count is generally less than 1% and most often no reticulocytes are observed (Gasser, 1957; Hirst and Robertson, 1967). Although the white cell and platelet counts are most often normal, an occasional patient may have a mild leukopenia and/or thrombopenia (Hirst and Robertson, 1967). The distribution of white cells in the blood differential count is generally normal but occasional lymphocytosis and eosinophilia have been noted (Tsai and Levin, 1957; Hirst and Robertson, 1967).

The bone marrow most often has an almost complete absence of erythroblasts (Gasser, 1957; Jacobs *et al.*, 1959; Schmid *et al.*, 1965). However, in some cases that appear to have a similar pathogenesis and a similar response to the same therapeutic agents, a small number of early erythroblasts such as proerythroblasts and basophilic erythroblasts may be present (Eisemann and Dameshek, 1954; Gasser, 1957; Krantz and Kao, 1969; Wranne *et al.*, 1970; Böttiger and Rausing, 1972; Zaentz *et al.*, 1975). The bone marrow most often appears to have a normal cellularity because of a normal granulopoiesis and megakaryocytopoiesis (Gasser, 1957). Figure 1A shows a particle section of the bone marrow from a patient with PRCA. The cellular area is almost equal to the fat spaces and is within the normal range. However, the marrow particle smear (Fig. 1B) indicates that the cells were entirely granulocyte precursor cells and lymphocytes. In primary acquired PRCA the marrow cellularity may occasionally be increased due to a granulocytic or lymphocytic hyperplasia (Hirst and Robertson, 1967; Marmont *et al.*, 1975; Zaentz *et al.*, 1975). A diffuse lymphocytic infiltration of the marrow may be present, but on occasion there is an increased number of lymphocytic aggregates (Hirst and Robertson, 1967; Rogers *et al.*, 1968; Böttiger and Rausing, 1972; Marmont *et al.*, 1975).

These laboratory features are markedly different from those of aplastic anemia. Patients with aplastic anemia are usually pancytopenic at the time of examination and their bone marrows are markedly hypocellular with a depression of all hematopoietic cell lines (Van Der Weyden and Firkin, 1972). Differentiation of PRCA from aplastic anemia is of great importance due to the different therapeutic approaches that are currently used for these two conditions.

## 5.3.2. Other Laboratory Abnormalities

### 5.3.2.1. Roentgenographic

No specific roentgenographic findings are present other than those relating to the presence of a thymoma. Frontal views of the chest may be inadequate for visualization of a thymoma, since thymic enlargement may be concealed behind the heart and great vessels. Oblique views may be of some use in delineating thymic enlargement. Even better is lateral tomography which should be performed wherever possible in this condition because of the high association of PRCA with thymomas and because this procedure may reveal a thymoma not seen by other roentgenographic methods (Hirst and Robertson, 1967).

### 5.3.2.2. Immunologic

Chronic acquired PRCA has been associated with a number of abnormalities of the immune system (Rogers *et al.*, 1968). Thymomas have been reported in approximately half the patients with this disease (Jacobs *et al.*, 1959; Hirst and Robertson, 1967). Paraproteins (Voyce, 1963; Krantz and

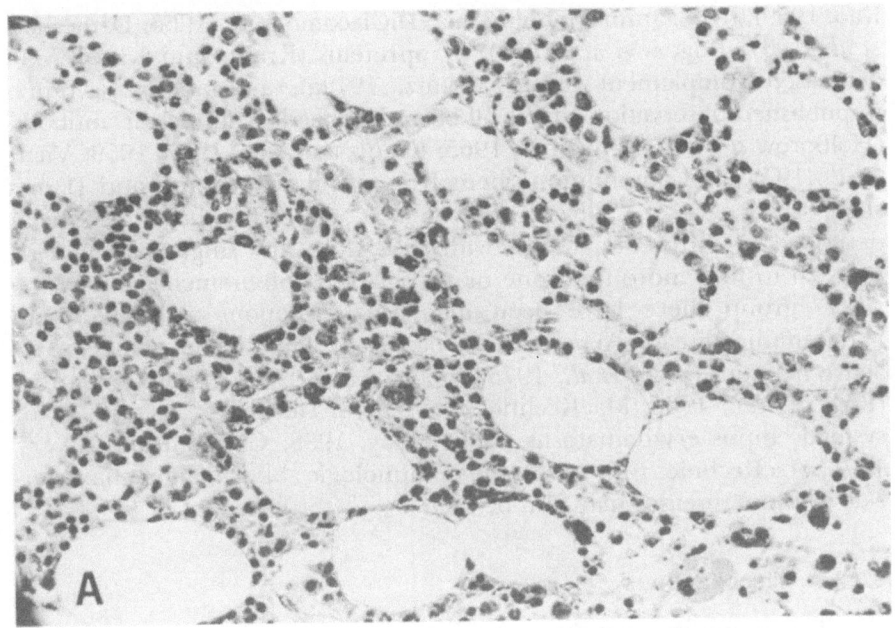

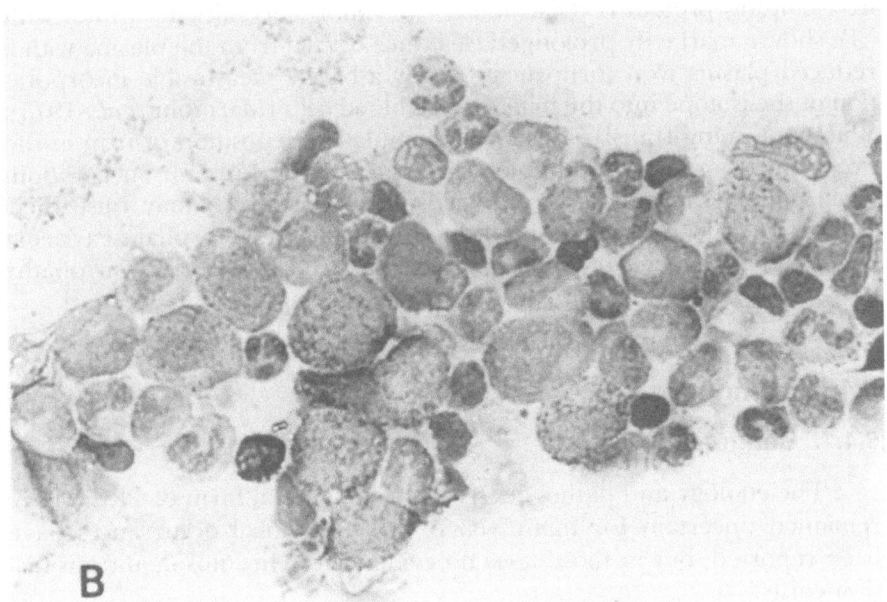

**Fig. 1.** Bone marrow in PRCA. (A) Particle section showing normal cellularity. (B) Particle smear showing absence of erythroblasts and predominance of granulocyte precursor cells and lymphocytes.

Kao, 1969), hypogammaglobulinemia (DiGiacomo *et al.*, 1966; Dameshek *et al.*, 1967; Rogers *et al.*, 1968), pyroproteins (Krantz and Kao, 1969), decreased complement levels (Krantz, 1972a), and anergy (Krantz, unpublished observations) have all been described. Antinuclear antibody (Holborow *et al.*, 1963; Barnes, 1965; Krantz and Kao, 1967, 1969; Vilan *et al.*, 1973) and autoimmune hemolytic anemia (Eisemann and Dameshek, 1954; Gasser, 1957; DiGiacomo *et al.*, 1966) have also been described in different patients with PRCA. In any single patient it is unusual to find more than one or two of these phenomena, but in the whole group there have been many manifestations associated with autoimmune disease. When PRCA occurs in conjunction with chronic active hepatitis (Sears *et al.*, 1975; Zaentz *et al.*, 1975), myasthenia gravis (Rogers *et al.*, 1968; MacKechnie *et al.*, 1973; DeSevilla *et al.*, 1975), or systemic lupus erythematosus (Doughaday, 1968; Cassileth and Myers, 1973; MacKechnie *et al.*, 1973), the immunologic abnormalities characteristic of those diseases may also be seen.

### 5.3.2.3. Miscellaneous

The serum iron concentration is increased as is the saturation of the iron binding protein (DiGiacomo *et al.*, 1966). Ferrokinetic studies with $^{59}$Fe show a markedly prolonged clearance of $^{59}$Fe from the plasma with a reduced plasma iron turnover and only a barely measurable incorporation of the isotope into the marrow and blood cells (Marmont *et al.*, 1975). With continuing transfusions and a cumulative deposition of iron in the liver, the laboratory findings of cirrhosis may be present. In addition, some patients acquire a chronic active hepatitis which may raise their serum glutamic oxalacetic transaminase and alkaline phosphatase (Zaentz *et al.*, 1975). Diabetes mellitus, cardiac arrhythmias, and cardiomyopathy may also be present from iron deposition in these tissues.

## 5.4. Pathogenesis

### 5.4.1. Congenital PRCA

The etiology and pathogenesis of the congenital form of PRCA have remained uncertain for many years. Twelve familial occurrences have been reported, but in most cases no evidence of chromosomal transmission exists.

Riboflavin deficiency, initiated experimentally, can produce an erythroid aplasia (Alfrey and Lane, 1970). This has prompted one group of investigators to evaluate riboflavin metabolism in congenital PRCA (Mentzer *et al.*, 1975). They found that the dietary intake of riboflavin and the plasma levels of riboflavin and flavine-adenine dinucleotide were normal in five of these patients. Nevertheless, the transport of riboflavin into their red cells *in vitro* was reduced and the total red cell flavins were lower. However, the precise relationship of these abnormalities to the anemia of these patients is unknown.

Erythropoietin production appears to be adequate in congenital PRCA as evidenced by an increased erythropoietin concentration in the urine and serum of these patients (Hammond *et al.*, 1968). The marrow cells of these patients have been cultured *in vitro* and their heme synthesis has been measured with and without erythropoietin (Freedman *et al.*, 1975; Ortega *et al.*, 1975). The percentage increase in heme synthesis produced by the hormone was greatly reduced or absent compared to normal marrows. In one patient the response of heme synthesis *in vitro* to erythropoietin became normal after a spontaneous remission (Freedman *et al.*, 1975).

The marrow cells of these patients have also been cultured in a plasma clot system where normal marrow cells produce erythroid colonies in the presence of erythropoietin (Freedman *et al.*, 1976). The number of erythroid colonies produced by the marrow of two patients with congenital PRCA was greatly reduced, indicating that the erythropoietin-responsive cells that gave rise to these colonies were either reduced in number or were unable to respond to erythropoietin in this disease. The marrows of two patients receiving prednisone and producing erythroblasts had a normal number of erythroid colonies. Nandrolone decanoate produced a 38% increase in the number of erythroid colonies drawn from normal marrow cells *in vitro*, but was completely ineffective when added to the marrow cells of patients with congenital PRCA.

The existence of a plasma inhibitor of erythropoiesis in these patients is uncertain. One group of investigators reported that the serum of some of these patients reduced the effect of erythropoietin on heme synthesis *in vitro* by the patients' marrow cells and normal marrow cells (Ortega *et al.*, 1975). However, two other groups were unable to demonstrate such an inhibitor (Geller *et al.*, 1975; Freedman *et al.*, 1975) and no serum inhibitor of erythroid colony growth could be demonstrated in the patients' sera when they were cultured with normal marrow cells (Hoffman *et al.*, 1976; Freedman *et al.*, 1976).

Recently, Hoffman *et al.* (1976) cultured normal marrow cells in the plasma clot system with either peripheral blood lymphocytes from normal donors or blood lymphocytes from patients with congenital PRCA. These lymphocytes had been purified on Ficoll-Hypaque density gradients. The number of erythroid colonies from the normal marrow cells was either not affected by the blood lymphocytes from the normal donors or was increased. However, the blood lymphocytes from four patients with congenital PRCA caused a marked reduction (54–95%) in the number of erythroid colonies. These results indicated that the blood lymphocytes of patients with congenital PRCA may have a role in suppressing marrow cell erythropoiesis of these patients. It should be noted, however, that the culture of autologous lymphocytes with marrow cells from patients with this disease was not reported and that further work is still necessary to determine if this is an autoimmune effect. Nevertheless, these experiments suggest that cellular immune processes may play a role in the pathogenesis of congenital PRCA rather than humoral immunity, which appears to be related to the pathogenesis of acquired PRCA.

### 5.4.2. Acquired PRCA

#### 5.4.2.1. Immunoglobulin Inhibitors of Marrow Erythroid Cells

The presence of a wide variety of associated immunologic abnormalities (see Section 5.3.2.2) and the high incidence of thymomas in patients with acquired PRCA suggested to several investigators that this disorder might have an immunologic pathogenesis. Jepson and Lowenstein (1966) administered plasma from two patients with PRCA to mice and found that the plasma depressed their erythropoiesis. Barnes (1966) presented preliminary evidence from cell culture experiments that patients with thymomas and refractory anemia had a serum immunoglobulin inhibitor of human marrow cell growth and proliferation. Field *et al.* (1968) also described a mouse stem cell suppressing factor in the serum of a patient with PRCA, thymoma, and Hodgkin's disease. In addition, many patients with acquired PRCA have responded to corticosteroids, cytotoxic drugs, and, occasionally, splenectomy, which have in common an immunosuppressive capacity and have been frequently utilized in autoimmune diseases (see Section 5.5.2.2).

Recent investigation into this disease has provided additional evidence that in some cases humoral immunity may be responsible for the reduced number of erythroblasts. The basis of many of these studies has been a cell culture system in which marrow cells respond to the addition of erythropoietin *in vitro* with an increase in hemoglobin synthesis (Krantz *et al.*, 1963). Human marrow cells are incubated at 37°C in a tissue culture solution containing normal human plasma. At daily time intervals, $^{59}Fe$, as $^{59}FeCl_3$ bound to transferrin, is added to the cultures. The $^{59}Fe$ is incorporated into hemoglobin and 4 hr later the marrow cells are lysed and heme is extracted for a measurement of its radioactivity. It has been shown that the heme radioactivity is equivalent to hemoglobin radioactivity (Gallien-Lartigue and Goldwasser, 1964) and that the addition of erythropoietin to cultures of normal human marrow cells produces a large increase in the rate of hemoglobin synthesis after 3 days of incubation (Krantz, 1965).

Marrow cells from eight patients with PRCA were studied in this way (Krantz and Kao, 1967, 1969; Safdar *et al.*, 1970; Krantz, 1972a, 1974; Krantz *et al.*, 1973). In five cases the addition of erythropoietin resulted in a three- to sixfold increase in the rate of heme synthesis above the original rate. In another similar case the increase in the rate of heme synthesis was accompanied by the appearance of increased erythroblasts *in vitro* with the development of more mature polychromatophilic erythroblasts (Zaentz *et al.*, 1975). In the remaining three cases heme synthesis either decreased or had an increase of less than twofold. This large increase in the rate of heme synthesis *in vitro*, above the original rate, could be explained by postulating either an inhibitor in the patient's body, from which the cells were freed, or a necessary new ingredient in the culture medium which the patient's body lacked. To distinguish between these alternatives, four of the five marrows which had a large response to the addition of erythropoietin *in vitro* were incubated in a balanced salt solution with only a little of the patient's plasma, containing antibiotics, heparin, and erythropoietin. The rate of heme synthesis of these marrows responded to erythropoietin with a 1.5- to 5.5-fold increase after 3 days of cell culture (Krantz, 1974). Since little had been added to the cells which could create such an increase it appeared that removing the marrow cells from the patients had freed them fron an inhibitor of heme synthesis. It should be added that all these patients had large amounts of erythropoietin in their blood and that many had previously received antibiotics for infections.

To demonstrate an inhibitor in these patients one of the patient's marrows was cultured with increasing concentrations of his own plasma or increasing concentrations of normal plasma, and the rate of heme synthesis was measured 3 days later (Krantz and Kao, 1967). Increased concentrations of the patient's plasma greatly inhibited the rate of heme synthesis of his own marrow cells compared to normal plasma (Fig. 2A). Furthermore, high concentrations of the patient's plasma prevented the large increase in heme synthesis that occurred when the patient's own marrow cells were incubated *in vitro* with erythropoietin (Krantz and Kao, 1967). These experiments indicated that the inhibition was not due to histocompatibility factors since a completely autologous system was being used. In addition, a similar inhibition was evident when the same plasmas were used with normal marrow cells (Fig. 2B). Of the eight patients whose marrows were studied and reported herein, six had plasmas that inhibited hemoglobin synthesis by normal marrow cells.

Because this inhibitor might be an antibody, the IgG-globulins from seven of these patients and from normal donors were purified. After

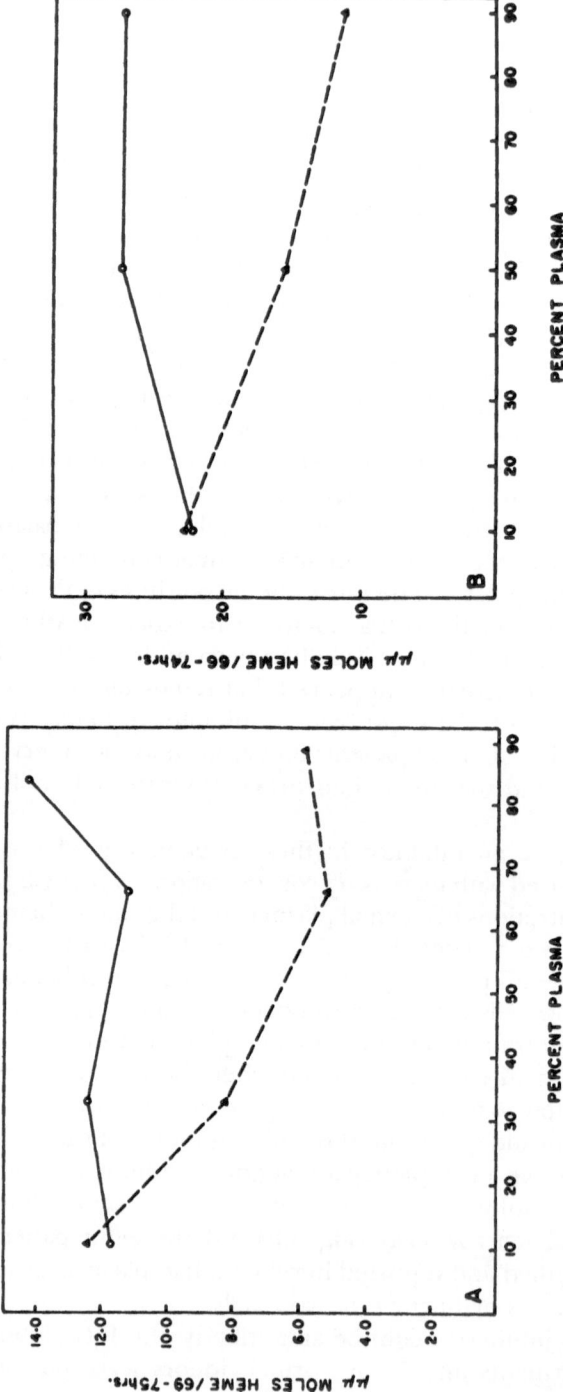

**Fig. 2.** Effect of concentration of patient's plasma and normal plasma on heme synthesis by (A) patient's marrow and (B) normal marrow. Cultures were started in a total volume of 1.0 ml medium which consisted of NCTC-109 and either the patient's plasma (–––) or normal plasma (———). $^{59}$Fe was added after 3 days of prior incubation for a period of 6 hr before extracting heme. (From Krantz and Kao, 1967, with the permission of the authors and publisher.)

ammonium sulfate precipitation and DEAE-cellulose chromatography the IgG-globulins were free of impurities on immunoelectrophoresis. Six of the IgG-globulins were incubated with normal marrow cells and inhibited the rate of heme synthesis by those cells *in vitro* when compared to normal IgG-globulins (Krantz, 1974). One of those patients had multiple blood samples drawn during a course of treatment with prednisone and cyclophosphamide and throughout a period of remission of the disease (Krantz *et al.*, 1973). The IgG-globulins of three blood samples drawn while the patient had PRCA markedly inhibited the rate of heme synthesis of his own marrow cells obtained after he was in remission and had many marrow erythroblasts (Fig. 3A). The IgG-globulins of two blood samples drawn during a posttreatment period had a greatly reduced inhibitory capacity, and this was associated with the appearance of increased reticulocytes in the patient's blood and the ability to sustain his own hematocrit (Fig. 3A). A similar effect of the patient's IgG-globulins was demonstrated when normal marrow cells were used *in vitro* (Fig. 3B). In both cases physiologic concentrations of IgG-globulins were utilized.

A serum IgG-globulin inhibitor to marrow erythropoiesis has also been demonstrated in the plasma of a PRCA patient with a thymoma, by studying the effect of the plasma on mouse erythropoiesis (Al-Mondhiry

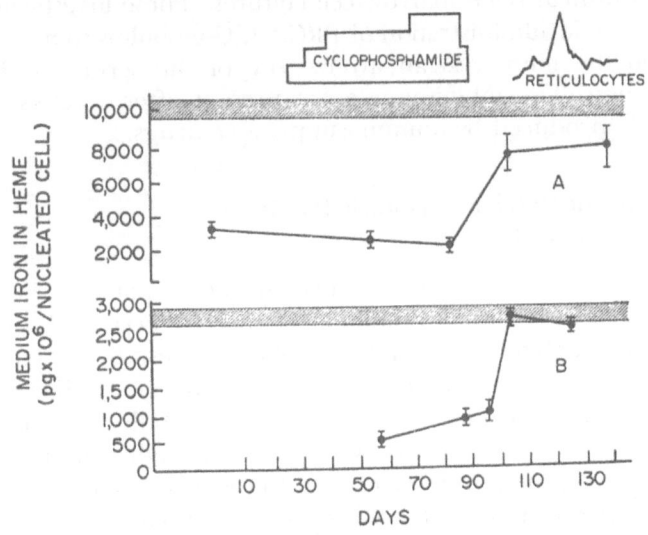

**Fig. 3.** Effect of patient's γG-globulins on heme synthesis by (A) patient's posttreatment marrow cells or (B) normal marrow cells. Marrow cultures were begun with γG-globulins present that were previously extracted from patient's plasma obtained at the days cited during treatment. After 44 hr of incubation $^{59}$Fe was added and 24 hr later heme was extracted. The shaded areas show the mean ± SEM for 20 cultures incubated with medium without added γG-globulins. (From Krantz *et al.*, 1973, with the permission of the authors and publisher.)

*et al.*, 1971). This patient, like those already described, had large amounts of erythropoietin in the plasma and urine. Both the patient's plasma and IgG-globulin fraction depressed [59]Fe incorporation into new mouse red cells. After thymectomy of the patient, a remission of the disease occurred and the plasma inhibitor no longer was present. No inhibitory activity was found in a saline extract of the thymoma in this patient or a subsequent patient (Jepson and Vas, 1974). Zalusky *et al.* (1973) have also shown that the serum and IgG-globulins of a patient with marked erythroid hypoplasia suppressed erythropoiesis in normal mice and heme synthesis in rat and human bone marrow cells *in vitro*. Chronic administration of the patient's serum to mice resulted in an anemia with a concomitant increase in the mouse's erythropoietin level. This patient also had large amounts of erythropoietin present and the patient's inhibitor did not behave like an antibody to erythropoietin since it did not appear to neutralize the hormone. The inhibitor was not absorbed by human or rat red cells or marrow from hypertransfused rats whose erythropoiesis was greatly suppressed. It was absorbed by normal rat marrow cells, however, indicating that the inhibitor might act directly on early erythroid cells. Marmont *et al.* (1975) also have demonstrated IgG-globulin inhibitors to marrow erythroid cells in the sera of patients with PRCA using normal mice, plethoric mice, and human bone marrow cell cultures. These investigators found that the chronic administration of PRCA IgG-globulins to mice produced anemia in the mice with an inverse rise of the serum erythropoietin concentration. The inhibitor was not present after a remission of the disease was produced by immunosuppressive drugs.

### 5.4.2.2. Immunoglobulins Cytotoxic for Marrow Erythroblasts

These experiments demonstrated that some patients with acquired PRCA had an IgG-globulin inhibitor of marrow erythroid cells in their plasma. The inhibitor reduced hemoglobin synthesis by the patient's own marrow cells *in vitro* and inhibited mouse erythropoiesis while erythropoietin levels remained quite high. The inhibitor could be producing this effect on the marrow cells in several ways. It might suppress new erythroblast development by interfering with the action of erythropoietin on the early, less differentiated, erythropoietin-responsive cells that develop into erythroblasts. The IgG-globulins could also have a cytotoxic effect on the already differentiated erythroblasts, producing erythroblast injury and death. It has been shown that cytotoxic effects of antibodies on cells produce a reduction in protein synthesis that parallels the cytotoxic injury as measured by trypan blue exclusion (Schecter *et al.*, 1974). In addition, Böttiger and Rausing (1972) studied a patient with PRCA whose marrow still had some erythroblasts and demonstrated fragmentation of the erythroblasts by electron microscopy.

A system capable of detecting cytotoxic injury to erythroblasts was developed to test the latter possibility (Krantz et al., 1973). Normal human marrow cells were incubated with NCTC-109 and human plasma to which $^{59}FeCl_3$ had been added. The incubation was carried out for 24 hr at 37°C in a 5% $CO_2$ atmosphere, and then the cells were washed extensively with a balanced salt solution to free them of the unincorporated radioisotope. It had previously been demonstrated that erythroblasts made most of the newly synthesized hemoglobin in the bone marrow (Thorell, 1947; Kailis and Morgan, 1974; Denton et al., 1975) and that under these conditions 100% of the erythroblasts were radioactive (Lau et al., 1970). The marrow cells with radioactive erythroblasts were then mixed with PRCA plasma, or IgG-globulins plus normal plasma, and were incubated for an additional 20–25 hr at 37°C in a 5% $CO_2$ atmosphere. After this, the cell suspensions were centrifuged and the supernatants were removed and counted. The amount of $^{59}Fe$ in the supernatant medium was shown to be proportional to the release of radioactive heme or hemoglobin from the marrow cells and was expressed as a release index (RI):

$$RI = \frac{\text{radioactivity of the supernatant}}{\text{total radioactivity}} \times 100$$

Using this system, a PRCA patient's pretreatment and posttreatment plasmas were incubated with the patient's $^{59}Fe$-labeled, posttreatment, highly erythropoietic bone marrow cells in vitro. The pretreatment plasma produced a release of $^{59}Fe$ into the medium that was twice as great as the posttreatment plasma or normal plasma, which were both similar. In addition, the patient's pretreatment IgG-globulins produced a 43% increase in the release of $^{59}Fe$ from his posttreatment marrow cells compared to his posttreatment IgG-globulins, and this effect was abolished by preincubation of the IgG-globulins with rabbit antibody to human IgG-globulins (Table IV). No effect of the patient's pretreatment IgG-globulins was observed on $^{51}Cr$-labeled lymphocytes or $^{51}Cr$-labeled marrow cells which contained 100-fold excess of $^{51}Cr$-labeled erythrocytes. These experiments demonstrated that the IgG-globulins of a patient with PRCA had a selective cytotoxicity for the patient's own erythroblasts and indicated that the erythroblastopenia of some patients with this disease might be due to antibodies or immune complexes that damage the erythroblasts and produce a premature demise of these particular cells. Although this patient had multiple blood transfusions and might have acquired antibodies to transfused cells the particular effect demonstrated here could not be due to histocompatibility factors since a completely autologous system was used. The demonstration of cytotoxicity for erythroblasts did not exclude

**Table IV.** Effect of RAHγGG[a] on Erythroblast Cytotoxicity Produced by Patient's γG-Globulins

| Cultures[b] No. | γG-Globulins (8.4 mg/ml) | Medium $^{59}$Fe (cpm) | Cell $^{59}$Fe (cpm) | $^{59}$Fe RI |
|---|---|---|---|---|
| 4 | Pretreatment | 3292 ± 77 | 7538 ± 130 | 30.4 ± 0.76 (<0.01) |
| 4 | Posttreatment | 2298 ± 26 | 8465 ± 52 | 21.4 ± 0.28 |
| 4 | Pretreatment plus RAHγGG | 2349 ± 69 | 8374 ± 108 | 21.9 ± 0.58 |
| 4 | Posttreatment plus RAHγGG | 2323 ± 68 | 8509 ± 217 | 21.4 ± 0.53 |

Mean values ± SEM are shown. $P$ values are shown in parentheses in between corresponding RI measurements if $P < 0.05$.
[a]RAHγGG: rabbit anti-human γG-globulin.
[b]Patient's posttreatment marrow cells labeled with $^{59}$Fe were incubated for 25 hr with patient's γG-globulins. Cells and supernatants were then separated and counts per minute measured. (Modified from Krantz *et al.*, 1973, with the permission of the authors and publisher.)

the possibility that reticulocytes, or the early erythropoietin-responsive cells that precede the erythroblasts, might also be injured by similar factors. Nor did it exclude the possibility that the receptors of the erythro-poietin-responsive cells for erythropoietin or transferrin might be blocked by similar factors, in some patients, producing an interference with the action of the hormone in promoting differentiation of these cells into erythroblasts.

In an effort to elucidate the mechanism of the cytotoxicity for ery-throblasts, the two-stage procedure devised by Amos and his co-workers (1969) for the detection of cytotoxicity for lymphocytes was adopted for use with marrow cells (Zaentz and Krantz, 1973). The $^{59}$Fe-labeled mar-row cells were first incubated for 1 hr at 37°C with PRCA or normal plasmas that had been heat-treated at 56°C for 1 hr to inactivate comple-ment. This first-stage mixture was then centrifuged and the supernatants were removed for the measurement of radioactivity. No difference was apparent. Fresh frozen normal human plasma was added to the cells and the second stage mixture was incubated for an additional 20 hr at 37°C in a 5% $CO_2$ atmosphere. The amount of radioactivity released into the second-stage supernatants was measured and was again expressed as a release index. Four out of seven PRCA plasmas produced an increased release of $^{59}$Fe into the second-stage supernatants when compared to normal plasmas. These same four plasmas had previously been shown to inhibit heme synthesis by marrow cells *in vitro* (Krantz, 1972a,b). PRCA IgG-globulins in the first stage produced a similar result. However, PRCA plasmas in the first stage were ineffective when the second-stage fresh frozen plasma was treated by a variety of methods that reduced complement activity: heat treatment at 56°C for 1 hr; pretreatment of the second-stage plasma with Suramin, a competitive inhibitor of the complement system; pretreatment with Zymosan, which depletes the plasma of complement components C3 and C5–C9; and treatment with sodium ethyleneglycoltetraacetic acid (EGTA), which binds calcium and inhibits the classic complement pathway. This dependence on PRCA IgG-globulins in the first stage and on complement in the second stage for cytotoxicity indicated that the cytotoxic factor was either an antibody or an immune complex. Like the preceding experiments using a single-stage cytotoxicity test, no increased cytotoxicity for $^{51}$Cr-labeled red cells from the same donors was observed.

Most of the patients with PRCA have had multiple blood transfusions and may have acquired antibodies to heterologous cells. To test the possibility that the multiple transfusions which these patients received might be responsible for the presence of complement-dependent cytotoxic antibodies to erythroblasts, a series of plasmas was obtained from other patients who had received a minimum of 10 transfusions over the previous 12 months. These plasmas were tested for cytotoxicity to erythroblasts in this system (Zaentz and Krantz, 1973). One of 11 such plasmas had significant cytotoxic activity. This plasma was obtained from a patient who was rejecting a renal transplant and had evidence of marrow failure at the time the sample was obtained. Further investigation is still needed to determine if these complement-dependent antibodies are acquired from multiple transfusions or if they are autoimmune and pathogenetic.

Recently, a similar but more sensitive system for the detection of complement-dependent cytotoxic antibodies to erythroblasts has been developed in which the radioactive marrow cells were first pretreated with glutathione to increase their sensitivity to complement (Zaentz et al., 1977). With this system, larger release indices were detected with some PRCA plasmas and cytotoxicity to erythroblasts could be detected with additional PRCA plasmas that did not affect untreated marrow cells (Fig. 4). Utilizing this method two PRCA plasmas that were cytotoxic for erythroblasts when tested on normal marrow cells, were not cytotoxic when incubated with the patients' own $^{59}$Fe-labeled marrow cells obtained when the patients were in remission and had many erythroblasts present (Krantz, 1977). In addition, two patients who received multiple transfusions, but did not have a refractory anemia, also had plasmas that were cytotoxic for erythroblasts (Krantz, 1977). This particular system may be detecting antibodies that have been acquired and are not autoimmune or pathogenetic. To avoid the problem of acquired antibodies and to confine the investigation of the pathogenesis of PRCA to autoimmune factors it may now be necessary to work with completely autologous systems.

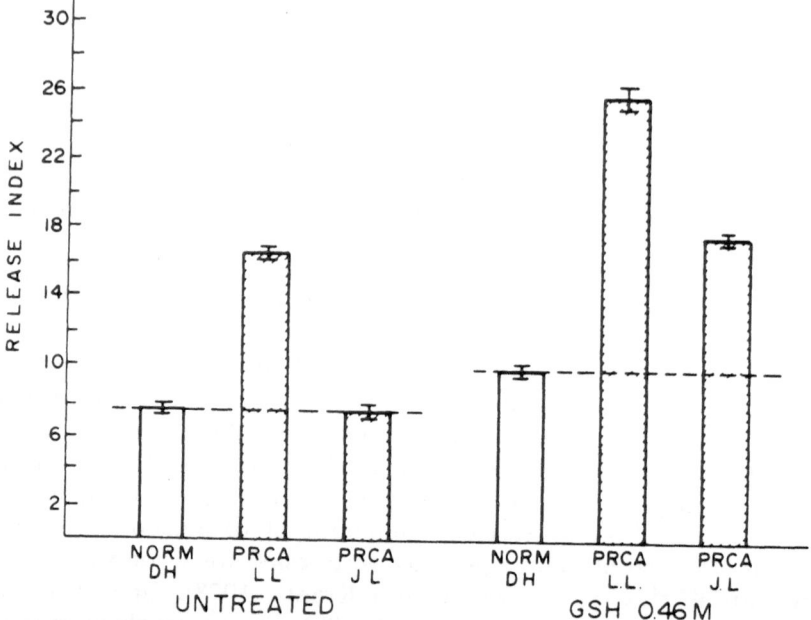

**Fig. 4.** $^{59}$Fe release indices resulting from incubation of normal (NORM) and PRCA plasmas with labeled human marrow cells from the same donor, which were untreated or treated with glutathione (GSH). Both patients had PRCA for more than a year and had received multiple blood transfusions. (From Zaentz *et al.*, 1977, with permission of the authors and publisher.)

### 5.4.2.3. Immunoglobulins That Inhibit Erythropoietin-Responsive Cells

It is also possible that an inhibitor of the marrow erythroid cells might act by interfering with further differentiation of the early erythropoietin-responsive cells (ERC) to the well-developed erythroblasts. It has been shown in other systems that inhibitors may interfere with target cell receptors, and thereby prevent the binding of a hormone to its target tissue (Carnegie and Mackay, 1975; Kahn *et al.*, 1976; Mittag *et al.*, 1976; Shiu and Friesen, 1976). Shiu and Friesen (1976) have demonstrated that a guinea pig antiserum selectively inhibited the binding of prolactin to mammary gland receptors, and reduced the prolactin-mediated incorporation of leucine into casein as well as the transport of aminoisobutyric acid. Mittag *et al.* (1976) have studied the sera of patients with myasthenia gravis and in many cases found anti-acetylcholine-receptor immunoglobulins, while other investigators have shown that antibodies against purified acetylcholine receptor can paralyze inoculated rabbits (Patrick and Lindstrom, 1973). In acquired acanthosis nigricans with insulin-resistant diabetes mellitus, antibodies to the insulin receptor of cultured human lymphoblastoid cells have been demonstrated (Kahn *et al.*, 1976). While antibodies to the erythropoietin receptor might block differentiation of the ERC, antibodies could also occur to other receptors, such as the transferrin receptor, that might block erythroblast development even when the primary signal to differentiation from the hormone had been received. It is also possible that a cytotoxic effect on the ERC could result from antibody activity, thereby reducing the number of these cells.

Recently a PRCA serum that had an IgG-globulin inhibitor of hemoglobin synthesis by normal human marrow cells, was shown to inhibit erythroid colony development in a plasma clot culture system (Browman et al., 1977). In the latter culture system, human marrow cells are seeded at a low concentration and, in the presence of erythropoietin, erythroid colonies develop from a precursor cell (Tepperman et al., 1974). When normal serum was replaced by PRCA serum a marked reduction in the number of erythroid colonies occurred either from autologous PRCA marrow cells or normal marrow cells (Browman et al., 1977; Freedman et al., 1976; Hoffman et al., 1976). It was concluded that the serum inhibitor acted at a progenitor cell level to block differentiation of these cells into new erythroblasts. Since complement was absent in this system it was unlikely that the inhibitory effect was due to immune cytolysis (Browman et al., 1977). It should be noted, however, that purified IgG-globulins were not actually added to the clot culture system. In addition, the PRCA serum replaced normal serum and it is still possible that the reduced number of erythroid colonies resulted from a deficiency of the PRCA serum rather than the presence of an inhibitor or that the inhibitor was directed against the hormone rather than the cells. Further investigation is necessary to delineate fully the mechanism of this interesting effect, but the possibility of an immunoglobulin inhibitor of the ERC is suggested by this preliminary work. Thus, it is possible that two types of inhibition of marrow erythroid cells may occur in PRCA: (a) inhibition by immunoglobulins cytotoxic for marrow erythroblasts, and (b) inhibition by immunoglobulins that inhibit the ERC either by blocking a critical cell receptor or through cytotoxicity.

### 5.4.2.4. Immunoglobulin Inhibitors of Erythropoietin

In contrast to many of these patients with PRCA are two individuals that have been described in whom the serum or urinary erythropoietin levels were greatly depressed for the degree of anemia (Jepson and Lowenstein, 1968; Peschle et al., 1975). The patient described by Jepson and Lowenstein (1968) had an aplastic marrow and not a red cell aplasia, no detectable urinary erythropoietin, and an apparent IgG-globulin inhibitor of normal erythropoietin. The second patient was studied in much greater detail (Peschle et al., 1975). This patient had a depressed serum erythropoietin level. When the patient's IgG-globulins were incubated with erythropoietin the latter was neutralized. Additional incubation with goat anti-human $\gamma$-globulin to remove the inhibitor from the serum did not restore the erythropoietin activity, as it did when patients' IgG-globulin inhibitors to marrow cells were incubated with the same goat anti-human $\gamma$-globulin antibody. This indicated that in the former case the inhibitor might be attached to erythropoietin, whereas in the latter case it was distinct and separable from the hormone. Furthermore, the patient's serum erythropoietin activity was increased by acidification and boiling which denatures IgG-globulins, but not erythropoietin. After successful immunosuppressive treatment of this patient, the inhibitor to the hormone was not present and erythropoietin levels were increased. This type of PRCA, which occurs with an IgG-globulin inhibitor of erythropoietin, was termed PRCA type B in contrast to the cases that had an inhibitor to the marrow cells and were termed PRCA type A. It is possible that the type A patients may be subdivided into two groups: $A_1$ with cytotoxic antibody to erythroblasts and $A_2$ with an inhibitor to ERC development.

Although inhibition of marrow erythroid cells or erythropoietin by IgG-globulins may be pathogenetic for PRCA in some cases, other mechanisms for the disease might also exist. It is possible that cellular immunity may play a role in this disease. Zanjani et al. (1975) have shown that the lymphocytes of a patient with variable immunodeficiency and a steroid-responsive PRCA in remission, inhibited erythroid colony formation by human marrow cells in vitro. Lymphocytes from normal donors did not do this, but the result of incubating PRCA lymphocytes in a completely autologous system was not reported. It is also possible that antibody-dependent cellular cytotoxicity might play a role in this condition. This is an immune mechanism in which antibody-coated cells are damaged by attack lymphocytes (Ortiz de Landazuri et al., 1974). In addition, nonimmune mechanisms, such as acquired metabolic deficiencies, might occur which could produce this disease since riboflavin deficiency has been associated with PRCA (Alfrey and Lane, 1970). There remains a group of PRCA patients in whom no inhibitors or metabolic deficiencies have been demonstrated. The pathogenesis of the disease in these patients is unknown, and such cases have been termed "idiopathic."

## 5.5. Treatment

### 5.5.1. Congenital PRCA

Corticosteroid therapy has been used on an empiric basis to treat the congenital form of PRCA after transfusion of any necessary red cells (Gasser, 1951, 1957). Most patients with this disease if diagnosed and treated early will respond to this form of treatment. In the series of patients reported by Allan and Diamond (1961), 11 out of 13 consecutive infants treated with corticosteroids responded with increased erythropoiesis. These patients frequently relapsed, especially after infection, and many needed temporary reinstitution of corticosteroids. Some children are dependent on the chronic administration of extremely small amounts of corticosteroids, such as 5 mg/day of prednisone, for the maintenance of their erythropoiesis. Infants who were treated immediately after the disease was recognized responded better than those with long-standing disease. In the series of Allan and Diamond (1961), patients who responded to corticosteroids had an average duration of disease of 7 months whereas nonresponding patients had an average duration of disease of 7 years. None of the patients whose disease already was present for 3 years responded to corticosteroids.

The reason for the success of this form of therapy in congenital PRCA is unknown. The recent work of Hoffman *et al.* (1976) suggests that peripheral blood lymphocytes may play a role in the pathogenesis of the condition. If cellular immunity is responsible for the reduced erythropoiesis, this could provide an explanation for the favorable effect of corticosteroids which produce a lymphopenia and are immunosuppressive. One 15-month-old child has been described who responded to treatment with 6-mercaptopurine (Siegler *et al.*, 1970), but an immune pathogenesis was not demonstrated in that case. Another 5-year-old child also responded to 6-mercaptopurine and prednisone, but he probably had an acquired PRCA (Wranne *et al.*, 1970).

### 5.5.2. Acquired PRCA

The initial therapy of acquired PRCA consists of supporting the patient with transfusions of packed red blood cells while initiating a search for any possible underlying cause for the condition. If the red cell aplasia is uncomplicated by hemolysis or hemorrhage, these patients generally require an average of 1 unit of red cells per week to maintain a hemoglobin range of 9–12 g/100 ml. Many of the cases of PRCA appear to be secondary to infections or drugs, and because they may be acute and self-limited, any additional treatment may be delayed for 1–2 months. The "aplastic" crisis of hemolytic anemia is also usually self-limited (see Section 5.2.3). A history of infection or drug ingestion is helpful, and any drug that the patient is taking that might be related to the PRCA should be discontinued.

Four cases of PRCA with folate or vitamin $B_{12}$ deficiency plus either severe malnutrition, alcoholism, hypothyroidism, or pregnancy have been reported; in these cases the anemia responded to folic acid or vitamin $B_{12}$, plus additional therapy for the accompanying disorders (Pezzimenti and Lindenbaum, 1972). Serum folate and $B_{12}$ levels should be measured and if they are low, treatment for 1–2 weeks should be initiated. In most cases, however, treatment with different hematinics such as vitamin $B_{12}$, folic acid, pyridoxine, and liver extract has not been successful (Roland, 1964).

When PRCA occurs in association with severe renal failure, a remission of the anemia may be dependent on the results of the treatment of the primary disorder (Gasser, 1957). The PRCA that may occur with systemic lupus erythematosus, or with neoplasms other than the thymoma, is often chronic and best treated like a chronic acquired primary PRCA. Many of these patients have had a response to corticosteroids (Table II).

### 5.5.2.1. Thymectomy

If a resectable thymoma is found, the tumor should be excised. When PRCA occurs with a thymoma removal of the tumor has resulted in a remission of the disease in 29% of the cases (Jacobs *et al.*, 1959) and has improved the response rate to corticosteroids in others (Roland, 1964; Hirst and Robertson, 1967). One patient responded to an androgenic steroid after resection of a thymoma (Hirst and Robertson, 1967). Most patients did not respond to corticosteroids unless the thymoma was first resected (Roland, 1964; Hirst and Robertson, 1967). Only one out of nine patients with a thymoma responded to corticosteroids without prior removal of the thymoma (Hirst and Robertson, 1967). Irradiation of the thymoma has generally not produced a remission of the PRCA (Roland, 1964). However, one patient with PRCA, Hodgkin's disease, and a thymoma had a remission of the PRCA after the thymoma was irradiated (Field *et al.*, 1968), and several patients responded to corticosteroids after their thymomas were treated with irradiation (Roland, 1964; Hamilton and Conley, 1969). One patient with PRCA and a thymoma responded to cyclophosphamide and prednisone with a remission of the anemia, after refusing excision of the tumor (Marmont *et al.*, 1975). Therefore, if a thymoma is present in a patient with PRCA it should be excised because of the high remission rate and the possibility of malignancy. If it cannot be excised, it should either be irradiated, a treatment that may have to be followed by corticosteroid therapy, or the patient should receive cyclophosphamide and corticosteroids in combination.

One elective resection of a normal thymus gland in a patient with primary acquired PRCA has been reported (Soulter and Emerson, 1960). A brief increase in reticulocytes occurred, but no remission of the disease followed. This patient eventually died of acute leukemia. We have performed a similar elective thymectomy in a patient with PRCA who did not respond to corticosteroids and cyclophosphamide, splenectomy, or androgenic steroids, but no erythropoietic response was noted months later (Krantz and Zaentz, unpublished observations).

### 5.5.2.2. Immunosuppressive Drugs

Patients who are still transfusion dependent after 1–2 months and in whom no cause for the condition can be detected have a chronic acquired primary PRCA. Since some of these cases are associated with the presence of immunoglobulin inhibitors of erythroid cells, or of erythropoietin, a trial of immunosuppressive therapy should be considered. Immunosuppressive drugs have been effective in some of these cases even when no immunoglobulin inhibitor could be demonstrated (Zaentz et al., 1977), so we believe that a careful trial of this type of therapy is warranted even when the precise pathogenesis has not been revealed. Corticosteroids alone (Gasser, 1957; Tsai and Levin, 1957; Roland, 1964; Schmid et al., 1965) or cytotoxic immunosuppressive drugs such as 6-mercaptopurine (Krantz and Kao, 1967), azathioprine (Böttiger and Rausing, 1972), or cyclophosphamide (Krantz and Kao, 1969; Vilan et al., 1973) have produced remissions of this disease. In addition, combinations of cyclophosphamide and prednisone (Krantz et al., 1973; Zaentz et al., 1976) or cyclophosphamide and antilymphocyte globulin have been effective (Krantz, 1972; Marmont et al., 1975; Peschle et al., 1975). In children or patients of childbearing age, high daily doses (40–60 mg/day) of prednisone should be administered first as a single agent to try to avoid the mutagenic effects and possible sterility that may result from cytotoxic immunosuppressive agents (Fairley et al., 1972; Udall et al., 1972). In older patients combined therapy with prednisone and a cytotoxic immunosuppressive drug would be our treatment of choice since such combined therapy should have a high degree of therapeutic effectiveness while permitting a decrease in the prednisone dosage to a level with fewer side effects.

At least nine adult patients with PRCA have now been reported who have responded to treatment with 6-mercaptopurine, azathioprine, cyclophosphamide, or cyclophosphamide plus prednisone with a remission of the disease (Krantz and Kao, 1967, 1969; Safdar et al., 1970; Böttiger and Rausing, 1972; Krantz et al., 1973; Vilan et al., 1973; Krantz, 1974; Marmont et al., 1975; Zaentz et al., 1976). The number of failures with these drugs is harder to ascertain, but in our series three of eight consecutive patients treated with these agents did not have a remission of their disease (Krantz, 1974). With some patients an increase in blood reticulocytes 1–8 weeks after starting therapy was the first indication of a response (Krantz and Kao, 1967; Safdar et al., 1970; Böttiger and Rausing, 1972;

Vilan *et al.*, 1973; Hartmann and Krantz, 1974; Marmont *et al.*, 1975). In Fig. 5 is shown the course of a 43-year-old white male who had primary PRCA for 2 years. The figure shows that this patient had no blood reticulocytes and his packed cell volume declined and had to be restored with red cell transfusions every 2–3 weeks. The patient was begun on prednisone 30 mg/day, and cyclophosphamide 100 mg/day. We generally begin cyclophosphamide therapy at 50 mg/day, but this patient previously had a short course of the drug which indicated that he was not overly sensitive to 100 mg/day. The cyclophosphamide was gradually increased in stepwise increments and 40 days after beginning treatment the first increase in reticulocytes was noted. The cyclophosphamide and prednisone were continued until the patient could sustain his own hematocrit and were then discontinued. This patient is presented as an example of one type of response, an initial increase in reticulocytes, observed with immunosuppressive drugs. In his case, the precise role of each of the two drugs was not ascertained. However, other patients, have responded in a similar manner to cyclophosphamide or azathioprine alone (Vilan *et al.*, 1973; Böttiger and Rausing, 1972), or to 6-mercaptopurine with a small amount of prednisone, or to cyclophosphamide with a small amount of prednisone, when prior high doses of prednisone were ineffective (Krantz and Kao, 1967, 1969; Safdar *et al.*, 1970).

In some patients with PRCA, however, the drugs were administered for 2–3 months with a gradual increase in the dose of the cytotoxic immunosuppressive agent and no increase in reticulocytes occurred (Krantz and Kao, 1969; Krantz *et al.*, 1973; Marmont *et al.*, 1975). The drugs were then continued and slowly increased until marrow toxicity occurred as judged by a white cell count of 2000 cells/$\mu$l, or a platelet count of 80,000–90,000/$\mu$l. The drugs were then discontinued and marrow recovery generally occurred in 3–5 weeks. This was the maximum amount of the cytotoxic drug the patients could tolerate and with marrow recovery there often occurred a reticulocytosis and the capacity to sustain a normal hematocrit. Because these drugs can greatly depress the white cell and platelet concentrations it is necessary to obtain complete blood counts initially every week, and later every 2 weeks, to avoid overtreatment or extreme marrow toxicity.

Horse antihuman thymocyte or lymphocyte $\gamma$-globulin has been administered to patients with PRCA in combination with cyclophosphamide or corticosteroids and appears to have been of help in two patients although it was associated with serum sickness in a third (Krantz, 1972; Marmont *et al.*, 1975; Peschle *et al.*, 1975). Antilymphocyte globulin is very variable, however, in its therapeutic effectiveness and in its toxicity, and is only available as a research drug at the present time. Until a more standardized product is available and more experience is gained with its

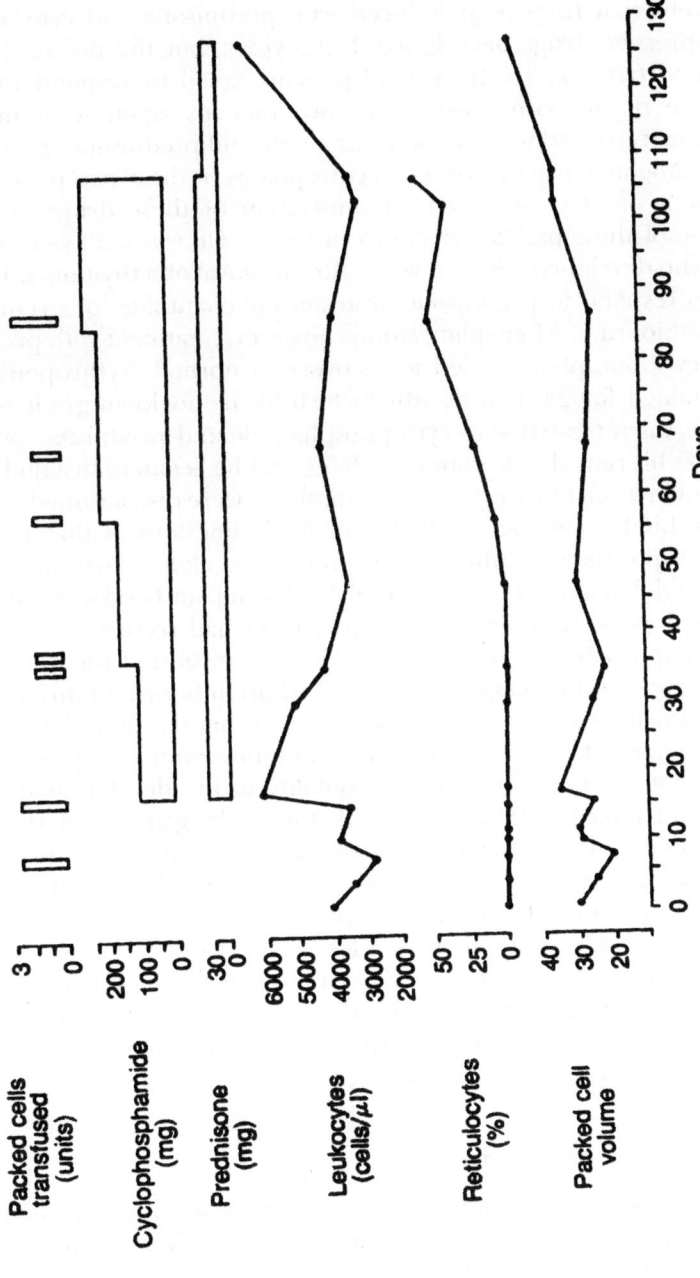

**Fig. 5.** Prednisone–cyclophosphamide treatment of pure red cell aplasia of 2 years' duration in a 43-year-old man. Patient needed frequent red cell transfusions during first 40 days of treatment to maintain packed cell volume. Reticulocytes in blood increased to substantial number before evidence of marrow toxicity appeared and were the indication for terminating cyclophosphamide treatment. (From Hartmann and Krantz, 1974, with permission of the authors and publisher.)

use, it should be restricted to very refractory cases and used under carefully controlled conditions.

Remissions that have been induced with prednisone and cytotoxic immunosuppressive drugs have lasted 1–3½ years, but the disease has often returned (Krantz, 1974). Several patients failed to respond to a second course of the same drugs, but two patients again went into remission when retreated with cyclophosphamide and prednisone (Zaentz et al., 1976). Maintenance of normal erythropoiesis in these two patients was dependent on the continued administration of these drugs. The course of one of these patients is shown in Fig. 6. He was a 50-year-old white male who developed PRCA 2 years after removal of a thymoma. He had failed to respond to prednisone, testosterone enanthate, or prednisone with azathioprine. After splenectomy, however, treatment with prednisone and cyclophosphamide led to recovery of normal erythropoiesis that was sustained for 24 months, after which his hemoglobin gradually declined. He was retreated with cyclophosphamide and prednisone and within 3 weeks his reticulocyte count was 8.5% and he began to sustain his own hemoglobin level. Once again the medications were discontinued. Six months later his hemoglobin again began to decline and at that time normal erythropoiesis was induced with prednisone alone. Two months later his hemoglobin again had fallen to 6.4 g/100 ml, and cyclophosphamide and prednisone were restarted. This patient had recurrent PRCA that returned approximately every 6 months. A remission of the disease was then reinduced with cyclophosphamide and prednisone and this time he was maintained on 15 mg of prednisone every other day and 50 mg of cyclophosphamide a day. He then remained in remission for 2½ years.

Were it not for the increased susceptibility to the development of malignancy and infection that occurs with the prolonged use of these drugs, we would consider maintaining all PRCA patients on cytotoxic immunosuppressive drugs for a period of time after induction of a remission. It is possible, however, that patients treated earlier in the course of the disease, or patients with a less severe form of the disease, might not have the same incidence of recurrence as these patients who had a very severe, chronic PRCA. Since the risk-to-benefit ratio of such maintenance therapy is unknown a study randomizing maintenance and nonmaintenance therapy is greatly needed.

### 5.5.2.3. Splenectomy; Androgens

Those patients who do not respond to immunosuppressive drugs may have a remission following splenectomy. Although some patients with PRCA fail to respond to splenectomy (Jacobs et al., 1959; Schmid et al., 1965; Hirst and Robertson, 1967; Krantz and Kao, 1967, 1969), in at

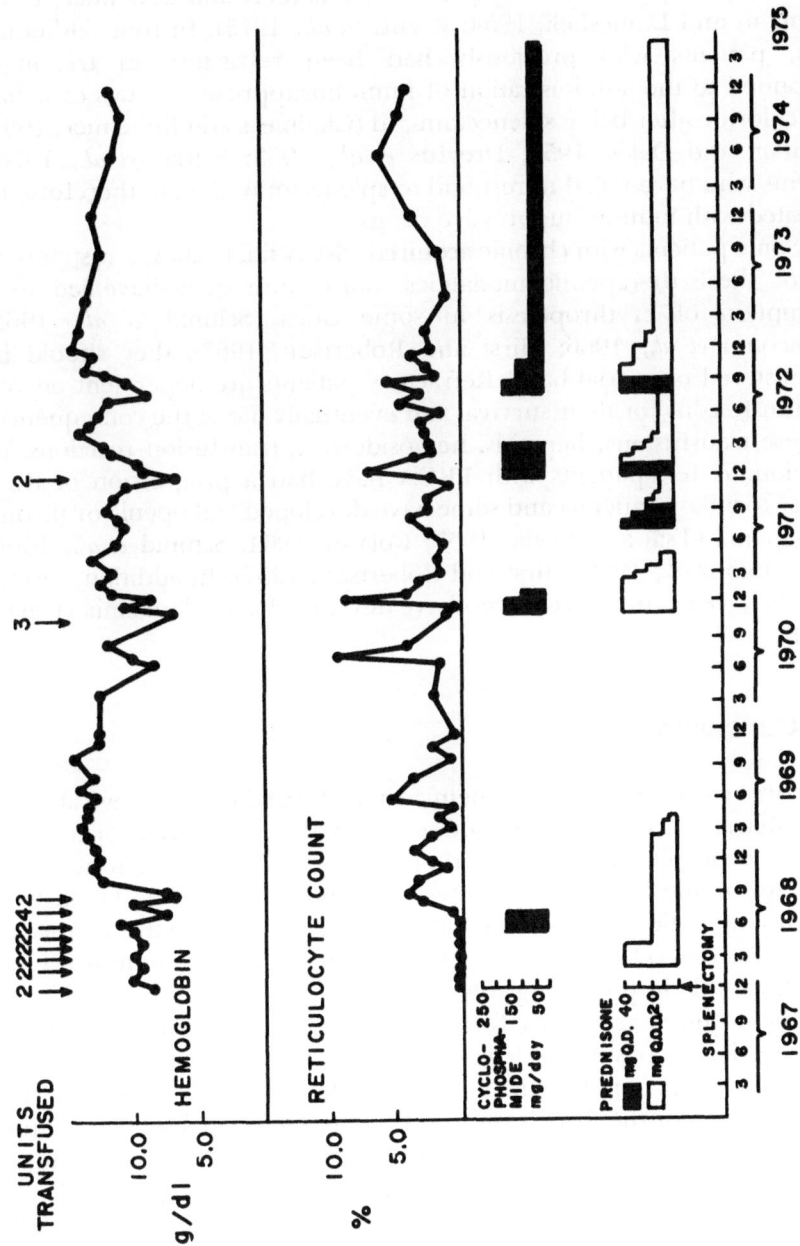

**Fig. 6.** Clinical progress of a patient with PRCA. (From Zaentz *et al.*, 1976, with permission of the authors and publisher.)

least five adults the procedure has been followed by a resumption of normal erythropoiesis (Loeb *et al.*, 1953; Chalmers and Boheimer, 1954; Eisemann and Dameshek, 1954; Zaentz *et al.*, 1975). In four additional cases, patients who previously had been refractory to treatment responded to the administration of immunosuppressive drugs or cobaltous chloride after being splenectomized (Chalmers and Boheimer, 1954; Fountain and Dales, 1955; Dreyfus *et al.*, 1963; Safdar *et al.*, 1970). Patients who have failed to respond to splenectomy should, therefore, be retreated with immunosuppressive drugs.

Some patients with chronic acquired PRCA fail to show a response to any of these therapeutic modalities. Since androgens have led to a resumption of erythropoiesis in some cases (Schmid *et al.*, 1965; DiGiacomo *et al.*, 1966; Hirst and Robertson, 1967), they should be administered on a trial basis. Refractory patients are dependent on red cell transfusions for their survival and eventually die of the consequences of these transfusions: hepatitis, hemosiderosis, transfusion reactions, or infection. A few patients with PRCA have had a progression of their disease to aplastic anemia and some have developed leukopenia or thrombocytopenia (Tsai and Levin, 1957; Roland, 1964; Schmid *et al.*, 1965; DiGiacomo *et al.*, 1966; Hirst and Robertson, 1967). In addition, several patients have been reported who have developed acute leukemia (Pierre, 1974).

## 5.6. Conclusion

Pure red cell aplasia is an anemia characterized by a selective absence of the marrow erythroid cells. Both congenital and acquired forms exist, with the congenital variety occurring during the first 18 months of life and often remitting with corticosteroid administration. The blood lymphocytes of patients with congenital PRCA depress erythropoiesis by normal marrow cells *in vitro,* suggesting that cellular immune processes may play a role in producing this condition.

The acquired secondary form of PRCA has occurred in association with infection, exposure to drugs or chemicals, or hemolytic anemia. In these cases it is generally acute and self-limited; it usually subsides as the infection clears or the drug is removed. It has also occurred in association with severe renal failure, severe nutritional deficiency, systemic lupus erythematosus, rheumatoid arthritis, and a variety of neoplasms. In the first two instances remission of the PRCA may be dependent on successful treatment of the primary disorder. In the remainder, excluding cases with thymomas, the PRCA is best treated like an acquired primary PRCA and often responds to corticosteroids. PRCA has a very high association with thymomas and remits in 29% of these cases where the thymoma is resected. Thus, thymectomy is recommended wherever a thymic tumor has been demonstrated.

In the remaining cases of acquired primary PRCA the disease tends to be chronic and in some cases may have an immune pathogenesis. IgG-globulin inhibitors of the marrow cells and of erythropoietin have been demonstrated. In the former case, a patient's own IgG-globulins may produce a marked decrease of hemoglobin synthesis by his marrow cells and may be cytotoxic to his own erythroblasts as demonstrated by the release of $^{59}$Fe-labeled hemoglobin from the cells into the surrounding medium. In some cases the plasma of these patients inhibits the erythropoietin-responsive cells of normal or autologous bone marrows from further erythroid development. Patients with immunoglobulin inhibitors of the marrow erythroid cells generally have high erythropoietin levels. Where inhibitors to erythropoietin have been demonstrated, the patient's IgG-globulins have neutralized the hormone and these patients have had very low erythropoietin levels.

Other immune pathogenetic mechanisms could also be present in acquired PRCA, but remain to be demonstrated. It is possible that cellular immunity or antibody-dependent cellular cytotoxicity may have a role in this disease. As the methods for studying PRCA have become more developed, increased sensitivity may be revealing antibodies to erythroblasts that are acquired from multiple transfusions and that may necessitate the use of completely autologous systems to study the pathogenesis of this disease.

The demonstration of immune inhibitors of erythropoiesis in this disease has led to its successful treatment, in some cases, with immunosuppressive drugs such as cyclophosphamide, 6-mercaptopurine, or antilymphocyte globulin, with or without corticosteroids. In addition, splenectomy may be of benefit in some cases. To study PRCA a model system involving erythropoietin-responsive cells, erythroblasts, and the hormone erythropoietin exists. With this system it may be possible to distinguish several immune pathogenetic mechanisms for the PRCA. Hopefully, this knowledge may then be applied to the study of aplastic anemia where the pluripotential colony-forming cells could be injured by a similar mechanism, but where a model system for the factors that control the development of this cell is still undeveloped. The experimental techniques designed to study PRCA provide a means for investigating an immune pathogenesis in a wide range of "refractory anemias" or "marrow failures" and may define a broader category of anemia due to immune injury of marrow cells.

# References

Abeloff, M. D., and Waterbury, L., 1974, Pure red cell aplasia and chronic lymphocytic leukemia, *Arch. Intern. Med.* **134**:721.

Alfrey, C. P., and Lane, M., 1970, The effect of riboflavin deficiency on erythropoiesis, *Semin. Hematol.* **7**:49.

Allan, D. M., and Diamond, L. K., 1961, Congenital (erythroid) hypoplastic anemia, *Am. J. Dis. Child.* **102**:416.

Al-Mondhiry, H., Zanjani, E. D., Spivack, M., Zalusky, R., and Gordon, A. S., 1971, Pure red cell aplasia and thymoma: Loss of serum inhibitor of erythropoiesis following thymectomy, *Blood* **38**:576.

Amos, D. B., Bashir, H., Boyle, W., MacQueen, M., and Tiilikainen, A., 1969, A simple microcytotoxicity test, *Transplantation* **7**:220.

Barnes, R. D., 1965, Thymic neoplasms associated with refractory anemia, *Guys Hosp. Rep.* **114**:73.

Barnes, R. D., 1966, Refractory anemia with thymoma, *Lancet* **2**:1464.

Battle, J. D., Hewlett, J. S., and Hoffman, G. C., 1963, Prolonged erythroid aplasia in chronic lymphocytic leukemia, *Ann. Intern. Med.* **58**:731.

Böttiger, L. E., and Rausing, A., 1972, Pure red cell anemia: Immunosuppressive treatment, *Ann. Intern. Med.* **76**:593.

Bouroncle, B. A., 1964, Familial crisis in hereditary spherocytosis, *Am. Med. Wom. Assoc. J.* **19**:1045.

Bove, J. R., 1956, Combined erythroid hypoplasia and symptomatic hemolytic anemia, *N. Engl. J. Med.* **255**:135.

Brafield, A. J. E., and Verbov, J., 1966, A case of thrombocythaemia with red cell aplasia, *Postgrad. Med. J.* **42**:525.

Brittingham, T. E., Lutcher, C. L., and Murphy, D. L., 1964, Reversible erythroid aplasia induced by diphenylhydantoin, *Arch. Intern. Med.* **113**:764.

Browman, G. P., Freedman, M. H., Blajchman, M. A., and McBride, J. A., 1977, A complement independent erythropoietic inhibitor acting on the progenitor cell in refractory anemia, *Am. J. Med.* **61**:572.

Carnegie, P. R., and Mackay, I. R., 1975, Vulnerability of cell-surface receptors to autoimmune reactions, *Lancet* **2**:684.

Cassileth, P. A., and Myers, A. R., 1973, Erythroid aplasia in systemic lupus erythematosis, *Am. J. Med.* **55**:706.

Chalmers, J. N. M., and Boheimer, K., 1954, Pure red-cell anaemia in patients with thymic tumours, *Br. Med. J.* **2**:1514.

Chernoff, A. I., and Josephson, A. M., 1951, Acute erythroblastopenia in sickle cell anemia and infectious mononucleosis, *Am. J. Dis. Child.* **82**:310.

Clarkson, B., and Prokop, D. J., 1958, Aregenerative anemia associated with benign thymoma, *N. Engl. J. Med.* **259**:253.

Cornet, A., Cornu, P., Barbier, J. P., Favriel, J. M., and Massouline, G., 1974, A case of reversible erythroblastopenia due to thiamphenicol, *Sem. Hop. Paris* **50**:1567.

Dameshek, W., Brown, S. M., and Rubin, A. D., 1967, "Pure" red cell anemia (erythroblastic hypoplasia) and thymoma, *Semin. Hematol.* **4**:222.

Davis, L. J., Kennedy, A. C., Baikie, A. G., and Brown, A., 1952, Hemolytic anemias of various types treated with ACTH and cortisone, *Glasgow Med. J.* **33**:263.

Denton, M. J., Spencer, N., and Arnstein, H. R. V., 1975, Biochemical and enzymic changes during erythrocyte differentiation. The significance of the final cell division, *Biochem. J.* **146**:205.

DeSevilla, E., Forrest, J. V., Zivnuska, F. R., and Sagel, S. S., 1975, Metastatic thymoma with myasthenia gravis and pure red cell aplasia, *Cancer* **36**:1154.

Diamond, L., and Blackfan, K. D., 1938, Hypoplastic anemia, *Am. J. Dis. Child.* **56**:464.

Diamond, L. K., Allen, D. M., and Magill, F. B., 1961, Congenital (erythroid) hypoplastic anemia, *Am. J. Dis. Child.* **102**:403.

DiGiacomo, J., Furst, S. W., and Nixon, D. D., 1966, Primary acquired red cell aplasia in the adult, *J. Mt. Sinai Hosp., N.Y.* **33**:382.

Doughaday, W. H., 1968, Lupus erythematosus with severe anemia, selective erythroid hypoplasia and multiple red blood cell isoantibodies, *Am. J. Med.* **44**:590.

Dreyfus, B., Aubert, P., Patte, D., and LeBolloc'h Combrisson, A., 1963, Erythroblastopenic chronique decouverte aprés une thymectomie, *Nouv. Rev. Fr. Hematol.* **3**:765.

Eisemann, G., and Dameshek, W., 1954, Splenectomy for "pure red-cell" hypoplastic (aregenerative) anemia associated with autoimmune hemolytic disease. Report of a case, *N. Engl. J. Med.* **251**:1044.

Entwistle, C. C., Fentem, P. H., and Jacobs, A., 1964, Red-cell aplasia with carcinoma of the bronchus, *Br. Med. J.* **2**:1504.

Fairley, K. F., Barrie, J. U., and Johnson, W., 1972, Sterility and testicular atrophy related to cyclophosphamide therapy, *Lancet* **1**:568.

Field, E. O., Caughi, M. N., Blackett, N. M., and Smithers, D. W., 1968, Marrowsuppressing factors in the blood in pure red-cell aplasia, thymoma and Hodgkin's disease, *Br. J. Haematol.* **15**:101.

Fountain, J. R., and Dales, M., 1955, Pure red cell aplasia successfully treated with cobalt, *Lancet* **1**:541.

Foy, H., and Kondi, A., 1961, Pure red-cell aplasia in marasmus and kwashiorkor treated with riboflavin, *Br. Med. J.* **1**:397.

Freedman, M. H., Amato, D., and Saunders, E. F., 1975, Haem synthesis in the Diamond–Blackfan syndrome, *Br. J. Haematol.* **31**:515.

Freedman, M. H., Amato, D., and Saunders, E. F., 1976, Erythroid colony growth in congenital hypoplastic anemia, *J. Clin. Invest.* **57**:673.

Gallien-Lartigue, O., and Goldwasser, E., 1964, Hemoglobin synthesis in marrow cell culture: The effect of rat plasma on rat cells, *Science* **145**:277.

Gasser, C., 1949, Akute Erythroblastopenie: Zehn Fälle aplasticher Erythroblastenkrisen mit Riesenproerythroblasten bei allergischotischen Zustandsbidern, *Helv. Paediatr. Acta* **4**:107.

Gasser, C., 1951, Aplastiche Anämie (chronische Erythroblastophthise) und Cortison, *Schweiz, Med. Wochenschr.* **81**:1241.

Gasser, C., 1957, Aplasia of erythropoiesis: Acute and chronic erythroblastopenia or pure (red cell) aplastic anemia in childhood, *Pediatr. Clin. N. Am.* **4**:445.

Geller, G., Krivit, W., Zalusky, R., and Zanjani, E. D., 1975, Lack of erythropoietic inhibitory effect of serum from patients with congenital pure red cell aplasia. *J. Pediatr.* **86**:198.

Gilbert, E. F., Harley, J. B., Anido, V., Mengoli, H. F., and Hughes, J. T., 1968, Thymoma, plasma cell myeloma, red cell aplasia and malabsorption syndrome, 1968, *Am. J. Med.* **44**:820.

Goodman, S. B., and Block, M. H., 1964, A case of red cell aplasia occurring as a result of anti-tuberculosis therapy, *Blood* **24**:616.

Green, P., 1958, Aplastic anemia associated with thymoma, *Can. Med. Assoc. J.* **78**:419.

Hamilton, Jr., C. R., and Conley, C. L., 1969, Pure red cell aplasia and thymoma, *Johns Hopkins Med. J.* **125**:262

Hamilton, P. J., Dawson, A. A., and Galloway, W. H., 1974, Congenital erythroid hypoplastic anemia in mother and daughter, *Arch. Dis. Child.* **49**:71.

Hammond, D., Shore, N., and Movassaghi, N., 1968, Production, utilization and excretion of erythropoietin. I. Chronic anemias. II. Aplastic crisis. III. Erythropoietic effects of normal plasma, *Ann. N.Y. Acad. Sci.* **149**:516.

Hartmann, R. C., and Krantz, S. B., 1974, Paroxysmal nocturnal hemoglobinuria and pure red cell aplasia. Two rare anemias with immunologic implications, *Postgrad. Med.* **55**:141.

Hirst, F., and Robertson, T. I., 1967, The syndrome of thymoma and erythroblastopenic anemia, *Medicine* **46**:225.

Hoffman, R., Zanjani, E. D., Vila, J., Zalusky, R., Lutton, J. D., and Wasserman, L. R., 1976, Diamond–Blackfan syndrome: Lymphocyte-mediated suppression of erythropoiesis, *Science* **193**:899.

Holborow, E. J. Asherson, G. L., Johnson, G. D., Barnes, R. D. S., and Carmichael, D. S., 1963, Antinuclear factor and other antibodies in blood and liver diseases, *Br. Med. J.* **1**:656.

Hughes, D. W. O'G., 1961, Hypoplastic anemia in infancy and childhood: Erythroid hypoplasia. *Arch. Dis. Child.* **36**:349.

Hunt, F. A., and Lander, C. M., 1975, Successful use of combination chemotherapy in pure red cell aplasia associated with malignant lymphoma, of histiocytic type, *Aust. N.Z. J. Med.* **5**:469.

Hunter, R. E., and Hakami, N., 1972, The occurrence of congenital hypoplastic anemia in half brothers, *J. Pediatr.* **81**:346.

Ibrahim, J. M., Raustron, J., and Booth, J., 1966, A case of red cell aplasia in a Negro child, *Arch. Dis. Child.* **41**:213.

Jacobs, E. M., Hutter, R. V. P., Pool, J. L., and Ley, A. B., 1959, Benign thymoma and selective erythroid aplasia of the bone marrow, *Cancer* **12**:47.

Jepson, J. H., and Lowenstein, L., 1966, Inhibition of erythropoiesis by a factor present in plasma of patients with erythroblastopenia, *Blood* **27**:425.

Jepson, J. H., and Lowenstein, L., 1968, Panhypoplasia of the bone marrow. I. Demonstration of a plasma factor with anti-erythropoietin-like activity, *Can. Med. Assoc. J.* **99**:99.

Jepson, J. H., and Vas, M., 1974, Decreased *in vivo* and *in vitro* erythropoiesis induced by plasma of 10 patients with thymoma, lymphosarcoma or idiopathic erythroblastopenia, *Cancer Res.* **34**:1325.

Jurgensen, J. C., Abraham, J. P., and Hardy, W. W., 1970, Erythroid aplasia after halothane hepatitis. Report of a case, *Am. J. Dig. Dis.* **15**:577.

Kahn, C. R., Flier, J. S., Bar, R. S., Archer, J. A., Gordon, P., Martin, M. M., and Roth, J., 1976, The syndromes of insulin resistance and acanthosis nigricans, *N. Engl. J. Med.* **294**:739.

Kailis, S. G., and Morgan, E. H., 1974, Transferrin and iron uptake by rabbit bone marrow cells *in vitro*, *Br. J. Haematol.* **28**:37.

Kark, R. M., 1937, Two cases of aplastic anemia, *Guys Hosp. Rep.* **87**:343.

Kaznelson, P., 1922, Zur Entstehung der Blutplättchen. Verhandl. deutsch. Gesellsch. inn., *Med. Kong.* **34**:557.

Kho, J. K., Odang, O., Thajeb, S., and Markum, A. H., 1962, Erythroblastopenia (pure red cell aplasia) in childhood in Djakarta, *Blood* **19**:168.

Krantz, S. B., 1965, The effect of erythropoietin on human bone marrow cells *in vitro*, *Life Sci.* **4**:2393.

Krantz, S. B., 1972a, Studies on red cell aplasia. III. Treatment with horse anti-human thymocyte gamma globulin, *Blood* **39**:347.

Krantz, S. B., 1972b, Studies on red cell aplasia. IV. Treatment with immunosuppressive drugs, *in International Conferences on Hematopoiesis. I. Regulation of Erythropoiesis* (A. S. Gordon, M. Condorelli, and C. Peschle, eds.), pp. 312–330, Il Ponte, Rome, Italy.

Krantz, S. B., 1974, Pure red-cell aplasia, *N. Engl. J. Med.* **291**:345.

Krantz, S. B., 1977, Implications of studies on pure red cell aplasia (PRCA) for the study of aplastic anemia, *in Aplastic Anemia* (S. Hibino, F. Takaku, and N. T. Shahidi, eds.), Tokyo University Press, Tokyo, Japan, in press.

Krantz, S. B., and Kao, V., 1967, Studies on red cell aplasia. I. Demonstration of a plasma inhibitor to heme synthesis and an antibody to erythroblast nuclei, *Proc. Nat. Acad. Sci. U.S.A.* **58**:493.

Krantz, S. B., and Kao, V., 1969, Studies on red cell aplasia. II. Report of a second patient with an antibody to erythroblast nuclei and a remission after immunosuppressive therapy, *Blood* **34**:1.

Krantz, S. B., Gallien-Lartique, O., and Goldwasser, E., 1963, The effect of erythropoietin upon heme synthesis by marrow cells *in vitro*, *J. Biol. Chem.* **238**:4085.

Krantz, S. B., Moore, W. H., and Zaentz, S. D., 1973, Studies on red cell aplasia. V. Presence of erythroblast cytotoxicity in IgG-globulin fraction of plasma, *J. Clin. Invest.* **52**:324.

Lau, P., Cornwell III, G. G., and Williams, W. J., 1970, Mucopolysaccharide synthesis by human bone marrow in short-term suspension cultures, *J. Lab. Clin. Med.* **76**:739.

Lawton, J. W. M., Aldrich, J. E., and Turner, T. L., 1974, Congenital erythroid hypoplastic anemia: Autosomal dominant transmission, *Scand. J. Haematol.* **13**:276.

Loeb, V., Moore, C. B., and Dubach, R., 1953, The physiologic evaluation and management of chronic bone marrow failure, *Am. J. Med.* **15**:499.

MacIver, J. E., 1961, The aplastic crisis in sickle cell anemia, *Lancet* **1**:1086.

MacKechnie, H. L. N., Squires, A. H., Platts, M., and Pruzanski, W., 1973, Thymoma, myasthenia gravis, erythroblastopenic anemia, and systemic lupus erythematosus in one patient, *Can. Med. Assoc. J.* **109**:733.

Marmont, A., Peschle, C., Sanguineti, M., and Condorelli, M., 1975, Pure red cell aplasia (PRCA). Response of three patients to cyclophosphamide and/or antilymphocyte globulin (ALG) and demonstration of two types of serum IgG inhibitors to erythropoiesis, *Blood* **45**:247.

McGrath, B. P., Ibels, L. S., Raik, G., Hargrave, M., Mahoney, J. F., and Stewart, J. H., 1975, Erythroid toxicity of azathioprine: Macrocytosis and selective marrow hypoplasia, *Q. J. Med.* **44**:57.

Mentzer, W. C., Wang, W. C., and Diamond, L. K., 1975, An abnormality of riboflavin metabolism in congenital hypoplastic anemia, *Blood* **46**:1005.

Meyer, L. M., and Bertcher, R. W., 1960, Acquired hemolytic anemia and transient erythroid hypoplasia of the bone marrow, *Am. J. Med.* **28**:406.

Mielke, H. G., 1958, Aplastische Anämie (erythroblastophthise) nach INH-behandlung, *Folia Haematol. (Frankfort, New Ed.)* **2**:1.

Mitchell, A. B. S., Pinn, G., and Pegrum, G. D., 1971, Pure red cell aplasia and carcinoma, *Blood* **37**:594.

Mittag, T., Kornfeld, P., Tormay, A., and Woo, C., 1976, Anti-acetylcholine receptor factors in myasthenia gravis, *N. Engl. J. Med.* **294**:691.

Ortega, J. A., Shore, N. A., Dukes, P. P., and Hammond, D., 1975, Congenital hypoplastic anemia. Inhibition of erythropoiesis by sera from patients with congenital hypoplastic anemia, *Blood* **45**:83.

Ortiz de Landazuri, M., Kedar, E., and Fahey, J. L., 1974, Antibody-dependent cellular cytotoxicity to a syngeneic gross virus-induced lymphoma, *J. Nat. Cancer Inst.* **52**:147.

Pasternack, A., and Wahlberg, P., 1967, Bone marrow in acute renal failure, *Acta Med. Scand.* **181**:505.

Patrick, J., and Lindstrom, J., 1973, Autoimmune response to acetylcholine receptor, *Science* **180**:871.

Peschle, C., Marmont, A. M., Marone, G., Genovese, A., Sasso, G. F., and Condorelli, M., 1975, Pure red cell aplasia: Studies on an IgG serum inhibitor neutralizing erythropoietin, *Br. J. Haematol.* **30**:411.

Pezzimenti, J. F., and Lindenbaum, J., 1972, Megaloblastic anemia associated with erythroid hypoplasia, *Am. J. Med.* **53**:748.

Pierre, R. V., 1974, Preleukemic states. *Semin. Hematol.* **11**:73.

Recker, R. R., and Hynes, H. E., 1969, Pure red blood cell aplasia associated with chlorpropamide therapy, *Arch. Intern. Med.* **123**:445.

Rogers, B. H. G., Manaligod, J. R., and Blazek, W. V., 1968, Thymoma associated with pancytopenia and hypogammaglobulinemia: Report of a case and review of the literature, *Am. J. Med.* **44**:154.

Roland, A. S., 1964, The syndrome of benign thymoma and primary aregenerative anemia. An analysis of 43 cases, *Am. J. Med. Sci.* **247**:719.

Rosner, P., and Hausser, E., 1964, Les erythroblastopenies pures. A propos d'un cas d'erythroblastopénie pure primitive de l'adulte, *Presse Med.* **72**:3275.

Safdar, S. H., Krantz, S. B., and Brown, E. B., 1970, Successful immunosuppressive treatment of erythroid aplasia appearing after thymectomy, *Br. J. Haematol.* **19**:435.

Sallan, S. E., and Buchanan, G. R., 1977, Selective erythroid aplasia during therapy for acute lymphoblastic leukemia, *Pediatrics* (in press).

Schecter, B., Sachs, D. H., and Terry, W. D., 1974, Suppression of protein synthesis as a measure of humoral and cellular cytotoxicity, *Transplantation* **18**:267.

Schmid, J. R., Kiely, J. M., Pease, G. L., and Hargraves, M. M., 1963, Acquired pure red cell agenesis. Report of 16 cases and review of the literature, *Acta Haematol.* **30**:255.

Schmid, J. R., Kiely, J. M., Harrison, E. G., Mayrd, E. D., and Pease, G. L., 1965, Thymoma associated with pure red cell agenesis. Review of the literature and report of four cases, *Cancer* **18**:216.

Sears, D. A., George, J. N., and Gold, M. S., 1975, Transient red cell aplasia in association with viral hepatitis, *Arch. Intern. Med.* **135**:1585.

Sharff, O., and Neumann, H., 1944, Über eine seltene Form von Knochenmark-schädigung durch Salvarsan, *Med. Klin.* **40**:500.

Shiu, R. P. C., and Friesen, H. G., 1976, Blockade of prolactin action by an antiserum to its receptors, *Science* **192**:259.

Siegler, J., Bognar, I., and Keleman, K., 1970, Genesung einer isolierten chron-ischen Erythrozytenaplasie während einer Behandlung mit 6-Merkaptopu-rin, *Kinderaerztl. Prax.* **38**:145.

Singer, K., Motulsky, A. G., and Wile, S. A., 1950, Aplastic crisis in sickle cell anemia. A study of its mechanism and its relationship to other types of hemolytic crises, *J. Lab. Clin. Med.* **35**:721.

Soulter, L., and Emerson, C. P., 1960, Elective thymectomy in the treatment of aregenerative anemia associated with monocytic leukemia, *Am. J. Med.* **28**:609.

Stephens, M. E. M., 1974, Transient erythroid hypoplasia in a patient on long-term co-trimoxazole therapy, *Postgrad. Med. J.* **50**:235.

Stohlman, F., Quesenberry, P. J., Howard, D., Miller, M. E., and Schur, P., 1971, Erythroid aplasia. An autoimmune complication of chronic lymphocytic leukemia, *Clin. Res.* **19**:566.

Strauss, A. M., 1943, Erythrocyte aplasia following sulfathiazole, *Am. J. Clin. Pathol.* **13**:249.

Swineford, O., Curry, J. C., and Cumbia, J. W., 1958, Phenylbutazone toxicity: Depression of erythropoiesis. A case report, *Arthritis Rheum.* **1**:174.

Tatarsky, I., 1972, Transient erythroid hypoplasia in chronic lymphatic leukemia, *N. Istanbul Contrib. Clin. Sci.* **10**:130.

Tepperman, A. D., Curtis, J. E., and McCulloch, E. A., 1974, Erythropoietic colonies in cultures of human marrow, *Blood* **44**:659.

Thorell, B., 1947, Studies of the formation of cellular substances during blood cell production, *Acta. Med. Scand.* **129** (Suppl. 200):1.

Tsai, S. Y., and Levin, W. C., 1957, Chronic erythrocytic hypoplasia in adults. Review of the literature and report of a case, *Am. J. Med.* **22**:322.

Udall, P. R., Kerr, D. N. S., and Tacchi, D., 1972, Sterility and cyclophosphamide, *Lancet* **1**:568.

Van Der Weyden, M., and Firkin, B. G., 1972, The management of aplastic anaemia in adults (annotation), *Br. J. Haematol.* **22**:1.

Vilan, J., Rhyner, K., and Ganzoni, A., 1973, Pure red cell aplasia. Successful treatment with cyclophosphamide, *Blut* **26**:27.

Voyce, M. A., 1963, A case of pure red cell aplasia successfully treated with cobalt, *Br. J. Haematol.* **9**:412.

Wranne, L., Bonnevier, J. O., Killander, A., and Killander, J., 1970, Pure red-cell anemia with pro-erythroblast maturation arrest, *Scand. J. Haematol.* **7**:73.

Yunis, A. A., Arimura, G. K., Lutcher, C. L., Blasquez, J., and Halloran, M., 1967, Biochemical lesion in dilantin-induced erythroid aplasia, *Blood* **30**:587.

Zaentz, S. D., and Krantz, S. B., 1973, Studies on pure red cell aplasia. VI. Development of two-stage erythroblast cytotoxicity method and role of complement, *J. Lab. Clin. Med.* **82**:31.

Zaentz, S. D., Krantz, S. B., and Sears, D. A., 1975, Studies on pure red cell aplasia. VII. Presence of proerythroblasts and response to splenectomy. A case report, *Blood* **46**:261.

Zaentz, S. D., Krantz, S. B., and Brown, E. B., 1976, Studies on pure red cell aplasia. VIII. Maintenance therapy with immunosuppressive drugs, *Br. J. Haematol.* **32**:47.

Zaentz, S. D., Luna, J. A., Baker, A. S., and Krantz, S. B., 1977, Detection of cytotoxic antibody erythroblasts, *J. Lab. Clin. Med.* (in press).

Zalusky, R., Zanjani, E. D., Gidari, A. S., and Ross, J., 1973, Site of action of a serum inhibitor of erythropoiesis, *J. Lab. Clin. Med.* **81**:867.

Zanjani, E. D., Litwin, S. D., and Zalusky, R., 1975, Impairment of erythroid colony (EC) formation by lymphocytes from patients with variable immunodeficiency (VID), *Blood* **46**:1038.

# 6

# Neutrophil Function: Normal and Abnormal

## Thomas P. Stossel and Harvey J. Cohen

Intense interest in normal and abnormal neutrophil function has generated an immense outpouring of publications describing experiments and observations concerning this fascinating cell. Fortunately, comprehensive reviews have kept pace with this ground swell and provide historical perspective, diverse viewpoints, and compendia of emerging data and ideas (Bellanti and Dayton, 1975; Cline *et al.*, 1974; Humbert *et al.*, 1975; Lichtman, 1975; Stossel, 1974; Baehner, 1974). The principal intent of this chapter is to provide not another compendium but a critical appraisal of some recent directions in research concerning normal and abnormal neutrophil function. Our approach is to discuss recent developments in aspects of arbitrarily defined functions of the mature neutrophil: locomotion, ingestion, degranulation, oxidative metabolism, and microbicidal activity. Their artificial boundaries are mere conveniences for presentation. Many of the mechanisms underlying the functions discussed are similar, which will be apparent from the repetition that this approach requires. In focusing on neutrophil function, we must neglect the important subjects of the neutrophil's production and life cycle and the growing field of neutrophil transfusion. We direct interested readers to recent reviews (Stanley *et al.*, 1975; Herzig and Graw, 1975; Boggs, 1974; Higby and Henderson, 1975).

---

THOMAS P. STOSSEL • Medical Oncology Unit, Massachusetts General Hospital, Boston, Massachusetts 02114. HARVEY J. COHEN • Division of Hematology–Oncology, Children's Hospital Medical Center, Boston, Massachusetts 02115.

## 6.1. Some General Comments Concerning Normal and Abnormal Neutrophil Function

All now agree with Metchnikoff's (1887) idea that neutrophils help protect the host against microbial infection and mediate inflammation. However, the expectation that observations of humans and animals with congenital and acquired disorders involving neutrophils would produce information on the mechanism of these processes has not been entirely fulfilled, because few functional disorders of phagocytic cells limit themselves to neutrophils alone. Exactly where the neutrophil fits in the total picture is still not clear. Individuals with numerical deficiencies of neutrophils often have either a diminution or increase in mononuclear phagocytes (Pincus *et al.*, 1976), and inflammation occurs in the setting of neutropenia (Ortel and Newcombe, 1974). However, a few generalizations are possible. Neutrophil deficiency or dysfunction appears to predispose to infections of the skin, lungs, and gastrointestinal tract. The offending organisms tend to be "low grade" pathogens, *Staphylococcus aureus*, anaerobic microbes, and gram-negative enteric flora (Pincus *et al.*, 1976; Kostman, 1975). The observations are consistent with the inferential idea that the neutrophils, as the most mobile and invasive phagocytes, defend against pathogens residing at tissue interfaces with the environment, the skin, the lung, and the gut. These thoughts are relevant to the clinical importance of neutrophil dysfunction. Even if clinical disorders of neutrophil function have not completely elucidated the role of the neutrophil, they have unquestionably contributed to the understanding of normal neutrophil function and will continue to provide this kind of understanding.

## 6.2. The Humoral Dimension of Neutrophil Function

### 6.2.1. Factors with Chemotactic Activity for Neutrophils

The list of chemotactic factors, defined as substances which attract neutrophils, continues to grow (Table I) (reviewed by Ward, 1974; Gallin and Wolff, 1975). Among new additions are some nonprotein factors. These include products of lipid peroxidation (Turner *et al.*, 1975) and *N*-formylated methionyl oligopeptides (Schiffman *et al.*, 1975a). The importance of these compounds as chemotactic factors is that their mechanisms of action may be easier to define than those of proteins. In particular, the

**Table I.** Chemotactic Factors and Chemotactic Factor Inhibitors

| Factors | Inhibitors |
| --- | --- |
| Proteins | C3a inactivator |
|   Complement fragments | "Chemotactic factor inhibitors" increased in: |
|     C3a |   Hodgkin's disease (Ward and Berenberg, 1974) |
|     C5a |   Sarcoidosis (Maderazo et al., 1976) |
|     C567 |   Patients with leukocytosis and anergy (Van Epps et al., 1974) |
|   Alternate pathway intermediates |   Alcoholic cirrhosis (Van Epps et al., 1975; Maderazo et al., 1975) |
|   Coagulation proteins |   Cancer (Brozna and Ward, 1975) |
|   Plasminogen activator |   Viral diseases (Anderson et al., 1974) |
|   Fibrinopeptide B |   "Lymphokines" (Weisbart et al., 1975) |
|   Prekallikrein | |
|   Other proteins | |
|     Random coil proteins (e.g., casein) Wilkinson and McKay, 1974) | |
|     IgG hydrolysis products (Nishiura et al., 1976) | |
|     Cell-bound antigen (Jensen and Esquenazi, 1975) | |
| Lipids and other molecules | |
|   Products of lipid peroxidation (Turner et al., 1975) | |
|   Prostaglandins (Higgs et al., 1975) | |
|   Bacterial filtrate factors | |
|   Formyl-methionyl peptides (Schiffman et al., 1975a) | |
|   Cyclic purine nucleotides (Gamow and Barnes, 1974) | |
|   Transfer factor (Gallin and Kirkpatrick, 1974) | |
|   Lymphokines | |

oligopeptides demonstrate large differences in dose–effectiveness, depending on their primary structure. There is some evidence as well that the chemotactic activity in bacterial culture filtrates may reside in similar compounds (Schiffman *et al.*, 1975b).

Concerning protein chemotactic factors, most attention continues to focus on complement fragments. More experiments have confirmed the capacity of neutrophil granule-associated proteases to generate chemotactically active products from complement components (Venge and Olsson, 1975; Goldstein and Weissman, 1974). Activated proteins of the alternate complement pathway were said to have chemotactic activity (Ruddy *et al.*, 1975). The observation that serum from genetically C5-deficient humans, activated with endotoxin or aggregated IgG, had diminished chemotactic activity relative to activated normal serum and was correctable by addition of purified C5 provided further support for the strong circumstantial evidence that a fragment of C5 is an important serum chemotactic factor (Rosenfeld *et al.*, 1976). The finding that activated serum from a patient with hereditary C7 deficiency also had diminished chemotactic activity (Boyer *et al.*, 1975) is consistent with the previously held idea that the C567 complex is chemotactic for neutrophils.

With respect to noncomplement proteins with chemotactic effects, a novel concept supported by some experiments is that an antigen gradient can attract phagocytes that have specific antibody bound to their membranes (Jensen and Esquenazi, 1975). Further work on chemotactic fragments generated by the blood coagulation system suggested that fibrinopeptide B is the major active principle (Richardson *et al.*, 1976; Stecher, 1975). The common denominator of this myriad of proteins which can attract neutrophils remains unknown. The suggestion that random coil proteins are active because of exposed hydrophobic groups is a tenable beginning (Wilkinson and McKay, 1974).

## 6.2.2. Inhibitors of Chemotactic Activity

The list of serum factors which inhibit the generation of chemotactic factors or which inactivate formed chemotactic agents has kept up with the proliferation of known chemotactic factors (Table I) (reviewed by Ward *et al.*, 1974). Wagner *et al.* (1974) reported that IgM rheumatoid factor competes with other activators for serum complement components, thereby preventing the generation of chemotactic activity. Otherwise, the detailed molecular nature of various chemotactic factor inhibitors of serum (Till and Ward, 1975) which appear to become hyperactive in a surprisingly large number of diseases remains to be defined. The role of these inhibitors in the clinical manifestations of these diseases is also not clear.

### 6.2.3. Opsonins

More and more investigations of the interactions between microorganisms and serum support earlier work providing that antibody and complement either alone or in combination are the important opsonins (agents which bind to objects thereby increasing the rate at which phagocytes ingest them) of serum for neutrophils (reviewed by Stossel, 1975) (Table II). Either the classical or alternate complement pathways or both participate in complement-mediated opsonization by depositing a fragment of C3 on the surface of the target particle. Reconstitution of the opsonic power of the alternate pathway with purified proteins remains elusive. Most studies have relied on addition of magnesium plus the calcium chelator EGTA to serum to assess the role of the alternate pathway because of its alleged independence from calcium in its activity. These kinds of experiments are hazardous because the equilibria of free and bound divalent ions are difficult to control. Furthermore, the soaplike surfaces of microorganisms may contribute large quantities of bound calcium to the system, and this dimension has not been controlled. The molecular basis by which opsonins elicit recognition by neutrophils remains unknown. IgG is the major class of opsonically active antibody, and except for recent work showing that intact IgG binds more efficiently to neutrophils than Fc fragments (Lawrence et al., 1975), knowledge of its mechanism of action on neutrophils has advanced little. Information exists as to the stability and structure of the opsonic fragment of C3 (Stossel el al., 1975), but the particle binding or opsonic effector sites of the molecule have not yet been defined.

Since the description of the major serum opsonic defects associated with hereditary or acquired deficiency of serum C3 or of proteins which are involved in the activation of C3 (reviewed by Alper et al., 1975), no new reports correlating well-defined serum opsonic abnormalities with human disease have appeared. Defective serum opsonic activity was demonstrated in complement-depleted sera of patients with systemic lupus erythematosus (Jasin et al., 1974) and in patients with either serious sepsis with gram negative microorganisms or in patients with severe thermal burns and possible complement abnormalities (Bjornson and Alexander, 1974; Weinstein and Young, 1976).

### 6.2.4. Other Serum Factors

Agents in serum may modulate neutrophil responses to the major chemotactic factors and opsonins. The inhibitor of the first component of complement was reported to increase the chemotactic responsiveness of neutrophils to the C5 chemotactic fragment (Smith et al., 1975; Goetzl, 1975), whereas the serum protease inhibitor α-1-antitrypsin was found to

**Table II.** Summary of Some Recent Studies of the Role of Serum Opsonins for the Ingestion of Various Microorganisms by Neutrophils

| Microorganism | Findings | Reference |
|---|---|---|
| *Bacteroides fragilis* | Ingestion promoted by fresh serum | Casciato *et al.*, 1975 |
| *Shigella* species | IgG antibody, not IgM or IgA, promoted ingestion of some strains alone. IgM antibody plus fresh serum opsonized all strains. Chelator studies suggested alternate complement pathway involved | Reed, 1975 |
| Group A streptococci | Type-specific antibody plus fresh serum appear to be required for phagocytosis | Matthews *et al.*, 1974 |
| *Francisella tularensis* | Immune serum required for phagocytosis | Proctor *et al.*, 1975 |
| *Serratia marcescens* | Chelator and reduction studies suggest fresh preimmune serum opsonizes via alternate pathway, immune serum opsonizes via classical or alternate pathways | Simberkoff *et al.*, 1976 |
| *Streptococcus fecalis* | | |
| *Pneumococci pneumoniii* | | |
| *Staphylococcus albus* | Chelator studies suggest opsonization by fresh serum via alternate pathway | |
| *Staphylococcus aureus* | Chelator studies suggest opsonization by fresh serum only via classical pathway. Heat-stable opsonic activity against cell wall mucopeptide in patients infected with the organism | Forsgren and Quie, 1974 |
| | | Humphreys *et al.*, 1974 |
| *Pseudomonas aeruginosa* | Chelator studies suggest opsonization by fresh serum via both pathways. Patients with pseudomonas infections have heat-stable (antibody?) opsonins | Bjornson and Michael, 1974 |
| | | Forsgren and Quie, 1974 |
| *Cryptoccocus neoformans* | Studies with normal, C4-deficient, and heated sera suggest both complement pathways opsonize | Crowder *et al.*, 1974 |
| | | Diamond *et al.*, 1974 |
| *Neisseria gonorrhoeae* | Virulent strains not opsonized by fresh serum. Avirulent strains opsonized by fresh serum. Nature of serum interactions not defined | Gibbs and Roberts, 1975 |
| | | Dilworth *et al.*, 1975 |

diminish chemotactic responsiveness while enhancing random locomotion (Goetzl, 1975). Normal human serum, depending on its concentration and on the manner of exposure to cells, or chemotaxis-activating agents, or both, can enhance or inhibit neutrophil locomotion in a complex way (Keller *et al.*, 1974).

A serum protein fraction which acts on antibody- or complement-reacted erythrocytes to increase their ingestibility by human neutrophils was recently discovered (Gigli *et al.*, 1976). Human but not ovine lysozyme was claimed to enhance phagocytosis by human neutrophils by an action on the cell (Klockars and Roberts, 1976). Many publications from one group (reviewed by Najjar, 1975) concern the putative phagocytosis-enhancing action of a tetrapeptide derived from serum immunoglobulin. The tetrapeptide is claimed also to act on the cell, and the immunoglobulin is said to be produced by the spleen. Erp and Fahrney (1975) reported that an immunoglobulin fraction of bovine serum modestly enhanced phagocytosis of opsonized heat-killed *S. aureus* by bovine neutrophils, but that the tetrapeptide fragment was relatively inactive. Furthermore, splenectomy had no influence on the phagocytosis-enhancing effect of the serum fractions. These discrepancies may resolve when a technique other than enumeration of "ingested" particles viewed with the light microscope is used to assay the rate of phagocytosis. Serum from persons with infectious or other inflammatory diseases enhanced the adherence of neutrophils to foreign surfaces (Lentnek *et al.*, 1976).

## 6.3. The Cellular Dimension of Neutrophil Function

Many aspects of neutrophil function have common features. Locomotion, ingestion, lysosomal fusion with the plasmalemma, and oxygen metabolism are activated by initial membrane contact with diverse stimuli. The various functions are susceptible to similar kinds of perturbation by drugs and other agents. Reversible adhesion to a substrate is required for locomotion and to a particle for ingestion. Pseudopod movements characterize locomotion and ingestion. Membrane fusion is involved in closure of the phagocytic vacuole during ingestion and in the degranulation process which occurs during ingestion and even during locomotion. These similarities should simplify elucidation of underlying mechanisms, but unique features of the different functions often confound the common themes.

### 6.3.1. Structure and Metabolism of Neutrophils

Analysis of the anatomy and metabolism of neutrophils independently of specific functions can shed light on the functions.

Still no convincing preparation of a neutrophil plasma membrane in good yield has been produced, which is unfortunate in view of the importance of this structure for neutrophil functions. A detailed examination of guinea pig neutrophils showed that 5'-nucleotidase and other phosphohydrolases are ectoenzymes, potentially useful as markers for a definitive plasma membrane isolation (DePierre and Karnovsky, 1974). The histochemical demonstration of ricin bound to rabbit granule membranes suggests that lectin binding may not be a reliable marker for plasmalemma isolation (Feigenson et al., 1975).

There has been progress in definition of cytoplasmic "contractile" proteins which may be relevant for various neutrophil functions. Early crude "actomyosin" preparations have given way to the definitive isolation of actin and myosin molecules from neutrophils of various species; the properties and interactions of these molecules have been examined (Stossel and Pollard, 1973; Takeuchi et al., 1975; Boxer and Stossel, 1976). As in other nonmuscle cells, actin comprises a major fraction (about 10%) of the total cell protein, and the actin : myosin ratio is much higher than that of skeletal muscle. Reversible interconversions between the monomeric and filament are states of actin and may influence the consistency of cytoplasm and control the location of movement. A high molecular weight "actin binding protein" which regulates the consistency of actin has been isolated from human neutrophils as well as other cell types (Boxer and Stossel, 1976). Cytochalasin B, the fungal metabolite that alters many neutrophil functions (see later), has recently been shown to diminish the gel state of cytoplasmic actin by interfering with its interaction with the actin binding protein of macrophages (Hartwig and Stossel, 1976). By analogy from skeletal muscle physiology, myosin in neutrophils could generate neutrophil movements. Purified neutrophil myosin has been shown to cause the aggregation of actin gels prepared from purified neutrophil proteins in the presence of $Mg^{2+}$ and ATP. Antiserum against neutrophil myosin inhibited this aggregation (Boxer and Stossel, 1976).

Centriolar microtubules of neutrophils continue to be a source of fascination, but have only been examined morphologically (Hoffstein et al., 1974). Intermediate (10 nm) filaments are also prominent components of the neutrophil cytocenter and deserve biochemical attention.

The granules of neutrophils are still being sorted into classes according to density, morphology, and enzyme content (Bainton, 1975). Earlier emphasis on animal neutrophils is shifting to the human cells and confirms that there is considerable heterogeneity among animal species with respect to the character of neutrophil granules (Rausch and Moore, 1975), especially with respect to the secondary or specific granule. For example, alkaline phosphatase is not localized to the specific granule of human neutrophils as it is to that of rabbit or guinea pig neutrophils (Avila and Convit, 1974; Bretz and Baggiolini, 1974; Spitznagel et al.,

1974). However, the primary or azurophil granule, the granule produced first in myeloid development and which contains myeloperoxidase and lysosomal hydrolases, is relatively consistent among species in its composition.

The neutral proteases of neutrophil granules have received much attention because of their potential as mediators of inflammatory disease. Most of the enzymes reside in primary granules and are collagenaselike, elastaselike, and chymotrypsinlike. Complement components, cartilage proteoglycan, and fibrinogen are demonstrated and possibly physiologically relevant target proteins of these hydrolases (DeWald et al., 1975; Baugh and Travis, 1976; Kopitar and Lebez, 1975; Janoff et al., 1976; Venge and Olsson, 1975; Ohlsson and Olsson, 1974; Dubin et al., 1976; Plow and Edginton, 1975; Goldstein and Weissman, 1974). α-1-Antitrypsin and α-2-macroglobulin are natural serum inhibitors of neutrophil proteases. Other neutrophil granule-associated enzymes or activities which have been scrutinized recently include a phospholipase $A_2$ activity (Franson et al., 1974) and a ribonuclease activity specific for secondary esters of uridine-3-phosphate (Reddi, 1976).

Relatively little recent work has been devoted to the metabolism of neutrophils. Two enzymes of glycogen metabolism, glycogen synthetase and glycogen phosphorylase, were purified from human neutrophils and the enzymatic mechanism of the former enzyme was analyzed (Plesner et al., 1974; Sørensen and Wang, 1975). Careful characterization of insulin binding catabolism and effects on glycolysis by neutrophils has been done (LeRoux et al., 1975; Fussganger et al., 1976). Extracellular calcium was shown to enhance lactate production by a variety of neutrophil preparations (Elliot et al., 1975), but understanding of the regulation of carbohydrate metabolism in neutrophils remains incomplete.

Craddock et al. (1974) provided further weight to preexisting evidence that intermediary metabolism and maintenance of cellular energy in the form of ATP are relevant to neutrophil function by demonstrating that neutrophils of phosphate-depleted dogs and humans had low ATP levels and were impaired in chemotactic responsiveness and ingestion. Strauss et al. (1974) showed that human neutrophils with a defect of the glycolytic pathway, a deficiency of phosphoglycerate kinase activity, can maintain normal function presumably by supplying ATP via oxidative phosphorylation.

Comprehension of protein turnover and of lipid and nucleic acid metabolism in neutrophils is rudimentary. Protein (histone) kinases and phosphatases of human neutrophils were partially characterized, although their natural substrates were not identified (Tsung et al., 1975). Mature neutrophils were shown to have active nucleotide deaminase activity, a potentially important finding for the study of certain anticancer agents (Chabner et al., 1974). The fatty acid composition of purified human neutrophils was reported (Stossel *et al.*, 1974) as was evidence for triglyceride fatty acid synthesis from glucose via glycerol (Burns *et al.*, 1976). This information may be relevant to future studies of lipid alterations in response to neutrophil functions.

### 6.3.2. Neutrophil Locomotion

There have been some interesting additions to the already extensively described phenomenology of neutrophil locomotion (reviewed by Ramsey, 1974a). One is the finding that molecules on the surface of neutrophils which bind fluorescein isothiocyanate are swept to the trailing knob or tail of a locomoting neutrophil and subsequently shed or interiorized (Ryan *et al.*, 1974). A second is that neutrophils deviate little from the path toward the source of a chemotactic factor, implying that the factor-sensing mechanism is spatial rather than temporal, i.e., the cell senses the gradient continuously rather than sequentially (Zigmond, 1974; Ramsey, 1974b). A third is that exposure to chemotactic factors reduces the net negative charge of neutrophils (Gallin *et al.*, 1975). A fourth is that chemotactic factors induce the secretion of lysosomal enzymes by substrate-attached neutrophils (Becker *et al.*, 1974; Showell *et al.*, 1976; Wilkinson and McKay, 1974). It has been suggested that lysosomal secretion during locomotion is a concomitant of plasma membrane replacement by secretory vesicles to compensate for loss of membrane by endocytosis and shedding at the tail, and that the removal of membrane is a mechanism for destroying "chemotactic memory," permitting interaction and membrane gradient establishment by new sources. It is also a mechanism for destroying adhesion points between the membrane and the substrate of the chemotactic factor (Stossel, 1977).

The idea that contractile proteins, microtubules, and other filamentous structures are involved in neutrophil locomotion continues to be attractive. The evidence for the role of contractile proteins is circumstantial: (a) Actin-containing microfilaments are concentrated in the anterior lamellipod and the zone of cell–substrate attachment (Stossel, 1977). (b) Cytochalasin B inhibits locomotion and induces neutrophil shrinkage at concentrations which inhibit actin gel formation (Hsu and Becker, 1975; Hartwig and Stossel, 1976). (c) Human neutrophils containing a dysfunctional actin were unable to locomote *in vitro* or *in vivo* (Boxer *et al.*, 1974). Monomeric actin in extracts of neutrophils from an infant with recurrent pyogenic infections failed to polymerize in the presence of salt concentrations which polymerized normal neutrophil actin. The evidence for the participation of other cytoskeletal elements is weaker. Electron micrographs of neutrophils exposed to chemotactic factors were reported to show more centriolar microtubules than micrographs of neutrophils at rest (Gallin and Rosenthal, 1974). Drugs which react with tubulin, the subunit protein of microtubules, e.g., colchicine, vinblastine, and griseo-fulvin, have been reported to inhibit neutrophil locomotion toward chem-otactic factors by some (Bandmann *et al.*, 1974). but not all investigators (Ryan *et al.*, 1974; Ramsey, 1974a). In any case, the site of action of these drugs in intact cells is moot.

Extensive and sometimes contradictory data continue to accrue con-cerning the effects of monovalent and divalent ions, ionophores, and a variety of drugs on locomotion and chemotaxis by neutrophils (Goetzl *et al.*, 1974; Sandler *et al.*, 1975; Estensen *et al.*, 1976; Rivkin *et al.*, 1975; Gallin and Rosenthal, 1974; Becker *et al.*, 1974; Wilkinson, 1975; Woodin *et al.*, 1975; Hawley and Gordon, 1976). When the mechanisms of loco-motion are known, the effects of these agents will be understood.

More diseases have been added to the list of disorders in which neutrophil responsiveness to chemotactic factors was depressed (reviewed by Gallin and Wolff, 1975). These include Down's syndrome (Khan *et al.*, 1975), influenza (Larson and Blades, 1976), thermal burns (Warden *et al.*, 1974), and a heterogeneous collection of some familial syndromes, associ-ated with eczema, variably severe pyogenic infections, and elevated serum IgE levels (Pincus *et al.*, 1975; Van Scoy *et al.*, 1975). To be explained is why the chemotactic defects associated with these dermatoses can some-times be detected only in neutrophils obtained from fresh and not stored blood and why many individuals with eczema and elevated IgE levels do not have abnormalities of chemotaxis. However, unraveling of the mecha-nism behind these syndromes may shed some light on the nature of chemotactic responses. Craddock *et al.* (1976) reported that neutrophils of patients with paroxysmal nocturnal hemoglobinuria had impaired chemo-tactic activity. The defect was ascribed to the complement-mediated mem-brane damage which characterizes this disease, although critical proof of this and a description of the type of structural damage were not provided. The study of Dale *et al.* (1974) added important new information con-cerning the well-described effect of corticosteroids on inhibition of neu-trophil emigration from the blood into tissues. Daily, but not every other day administration of the drug inhibited neutrophil migration into Rebuck windows. However, the basic mechanism of the steroid effect still is not known.

### 6.3.3. Ingestion

An important study of phagocytosis by human neutrophils empha-sized the complexity of the recognition mechanism (Davies *et al.*, 1975). It showed that when neutrophils and polystyrene beads were suspended in buffered salt solution, "phagocytosis" could not be evaluated because of nonspecific clumping of beads and cells. Coating of the beads with a monolayer of human IgG decreased the very negative net bead surface charge (a maneuver historically believed to *promote* ingestion) but in fact *reduced* real and apparent ingestion. In fresh human serum true ingestion of IgG-coated beads increased, implying deposition of opsonically active C3 on the bead surface (although this was not proven). The findings emphasize the role of subtle surface alterations on recognition of particles by neutrophils and the problems in quantifying true ingestion. The manner in which "opsonic" molecules are organized on the particle surface, the amount of opsonin deposited, the type of cell exposed to the particles, and other factors influence the results. Much continues to be written about the role of neutrophil membrane "receptors" for the Fc region of IgG and opsonically active C3 (erroneously referred to as C3b). Little is known about the molecular basis for such "receptors." For example, the willingness of different neutrophil preparations to ingest IgG-coated erythrocytes was automatically ascribed to the degree of expression of IgG "receptors" on the responsive and nonresponsive neutrophils (Zipursky and Brown, 1974), when the capacity to ingest the erythrocytes could reside in other factors. As another example, the inhibition of neutrophil phagocytosis but not attachment (assessed by light microscopy) of C3-coated erythrocytes by anti-IgG Fab fragments was taken as evidence that the IgG "receptor" mediates particle ingestion whereas the C3 "receptor" mediates attachment (Mantovani, 1975). Aside from the technical difficulties associated with assaying "ingestion" and "attachment" morphologically, the study suffers from the failure to recognize that the complex aggregate of IgG–anti-IgG might have nonspecific inhibiting effects on phagocytosis.

It is reasonable that IgG and opsonically active C3 might act independently or synergistically to enhance the ingestion of objects by neutrophils. Some workers have proposed that C3 only promotes "binding" whereas IgG or some other factor is required for ingestion (Scribner and Fahrney, 1976). This conclusion is contradicted by kinetic studies (Stossel, 1973) and by the observation that C3 is opsonic for otherwise noningestible objects in agammaglobulinemic serum (Stossel *et al.*, 1973; Jasin 1972).

There is evidence for the participation of contractile proteins in ingestion by neutrophils: (a) Actin-containing microfilaments are prominent in pseudopodia surrounding particles. (b) Cytochalasin B inhibits phagocytosis by neutrophils. (c) The neutrophils with dysfunctional actin described by Boxer *et al.* (1974) were markedly deficient in their ability to ingest opsonized particles.

### 6.3.4. Degranulation

The study of granule fusion with the plasma membrane, originally focused on the secretion of granules into phagosomes, has broadened to encompass granule secretion into the extracellular medium during neutrophil locomotion, interaction with certain surfaces, and even of interaction with immune complexes and other surface-active agents. The rather meager amounts of granule enzymes released extracellularly can be increased by exposing the cells to cytochalasin B (Zurier *et al.*, 1973). This fact and the observation that the neutrophils with dysfunctional actin described by Boxer *et al.* (1974) secreted supernormal quantities of granule-associated enzymes into phagosomes and into the extracellular medium are consistent with the idea supportable by impressions from morphology that a peripheral cytoplasmic actin gel may regulate the access of granules to the plasma membrane. In general, the enzymes of specific granules are more efficiently or even selectively released from stimulated neutrophils (Goldstein *et al.*, 1975; White and Estensen, 1974). Whether this granule class is really more labile, under different regulation with respect to its fusion mechanism, or whether its numerical dominance causes its release to be preferentially detectable is not entirely clear. The "secretory" neutrophil has been used extensively as a model for probing the mechanism of degranulation with various drugs and other agents (Weissman *et al.*, 1975; Henson and Oades, 1975). β-Adrenergic agonists have been reported to inhibit granule enzyme release concomitantly with their elevation of neutrophil adenosine 3',5'-monophosphate levels, whereas cholinergic agents, shown to increase neutrophil guanosine 3',5'-monophosphate levels, enhance release of granule enzymes (Zurier *et al.*, 1973; Ignarro *et al.*, 1974; Hawkins, 1974). Similar effects of these agents on neutrophil locomotion, ingestion, and adhesion to surfaces have been reported, suggesting that the mechanisms of these acts may be relatively similar (Rivkin *et al.*, 1975; Stossel, 1975; Bryant and Sutcliffe, 1974). On the other hand, extracellular magnesium ions are more potent promoters of adhesion, ingestion, and locomotion than calcium ions (reviewed by Becker, 1974; Stossel, 1975), whereas magnesium ions were reported to inhibit granule enzyme secretion by human neutrophils, and calcium ions promoted secretion (Goldstein *et al.*, 1974; Smith and Ignarro, 1975). Needless to say, the sites of action of these agents and the interrelationships of the various neutrophil functions remain obscure and will be integrated when the molecular mechanism of degranulation is clarified.

### 6.3.5. The Chediak–Higashi Syndrome

The number of neutrophil abnormalities which characterize this disease has grown markedly (Table III). Despite its rarity in man, its complexity, and its lack of a proven unifying concept to explain this complexity, the Chediak–Higashi syndrome is an excellent model for the investigation of the cellular dimension of neutrophil function because of the many strains of animals which have a similar genetic disease.

**Table III.** Abnormalities of Neutrophil Function in the Chediak–Higashi Syndrome

| |
|---|
| Giant lysosomes containing enzymes associated with azurophil granules |
| Neutropenia |
| Impaired chemotactic responsiveness |
| Increased rate of phagocytosis |
| Giant granules fuse belatedly with phagosomes |
| Total azurophil granule enzyme content occasionally reduced |
| Increased resting rate of oxygen consumption, [1-$^{14}$C]glucose oxidation, protein iodination, nitroblue tetrazolium reduction |
| Increased tendency to "cap" bound concanavalin A |

Recent studies have yielded exciting results, the meaning of which still requires sorting out. The recent finding that neutrophils of mice and humans with the Chediak–Higashi syndrome have an increased tendency to "cap" the lectin concanavalin A (Oliver et al., 1975) suggests increased membrane activity of the affected cells. This conclusion is consistent with earlier work demonstrating high resting levels of oxygen metabolism and supernormal rates of phagocytosis by Chediak–Higashi neutrophils. The observations that giant granules appear early in myeloid development (Oliver and Essner, 1975) and the demonstration that membrane stimulation and granule fusion are coupled events suggest that chronic membrane perturbation (and possibly endocytosis) may promote fusion of granules to form the characteristic giant lysosomes. This hypothesis implies that regulation of membrane activation is faulty in the Chediak–Higashi syndrome. However, colchicine (Oliver et al., 1975) and agents that oxidize cellular SH groups (Oliver et al., 1976) enhancee concanavalin-A-induced neutrophil cap formation. Both agents inhibit microtubule polymerization. Invoking other studies showing that concanavalin A apparently promotes microtubule asssembly in normal neutrophils (Hoffstein et al., 1976), various investigators proposed that a disorder of microtubule polymerization may be the basis of the cellular abnormalities in the Chediak–Higashi syndrome. Direct biochemical proof of this hypothesis is awaited. Oliver and Zurier (1976) have also reported that the cholinergic agent, carbamylcholine, causes reduction in size of the giant granules of cultivated Chediak–Higashi syndrome fibroblasts and mononuclear phagocytes of mice and of cultured monocytes of man. Administration of carbamylcholine to the mice was also reported to reduce the number of giant granule-containing leukocytes in their blood. These drugs also improved chemotactic responsiveness, lysosomal enzyme secretion, and bactericidal activity of human Chediak–Higashi neutrophils in vitro (Boxer et al., 1977). In the absence of more information, speculation on how carbamylcholine might work in this setting could be endless. Of greater importance is the theoretical clinical spin-off of the observation. Unfortunately, treatment of two human patients with the Chediak–Higashi syndrome with carbamylcholine failed to influence the number, morphology or function of their neutrophils (Buchanan, unpublished observation; Boxer, unpublished observation). Boxer *et al.* (1976) reported that administration of ascorbic acid to a patient with the Chediak–Higashi syndrome caused the patient's neutrophils to improve their locomotion, secretion, and bactericidal activity, although granule morphology was not altered. Ascorbic acid also lowered astoundingly high cyclic AMP levels measured in the cells. Clearly, before this explosion of fascinating information can be clarified, confirmation as well as new insights will be required.

## 6.4. Oxygen Metabolism and Microbicidal Activity

Following and/or coincident with ingestion of microorganisms by phagocytic cells, bactericidal action occurs which usually results in the killing of the ingested organism within 5–20 min (Wilson *et al.*, 1957). The biochemical events that accompany this process are only now beginning to be understood. Alterations in oxygen metabolism and its relationship to bacterial killing have received much attention since the study of Sbarra and Karnovsky (1959) demonstrated a cyanide-insensitive burst of oxygen consumption occurring during ingestion of particles by granulocytes. Although it is true that oxygen-independent bactericidal mechanisms exist in polymorphonuclear leukocytes,* it is felt by most people that they play only a minor, if any, role in the host defense mechanisms against invasion. The acid pH of phagocytic vesicles may only serve to keep the oxidative enzymes at their pH optima (DeChatelet *et al.*, 1975). The hydrolytic enzymes present in neutrophil lysosomes may be more involved in digestion which follows the bactericidal event (Elsbach, 1973). Since it has been shown that totally anaerobic polymorphonuclear leukocytes are capable of effectively killing a few strains of bacteria (Mandell, 1974), there may be some role for nonoxidative mechanisms of bactericidal action. However, based on many clinical and laboratory investigations, it is believed that mechanisms involving oxygen metabolites contribute much more to the killing of microorganisms by phagocytic cells.

Recently, with the advent of methods to detect and quantify products of oxygen metabolism, much insight has been gained into potential mech-

---

*Proposed mechanisms include: acid pH, lysozyme, cationic bactericidal and fungicidal substances (Lehrer, 1972; Spitznagel *et al.*, 1974) and a bacterial permeability-inducing material (Weiss *et al.*, 1976). More information on these systems is needed.

anisms of oxidative bactericidal activity. The metabolites currently being investigated include superoxide, hydrogen peroxide, hydroxyl radical, and singlet oxygen. Each metabolite has been implicated in the process of bacterial killing either directly or indirectly.

The use of superoxide dismutase, an enzyme that catalyzes the conversion of two molecules of superoxide to one molecule each of oxygen and hydrogen peroxide, first described by McCord and Fridovich (1969), has contributed much to the investigation of this one-electron reduction product of oxygen. Utilizing their technique for following superoxide production (i.e., superoxide dismutase inhibitable $Fe^{3+}$-cytochrome $c$ reduction), Babior et al. (1973) showed that granulocytes stimulated to undergo phagocytosis aerobically produced superoxide but none was detected in the absence of oxygen (Curnutte and Babior, 1975) or granulocytes from patients with chronic granulomatous disease (Curnutte et al., 1974) where previous studies had shown a defect in the oxidative burst (Holmes et al., 1967). Early investigations led to the conclusion that superoxide by itself was responsible for the killing of bacteria by neutrophils (Babior et al., 1973). However, recent reports have demonstrated that superoxide is most probably only indirectly responsible for the bactericidal activity of leukocytes (Johnston et al., 1975).

Superoxide is the first oxygen reduction product, and recent data by Root and Metcalf (1976) and Roos et al. (1976) show that most if not all the hydrogen peroxide produced by cells undergoing phagocytosis is formed from superoxide.

Owing to its oxidation reduction potential, superoxide can be either a reductant or an oxidant. In both its enzyme-catalyzed and spontaneous dismutation it serves as both. Studies examining the effect of superoxide dismutase on hydrogen peroxide production by phagocytic cells neglect the fact that superoxide may be a reductant under phagocytic conditions and that the increased rate of hydrogen peroxide production reported in the presence of superoxide dismutase-coated particles (Baehner et al., 1975) may reflect a change in the fate of superoxide from a reductant to both a reductant and oxidant. It has recently been determined that the oxidation–reduction potential of superoxide makes it more likely to act as a reductant. This view is consistent with the data reported by Baehner et al. (1975) which show that in the presence of dismutase-coated particles not only was hydrogen peroxide production increased, but so was oxygen consumption. Their explanation of dismutase causing a more rapid accumulation of hydrogen peroxide by converting superoxide into it would predict a decrease in oxygen consumption since for every molecule of hydrogen peroxide produced, a molecule of oxygen would be regenerated. McCord and Fridovich (1969) showed that the rate of hydrogen peroxide production from superoxide in the xanthine–xanthine oxidase system is unaffected by superoxide dismutase. Experiments in this laboratory on the xanthine–xanthine oxidase system at pH levels between 5 and 11 and at various fluxes of superoxide, showed no effect of superoxide dismutase on the rate of hydrogen peroxide production despite complete inhibition of superoxide-dependent cytochrome $c$ reduction.

The basic problem with the assays which depend on cytochrome $c$ reduction for measuring superoxide production by cells is that being a protein, cytochrome $c$ does not enter the cell and what is therefore measured is only the superoxide released into the extracellular fluid. That there is superoxide generated during phagocytosis which is not detected by this assay was shown by Root and Metcalf (1976) using cytochalasin B which inhibits ingestion of particles but not their attachment to phagocytic cells. Although ingestion of opsonized bacteria was inhibited greater than 50% by cytochalasin B, superoxide and hydrogen peroxide generation was stimulated two- to threefold, and only under these circumstances could most of the oxygen consumed be accounted for by superoxide production.

Nitroblue tetrazolium (NBT) reduction may offer a better approach toward the quantitation of superoxide generation. The reduction of NBT to formazan by phagocytic cells has been used to examine oxidative metabolism by leukocytes (Baehner and Nathan, 1967). It is known that superoxide can reduce NBT. Although superoxide dismutase can only partially inhibit NBT reduction by phagocytic cells, Baehner *et al.* (1976) have recently shown that NBT reduction does not occur in neutrophils which undergo phagocytosis anaerobically, despite enhanced ingestion of particles. Therefore, it is probably true that all NBT reduction in intact neutrophils occurs by way of superoxide and that the inability of superoxide dismutase to inhibit this reduction completely is due to the fact that NBT can enter parts of the cell not accessible to the enzyme.

Hydrogen peroxide—the two-electron product of oxygen consumption—has also received much study. A continuous method for hydrogen peroxide production by phagocytic cells has recently been developed (Root *et al.*, 1975). It utilizes the fact that scopoletin, a fluorescent compound, can be oxidized by hydrogen peroxide in the presence of horseradish peroxidase to a nonfluorescing compound. This assay allows for continuous monitoring, but because it employs a protein for detection, only extracellular hydrogen peroxide can be measured. In addition, since the enzyme is inhibited by cyanide and azide, the effects of these and certain other metabolic inhibitors cannot be investigated. Roos *et al.* (1976), using a more quantitative method for total hydrogen peroxide detection, found that in the presence of cytochalasin B all the hydrogen peroxide produced can be accounted for as coming from superoxide.

Studies relating oxygen consumption, superoxide production, and hydrogen peroxide production, however, have inherent problems. The most notable problem is to determine the proper stoichiometry of the reactions. Since superoxide can act as either an oxidant or reductant, or both, the ratio of superoxide generated to oxygen consumed is going to vary depending on the fate of the superoxide produced. Hydrogen peroxide can act as an oxidant or be "dismutated" by catalase so that the ratio of hydrogen peroxide generated to oxygen consumed may also vary, depending on its fate. Despite these problems, it is probably true that the respiratory burst occurring during phagocytosis involves a two-step reduction of oxygen, first to superoxide then to hydrogen peroxide.

Superoxide, hydrogen peroxide, hydroxyl radical, and singlet oxygen have been implicated as substances which kill bacteria. Johnston *et al.* (1975) have shown a moderate effect of superoxide dismutase bound to latex particles in preventing the killing of certain species of bacteria by granulocytes. A similar diminution was seen with catalase and free racical scavengers such as benzoate and mannitol. They concluded that superoxide, hydrogen peroxide, and hydroxyl free radical were all involved either directly or indirectly in the bactericidal activity of neutrophils. A role for singlet oxygen in killing bacteria was postulated by Krinsky (1974) to explain the finding that the presence of a carotenoid, a scavenger of singlet oxygen, in a bacteria protected it against the bactericidal action of neutrophils. Singlet oxygen production by granulocytes resulting in chemiluminescence can also be inhibited by superoxide dismutase, indicating a relationship between superoxide and singlet oxygen (Rosen and Klebanoff, 1976).

The work of Klebanoff and Hamon (1972) demonstrates that hydrogen peroxide in conjunction with halide ions, in the presence of myeloperoxidase, kills phagocytized bacteria. There is little doubt that this mechanism is operative in normal cells; however, the effects of scavengers of superoxide, singlet oxygen, and free radicals on bacterial killing indicate that more than one mechanism exists for oxygen-mediated neutrophil defense against microorganisms.

That superoxide and other oxygen metabolites generated by granulocytes are not innocuous to the cell itself was shown by Salin and McCord (1975). Resting granulocytes survive 36 hr of incubation at 37°C. However, 90% of cells which have phagocytized bacteria are dead within 36 hr. Superoxide dismutase, catalase, and free radical scavengers protect against this loss of viability. They concluded that hydroxyl radical produced by the interaction of superoxide and hydrogen peroxide (Haber–Weiss reaction) (Haber and Weiss, 1934) leads to the ultimate death of granulocytes. This death with the concomitant release of hydrolytic enzymes and chemotactic factors may play a role in perpetuating the inflammatory process. Superoxide dismutase has in addition been noted to have *in vivo* antiinflammatory properties (Lund-Olesen and Menander, 1974).

Curnutte *et al.* (1975) have shown that a particulate fraction made from human leukocytes which had ingested opsonized zymosan caused superoxide generation in the presence of reduced pyridine nucleotides. Very little activity was found from resting granulocytes and no detectable superoxide was produced by particles from granulocytes of patients with chronic granulomatous disease. Hohn and Lehrer (1975) made very similar observations looking at the oxidation of reduced pyridine nucleotides. However, they used manganous ion in their assays which has recently been shown to stimulate a superoxide-dependent, nonenzymatic oxidation of NADPH (Curnutte *et al.*, 1976).

The nature and localization of the enzyme activity responsible for the oxidation of pyridine nucleotides and the generation of superoxide are as yet unknown. Rossi and his associates have argued for an NADPH oxidase localized to the granular fraction of the cell (Patriarca *et al.*, 1973). Baehner and Karnovsky (1968) postulated that it is an NADH oxidase activity localized in the soluble portion of the cell. It has been postulated that a plasma membrane oxidase is responsible for the respiratory burst (Root and Stossel, 1974). Briggs *et al.* (1975) demonstrate evidence for a plasma membrane NADH oxidase in granulocytes stimulated to undergo phagocytosis. Their use of extracellular nucleotides, however, does not avoid the pitfall of relative permeability affecting the results obtained. It is most likely that the enzyme responsible for the oxidase activity uses both pyridine nucleotides as substrates depending on the conditions of pH and concentration and that where the enzyme is found may depend on the procedures used to stimulate the cells and to isolate the subcellular fractions. Unfortunately, the preparations used to assay for activity are not pure and contain granules, membranes, and other cell constituents. Using a particle preparation, Babior (personal communication) has found that there is a loss of activity in the presence of Triton X-100 but that this activity can be restored with the addition of FAD but not FMN. It is likely, therefore, that the oxidase is a flavoprotein, as are other superoxide-generating enzymes. Unfortunately, since the preparation used is heavily contaminated by many organelles, a precise interpretation of these results is not possible. Goldstein *et al.* (1977) provided more evidence that the neutrophil superoxide-generating system is an ectoenzyme by demonstrating inhibition of its activity by means of a nonpenetrating drug, the diazo salt of sulfanilic acid.

ACKNOWLEDGMENTS

This work was supported by USPHS grants HL-19499 and AI-08173 and an Established Investigatorship of the American Heart Association (to T.P.S.).

# References

Alper, C. A., Stossel, T. P., and Rosen, F. S., 1975, Genetic defects affecting complement and host resistance to infection, in *The Phagocytic Cell and Host Resistance* (D. Dayton and G. Bellanti, eds.), pp. 127–141, Raven Press, New York.

Anderson, R., Sher, R., and Rabson, A. R., 1974, Defective chemotaxis in measles patients, *S. Afr. Med. J.* **48**:1819.

Avila, J. L., and Convit, J., 1974, Studies on human polymorphonuclear leukocyte enzymes III. Differential activation of primary and specific granules by phospholipase C and deoxycholate, *Biochim. Biophys. Acta* **345**:11.

Babior, B. M., Kipnes, R. S., and Curnutte, J. T., 1973, Biological defense mechanisms. The production by leukocytes of superoxide, a potential bactericidal agent, *J. Clin. Invest.* **52**:741.

Baehner, R. L., 1974, Molecular basis for functional disorders of phagocytes, *J. Pediatr.* **84**:317.

Baehner, R. L., and Karnovsky, M. L., 1968, Deficiency of reduced nicotinamide-adenine dinucleotide oxidase in chronic granulomatous disease, *Science* **162**:1277.

Baehner, R. L., and Nathan, D. G., 1967, Quantitative nitroblue tetrazolium test in chronic granulomatous disease, *N. Engl. J. Med.* **278**:971.

Baehner, R. L., Murrmann, S. K., Davis, J., and Johnston, R. B., 1975, The role of superoxide anion and hydrogen peroxide in phagocytosis. Associated oxidative metabolic reaction, *J. Clin. Invest.* **56**:571.

Baehner, R. L., Boxer, L. A., Davis, J., 1976, The biochemical basis of nitroblue tetrazolium reduction in normal human and chronic granulomatous disease polymorphonuclear leukocytes, *Blood* **48**:309.

Bainton, D. F., 1975, Neutrophil granules, *Br. J. Haematol.* **29**:17.

Bandmann, U., Rydgren, L., and Norberg, B., 1974, The difference between random movement and chemotaxis, *Exp. Cell Res.* **88**:63.

Baugh, R. J., and Travis, J., 1976, Human leukocyte granule elastase: Rapid isolation and characterization, *Biochemistry* **15**:836.

Becker, E. L., Showell, H. J., Henson, P. M., and Hsu, L. S., 1974, The ability of chemotactic factors to induce lysosomal enzyme release I. The characteristics of the release, the importance of surfaces and the relation of enzyme release to chemotactic responsiveness, *J. Immunol.* **112**:2047.

Bellanti, J. A., and Dayton, D. H. (eds.), 1975, *The Phagocytic Cell in Host Resistance*, Raven Press, New York.

Bjornson, A. B., and Alexander, J. W., 1974, Alterations of serum opsonins in patients with severe thermal injury, *J. Lab. Clin. Med.* **83**:372.

Bjornson, A. B., and Michael, J. G., 1974, Factors in human serum promoting phagocytosis of *Pseudomonas aeruginosa*. I. Interaction of opsonins with the bacterium, *J. Infect. Dis.* **130** (Suppl.):119–125.

Boggs, D. R., 1974, Transfusion of neutrophils as prevention or treatment of infection in patients with neutropenia, *N. Engl. J. Med.* **290**:1055.

Boxer, L. A., and Stossel, T. P., 1976, Interactions of actin, myosin and an actin-binding protein of chronic myelogenous leukemia granulocytes, *J. Clin. Invest.* **57**:964.

Boxer, L. A., Hedley-Whyte, E. T., and Stossel, T. P., 1974, Neutrophil actin dysfunction and abnormal neutrophil behavior, *N. Engl. J. Med.* **293**:1093.

Boxer, L. A., Wanatabe, A. M., Rister, M., Besch, H. R., Allen, J., and Baehner, R. L., 1976, Correction of leukocyte function in Chediak–Higashi syndrome by ascorbate, *N. Engl. J. Med.* **295**:1041.

Boxer, L. A., Rister, M., Allen, J. M., and Baehner, R. L., 1977, Improvement of Chediak–Higashi leukocyte function by cyclic guanosine monophosphate, *Blood* **49**:9.

Boyer, J. T., Gall, E. P., Normal, M. E., Nilsson, U. R., and Zimmerman, T. S., 1975, Hereditary deficiency of the seventh component of complement, *J. Clin. Invest.* **56**:905.

Bretz, U., and Baggiolini, M., 1974, Biochemical and morphological characterization of azurophil and specific granules of human neutrophilic polymorphonuclear leukocytes, *J. Cell Biol.* **63**:251.

Briggs, R. T., Drath, D. B., Karnovsky, M. L., and Karnovsky, M. J., 1975, Localization of NADH oxidase on the surface of human polymorphonuclear leukocytes by a new cytochemical method, *J. Cell Biol.* **67**:566.

Brozna, J. P., and Ward, P. A., 1975, Antileukotactic properties of tumor cells, *J. Clin. Invest.* **56**:616.

Bryant, R. E., and Sutcliffe, M. C., 1974, The effect of $3',5'$-adenosine monophosphate on granulocyte adhesion, *J. Clin. Invest.* **54**:1241.

Burns, C. P., Welshman, I. R., and Spector, A. A., 1976, Differences in free fatty acid and glucose metabolism of human blood neutrophils and lymphocytes, *Blood* **47**:431.

Casciato, D. A., Rosenblatt, J. E., Goldberg, L. S., and Bluestone, R., 1975, *In vitro* interaction of *Bacteroides fragilis* with polymorphonuclear leukocytes and serum factors, *Infect. Immunol.* **11**:337.

Chabner, B. A., Johns, D. G., Coleman, C. N., Drake, J. C., and Evans, W. H., 1974, Purification and properties of cytidine deaminase from normal and leukemic granulocytes, *J. Clin. Invest.* **53**:922.

Cline, M. J., Craddock, C. G., Gale, R. P., Golde, D. W., and Lehrer, R. I., 1974, Granulocytes in human disease, *Ann. Intern. Med.* **81**:801.

Craddock, P. R., Yawata, Y., Van Santen, L., Giberstadt, S., Silvis, S., and Jacob, H. S., 1974, Acquired phagocytic dysfunction. A complication of parenteral hyperalimentation, *N. Engl. J. Med.* **290**:1403.

Craddock, P. R., Fehr, J., and Jacob, H. S., 1976, Complement-mediated granulocyte dysfunction in paroxysmal nocturnal hemoglobinuria, *Blood* **47**:931.

Crowder, J. G., Devlin, H. R., Fisher, M., and White, A., 1974, Heat-stable opsonins in sera of patients with *Pseudomonas* infections, *J. Lab. Clin. Med.* **83**:853.

Curnutte, J. T., and Babior, B. M., 1975, Effects of anaerobiosis and inhibitors of $O_2$-production by human granulocytes, *Blood* **45**:851.

Curnutte, J. T., Whitten, D. M., and Babior, B. M., 1974, Defective superoxide generation by granulocytes from patients with chronic granulomatous disease, *N. Engl. J. Med.* **290**:593.

Curnutte, J. T., Kipnes, R. S., and Babior, B. M., 1975, Defect in pyridine nucleotide-dependent superoxide production by a particulate fraction from granulocytes of patients with chronic granulomatous disease, *N. Engl. J. Med.* **293**:628.

Curnutte, J. T., Karnovsky, M. L., and Babior, B. M., 1976, Manganese-dependent NADPH oxidation by granulocyte particles: The role of superoxide and the nonphysiological nature of the manganese requirement, *J. Clin. Invest.* **57**:1059.

Dale, D. C., Fauci, A. S., and Wolff, S. M., 1974, Alternate-day prednisone. Leukocyte kinetics and susceptibility to infections, *N. Engl. J. Med.* **291**:1154.

Davies, W., Thomas, M., Linkson, P., and Penny, R., 1975, Phagocytosis and the gamma globulin monolayer: Analysis by particle electrophoresis, *J. Reticuloendothel. Soc.* **18**:136.

DeChatelet, L. R., McPhail, L. C., Mullikan, D., and McCall, C. E., 1975, An isotopic assay for NADPH oxidase activity and some characteristics of the enzyme from human polymorphonuclear leukocytes, *J. Clin. Invest.* **55**:714.

DePierre, J. W., and Karnovsky, M. L., 1974, Ectoenzymes of the guinea pig polymorphonuclear leukocyte II. Properties and suitability as markers for the plasma membrane, *J. Biol. Chem.* **248**:7121.

Dewald, B., Rindler-Ludwig, R., Bretz, U., and Baggiolini, M., 1975, Subcellular localization and heterogeneity of neutral proteases in neutrophilic polymorphonuclear leukocytes, *J. Exp. Med.* **141**:709.

Diamond, R. D., May, J. E., Kane, M. A., Frank, M. M., Bennet, J. E., 1974, The role of the classical and alternate complement pathways in host defenses against *Cryptococcus neoformans* infection, *J. Immunol.* **112**:2260.

Dilworth, J. A., Hendley, J. O., and Mandell, G. L., 1975, Attachment and ingestion of gonococci by human neutrophils, *Infect. Immunol.* **11**:512.

Dubin, A., Koj, A., and Chudzik, J., 1976, Isolation and some molecular parameters of elastase-like neutral proteinases from horse blood leukocytes, *Biochem. J.* **153**:389.

Elliot, C. G., Maung, U. C., and Crozier, M. J., 1975, The influence of preparative techniques on glycolytic metabolism in resting leukocytes, *Exp. Cell Res.* **92**:412.

Elsbach, P., 1973, On the interaction between phagocytes and microorganisms, *N. Engl. J. Med.* **289**:846.

Erp, E. E., and Fahrney, D., 1975, Chromatographic characterization and opsonic activity of bovine erythrophilic and leukophilic $\gamma$-globulins, *Arch. Biochem. Biophys.* **168**:1.

Estensen, R. D., Reusch, M. E., Epstein, M. L., and Hill, H. R., 1976, Role of $Ca^{2+}$ and $Mg^{2+}$ in some human neutrophil functions as indicated by ionophore A23187, *Infect. Immunol.* **13**:146.

Feigenson, M. E., Schnebli, H. P., and Baggiolini, M., 1975, Demonstration of ricin-binding sites on the outer face of azurophil and specific granules of rabbit polymorphonuclear leukocytes, *J. Cell Biol.* **66**:183.

Forsgren, A., and Quie, P. G., 1974, Influence of the alternate complement pathway on opsonization of several bacterial species, *Infect. Immunol.* **10**:402.

Franson, R., Patriarca, P., and Elsbach, P., 1974, Phospholipid metabolism by phagocytic cells. Phospholipases $A_2$ associated with rabbit polymorphonuclear leukocyte granules, *Lipid Res.* **15**:380.

Fussganger, R. D., Kahn, C. R., Roth, J., and DeMeyts, P., 1976, Binding and degradation of insulin by human peripheral granulocytes. Demonstration of specific receptors with high affinity, *J. Biol. Chem.* **251**:2761.

Gallin, J. I., and Kirkpatrick, C. H., 1974, Chemotactic activity in dialyzable transfer factor, *Proc. Nat. Acad. Sci. U.S.A.* **71**:498.

Gallin, J. I., and Rosenthal, A. S., 1974, The regulatory role of divalent cations in human granulocyte chemotaxis: Evidence for an association between calcium exchanges and microtubule assembly, *J. Cell Biol.* **62**:594.

Gallin, J. I., and Wolff, S. M., 1975, Leucocyte chemotaxis: Physiological considerations and abnormalities, *Clin. Haematol.* **4**:567.

Gallin, J. I., Durocher, J. R., and Kaplan, A. P., 1975, Interaction of leukocyte chemotactic factors with the cell surface I. Chemotactic factor-induced changes in human granulocyte surface charge, *J. Clin. Invest.* **55**:967.

Gamow, E., and Barnes, F. S., 1974, Chemotactic responses of human polymorphonuclear leukocytes to cyclic GMP and other compounds, *Exp. Cell Res.* **87**:1.

Gibbs, D. L., and Roberts, R. B., 1975, The interaction *in vitro* between human polymorphonuclear leukocytes and *Neisseria gonorrhoeae* cultivated in the chick embryo, *J. Exp. Med.* **141**:155.

Gigli, I., Wintroub, B. U., and Goetzl, E. J., 1976, A phagocytosis-enhancing factor in human plasma, *Immunology* **30**:915.

Goetzl, E. J., 1975, Modulation of human neutrophil polymorphonuclear leucocyte migration by human plasma α-globulin inhibitors and synthetic esterase inhibitors, *Immunology* **29**:163.

Goetzl, E. J., Wasserman, S. I., Gigli, I., and Austen, K. F., 1974, Enhancement of random migration and chemotactic response of human leukocytes by ascorbic acid, *J. Clin. Invest.* **53**:813.

Goldstein, I. M., and Weissman, G., 1974, Generation of C5-derived lysosomal enzyme-releasing activity (C5a) by lysates of leukocyte lysosomes, *J. Immunol.* **113**:1583.

Goldstein, I. M., Horn, J. K., Kaplan, H. B., and Weissman, G., 1974, Calcium-induced lysozyme secretion from human polymorphonuclear leukocytes, *Biochem. Biophys. Res. Commun.* **60**:807.

Goldstein, I. M., Hoffstein, S. T., and Weissman, G., 1975, Mechanisms of lysosomal enzyme release from human polymorphonuclear leukocytes. Effects of phorbol myristate acetate, *J. Cell Biol.* **66**:647.

Goldstein, I. M., Cerqueira, M., Lind, S., and Kaplan, H. B., 1977, Evidence that the superoxide-generating system of human leukocytes is associated with the cell surface, *J. Clin. Invest.* **59**:249.

Haber, F., and Weiss, J., 1934, The catalytic decomposition of hydrogen peroxide by iron salts, *Proc. Roy. Soc. Ser. A* **147**:332.

Hartwig, J. H., and Stossel, T. P., 1976, Interactions of actin, myosin and an actin-binding protein of rabbit pulmonary macrophages III. Effects of cytochalasin B, *J. Cell Biol.* **71**:295.

Hawkins, D., 1974, Neutrophilic leukocytes in immunologic reactions *in vitro*. III. Pharmacologic modulation of lysosomal constituent release, *Clin. Immunol. Immunopathol.* **2**:141.

Hawley, H. P., and Gordon, G. B., 1976, The effects of long chain-free fatty acids on human neutrophil function and structure, *Lab. Invest.* **34**:216.

Henson, P. M., and Oades, Z. G., 1975, Stimulation of human neutrophils by soluble and insoluble immunoglobulin aggregates. Secretion of granule constituents and increased oxidation of glucose, *J. Clin. Invest.* **56**:1053.

Herzig, G. P., and Graw, R. G., 1975, Granulocyte transfusion for bacterial infections, *Prog. Hematol.* **9**:207.

Higby, D. J., and Henderson, E. S., 1975, Granulocyte transfusion therapy, *Annu. Rev. Med.* **26**:289.

Higgs, G. A., McCall, E., and Youlten, L. J. F., 1975, A chemotactic role for prostaglandins released from polymorphonuclear leucocytes during phagocytosis, *Br. J. Pharmacol.* **53**:539.

Hoffstein, S., Zurier, R. B., and Weissmann, G., 1974, Mechanisms of lysosomal enzyme release from human leukocytes III. Quantitative morphologic evidence for an effect of cyclic nucleotides and colchicine on degranulation, *Clin. Immunol. Immunopathol.* **3**:201.

Hoffstein, S., Soberman, R., Goldstein, I., and Weissmann, G., 1976, Concanavalin A induces microtubule assembly and specific granule discharge in human polymorphonuclear leukocytes, *J. Cell. Biol.* **68**:781.

Hohn, D. C., and Lehrer, R. I., 1975, NADPH oxidase deficiency in X-linked chronic granulomatous disease, *J. Clin. Invest.* **55**:707.

Holmes, B. A., Page, A. R., and Good, R. A., 1967, Studies of the metabolic activity of leukocytes from patients with a genetic abnormality of phagocytic function, *J. Clin. Invest.* **46**:1422.

Hsu, L. S., and Becker, E. L., 1975, Volume changes induced in rabbit polymorphonuclear leukocytes by chemotactic factor and cytochalasin B, *Am. J. Pathol.* **81**:1.

Humbert, J. R., Miescher, P. A., and Jaffe, E. R. (eds.), 1975, *Neutrophil Physiology and Pathology*, Grune & Stratton, New York.

Humphreys, D. W., Wheat, L. J., and White, A., 1974, Staphylococcal heat-stable opsonins, *J. Lab. Clin. Med.* **84**:122.

Ignarro, L. J., Lint, T. F., and George, W. J., 1974, Hormonal control of lysosomal enzyme release from human neutrophils. Effect of autonomic agents on enzyme release, phagocytosis, and cyclic nucleotide levels, *J. Exp. Med.* **139**:1395.

Janoff, A., Feinstein, G., Malemud, C. J., and Elias, J. M., 1976, Degradation of cartilage proteoglycan by human leukocyte granule neutral proteases—A model of joint injury. I. Penetration of enzyme into rabbit articular cartilage and release of $^{35}SO_4$-labeled material from the tissue, *J. Clin. Invest.* **57**:615.

Jasin, H. E., 1972, Human heat-labile opsonins: Evidence for their mediation via the alternate pathway of complement activation, *J. Immunol.* **109**:26.

Jasin, H. E., Orozco, J. H., and Ziff, M., 1974, Serum heat-labile opsonins in system lupus erythematosus, *J. Clin. Invest.* **53**:343.

Jensen, J. A., and Esquenazi, V., 1975, Chemotactic stimulation by cell surface immune reactions, *Nature (London)* **256**:213.

Johnston, R. B., Keele, B. B., Misra, H. P., Lenmeyer, J. E., Webb, L. S., Baehner, R. L., and Rajagopalan, K. V., 1975, The role of superoxide anion generation in phagocytic bactericidal activity: Studies with normal and chronic granulomatous disease leukocytes, *J. Clin. Invest.* **55**:1357.

Keller, H. U., Hess, M. W., and Cottier, H., 1974, Inhibiting effects of human plasma and serum on neutrophil random migration and chemotaxis, *Blood* **44**:843.

Khan, A. J., Evans, H. E., Glass, L., Shin, Y. H., and Almonte, D., 1975, Defective neutrophil chemotaxis in patients with Down's syndrome, *J. Pediatr.* **87**:87.

Klebanoff, S. J., and Hamon, C. B., 1972, Role of myeloperoxidase-mediated antimicrobial systems in intact leukocytes, *J. Reticuloendothel. Soc.* **12**:170.

Klockars, M., and Roberts, P., 1976, Stimulation of phagocytosis by human lysozyme, *Acta Haematol.* **55**:289.

Kopitar, M., and Lebez, D., 1975, Intracellular distribution of neutral proteinases and inhibitors in pig leucocytes. Isolation of two inhibitors of neutral proteinases, *Eur. J. Biochem.* **56**:571.

Kostman, R., 1975, Infantile genetic agranulocytosis, *Acta Paediatr. Scand.* **64**:362.

Krinsky, N. I., 1974, Singlet excited oxygen as a mediator of the antibacterial action of leukocytes, *Science* **186**:363.

Larson, H. E., and Blades, R., 1976, Impairment of human polymorphonuclear leukocyte function by influenza virus, *Lancet* **1**:283.

Lawrence, D. A., Weigle, W. O., and Spiegelberg, H. L., 1975, Immunoglobulins cytophilic for human lymphocytes, monocytes and neutrophils, *J. Clin. Invest.* **55**:368.

Lehrer, R. I., 1972, Functional aspects of a second mechanism of candidacidal activity by human neutrophils, *J. Clin. Invest.* **51**:2566.

Lentnek, A. L., Schreiber, A. D., and MacGregor, R. R., 1976, The induction of augmented granulocyte adherence by inflammation. Mediation by a plasma factor, *J. Clin. Invest.* **57**:1098.

LeRoux, J. P., Marchand, J. C., Ha, R. T. H., and Cartier, P., 1975, The influence of insulin on glucose permeability and metabolism of human granulocytes, *Eur. J. Biochem.* **58**:367.

Lichtman, M. A. (ed.), 1975, Granulocyte and monocyte abnormalities, *Clin. Haematol.* **4**:485.

Lund-Olesen, K., and Menander, K. B., 1974, Orgotein: A new anti-inflammatory metalloprotein drug: Preliminary evaluation of clinical efficacy and safety in degenerative joint disease, *Curr. Ther. Res. Clin. Exp.* **16**:706.

Maderazo, E. G., Ward, P. A., and Quintiliani, R., 1975, Defective regulation of chemotaxis in cirrhosis, *J. Lab. Clin. Med.* **85**:621.

Maderazo, E. G., Ward, P. A., Woronick, C. L., Kubik, J., and DeGraff, Jr., A. C., 1976, Leukotactic dysfunction in sarcoidosis, *Ann. Intern. Med.* **84**:414.

Mandell, G. L., 1974, Bactericidal activity of aerobic and anaerobic polymorphonuclear neutrophils, *Infect. Immunol.* **9**:337.

Mantovani, B., 1975, Different roles of IgG and complement receptors in phagocytosis by polymorphonuclear leukocytes, *J. Immunol.* **115**:15.

Matthews, J. H., Klesius, P. H., and Zimmerman, R. A., 1974, Opsonin system of the group B streptococcus, *Infect. Immunol.* **10**:1315.

McCord, J. M., and Fridovich, I., 1969, Superoxide dismutase: An enzymic function for erythrocuprein (hemocuprein), *J. Biol. Chem.* **244**:5049.

Metchnikoff, E., 1887, Sur la lutte des cellules de l'organisme contre l'invasion des microbes, *Ann. Inst. Pasteur* **1**:321.

Najjar, V. A., 1975, Defective phagocytosis due to deficiencies involving the tetrapeptide, tuftsin, *J. Pediatr.* **87**:1121.

Nishiura, M., Matsumura, K., and Hayashi, H., 1976, The natural mediator for PMN emigration in inflammation VIII. Production of leucoegresin-like chemotactic factor in reversed passive arthus reactions in rats, *Immunology* **30**:521.

Ohlsson, K., and Olsson, I., 1974, The neutral proteases of human granulocytes. Isolation and partial characterization of granulocyte elastases, *Eur. J. Biochem.* **42**:519.

Oliver, C., and Essner, E., 1975, Formation of anomalous lysosomes in monocytes, neutrophils and eosinophils from bone marrow of mice with Chediak–Higashi syndrome, *Lab. Invest.* **32**:17.

Oliver, J. M., and Zurier, R. B., 1976, Correction of characteristic abnormalities of microtubule function and granule morphology in Chediak–Higashi syndrome with cholinergic agonists. Studies *in vitro* in man and *in vivo* in the beige mouse, *J. Clin. Invest.* **57**:1239.

Oliver, J. M., Zurier, R. B., and Berlin, R. D., 1975, Concanavalin A cap formation on polymorphonuclear leukocytes of normal and beige (Chediak–Higashi) mice, *Nature (London)* **253**:471.

Oliver, J. M., Albertini, D. F., and Berlin, R. D., 1976, Effects of glutathione-oxidizing agents on microtubule-dependent surface properties of human neutrophils, *J. Cell. Biol.* **71**:921.

Ortel, R. W., and Newcombe, D. A., 1974, Acute gouty arthritis and response to colchicine in the virtual absence of synovial-fluid leukocytes, *N. Engl. J. Med.* **290**:1363.

Patriarca, P., Cramer, R., Dri, P., Fant, L., Basford, R. E., and Rossi, F., 1973, NADPH oxidizing activity in rabbit polymorphonuclear leukocytes: Localization in azurophilic granules, *Biochem. Biophys. Res. Commun.* **53**:830.

Pincus, S. H., Thomas, I. T., Clark, R. A., and Ochs, H. D., 1975, Defective neutrophil chemotaxis with variant icthyosis, hyperimmunoglobulinemia E, and recurrent infections, *J. Pediatr.* **87**:908.

Pincus, S. H., Boxer, L. A., and Stossel, T. P., 1976, Chronic neutropenia in childhood. Analysis of 16 cases and a review of the literature, *Am. J. Med.* **61**:849.

Plesner, L., Plesner, I. W., and Esmann, V., 1974, Kinetic mechanism of glycogen synthase D from human polymorphonuclear leukocytes, *J. Biol. Chem.* **249**:1119.

Plow, E. G., and Edginton, T. S., 1975, An alternative pathway for fibrinolysis I The cleavage of fibrinogen by leukocyte proteases at physiologic pH, *J. Clin. Invest.* **56**:30.

Proctor, R. A., White, J. D., Ayala, E., and Canonico, P. G., 1975, Phagocytosis of *Francisella tularenses* by rhesus monkey peripheral leukocytes, *Infect. Immunol.* **11**:146.

Ramsey, W. S., 1974a, Leukocyte locomotion and chemotaxis, *Antibiot. Chemother.* **19**:179.

Ramsey, W. S., 1974b, Retraction fibers and leukocyte chemotaxis, *Exp. Cell Res.* **86**:184.

Rausch, P. G., and Moore, T. G., 1975, Granule enzymes of polymorphonuclear neutrophils: A phylogenetic comparison, *Blood* **46**:913.

Reddi, K. K., 1976, Human granulocyte ribonuclease, *Biochem. Biophys. Res. Commun.* **68**:1119.

Reed, W. P., 1975, Serum factors capable of opsonizing *Shigella* for phagocytosis by polymorphonuclear neutrophils, *Immunology* **28**:1051.

Richardson, D. L., Pepper, D. S., and Kay, A. B., 1976, Chemotaxis for human monocytes by fibrinogen-derived peptides, *Br. J. Haematol.* **32**:507.

Rivkin, I., Rosenblatt, J., and Becker, E. L., 1975, The role of cyclic AMP in the chemotactic responsiveness and spontaneous motility of rabbit peritoneal neutrophils. The inhibition of neutrophil movement and the elevation of cyclic AMP levels by catecholamines, prostaglandins, theophylline and cholera toxin, *J. Immunol.* **115**:1126.

Roos, D., HomaMüller, J. W. T., and Weening, R. S., 1976, Effect of cytochalasin B on the oxidative metabolism of human peripheral blood granulocytes, *Biochem. Biophys. Res. Commun.* **68**:43.

Root, R. K., and Metcalf, J., 1976, Initiation of granulocyte $O_2$- and $H_2O_2$ formation by stimulation of membrane phagocytic receptors, *Clin. Res.* **24**:352A.

Root, R. K., Metcalf, J., Oshino, N., and Chance, B., 1975, $H_2O_2$ release from human granulocytes during phagocytosis, *J. Clin. Invest.* **55**:945.

Root, R. K., and Stossel, T. P., 1974, Myeloperoxidase-mediated iodination by granulocytes. Intracellular site of operation and some regulating factors, *J. Clin. Invest.* **53**:1207.

Rosen, H., and Klebanoff, S. J., 1976, Chemiluminescence by granulocytes: Role of myeloperoxidase, singlet oxygen and superoxide anion, *Clin. Res.* **24**:353A.

Rosenfeld, S. I., Baum, J., Steigbigel, R. 1., and Leddy, J. P., 1976, Hereditary deficiency of the fifth component of complement in man II. Biological properties of C5-deficient human serum, *J. Clin. Invest.* **57**:1635.

Ruddy, S., Austen, K. F., and Geotzl, E. J., 1975, Chemotactic activity derived from interaction of factors D and B of the properdin pathway with cobra venom factor or C3b, *J. Clin. Invest.* **55**:587.

Ryan, G. B., Borysenko, J. Z., and Karnovsky, M. J., 1974, Factors affecting the redistribution of surface-bound concanavalin A on human polymorphonuclear leukocytes, *J. Cell Biol.* **62**:351.

Salin, M. L., and McCord, J. M., 1975, Free radicals and inflammation: Protection of phagocytosing leukocytes by superoxide dismutase, *J. Clin. Invest.* **56**:1319.

Sandler, J. A., Gallin, J. I., and Vaughan, M., 1975, Effects of serotonin, carbamylcholine, and ascorbic acid on leukocyte cyclic GMP and chemotaxis, *J. Cell Biol.* **67**:480.

Sbarra, A. J., and Karnovsky, M. L., 1959, The biochemical basis of phagocytosis I. Metabolic changes during the ingestion of particles by polymorphonuclear leukocytes, *J. Biol. Chem.* **234**:1355.

Schiffmann, E., Corcoran, B. A., and Wahl, S. M., 1975a, *N*-Formylmethionyl peptides as chemoattractants for leukocytes, *Proc. Nat. Acad. Sci. U.S.A.* **72**:1059.

Schiffmann, E., Showell, H. V., Corcoran, B. A., Ward, P. A., Smith, E., and Becker, E. L., 1975b, The isolation and partial characterization of neutrophil chemotactic factors from *Escherichia coli, J. Immunol.* **114**:1831.

Scribner, D. J., and Fahrney, D., 1976, Neutrophil receptors for IgG and complement: Their roles in the attachment and ingestion phases of phagocytosis, *J. Immunol.* **116**:892.

Showell, H., Freer, R., Zigmond, S., Schiffmann, E., Aswanikumar, S., Corcoran, B., and Becker, E. L., 1976, Structure–activity relations of synthetic peptides as chemotactic factors and inducers of lysosomal enzyme secretion for neutrophils, *J. Exp. Med.* **143**:1154–1169.

Simberkoff, M. S., Ricupero, I., and Rahal, Jr., J. J., 1976, Host resistance to *Serratia marcescens* infection: Serum bactericidal activity and phagocytosis by normal blood leukocytes, *J. Lab. Clin. Med.* **87**:206.

Smith, C. W., Hollers, J. C., Bing, D. H., and Patrick, R. A., 1975, Effects of human C1 inhibitor on complement-mediated human leukocyte chemotaxis, *J. Immunol.* **114**:216.

Smith, R. J., and Ignarro, L. J., 1975, Bioregulation of lysosomal enzyme secretion from human neutrophils: Roles of guanosine 3′,5′-monophosphate and calcium in stimulus–secretion coupling, *Proc. Nat. Acad. Sci. U.S.A.* **72**:108.

Sørensen, N. B., and Wang, P., 1975, Purification of glycogen phosphorylase by affinity chromatography on 5′-AMP sepharose, *Biochem. Biophys. Res. Commun.* **67**:883.

Spitznagel, J. K., Dalldorf, F. G., Leffell, M. S., Folds, J. D., Welsh, I. R. H., Cooney, B. S., and Martin, L. E., 1974, Character of azurophil and specific granules purified from human polymorphonuclear leukocytes, *Lab. Invest.* **30**:774.

Stanley, E. R., Hansen, G., Woodcock, J., and Metcalf, D., 1975, Colony stimulating factor and the regulation of granulopoiesis and macrophage production, *Fed. Proc.* **34**:2272.

Stecher, V. J., 1975, The chemotaxis of selected cell types to connective tissue degradation products, *Ann. N.Y. Acad. Sci.* **256**:177.

Stossel, T. P., 1973, Quantitative studies of phagocytosis: Kinetic effects of cations and heat-labile opsonin, *J. Cell. Biol.* **58**:346.

Stossel, T. P., 1974, Phagocytosis, *N. Engl. J. Med.* **290**:717, 774, 833.

Stossel, T. P., 1975, Phagocytosis: Recognition and ingestion, *Semin. Hematol.* **14**:83.

Stossel, T. P., 1977, Motile functions of phagocytic effector cells, *in Development of Host Defenses* (D. H. Dayton *et al.*, eds.), Raven Press, New York (in press).

Stossel, T. P., and Pollard, T. D., 1973, Myosin in polymorphonuclear leukocytes, *J. Biol. Chem.* **248**:8288.

Stossel, T. P., Alpec, C. A., and Rosen, F. S., 1973, Phagocytosis of paeaffin oil emulsified with bacterial lipopolysaccharide, *J. Exp. Med.* **137**:690.

Stossel, T. P., Mason, R. J., and Smith, A. L., 1974, Lipid peroxidation in human blood phagocytes, *J. Clin. Invest.* **54**:638.

Stossel, T. P., Field, R. J., Gitlin, J. D., Alper, C. A., and Rosen, F. S., 1975, The opsonic fragment of the third component of human complement (C3), *Exp. Med* **141**:1329.

Strauss, R. G., McCarthy, D. J., and Mauer, A. M., 1974, Neutrophil function congenital phosphorglycerate kinase deficiency, *J. Pediatr.* **85**:341.

Takeuchi, K., Shibata, N., and Senda, N., 1975, ATPase activity and filament formation of partially purified myosin from leukocytes, *J. Biochem.* **78**:93.

Till, G., and Ward, P. A., 1975, Two distinct chemotactic factor inactivators in human serum, *J. Immunol.* **114**:843.

Tsung, P.-K., Sakamoto, T., and Weissmann, G., 1975, Protein kinase and phosphatases from human polymorphonuclear leukocytes, *Biochem. J.* **145**:437.

Turner, S. R., Campbell, J. A., and Lynn, W. S., 1975, Polymorphonuclear leukocyte chemotaxis toward oxidized lipid components of cell membranes, *J. Exp. Med.* **141**:1437.

Van Epps, D. E., Palmer, D. L., and Williams, Jr., R. C., 1974, Characterization of serum inhibitors of neutrophil chemotaxis associated with energy, *J. Immunol.* **113**:189.

Van Epps, D. E., Strickland, R. G., and Williams, Jr., R. C., 1975, Inhibitors of leukocyte chemotaxis in alcoholic liver disease, *Am. J. Med.* **59**:200.

Van Scoy, R. E., Hill, H. R., Ritts, Jr., R. E., and Quie, P. G., 1975, Familial neutrophil chemotaxis defect, recurrent bacterial infections, mucocutaneous candidiasis, and hyperimmunoglobulinemia E, *Ann. Intern. Med.* **82**:765.

Venge, P., and Olsson, I., 1975, Cationic proteins of human granulocytes VI. Effects on the complement system and mediation of chemotactic activity, *J. Immunol.* **115**:1505.

Wagner, T., Abraham, G., and Baum, J., 1974, The roles of IgG, IgM, rheumatoid factor, and their complexes in the induction of polymorphonuclear leukocyte chemotactic factor from complement, *J. Clin. Invest.* **53**:1503.

Ward, P. A., 1974, Leukotaxis and leukotactic disorders, *Am. J. Pathol.* **77**:520.

Ward, P. A., and Berenberg, J. L., 1974, Defective regulation of inflammatory mediators in Hodgkin's disease. Supernormal levels of chemotactic factor inactivator, *N. Engl. J. Med.* **290**:76.

Ward, P. A., Data, R., and Till, G., 1974, Regulatory control of complement-derived chemotactic and anaphylatoxin mediators, *Prog. Immunol.* **2**:209.

Warden, G. D., Mason, Jr., A. D., and Pruitt, Jr., B. A., 1974, Evaluation of leukocyte chemotaxis *in vitro* in thermally injured patients, *J. Clin. Invest.* **54**:1001.

Weinstein, R. J., and Young, L. S., 1976, Neutrophil function in gram-negative rold bacteremia. The interaction between phagocytic cells, infecting organisms, and humoral factors, *J. Clin. Invest.* **58**:190.

Weisbart, R. H., Isaacson, J., Bluestone, R., and Goldberg, L. S., 1975, Human polymorphonuclear leukocyte migration inhibitory factor. Evidence for antigen dependency, *Immunology* **29**:223.

Weiss, J., Franson, R. C., Schmiedler, K., Elsbach, P., 1976, Reversible envelope effects during and after killing of *Escherichia coli* W by a highly-purified rabbit polymorphonuclea leukocyte fraction, *Biochim., Biophys. Acta.* **436**: 154.

White, J. G., and Estensen, R. D., 1974, Selective labilization of specific granules in polymorphonuclear leukocytes by phorbol myristate acetate, *Am. J. Pathol.* **75**:45.

Wilkinson, P. C., 1975, Leukocyte locomotion and chemotaxis. The influence of divalent cations and cation ionophores, *Exp. Cell Res.* **93**:420.

Wilkinson, P. C., and McKay, I. C., 1974, Recognition in leukocyte chemotaxis. Studies with structurally modified proteins, *Antibiot. Chemother.* **19**:421.

Wilson, A. T., Wiley, G. G., and Bruno, P., 1957, Fate of nonvirulent group A streptococci phagocytized by human and mouse neutrophils, *J. Exp. Med.* **106**:777.

Woodin, A. M., Poole, A. R., and Dunn, G. A., 1975, The effect of triisopropyl phosphate on the mobility of surface concanavalin A receptors and on the locomotion of polymorphonuclear leukocytes, *Exp. Cell Res.* **94**:292.

Zigmond, S. H., 1974, Mechanisms of sensing chemical gradients by polymorphonuclear leukocytes, *Nature (London)* **249**:450.

Zipursky, A., and Brown, E. J., 1974, The ingestion of IgG-sensitive erythrocytes by abnormal neutrophils, *Blood* **43**:737.

Zurier, R. B., Hoffstein, S., Weissmann, G., 1973, Cytochalasin B: Effect on lysosomal enzyme release from human leukocytes, *Proc. Nat. Acad. Sci. USA* **70**:844.

# Phagocytosis: Role of C3 Receptors and Contact-Inducing Agents

## Alfred G. Ehlenberger and Victor Nussenzweig

## 7.1. Introduction

The primary immunologic defense mechanism in man, as well as other vertebrates and invertebrates, is clearly phagocytosis. This fact is demonstrated by the rapidly fatal course which results when phagocytes are absent or severely depleted. In contrast, the absence of lymphocytes can be tolerated in man over a period of months or even years.

The mechanism whereby phagocytes recognize and ingest "foreign" particles remains one of the classic problems in biology. Some particles and bacteria can be ingested without opsonization, and it is clearly not an accident that these bacteria are generally nonpathogenic. Virulent bacteria, on the other hand, often require the effect of serum factors to promote their ingestion. Wright and Douglas (1903), who coined the term "opsonin" for these serum factors, also showed that (a) opsonins acted on the bacteria and not on leukocytes; and (b) opsonic activity in serum was heat labile and could be destroyed by heating the serum at 60°C for 15 min. This heat lability suggested that at least some serum opsonins were

ALFRED G. EHLENBERGER • Department of Psychiatry, Stanford University Medical Center, Palo Alto, California 94304. VICTOR NUSSENZWEIG • Department of Pathology, New York University School of Medicine, New York, New York 10016.

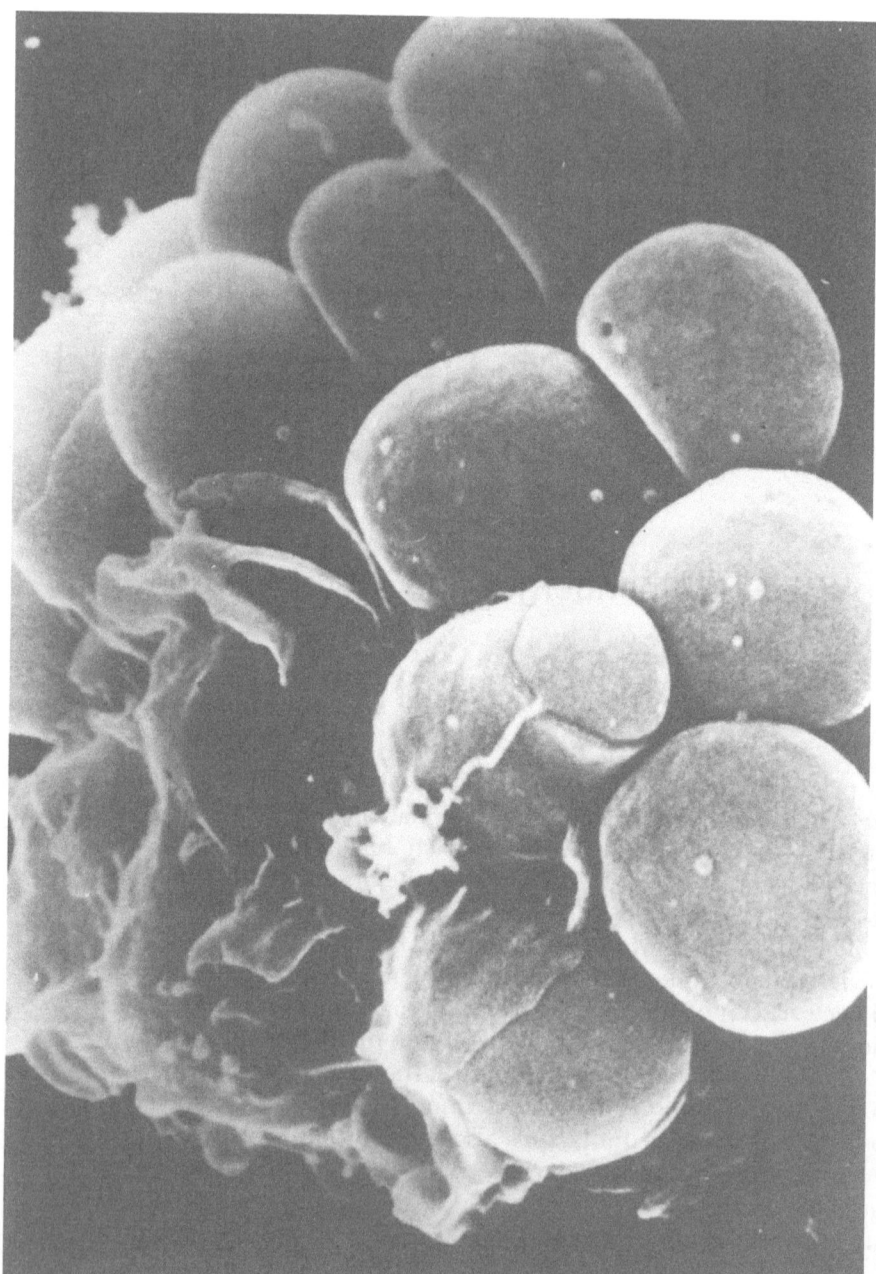

**Fig. 1.** Human monocyte ingesting opsonized sheep red cells. Red cells were initially bound to the monocyte through complement receptors. No ingestion occurred, however, even after 2 hr of incubation at 37°C. This photograph was taken 5 min after 0.1 µg/ml of IgG anti-sheep red cell antibody was added to the medium. (Courtesy of Dr. Jean-Paul Revel, California Institute of Technology.)

part of the complement system. This chapter will discuss the mechanism by which complement, and particularly C3, participates in the opsonization process.

The importance of C3 in defense mechanisms has been highlighted by the finding of patients with a hereditary deficiency in C3 (Alper *et al.*, 1972). These patients have repeated infections although they have normal levels of immunoglobulin and form antibodies to both thymus-dependent and -independent antigens (Rosen, 1975). Deficiencies in other complement components do not seem to cause this difficulty. This discovery correlates with the observation (Lay and Nussenzweig, 1968; Huber *et al.*, 1968; Ross *et al.*, 1973; Ehlenberger and Nussenzweig, 1975) that the so-called professional phagocytes (Rabinovitch, 1967a), i.e., monocytes, macrophages, and polymorphs, bear on their surfaces specific receptors for C3. Two different receptors for C3 products have been identified. The first recognizes cell-bound or fluid phase C3b, generated by the reaction between the C1,4,2 enzyme complex and C3. The second receptor recognizes C3d, a much smaller fragment, which remains on the cell after cleavage of C3b by a serum enzyme, C3b inactivator (Ruddy and Austen, 1971). Polymorphs, macrophages, and monocytes (as well as B lymphocytes) all bind C3b, but only lymphocytes and monocytes bind C3d (Eden *et al.*, 1973; Ross *et al.*, 1973; Ross and Polley, 1975; Ehlenberger and Nussenzweig, 1975; Griffin *et al.*, 1975a).

The exact mechanism whereby C3 and C3 receptors participate in opsonization remains controversial. This chapter will briefly review some of the classical and contemporary work on phagocytosis, and will also present some new data on the role of complement receptors in phagocytosis by human monocytes, human PMN, and both normal and "activated" macrophages from mouse peritoneal cavities. We will show that these data are all consistent with the idea that the complement receptor has the same function in all these various species and cell types, that is, that the complement receptor serves to establish an intimate contact between the surface of the phagocyte and the surface of the complement-coated particle. This contact, by itself, is not sufficient to induce phagocytosis. However, the establishment of such contact may be required for the phagocyte to recognize those surface moieties (such as particle-bound IgG) which do stimulate the ingestion process. The presence of complement on the particle may thus be a necessary condition for phagocytosis, but C3 by itself does not induce ingestion.

We will demonstrate that both C3b and C3d receptors exhibit this opsonic effect, and further that the opsonic action of C3–C3-receptor interaction can be mimicked by a variety of nonimmunologic physical agents which act by enhancing particle–phagocyte contact. These contact-inducing agents (CIA), like C3, markedly enhance the recognition of particle-bound IgG but, by themselves, do not induce ingestion. Further-more, the effect of these agents disappears when the particle is bound to the phagocyte by complement receptors. These results strongly suggest that the complement receptor itself functions as a contact-inducing agent.

## 7.2. Role of Contact and Surface Forces in Phagocytosis

We would first like to present briefly some of the theories and observations in which the role of physical forces or surface interactions between particle and phagocyte was considered relevant in the ingestion process. Before and early in the twentieth century Rhumbler (1898, 1914) had attempted to explain phagocytosis in terms of physical models. His work was carried forward and improved by several, including Fenn (1922), who postulated that one could explain phagocytosis as a physical process in terms of the surface tensions present at the particle–fluid, phagocyte–fluid, and particle–phagocyte interfaces. This view was widely held for many years, and it was considered that opsonins acted by altering these forces in a way which promoted ingestion. The longevity of this theory resulted in part from the fact that it explained everything in terms of forces which were generally not experimentally measurable and there-fore could not be tested. There is some current work, however, which relates particle ingestibility to surface forces measurable by the "contact angle" of liquids above a monolayer of these particles (Van Oss and Gillman, 1972).

The work of W. Barry Wood, Jr. (1946) in the late 1940s and 1950s, demonstrated in an experimental fashion the importance of the establish-ment of intimate contact in phagocytic recognition. Wood studied the ingestion of pneumococci by alveolar exudate cells *in vitro* and noted that the phagocytes were quite capable of ingesting these bacteria without opsonization when the phagocyte trapped the bacteria against a surface or against another phagocyte. Thus, these bacteria did not require opsoniza-tion to be recognized as "foreign," provided the phagocyte could press against the bacteria. This occurred most efficiently on a rough surface, such as was provided by alveolar tissue, but also could be provided on a number of artificial surfaces such as filter paper, cloth, and fiberglass. What these experiments showed, in effect, was that the recognition of ingestibility and subsequent interiorization of the particle required that some force be applied to approximate the surface of the bacteria and the surface of the phagocyte. When this force did not exist, the phagocyte was oblivious to the presence of the bacteria.

Rabinovitch (1967b) later divided phagocytosis into a two-stage pro-cess—first, particle attachment, and then interiorization. Again it was considered that the process of phagocytosis required that the phagocyte first establish contact with the particle before ingestion could occur.

More recently, the importance of surface interactions in phagocytosis has been highlighted by the "zipper theory" (Griffin *et al.*, 1975b), which claims that the ingestion process is a sequential linking up of ligands and receptors around the surface of the particle in a fashion much like the closing of a zipper. Thus, a particle will be ingested if it possesses ligands distributed over its entire surface and the phagocyte bears appropriate receptors for these ligands in a distribution which permits the sequential zippering process.

## 7.3. Role of C3 in Opsonization

The role of complement in opsonization has been debated since the original experiments showing the existence of heat-labile opsonins in serum. However, in 1931, Topley and Wilson stated, in a consensus view, that

> The very low concentration of the specific antibodies in normal serum necessitates the adjuvant action of a considerable amount of complement before its presence can be detected, so that the complementary action appears to dominate the picture. The high concentration of the specific antibody in an immune serum reduces the adjuvant action of the complement to a mere enhancement of an effect which takes place in its absence.

This view was reinforced by the work of Ward and Enders (1933), who investigated the ingestion of the pneumococcus by human peripheral blood phagocytes. These investigators compared the ingestion of pneumococci which had been opsonized by antibody alone, to the ingestion of pneumococci opsonized with both antibody and complement. It was clear to these authors that complement possessed an adjuvant or catalytic activity in the ingestion process. This activity was ascribed to a "speeding up" of the combination of antibody with its corresponding antigen, which was mediated by complement. In part, this view of complement as an adjuvant stemmed naturally from the sequence of events in the classical complement pathway, in that antibody must bind first in order to deposit complement. While Ward and Enders stated that "Muir's hypothesis, which states that complement alone can bring about phagocytosis, is untenable," experiments demonstrating the opsonic effect of complement deposition without the presence of opsonizing antibody could not be performed.

Further progress in understanding the role of serum opsonins became possible when modern chromatographic techniques permitted the isolation of complement components and the resolution of antibody into separate classes. It became clear that macrophages, monocytes, and neutrophils all bore receptors for the Fc fragment of IgG (Boyden, 1964; Berken and Benacerraf, 1966; Lo Buglio et al., 1967; Lay and Nussenzweig, 1968; Abramson et al., 1970) and that IgG directly stimulated both the attachment and interiorization of particles. IgM, it was found, was not recognized by these phagocytes (Abramson et al., 1970; Berken and Benacerraf, 1966; Huber and Fudenberg, 1968; Rabinovitch, 1967c) but could be used to deposit complement on the surface of test particles.

Receptors were also found for C3 on macrophages, PMN, and monocytes in various species (Lay and Nussenzweig, 1968; Nussenzweig et al., 1969; Huber et al., 1968) but the role of these complement receptors was not clear. Although the classical experiments of Gigli and Nelson (1968), as well as others (Shin et al., 1969; Johnston et al., 1969), showed that C3 was particularly important in the process of opsonization, it became clear that the effect of particle-bound C3, without IgG, was to induce binding without inducing ingestion. This fact has been demonstrated with human monocytes, mouse and human PMN, and mouse and human macrophages (Mantovani et al., 1972; Ross and Polley, 1974; Scribner and Fahrney, 1975; Ehlenberger and Nussenzweig, 1975; Mantovani, 1975). However, cooperation between C3 and IgG in opsonization is also well established in human, mouse, and guinea pig phagocytes (Huber et al., 1968; Mantovani et al., 1972; Ehlenberger and Nussenzweig, 1975; Scribner and Fahrney, 1975; Mantovani, 1975; Wellek et al., 1975). Recent experiments in our laboratory have confirmed and further quantitated this phenomenon. These experiments are performed according to the following basic protocol:

Sheep red cells (E) are sensitized with C3 using IgM anti-E and purified human complement components. In some experiments [125]I-labeled C3 was used to quantitate directly the number of C3 molecules per red cell. In experiments with mouse macrophages, C5-deficient mouse complement is used to opsonize with C3. After sensitization with C3, a known number of IgG molecules are bound to the red cells using an IgG preparation of a rabbit-anti-E serum, whose binding specificity was measured by labeling an aliquot with [125]I. We therefore have independent control of both IgG and C3 on the particle surface. These cells are designated EIgMC3·IgG. Red cells are also prepared using IgG alone (EIgG). A subscript indicates the number of IgG molecules bound per red cell—thus, $EIgMC3 \cdot IgG_{400}$ are red cells sensitized with C3 and an average of 400 molecules of IgG. The number of C3 molecules bound per red cell, when known, is also indicated in a subscript, for example, $EIgMC3d_{500} \cdot IgG_{600}$. The details of the preparation of EIgG and EIgMC3·IgG with human or mouse complement have been described in a previous work (Ehlenberger and Nussenzweig, 1976).

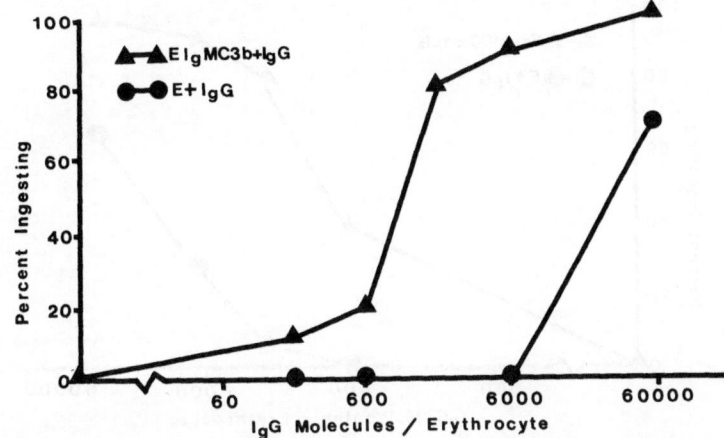

**Fig. 2.** Ingestion of EIgG and EIgMC3b·IgG by human PMN. Red cells were sensitized with IgG alone (EIgG) or with both C3b and IgG (EIgMC3b·IgG). Phagocytosis was assayed with the "overlay" technique. The figure shows the percentage of phagocytes ingesting red cells versus the number of IgG molecules bound per red cell.

The ingestion of EIgG is compared to ingestion of EIgMC3·IgG in Figures 2, 3, and 4 for monolayers of purified human polymorphs, human monocytes, and normal mouse macrophages, respectively. These experiments were carried out in "overlay" fashion; that is, monolayers of phagocytes are overlaid with a suspension of red cells and the suspension is allowed to settle down on the monolayer, producing a *saturating* concentration of particles on the phagocytes. After 30–45 min of incubation at 37°C, all external red cells are lysed by osmotic shock and the monolayers

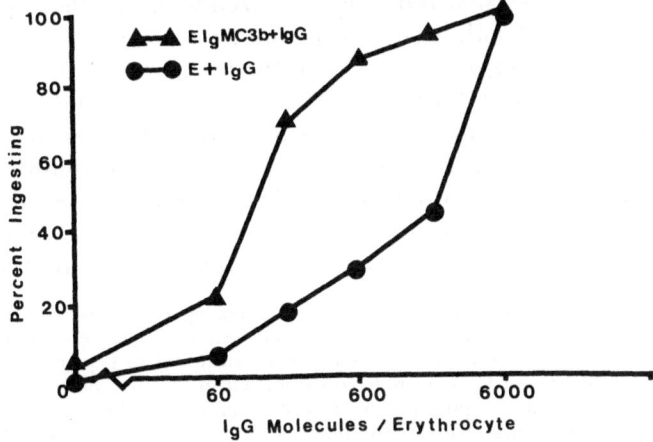

**Fig. 3.** Ingestion of EIgG and EIgMC3b·IgG by human monocytes, assayed with the "overlay" technique.

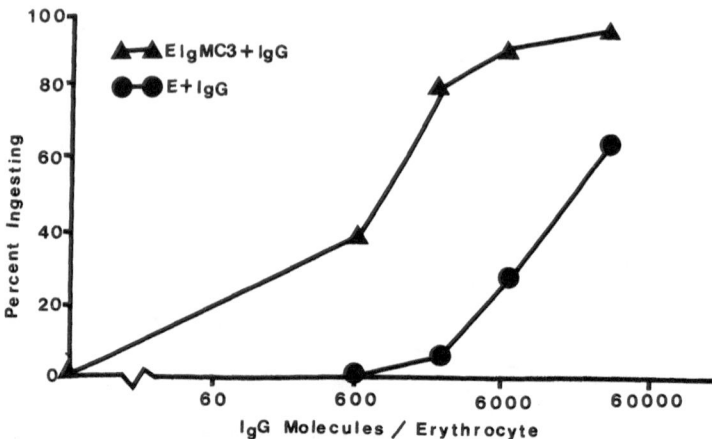

**Fig. 4.** Ingestion of EIgG and EIgMC3·IgG by normal mouse peritoneal macrophages. These experiments were also carried out in the "overlay fashion."

are fixed, stained, and examined for red cell ingestion. The osmotic lysis of external red cells does not affect leukocytes or ingested red cells, and one may thus distinguish absolutely between attached and ingested particles. The details of these techniques have been previously described (Ehlenberger and Nussenzweig, 1976).

The figures show the percentage of phagocytes ingesting red cells versus the number of IgG molecules used to sensitize E or EIgMC3. Similar behavior is shown by all three types of phagocytes: First, red cells sensitized with C3 alone (without IgG) are not ingested. In experiments with human phagocytes and labeled C3, up to 14,000 molecules of C3 could be attached to the red cell without inducing ingestion. In contrast, human monocytes ingested red cells opsonized with as little as 100 molecules of IgG.* Second, although C3 does not produce ingestion by itself, it tremendously enhances the sensitivity of the phagocyte to particle-bound IgG. In experiments with human PMN using labeled C3 and labeled IgG, opsonization with 1000 molecules of C3b and 2000 molecules of IgG proved more efficient at inducing phagocytosis than opsonization with 60,000 molecules of IgG without C3. Third, addition of C3 to a particle may cause that particle to be ingested, even though C3 does not mediate the process directly. When small amounts of IgG are present, the phago-

*The exquisite sensitivity of monocytes to IgG is probably responsible for the limited ingestion of EIgMC3b which did occur. Calculations indicated that contamination of the IgM anti-SRBC with as little as 0.1% IgG would be sufficient to explain this ingestion. Several lots of IgM proved to be frankly contaminated in that monocytes ingested both E "IgM" and E "IgM" C3b in significant amounts. We therefore used ingestion of EIgMC3b as a bioassay for the presence of IgG in the IgM preparations. Any lot which induced more than 5% of monocytes to ingest EIgMC3b or EIgM was discarded.

cyte apparently cannot recognize or respond without the synergistic effect C3 provides. Thus, addition of C3 to a red cell bearing a small amount of IgG will induce the ingestion of that red cell, but in an indirect fashion.

Red cells prepared with IgM, C1, C4, and C2 (but not C3) did not bind to the phagocytes nor was synergy with IgG observed with these cells. The effect was dependent on the presence of C3 on the red cells in sufficient quantities to produce binding and "rosette" formation (about 500–1000 C3 moieties per red cell were required). Deposition of C3 in amounts greater than this showed little further enhancement of phagocytosis.

It must be emphasized that these experiments were carried out under conditions in which the phagocytes were saturated with red cells and no shear forces existed between red cell and phagocyte. The effect of C3 is magnified if the red cell suspension is under agitation, as shown in the following experiment: Red cells were prepared, using $^{125}$I-C3 and purified C3b inactivator, so that about 500 *C3d* moieties were bound per red cell. After sensitization with C3d, various amounts of IgG were added. Red cells were also opsonized with just IgM and IgG. Phagocytosis of EIgMC3d$_{500}$·IgG and EIgM·IgG was compared under the following conditions, which we call phagocytosis in "suspension":

Test tubes, 12 × 100 mm, were filled with 4.0 ml of red cells suspended at $10^8$/ml. Coverslips, 9 mm × 21 mm, containing about 2 × $10^4$ monocytes were added and the test tubes were sealed. Continuous agitation was provided by inclining the test tubes at about 20° on an oscillating platform moving at about 60 strokes/min. The entire apparatus was placed in a 37°C incubator for 30 min. Quantitation of ingestion was then done as in the overlay situation.

This protocol may be analogous to the *in vivo* situation, where fixed phagocytes (e.g., in liver, spleen, and lymph node) are exposed to circulating, opsonized particles. Figure 5 compares ingestion with and without C3d under these conditions. The results are expressed in two indices of phagocytosis. One index is the percentage of cells which show ingestion at all, i.e., which have ingested one or more red cells. A second index is the percentage which have ingested three or more red cells. With these two indices, we give information both on the frequency of phagocytosis among the cell population and the frequency of phagocytes which show a large amount of ingestion. The results show that although C3d does not induce ingestion directly, the combined presence of 500 molecules of C3d and 600 molecules of IgG is much more effective at inducing ingestion than 10,000 molecules of IgG without C3d. Note also that ingestion of red cells coated with 600 molecules of IgG but without C3d does not occur. Further experiments with monocytes showed that C3b and C3d receptors had the same type of opsonic activity, both in "suspension" and "overlay"

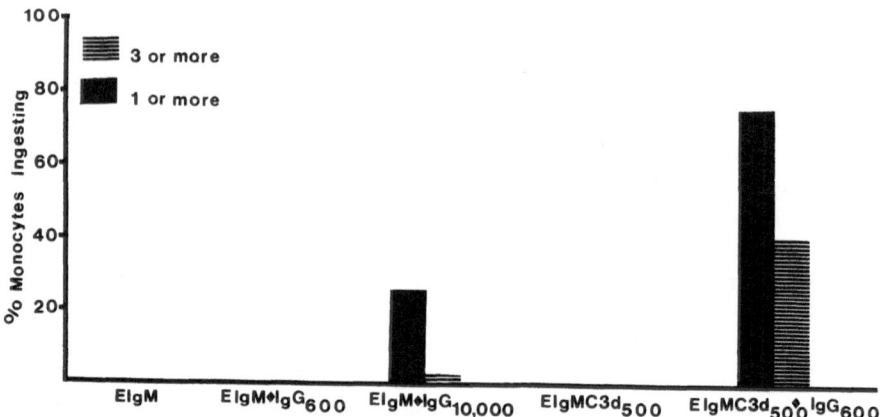

**Fig. 5.** Opsonic effect of C3d under "suspension" conditions. Note that ingestion of red cells opsonized with C3d (but not IgG) does not occur. However, opsonization with 500 molecules of C3d and 600 molecules of IgG (EIgMC3d$_{500}$·IgG$_{600}$) is much more effective than opsonization with 10,000 molecules of IgG alone. Both the percentage of monocytes ingesting at all (one or more red cells) and the percentage ingesting a large amount (three or more red cells) are presented.

conditions. Thus both C3b and C3d may act as opsonins, if the phagocyte has the appropriate receptor. PMN, which do not bear C3d receptors (Ross *et al.*, 1973), did not respond to C3d as an opsonin. This probably explains the findings of Gigli and Nelson (1968) and Stossel *et al.* (1975) on the effect of C3 inactivator on phagocytosis.

## 7.4. The Effect of Binding and Contact-Inducing Agents on Ingestion

Much of this enhancement of phagocytosis in the "suspension" situation can be explained by the binding of the particle to the phagocyte which is mediated by C3b and/or C3d receptors. This binding overcomes the shearing forces present between the particle and phagocyte which prevent ingestion. Furthermore, as the particles bind on the phagocyte surface, the effective particle concentration "seen" by the phagocyte rises tremendously. The local concentration of red cells in a "rosette" is about 2 × 10$^{10}$/ml. If the concentration of red cells in suspension is 10$^8$/ml, the formation of "rosettes" represents an increase of 200-fold in the concentration of particles on the phagocyte surface relative to the concentration in the medium.

However, overcoming shear forces and concentrating particles cannot be the only means by which complement receptors participate in phagocytosis, since the synergy effect, as we have shown, is also apparent in the "overlay" experiments in which phagocytes are saturated with particles not subject to agitation.

As we will now show, this synergistic effect with IgG under "overlay" conditions is also shown by a variety of nonimmunologic, physical agents which enhance contact between the red cell and the phagocyte. These contact-inducing agents (CIA) mimic the effect of C3–C3-receptor interaction in that (a) they do not, by themselves, cause particle ingestion, (b) they markedly (by 1000% or more) enhance the effect of particle-bound IgG, and (c) they may *appear* to induce ingestion when added to particles opsonized with small amounts of IgG.

The prototype of these CIA is high molecular weight dextran (dextran 110). This agent is known to agglutinate cells nonspecifically, probably by cross-linking (Brooks, 1973). In this way, dextran acts as a kind of artificial "receptor," in that it provides a surface structure linking one cell to another. The effect of dextran as an "opsonin" for human polymorphs, human monocytes, and mouse peritoneal macrophages is shown in Figs. 6, 7, and 8. The "opsonic" effect of dextran with human PMN was particularly dramatic (as Fig. 3 also shows, human PMN are particularly insensitive to particle opsonization with IgG alone). Even with 6000 molecules of IgG bound per red cell, no ingestion of EIgG occurs. Whereas dextran alone does not induce phagocytosis of E (or EIgMC3),

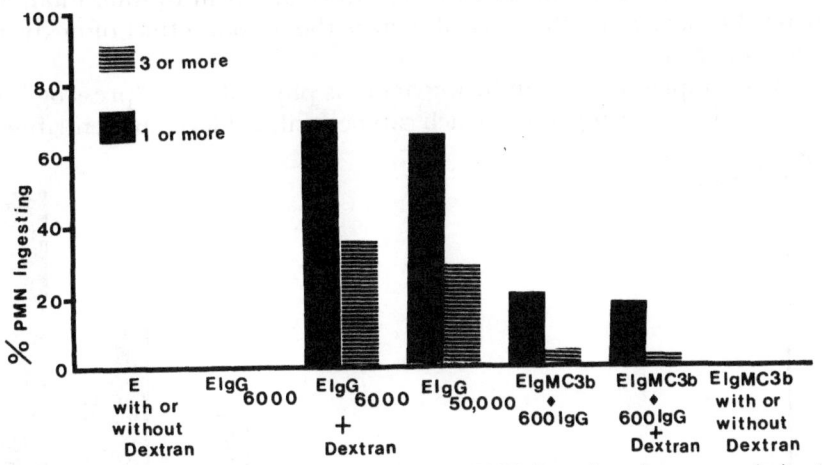

**Fig. 6.** Dextran 110 as an "opsonin" with human PMN. Experiments were carried out in "overlay" fashion. Red cells were suspended at $3 \times 10^8$/ml, and 0.1-ml aliquots were mixed with 0.1 ml of medium alone or medium containing 8% w/v Dextran 110. After mixing, the samples were immediately applied to coverslips containing PMN. Following incubation for 30 min, dextran and all free red cells were washed away in fresh medium. Osmotic lysis of external red cells was then used, as before, to quantitate ingestion. Although dextran does not induce ingestion of E or EIgMC3b, it does induce ingestion of EIgG$_{6000}$. However, the synergy of dextran and IgG disappears if the red cell also has C3b bound on its surface in sufficient quantities to mediate rosette formation.

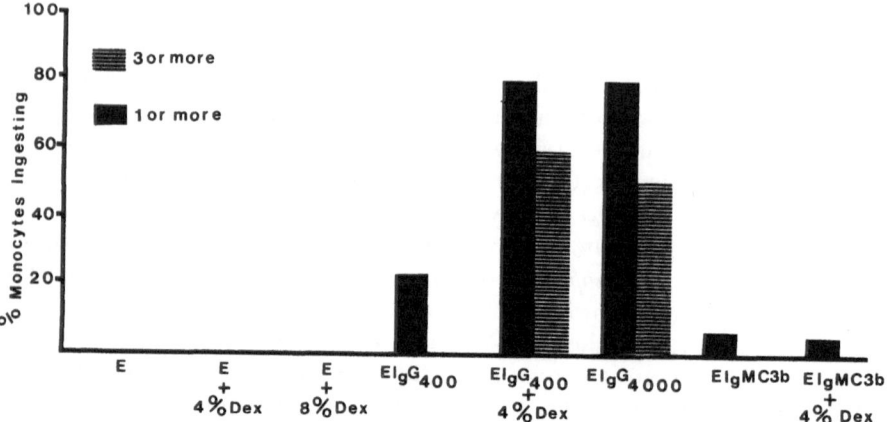

**Fig. 7.**  Opsonic effect of dextran with human monocytes. The protocol used is the same as mentioned with the PMN.

the presence of 4% Dextran 110 in the medium with $EIgG_{6000}$ induces more ingestion than opsonization with 60,000 molecules of IgG without dextran. Similar behavior is seen with monocytes and macrophages. The experiments also show that the synergistic effect of dextran with IgG disappeared when the red cell was bound to the phagocyte through C3 receptors. Thus, dextran mimics the effect of C3 in opsonization, and when C3 is present on the red cell surface the opsonic effect of dextran is no longer seen.

The simplest contact-inducing agent is physical force "pressing" particle and phagocyte together, which can be easily achieved by centrifuging

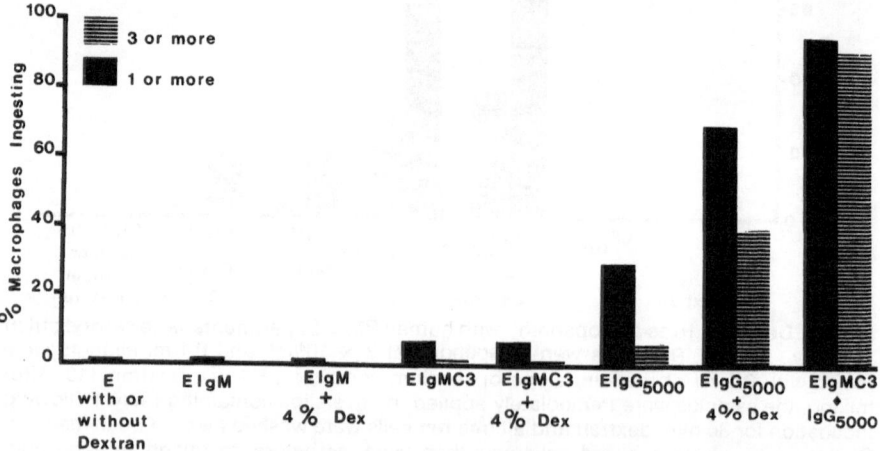

**Fig. 8.**  Opsonic effect of dextran with "normal" mouse peritoneal macrophages. Dextran does not induce ingestion of E, EIgM, or EIgMC3. Synergy of dextran with IgG was similar, but somewhat less than the synergy between cell-bound C3 and IgG.

the red cells onto the surface of the phagocyte. The enhanced contact this provides is probably analogous to the situation which occurred in Barry Wood's "surface phagocytosis," when the phagocyte would trap the particle against the alveolar tissue. The "opsonic" effect of centrifugation is shown in Fig. 9. Centrifugation, like opsonization with C3, does not induce phagocytosis of unsensitized red cells or of EIgMC3b. However, centrifugation enhances the sensitivity of the monocytes to particle-bound IgG by nearly tenfold. Also (data not shown) centrifugation did not enhance ingestion when C3b (or C3d) was present.

Enhancement of phagocytosis of EIgG could also be obtained by pretreating E with neuraminidase, a treatment that removes sialic acid residues and is known to decrease the surface charge of a cell (Seamen and Uhlenbruck, 1963). It has previously been shown that such treatment facilitates red cell agglutination (Uhlenbruck *et al.*, 1967) and T-cell rosette formation with E (Weiner *et al.*, 1973). Although large amounts of neuraminidase (1 unit/$10^9$ E) did not induce ingestion of E, even small amounts (0.01 unit/$10^9$ E) enhanced ingestion of EIgG. Protamine, a polycation with agglutinating properties, also had a similar effect, in that it enhanced ingestion of EIgG without inducing phagocytosis of unopsonized E. Polyanions, such as heparin, which do not have agglutinating properties, did not stimulate ingestion of EIgG. (In fact, they depressed EIgG ingestion somewhat.) The effect of polycations on the phagocytosis of bacteria was mentioned by Mudd *et al.* (1934) in their review on

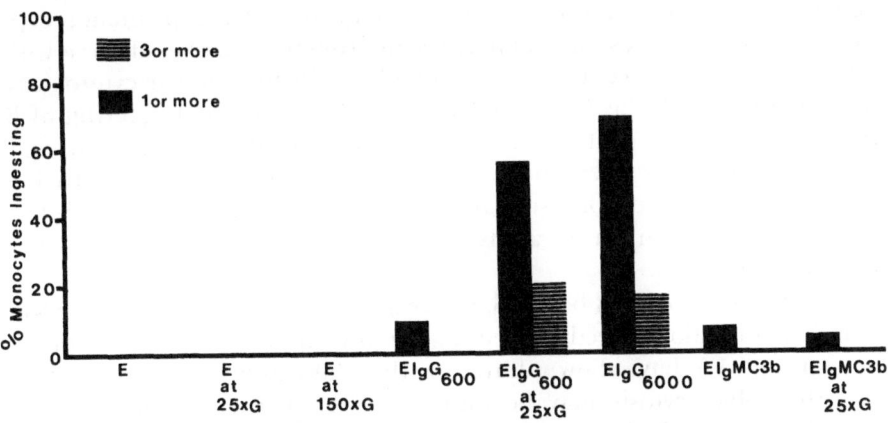

**Fig. 9.** Opsonic effect of centrifugation. In these experiments monolayers of phagocytes on 12-mm-round cover slips were placed in the bottom of 18-mm wells in tissue culture chambers. Red cells ($10^9$) opsonized in various ways were added in 1 ml of medium and the chambers sealed. The entire plate was centrifuged at 37°C for 20 min and then incubated for 20 min more at 37°C without centrifugation. Controls were incubated for 50 min at 37°C (the additional 10 min were to compensate for faster red cell settling under centrifugation). Ingestion was then quantitated as previously mentioned.

phagocytosis. Commenting on the work of Neufeld and Etinger-Tulczynska (1929), it was stated that "solutions of salts of polyvalent cations in certain ranges of concentrations both *agglutinated and caused phagocytosis\** of a virulent strain of pneumococci." Given our data, one may conjecture that these results and the phenomenon of "surface phagocytosis" of pneumococci are explainable in terms of the effects of contact-inducing agents.

The effects of these charge-altering agents suggest a mechanism to explain the need for enhanced contact in the recognition by phagocytes of those particle characteristics which mediate ingestion. Both of these agents alter cell charge, making them more positive. Most particles and cells carry an intrinsic negative surface charge (in fact, even an air bubble in saline picks up a net negative charge). Although the electric field surrounding a particle decays in exponential fashion, theoretical calculations on physiological saline have shown that the field is appreciable for 20, 30, or 40 Å (Eagland, 1975). Two such barriers (one on the phagocyte and one on the particle) may represent a considerable obstacle in the recognition of surface moieties by the phagocyte—an antibody molecule, for example, is about 100 Å long. Thus, electrostatic repulsion may act as an effective shield around particles, masking their surfaces from recognition. Both C3 and contact-inducing agents may act by overcoming this electrostatic shield and providing the intimate, surface-to-surface contact required for recognition of "foreign" or opsonic moieties such as IgG.

One may further speculate that this establishment of contact is a general problem in immunologic recognition. Indeed, complement receptors on B lymphocytes may serve the same function that we observe with phagocytes. Some recent data on antibody-mediated cellular cytotoxicity (Perlmann *et al.*, 1975; Lustig and Bianco, 1976) and the triggering of B cells by polyclonal activators (Möller and Coutinho, 1975) suggest this may be so. In both these phenomena, binding to C3 receptors apparently has an adjuvantlike function, similar to its role in phagocytosis. C3–C3-receptor interaction, in a variety of systems, seems not to trigger cell function directly.

Our data show that both C3 and contact-inducing agents may *appear* to induce ingestion directly, when ingestion without them is negligible or nonexistent. We have shown, however, that this can be an indirect effect, and that phagocytosis may be induced by triggering moieties on the particle surface which are effective only if contact is established. Claims that particle-bound C3 triggers the phagocytic act directly require the demonstration that the particle is not "intrinsically ingestible," and that interiorization will not occur if the particle and phagocyte are simply

*Italics mine.

approximated by physical means. Some of the findings which can be reinterpreted in the light of our observations are as follows.

1.   Gigli and Nelson (1968) studied the ingestion of red cells opsonized with antibody and purified guinea pig complement components by guinea pig neutrophils. This classical paper established the role of C3 as an opsonin. The authors postulated that C3b directly stimulated particle interiorization. However, in their experiments, both C3b and IgG were present on the red cells. It is therefore probable that ingestion was actually triggered by IgG present in insufficient amounts to mediate phagocytosis unless C3b was also present to induce particle binding.

2.   Stossel (1973) studied the ingestion of various lipid emulsions by human PMN and other phagocytes. Despite the available data on leukocyte complement receptors, these workers boldly suggested that deposition of C3 on particles enhanced their rate of ingestion *without* influencing the binding of these particles to the phagocytes, but rather by a direct opsonic effect. These conclusions were based on a mathematical analysis which treated phagocytosis as an enzyme–substrate reaction, and not on direct observation. This mathematical analysis has recently been criticized (Scribner and Fahrney, 1975). Furthermore, their data show that the particles used in these studies were ingested *even without C3* and therefore were "intrinsically ingestible." It is possible that C3 enhanced ingestion in these experiments by simply approximating particles and phagocytes. It should be stressed that these experiments were carried out under "suspension"-type conditions where we have demonstrated that the synergistic effect of C3 is crucial for efficient phagocytosis.

3.   It has been reported (Bianco *et al.*, 1975) that activated mouse macrophages ingest EIgMC3b, and it has been suggested that this occurs via an alteration in the function of the complement receptor. We have also investigated the ingestion of EIgMC3b by activated macrophages (macrophage activation was achieved, as in the original report, by intraperitoneal injection of thioglycollate medium) and the effect of contact-inducing agents in this system. Our results confirm that EIgMC3b are ingested by activated macrophages and that this ingestion provides a sensitive marker for macrophage activation. However, as Fig. 10 shows, EIgM are ingested in amounts comparable to EIgMC3b when contact is enhanced by the presence of Dextran 110 in the medium. As also shown by Bianco *et al.* (1975) activated macrophages ingest red cells opsonized with IgM without complement, although to a limited degree. Thus, EIgMC3b, with activated macrophages, do not meet the criteria previously mentioned to show phagocytosis directly via complement receptors, since IgM is a ligand capable of stimulating ingestion in these cells. The phenomenon of EIgMC3b ingestion is treated in greater depth in a subsequent publication (Ehlenberger and Nussenzweig, manuscript in preparation).

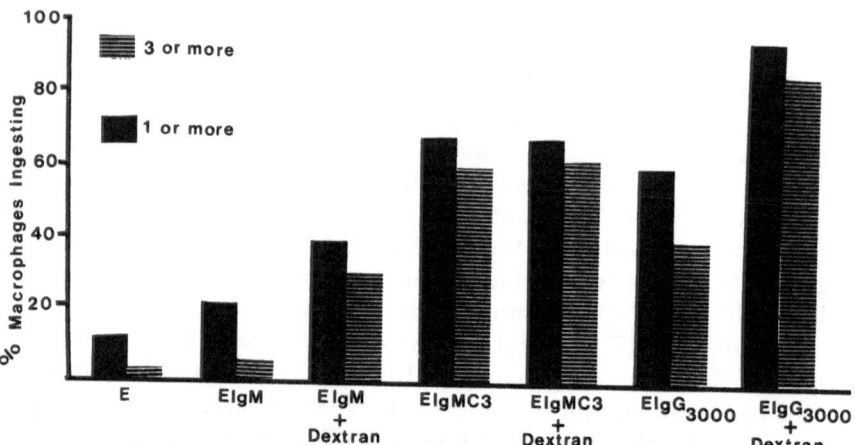

**Fig. 10.** Ingestion by activated macrophages. Experiments were carried out in "overlay" as previously described. In contrast with "normal" macrophages, 65% of "activated" macrophages ingested EIgMC3. The data also show, however, that EIgM were ingested by 40% of activated macrophages when contact was enhanced by dextran. Dextran also enhanced ingestion of EIgG, but had no effect on phagocytosis of EIgMC3.

In summary, we feel that the data strongly suggest that the complement receptors have the same function in all phagocytes; that is, they provide the contact between particle and phagocyte which is required for the recognition of those moieties which do stimulate the ingestion process. Data on B lymphocytes suggest a similar function in these cells for complement receptors. The establishment of an intimate contact between cell surfaces may be a general problem in the afferent and efferent branches of immunologic interaction, and the means by which cells establish this contact deserves careful study.

ACKNOWLEDGMENTS

The author gratefully acknowledges the guidance and inspiration of Dr. Victor Nussenzweig in this work. I also wish to thank Ms. Joanne Joseph for assistance in the preparation of the manuscript, and Ms. Jean Weiner and Ms. Gertrude Fastaia for assistance in the experiments.

This work was supported by grants AI-08499 and CA-16247, and NIH Training Grant 5 TO 5 GM 01668.

# References

Abramson, N., Gelfand, E. W., Jandl, J. H., and Rosen, F. S., 1970, The interaction between human monocytes and red cells: Specificity for IgG subclasses and IgG fragments, *J. Exp. Med.* **132**:1207.

Alper, C. A., Colten, H. R., Rosen, F. S., Rabson, A. R., Macnab, G. M., and Gear, J. S. S., 1972, Homozygous deficiency of C3 in a patient with repeated infections, *Lancet* **2**:1179.

Berken, A., and Benacerraf, B., 1966, Properties of antibodies cytophilic for macrophages, *J. Exp. Med.* **123**:119.

Bianco, C., Griffin, F. M., and Silverstein, S. C., 1975, Studies on the macrophage complement receptor: Alteration of receptor function upon macrophage activation, *J. Exp. Med.* **141**:1278.

Boyden, S. V., 1964, Cytophilic antibody in guinea pigs with delayed-type hypersensitivity, *Immunology* **7**:474.

Brooks, D. E., 1973, The effect of neutral polymers on the electrokinetic potential of cells and other charged particles, *J. Colloid Interface Sci.* **43**:714.

Eagland, D., 1975, The influence of hydration on the stability of hydrophobic colloidal systems, *in Water, A Comprehensive Treatise*, Vol. 5 (F. Franks, ed.), pp. 1–74, Plenum Press, New York.

Eden, A., Miller, G. W., and Nussenzweig, V., 1973, Human lymphocytes bear membrane receptors for C3b and C3d, *J. Clin. Invest.* **52**:3239.

Ehlenberger, A. G., and Nussenzweig, V., 1975, Synergy between receptors for Fc and C3 in the induction of phagocytosis by human monocytes and neutrophils, *Fed. Proc.* **34**:854.

Ehlenberger, A. G., and Nussenzweig, V., 1976, Identification of cells with complement receptors, *in In Vitro Methods in Cell-Mediated and Tumor Immunity*, Vol. II (B. R. Bloom and J. R. David, eds.), Academic Press, New York.

Fenn, W. O., 1921–1922, The theoretical response of living cells to contact with solid bodies, *J. Gen. Physiol.* **iv**:373.

Gigli, I., and Nelson, R. A., Jr., 1968, Complement-dependent immune phagocytosis. 1. Requirements for C'1, C'4, C'2, C'3, *Exp. Cell Res.* **51**:45.

Griffin, F. M., Bianco, C., and Silverstein, S. C., 1975a, Characterization of the macrophage receptor for complement and demonstration of its functional independence from the receptor for the Fc portion of immunoglobulin G, *J. Exp. Med.* **141**:1269.

Griffin, F. M., Jr., Griffin, J. A., Leider, J. E., and Silverstein, S. C., 1975b, Studies on the mechanism of phagocytosis. I. Requirements for circumferential attachment of particle-bound ligands to specific receptors on the macrophage plasma membrane, *J. Exp. Med.* **142**:1263.

Huber, H., and Fudenberg, H. H., 1968, Receptor sites on human monocytes for IgG, *Int. Arch. Allergy*, **34**:18.

Huber, H., Polley, M. J., Linscott, W. D., Fudenberg, H. H., and Müller-Eberhard, H. J., 1968, Human monocytes: Distinct receptor sites for the third component of complement and for immunoglobulin G, *Science* **162**:1281.

Johnston, R. B., Jr., Klemperer, M. R., Alper, C. A., and Rosen, F. S., 1969, The enhancement of bacterial phagocytosis by serum: The role of complement components and two co-factors, *J. Exp. Med.* **129**:1275.

Lay, W. H., and Nussenzweig, V., 1968, Receptors for complement on leukocytes, *J. Exp. Med.* **128**:991.

Lo Buglio, A. F., Cotran, R. S., and Jandl, J. H., 1967, Red cells coated with immunoglobulin G: Binding and sphering by mononuclear cells in man, *Science* **158**:1582.

Lustig, H. J., and Bianco, C., 1976, Antibody-mediated cell cytotoxicity in a defined system: Regulation by antigen, antibody, and complement, *J. Immunol.* **116**:253.

Mantovani, B., 1975, Different roles of IgG and complement receptors in phagocytosis by polymorphonuclear leukocytes, *J. Immunol.* **115**:15.

Mantovani, B., Rabinovitch, M., and Nussenzweig, V., 1972, Phagocytosis of immune complexes by macrophages. Different roles of the macrophage receptor sites for complement (C3) and for immunoglobulins (IgG), *J. Exp. Med.* **135**:780.

Möller, B., and Coutinho, A., 1975, Role of C'3 and Fc receptors in B-lymphocyte activation, *J. Exp. Med.* **141**:647.

Mudd, S., McCutcheon, M., and Lucké, B., 1934, Phagocytosis, *Physiol. Rev.* **14**:210.

Neufeld, F., and Etinger-Tulczynska, 1929, *Centralbl. F. Bakt. Orig.* **cxiv**:252.

Nussenzweig, V., Lay, W. H., and Miescher, P. A., 1969, γG and C' dependent receptor sites on leukocytes, in *Cellular Recognition* (R. T. Smith and R. A. Good, eds.), Appleton-Century-Crofts, New York.

Perlmann, P., Perlmann, H., and Müller-Eberhard, H. J., 1975, Cytolytic lymphocytic cells with complement receptors in human blood, *J. Exp. Med.* **141**:287.

Rabinovitch, M., 1967a, "Nonprofessional" and "professional" phagocytes: Particle uptake by L cells and by macrophages, *J. Cell. Biol.* **35**:108a (Abstract).

Rabinovitch, M., 1967b, The dissociation of the attachment and ingestion stages of phagocytosis by macrophages, *Exp. Cell. Res.* 46:19.

Rabinovitch, M., 1967c, Studies on the immunoglobulins which stimulate the ingestion of glutaraldehyde-treated red cells attached to macrophages, *J. Immunol.* **99**:1115.

Rhumbler, L., 1898, *Arch. F. Entwehlungsmech d. Organ.* **vii**:199.

Rhumbler, L., 1914, Das Protoplasma als physikalisches System, *Ergebn. Physiol.* **xiv**:474.

Rosen, F. S., 1975, Immunodeficiency, in *Immunogenetics and Immunodeficiency* (B. Benacerraf, ed.), pp. 229–257, University Park Press, Baltimore, Maryland.

Ross, G. D., and Polley, M. J., 1975, Human lymphocytes and granulocyte receptors for the fourth component of complement (C4) and the role of granulocyte receptors in phagocytosis, *Fed. Proc.* **33**:759 (Abstract).

Ross, G. D., and Polley, M. J., 1975, Specificity of human lymphocyte complement receptors, *J. Exp. Med.* **141**:1163.

Ross, G. D., Polley, M. J., Rabellino, E. M., and Grey, H. M., 1973, Two different complement receptors on human lymphocytes. One specific for C3b and one specific for C3b inactivator-cleaved C3b, *J. Exp. Med.* **138**:798.

Ruddy, S., and Austen, K. F., 1971, C3b inactivator of man. II. Fragments produced by C3b inactivator cleavage of cell bound or fluid phase C3b, *J. Immunol.* **107**:742.

Scribner, P. J., and Fahrney, D., 1975, Neutrophil receptors for IgG and complement: Their roles in the attachment and ingestion phases of phagocytosis, *J. Immunol.* **116**:892.

Seamen, G. V. F., and Uhlenbruck, G., 1963, The surface structure of erythrocytes from some animal sources, *Arch. Biochem. Biophys.* **100**:493.

Shin, H. S., Smith, M. R., and Wood, W. B., Jr., 1969, Heat-labile opsonins to pneumococcus. II. Involvement of C3 and C5, *J. Exp. Med.* **130**:1229.

Stossel, T. P., 1973, Quantitative studies of phagocytosis: Kinetic effects of cations and of heat-labile opsonin, *J. Cell Biol.* **58**:346.

Stossel, T. P., Field, R. J., Gitlin, J. D., Alper, C. A., and Rosen, F. S., 1975, The opsonic fragment of the third component of human complement (C3), *J. Exp. Med.* **141**:1329.

Topley, W. W. C., and Wilson, G. S., 1931, *in The Principles of Bacteriology and Immunology*, Vol. 1, William Wood, New York.

Uhlenbruck, G., Seamen, G. V. F., and Coombs, R. R. A., 1967, Factors influencing the agglutinability of red cells. III. Physicochemical studies on ox red cells of different classes of agglutinability, *Vox Sang.* **12**:240.

Van Oss, C. J., and Gillman, C. F., 1972, Phagocytosis as a surface phenomenon: I. Contact angles and phagocytosis of nonopsonized bacteria, *J. Reticuloendothel. Soc.* **12**:283.

Ward, H. K., and Enders, J. F., 1933, An analysis of the opsonic and tropic action of normal and immune sera based on experiments with the pneumococcus, *J. Exp. Med.* **57**:527.

Weiner, M. S., Bianco, C., and Nussenzweig, V., 1973, Enhanced binding of neuraminidase-treated sheep erythrocytes to human T lymphocytes, *Blood* **42**:939.

Wellek, B., Hahn, H., and Opferkuch, W., 1975, Quantitative contributions of IgG, IgM and C3 to erythrophagocytosis and rosette formation by peritoneal macrophages, and anti-opsonin activity of dextran sulfate 500, *Eur. J. Immunol.* **5**:378.

Wood, W. B., Jr., Smith, M. R., and Watson, B. W., 1946, Studies on the mechanism of recovery in pneumococcal pneumonia. IV. The mechanism of phagocytosis in the absence of antibody, *J. Exp. Med.* **84**:387.

Wright, A. E., and Douglas, S. R., 1903, An experimental investigation of the role of blood fluids in connection with phagocytosis, *Proc. Roy. Soc. Lond. B Biol. Sci.* **72**:357.

# Leukocyte 5'-Nucleotidase

## Maryrose Conklyn and Robert Silber

## 8.1. Introduction

The 5'-mononucleotides are dephosphorylated by the enzyme, 5'-ribonucleotide phosphohydrolase (EC 3.1.3.5), commonly known as 5'-nucleotidase (5'N). This enzyme was first described by Reis (1937, 1939) in heart and skeletal muscle and its specificity established histochemically for 5'-nucleotides by Gomori (1949a,b). The activity has since been described in many tissues (Drummond and Yamamoto, 1971). This review of 5'N in mammalian leukocytes is divided into two parts. The first part deals with its properties. Studies on the enzyme from sources other than leukocytes are included since much of the early knowledge was derived from other tissues. The second part, which discusses leukocyte 5'N, will attempt to resolve conflicting reports on the presence or absence of the enzyme in particular types of white cells. In addition, the effects of hematologic disorders on 5'N are summarized.

## 8.2. The Enzyme

### 8.2.1. The 5'N Reaction

The enzyme hydrolyzes the phosphate bond located on the fifth carbon of 5'-mononucleotides to yield inorganic phosphate (Pi) and the

MARYROSE CONKLYN and ROBERT SILBER • Department of Medicine, New York University Medical Center, New York, New York 10016.

appropriate nucleoside:

5′-Nucleotide → Nucleoside + Pi

In general, a higher reaction rate is observed with ribonucleotides than with deoxyribonucleotides (Hardonk, 1968).

*Assay.* The activity is quantitated by the amount of nucleoside or (more commonly) Pi liberated in the reaction. In view of the presence of nonspecific phosphatase, controls should contain other substances, such as 2′,3′-AMP. The dephosphorylation of AMP by nonspecific phosphatases may be diminished by the presence of an excess of another substrate for these enzymes. Belfield and Goldberg (1968) showed that the addition of excess β-glycerophosphate to the reaction mixture abolished the previously measurable hydrolysis of 2′,3′-AMP by alkaline phosphatases, while there was no effect on the hydrolysis of AMP. In addition, specific inhibitors for these phosphatases may also be used. The inclusion of sodium–potassium tartrate, an inhibitor for acid phosphatases (Marique and Hildebrand, 1973), is one example.

## 8.2.2. Properties of the Enzyme

### 8.2.2.1. Substrate Specificity

The specificity expressed by 5′-nucleotidase for the different 5′ nucleotides as substrates varies according to the tissue serving as the source of the enzyme and the species from which the sample is obtained (see Table I).

Several reports (Gough and Elves, 1967; Szmigielski *et al.*, 1967a) have stated that there is no 5′N in the human erythrocytes which is capable of using AMP as substrate. Subsequently, Paglia and Valentine (1975) established the presence of a 5′N in human erythrocytes. However, this enzyme hydrolyzes only the pyrimidine nucleotides. The finding that AMP, the substrate most commonly used in assays, is not hyrolyzed by this enzyme resolves the apparent contradiction.

### 8.2.2.2. pH Response

The optimum pH of 5′N may, like the substrate specificity, vary according to the source of the enzymes. In general it varies between 6.8 and 7.5 (Reis, 1937, 1951; Paglia and Valentine, 1975; Hill and Sammons, 1971; Pearse and Reis, 1952). In a study comparing 5′N levels in mouse and rat tissues, Hardonk (1968; Pearse and Reis, 1952) has shown the existence of two 5′Ns, one with maximal activity at pH 5.0 and the other at pH 7.0–7.5. The distribution of the acid nucleotidase differed from that of the neutral enzyme, and its localization resembled that of acid phosphatase.

**Table I.** Substrate Specificity of 5'N

| Source of enzyme | Substrate specificity of 5'N |
|---|---|
| Rat splenic red pulp (Hardonk, 1968) | AMP = IMP = UMP > dAMP = dCMP > UMP |
| Mouse splenic red pulp (Hardonk, 1968) | AMP = IMP = UMP = CMP = dAMP > dCMP |
| Guinea pig polymorphonuclear leukocytes (DePierre and Karnovsky, 1972) | AMP ≥ UMP > CMP > GMP > IMP |
| Human lymphocytes (Silber and Conklyn, unpublished) | AMP = CMP > IMP > GMP > dUMP > TMP |
| Human erythrocytes (Paglia and Valentine, 1975) | UMP > dUMP > CMP > dCMP > TMP |

### 8.2.2.3. Inhibitors and Activators

Ahmed and Reis (1958) studied the effects of different compounds on 5'N obtained from human aorta and human placenta. The results of their experiments showed that the activity of 5'N from the aorta increased by 12% in the presence of $Mg^{2+}$ and by 59% with $Mn^{2+}$. A variety of inhibitory effects by cations have been reported; these are summarized in Table II.

### 8.2.2.4. Effect of Detergents

In their studies on the solubilization of pig lymphocyte membranes, Allan and Crumpton (1971) noted an increase in 5'N activity in the presence of sodium deoxycholate, which was maximal at a concentration of 1%. A similar increase in 5'N activity by the addition of deoxycholate was reported by Nakamura (1976), working with enzyme purified from rat liver plasma membranes. Experiments using mouse L-1210 leukemic membranes as the source of enzyme (Silber and Conklyn, unpublished observations) showed a stimulation by Triton X-100. Stimulation of 5'N

**Table II.** Inhibition of 5'N by Cations

| Source of enzyme | % Inhibition of 5'N by | | | | |
|---|---|---|---|---|---|
| | $Ni^{2+}$ | $Co^{2+}$ | $Mn^{2+}$ | $Ca^{2+}$ | $Cu^{2+}$ |
| Aorta (Ahmed and Reis, 1958) | 96.8 | 75.8 | 80 | — | — |
| Placenta (Ahmed and Reis, 1958) | 100 | 66.9 | 97.0 | 7.5 | 59.3 |
| Sheep brain (Ipata, 1968) | 58.4 | 19.5 | 96.3 | 16.8 | 55.2 |

obtained from guinea pig leukocytes by detergents was also reported by
DePierre and Karnovsky (1974a).

### 8.2.2.5. Studies on Purified Preparations of 5'N

The enzyme 5'N has been purified by several investigators. Ipata
(1968) purified the enzyme from sheep brain. The molecular weight,
determined by Sephadex G-100 gel filtration and sucrose density gradients, was 134,000 and 142,000, respectively. The enzyme activity was
strongly but reversibly inhibited by the nucleotide triphosphate, ATP,
UTP, and CTP. This inhibition was both competitive and noncompetitive
in nature. Kinetic studies suggest there are two interacting inhibitor
binding sites on the enzyme molecule. The enzyme may be made insensitive to the presence of ATP and UTP but not to the inhibitory effect
of CTP. Slight inhibition of activity by UDP, ADP, and CDP was
noted.

Widnell (1974) has characterized a 5'N obtained from rat liver. This
purified enzyme has a molecular weight of approximately 85,000 as
determined by sodium dodecyl sulfate (SDS) acrylamide gel electrophoresis. Only one phospholipid was detected: sphingomyelin, which occurred
in amounts varying from 1 to 4 $\mu$mol lipid phosphate/mg protein. Complete removal of the sphingomyelin resulted in irreversible inactivation of
the 5'N activity. This enzyme hydrolyzed AMP, UMP, and CMP at the
same rate. The hydrolysis of GMP and IMP was one-half the rate
observed with the first three nucleotides. The following cations were
inhibitory at concentrations ranging from 0.1 to 4 mM: $Ca^{2+}$, $Fe^{2+}$, $Na^{2+}$,
$Cd^{2+}$, and $Zn^{2+}$. Only the effects of $Ca^{2+}$ and $Fe^{2+}$ could be neutralized by
excess $Mg^{2+}$.

Evans and Gurd (1973) used mouse liver plasma membranes solubilized in sarcosyl–tris buffer as the source of 5'N in their purification
procedure. The molecular weight determined by gel filtration was
140,000–150,000. The authors concluded that this 5'N was composed of
two active glycoproteins with a molecular weight of 70,000–75,000.
Contrary to Widnell's findings, Evans and Gurd could not demonstrate a
phospholipid dependency for enzyme activity nor detect any phospholipid
in their preparations. The finding of appreciable amounts of these lipids by
others was attributed to the use of ionic detergents.

### 8.2.3. Representative Methods Utilized in 5'N Assays

#### 8.2.3.1. Histochemistry

One of the most commonly quoted techniques for the histochemical
detection of 5'N activity is that of Wachstein and Meisel (1957). In this

method the phosphate liberated from the hydrolysis of the substrate AMP, immediately precipitates as lead phosphate, presumably at the site of the enzyme. Treatment with ammonium sulfide then forms the black precipitate lead sulfide, readily seen with light microscopy.

Although this assay is very simple and is commonly used as stated, the described method contains no inhibitors of nonspecific phosphatases. Several disadvantages of this technique have been described by Pearse (1968). Loss of enzyme during tissue preparation or fixation is one. In addition, the formation of precipitate may not necessarily occur at the true site of the enzyme. Diffusion of product and/or diffusion of the enzyme itself may result in the false localization of product. Spontaneous precipitation of the lead may result from the presence of phosphate from other sources. In spite of these, Pearse considers the lead phosphate technique as the method of choice for localization of 5'N.

### 8.2.3.2. Chemical Assays

Ipata (1968) couples the 5'N reaction with that of adenosine deaminase. This method involves two reactions. The first is the hydrolysis of AMP to adenosine and Pi. In the second, the adenosine formed is deaminated to inosine. The reaction is monitored by the decrease in optical density measured at 265 nm. In this method of Mitchell and Hawthorne (1965) the inorganic phosphate is measured by colorimetric estimation, most commonly by the procedure of Fiske and Subbarow (1925). DePierre and Karnovsky (1972) used [$^{32}$P]AMP as the substrate. The assay mixture also included 1 mM $p$-nitrophenyl phosphate, a nonspecific phosphatase inhibitor. After incubation at 37°C, 10% acid-washed Norit in 10% TCA is added to the assay solution. The Norit will bind any remaining [$^{32}$P]AMP but not $^{32}$Pi. After filtration of the assay solution, an aliquot is counted in a liquid scintillation counter. Quagliata $et\ al.$ (1974) use a similar system in human cells.

## 8.3. Studies on 5'N in Leukocytes

### 8.3.1. Distribution of the Enzyme in Leukocytes

#### 8.3.1.1. Animal Leukocytes

Granulocytes obtained from rabbit (Bainton and Farquhar, 1968a,b; Szmigielski $et\ al.$, 1966a; Oliver $et\ al.$, 1974), rat (Fritzson, 1967; Kolakowska-Polubiec $et\ al.$, 1970), and guinea pig (DePierre and Karnovsky, 1972) have demonstrated 5'N activity. The enzyme has also been reported in lymphocytes from L5178Y leukemic mice (Bosmann, 1972), from the lymph nodes of pigs (Allan and Crumpton, 1971, 1970; Ferber *et al.*, 1972), from the thymus and rat spleen (Misra *et al.*, 1974; Ladoulis *et al.*, 1974), in mouse lymphoblastic leukemic cell lines, and normal mouse lymphoid cells (Warley and Cook, 1973).

DePierre and Karnovsky (1974a) studied the enzyme levels of cell populations enriched with various types of guinea pig leukocytes. In that species, the polymorphonuclear leukocyte exhibited the highest level of 5'N activity. This level was 10 times higher than that measured in the guinea pig lymphocytes and eosinophils. There was barely detectable substrate hydrolysis by monocytes and no enzymatic action could be demonstrated in the erythrocytes.

### 8.3.1.2. Human Granulocyte 5'N

Publications on 5'N in human leukocytes present a more complicated and conflicting picture. The enzyme has been reported in lymphocytes by several workers (Marique and Hildebrand, 1973; Gough and Elves, 1967; Lopes *et al.*, 1973b; Demus, 1973) whereas Szmigielski *et al.* (1967a; Szmigielski, 1965) stated that 5'N was found in the granulocytes and not in the lymphocytes. A study on leukemic granulocytes and leukemic lymphocytes (Swendsied *et al.*, 1952) states that the enzyme is present in both types of cells. Strauss and Burrows (1975) examined human poly-morphonuclear leukocytes. After testing for activity in whole cells, homogenates, and membranes of these leukocytes, they concluded that little or no 5'N was to be found in human granulocytes. Because of the conflicting results in these reports, further discussion of these works is necessary.

Swendseid *et al.* (1952) published a report on nucleotidase activity in leukocytes obtained from the peripheral blood of patients with chronic forms of leukemia, either granulocytic or lymphocytic. They concluded that the nucleotidase activity in granulocytes was 10 times greater than that measured in lymphocytes. This enzyme had an optimal pH of 4.0 and was thus considered to be an acid phosphatase. They also noted that this nucleotidase was nonspecific. It dephosphorylated other mononucleotides such as 2'-AMP and 3'-AMP; in the case of 3'-AMP the rate was greater than the rate for AMP. In lymphocytes, at pH 4.0, the rates of phosphate liberation from these three different substrates were equal. This suggests that the enzyme activity measured in granulocytes and in lymphocytes at pH 4 was a nonspecific acid phosphatase and not 5'N. Further support for this interpretation is provided by the pH response of the granulocyte enzyme. The hydrolysis of AMP by the granulocyte enzyme decreased considerably above pH 5.0: Only 20% of the activity at pH 4 remains at pH 7.0. In contrast, the activity in the lymphocytes at pH 7.0 is 50% of that seen at pH 4.0. Subsequent studies suggest that the lymphocyte enzyme is 5'N; this point is now discussed.

Marique and Hildebrand (1973) published a study on leukocyte 5'N in 15 patients with chronic lymphocytic leukemia (CLL) and 6 patients with chronic myelogenous leukemia (CML). They confirmed the presence of an enzyme capable of hydrolyzing AMP at acid pH in the lymphocytes and the granulocytes. Their data showed this enzyme was inhibited by sodium–potassium tartrate, was not affected by the absence of $Mg^{2+}$, was able to hydrolyze $\beta$-glycerophosphate, and had a pH optimum of 5.0. Because of these findings, they considered this enzyme to be a nonspecific acid phosphatase. An "alkaline phosphatase" was detected in the lymphocytes of four patients with CLL and in the cells of one patient with CML which was $Mg^{2+}$ dependent, was not inhibited by sodium–potassium tartrate, and had an optimum pH of 7.5. This enzyme was considered to be a true 5'N.

In their survey of 5'N in human blood and bone marrow smears, Szmigielski et al. (1967a) used the lead phosphate precipitate histochemical technique. Their samples were fixed for 5 min in Formalin vapors at 4°C. They did not find any demonstrable 5'N activity in erythroblasts or lymphocytes. An enzyme activity was noted in reticuloendothelial cells, megakaryocytes, granulocytes, and granulocyte precursors. In order to test for the presence of any other active phosphatase, control smears were incubated in a medium using $\beta$-glycerophosphate in the place of AMP as the substrate. These controls were said to be negative. In a previous study (Szmigielski, 1965) this investigator reported that the percentage of 5'N-positive granulocytes in the peripheral blood smears of patients with acute infections was increased, a property well documented for alkaline phosphatase. He also noted that the increase in the percentage of positive granulocytes seemed to have a direct relationship to the severity of infection. The negative results obtained with $\beta$-glycerophosphate as a control are open to question since this compound is a known substrate for granulocyte alkaline phosphatase (Follette et al., 1959; Trubowitz et al., 1961). Furthermore, the failure to use 2',3'-AMP as a control makes it impossible to state that 5'N rather than some other phosphatase with a preference for AMP over $\beta$-glycerophosphate as substrate was actually the enzyme being measured.

Gough and Elves (1967) also used a similar histochemical technique to study 5'N in unfixed buffy coat smears of leukocytes from human peripheral blood. They found positive granules in neutrophils, macrophages, and a few lymphocytes. Two controls were included. In one assay the substrate was omitted from the reaction mixture. In the other control assay, $Ni^{2+}$ was added to inhibit 5'N. No positive cells were noted in the examination of these control smears. These two controls are inadequate.

The first will only determine if any spontaneous lead precipitation or precipitation by endogenous phosphate occurs. In the second, there is no evidence that the $Ni^{2+}$ is an inhibitor exclusively for 5'N, nor that it completely inhibits the human 5'N. The presence of this ion may adversely affect other enzymes reactive in this system. A third control assay containing another phosphate, such as 2',3'-AMP, was not included.

Strauss and Burrows (1975) presented evidence that very little or no 5'N exists in human granulocytes. The assay method was that of DePierre and Karnovsky (1974b) utilizing $^{32}P$-labeled AMP. These results have been confirmed by us using a similar isotope method or by a histochemical assay method (Silber and Conklyn, unpublished observations). In studies on human polymorphonuclear leukocytes, intact whole cell assays demonstrated barely detectable levels of enzyme activity. Homogenates of these granulocytes had a slightly increased activity. Plasma membranes prepared from the same cells demonstrated no activity. Simultaneous assays of intact and homogenized guinea pig polymorphonuclear cells showed marked 5'N activity.

Recent publications from two laboratories present data that may have some bearing on these conflicting conclusions. Using light and electron microscopy, Bainton and Farquhar (1968a,b) studied the enzymatic content of the azurophil and the specific granules of myelocytic cells in the bone marrow of New Zealand rabbits. They reported the presence of an acid nucleotidase in the azurophil granules. This enzyme was similar to that described by Swendseid et al. (1952). At pH 7.2, they found a 5'N localized in the specific granules. If their granules are assumed to be the source of the 5'N activity reportedly found in human granulocytes, a hypothesis may be formulated concerning the previously discussed results.

Strauss and Burrows (1975) found very low activity in the intact human polymorphonuclear cells. After homogenization of these leukocytes, there is a moderate increase in the 5'N activity. During homogenization of the granulocytes, lysis of some granules is likely to occur. This could result in an increase in the 5'N activity. The lack of detectable activity in preparations of plasma membranes supports the idea that the enzyme may be located in the interior of the granulocyte. Conceivably the activity detected by Szmigielski et al. (1967a) and Evans and Gough might be lysosomal enzyme (perhaps 5'N) which is exposed to substrate to which the cells become permeable after smearing or fixation. Alternatively, one must consider the possibility that these workers were not assaying 5'N since some appropriate controls were omitted in these studies.

The dramatic increase in the number of positive granulocytes during infections noted by Szmigielski (1965) needs an explanation. The normal percentage of "5'-nucleotidase" containing granulocytes was only 3–10%.

In the leukocytes of patients with various infections, as many as 64% were positive for the enzyme. As the infections subsided, the number of positive cells returned to normal levels. Pertinent to these observations by Szmigielski, is the work of Cohn and Hirsch (1960a,b). Using peritoneal exudate from New Zealand rabbits as the source of granulocytes, these workers (Cohn and Hirsch, 1960a) assayed for a variety of activities in the granules. One of the enzymes was a nucleotidase active at pH 4.0. Further studies (Hirsch and Cohn, 1960) showed that after phagocytosis, the polymorphonuclear cells are degranulated. The more particles phagocytized, the greater was the degree of degranulation. Their enzymes were released either into the cytoplasm or into the phagocytic vacuoles (Cohn and Hirsch, 1960b). The hydrolases were released more into the cytoplasm than into the vacuoles.

If the source of 5'N found in the human polymorphonuclear cells is the granules, then the increased lysis of these granules as a result of stimulated phagocytic activity resulting from the presence of infectious agents could result in activation and release of enzymes from the granules into the cytoplasm. This would lead to an increase in the number of cells expressing 5'N activity. The return to normal numbers of 5'N-positive cells may be an expression of decreased phagocytic activity.

There are also strong arguments to be made against the presence of a significant 5'N activity in human polymorphonuclear granulocytes. Demonstration of 5'N in the granules of rabbit polymorphs is not proof that the enzyme is present in similar structures of human granulocytes. Another factor to be considered is that the phosphorolysis of AMP in neutrophils is catalyzed by another enzyme, not a true 5'N. The lack of 2',3'-AMP controls from those studies reporting the presence of 5'N in neutrophils makes this an open question. Although further studies are necessary to resolve this problem, we favor the idea that human neutrophils lack significant levels of 5'N.

### 8.3.1.3. Lymphocyte 5'N

The presence of 5'N has been demonstrated in the plasma membranes of lymphocytes obtained from human tonsil tissue (Lopes *et al.*, 1973a; Demus, 1973), thymus (Allan and Crumpton, 1972), and peripheral blood (Lopes et al., 1973a). The enzyme has also been detected in undisrupted preparations of lymphocytes (Quagliata *et al.*, 1974).

### 8.3.1.4. Heterogeneity of 5'N

There is a wide range of lymphocyte 5'N activity from normal subjects although the level tends to be reproducible (±25%) for a given individual tested at different times (Silber *et al.*, 1975). A partial explanation for this observation was found in histochemical studies on human peripheral blood lymphocytes which indicate that 5'N is not present in all lymphocytes. There exist in each preparation of these cells from subpopulations of normal subjects, 5'N-positive (5'N+) lymphocytes which exhibit enzyme activity and 5'N-negative (5'N−) lymphocytes which show no activity. The percentage of 5'N+ lymphocytes determined histochemically is closely related to the level of specific activity measured by chemical methods. The correlation coefficient for the relationship between percent 5'N+ lymphocytes and the specific activity of 5'N in the same preparation was 0.94. It therefore appears that different ratios of 5'N+ to 5'N− lymphocytes are found in the circulation of normal subjects. Further characterization of these subpopulations is needed.

### 8.3.1.5. Relationship between T and B Cells and 5'N in Human Lymphocytes

A strong 5'N reaction has been noted in the germinal centers of human spleen (Gomori, 1949b), lymph nodes (Braunstein *et al.*, 1958, 1962), and tonsils (Kaiserling and Caesar, 1969). Muller-Hermelink *et al.* (1974) studied the relationship of T- and B-cell areas and their enzyme content in the white splenic pulp. An area was considered to contain B lymphocytes if EAC (erythrocytes coated with amboceptor) rosette formation occurred. If there was no rosette formation, it was assumed that the section contained predominantly T lymphocytes. Only the follicles and the germinal centers formed EAC rosettes. These areas also showed 5'-nuceotidase activity. The data showed that the B lymphocytes were situated in the follicles and the germinal centers and contained 5'-nucleotidase, whereas the T lymphocytes occupied the remaining areas of the splenic white pulp and did not demonstrate 5'-nucleotidase activity. Muller-Hermelink (1974) extended this study to human lymph nodes and tonsils. The results obtained using these tissues confirmed the findings in the spleen.

Although these conclusions may hold true for spleen and tonsil lymphocytes, studies from this laboratory have not shown such a correlation in blood lymphocytes (Quagliata *et al.*, 1974). Selective depletion of B or T lymphocytes from a mixed cell population failed to alter the 5'N specific activity. Furthermore, the 5'N content of lymphocytes from CLL patients showed no correlation with the percentage of B and T cells. In this study it was found that the 5'N levels in thymus tissues (95% T cells) was lower than in tonsils, which contain predominantly B cells. Allan and Crumpton (1972) had previously reported that plasma membranes from thymocytes had a lower 5'-nucleotidase activity than the plasma membranes of peripheral blood lymphocytes.

It may be possible that in the noncirculating T lymphocytes, the 5'N activity is indeed lower, but as these cells are released into the bloodstream, the 5'N is activated. An alternative explanation is that T lymphocytes located in structures such as spleen and lymph nodes do have a low 5'N not detected in the histochemical assay. Wachstein and Meisel (1957) reported considerable inactivation of this enzyme after Formalin fixation. In unpublished data Gerson and Silber have shown that fixation of L-1210 lymphocyte membranes with 10% formaldehyde inhibited the 5'N activity by 40%. In Muller-Hermelink's studies (1974) the sections were fixed in formol calcium. This may have partially inhibited the enzyme present in all the cells, thereby detecting activity in only those cells with a very high 5'N level.

## 8.3.2. Subcellular Localization of 5'N in Leukocytes

In the early 1970s, several investigators determined the 5'N characterized content of lymphocyte subcellular fractions from pig blood (Allan and Crumpton, 1971, 1970), rat spleen (Misra et al., 1974), as well as on human and rat thymocytes (Misra et al., 1974; Ladoulis et al., 1974). In several studies the highest specific activity of 5'-nucleotidase was found in the plasma membrane fractions of lymphocytes from calf mediastinum, pig mesenteric (Ferber et al., 1972), and human tonsil (Lopes et al., 1973a; Demus, 1973). However, the enzyme was also detected in other subcellular fractions. This finding was interpreted to indicate that 5'N may not be localized exclusively on the plasma membrane or that the other subcellular fractions are contaminated by the presence of plasma membranes. After one fractionation procedure, Warley and Cook (1973) found 40% of the total 5'-nucleotidase activity in the nuclear mitochondrial fraction and only 1.7% of the total activity in the plasma membrane fraction. They concluded that 5'-nucleotidase is not only in the plasma membrane but in the membranes from other organelles. In his study on the subcellular fractions of human tonsil lymphocytes, Demus (1973) also concluded that 5'-nucleotidase is present in the plasma membranes of lymphocytes but that it could not be said to be located there exclusively. In a recent study from this laboratory it was also found that the specific activity of 5'N in intact cells was equal to the activity of the homogenate, suggesting that most of the enzyme is on the external plasma membrane of these human lymphocytes (Quagliata et al., 1974).

A thorough study on the localization of 5'N in leukocytes has been made by DePierre and Karnovsky (1972, 1974a,b) using guinea pig polymorphonuclear leukocytes. In one of their experiments, the cells were treated with the diazonium salt of sulfanilic acid, a nonpenetrating reagent. In sonicated suspensions of leukocytes containing this salt, 5'N and lactate dehydrogenase, a cytoplasmic enzyme, were equally inhibited.

In intact cell suspensions containing the salt, lactic dehydrogenase activity was not affected, but the 5'N activity was inhibited by 90%. Therefore, it was concluded that at least the functional groups of the 5'N are located on the exterior aspect of the plasma membrane. When the nucleotidase reaction of intact cells was run to completion, approximately 99.3% of the $^{32}$Pi liberated was in the supernatant. The possibility that the substrate was hydrolyzed internally and the product was transported out of the cell still remained. A third experiment was designed to test this. The leukocytes were preloaded with $^{33}$Pi prior to assaying. If the substrate was hydrolyzed intracellularly and the product, Pi, transported extracellularly, then the supernatant would be expected to contain both $^{33}$Pi and $^{32}$Pi. The $^{32}$Pi was found in the supernatant whereas the $^{33}$Pi remained inside the leukocytes. The conclusion, based on the results of these three experiments, is that 5'N in guinea pig polymorphonuclear leukocytes is an ectoenzyme.

### 8.3.3. Studies of 5'N in Pathological Conditions

#### 8.3.3.1. Animal Studies

Szmigielski and his co-workers have published several studies on the effects of bacterial toxins on leukocyte 5'N in rabbits (1966a). Following the intravenous injection of *Streptococcus pyogenes, Escherichia coli, Klebsiella rhinoscleromatis,* and varous strains of staphylococci, 5'N and alkaline phosphatase activities were measured in the polymorphonuclear leukocytes of blood and bone marrow over a period of 16 days. In the animals injected with the staphylococcal and streptococcal bacteria, the percentage of blood and bone marrow demonstrating 5'N and alkaline phosphatase activities was increased. A more marked increase was noted in 5'N than in alkaline phosphatase activity. The rabbits injected with *E. coli* and *Klebsiella rhinoscleromatis* showed no significant changes in the two enzyme activities.

Intravenous injection of staphylococcal leukocidin, one of the bacterial toxins injurious to rabbit granulocytes, produced similar results (Szmigielski *et al.,* 1966b). Seventy-two hours after the injection, there was an increase in the number of leukocytes containing 5'N. A similar but less pronounced increase in alkaline phosphatase activity occurred. A rise in the percentage of cells exhibiting Na-K-ATPase was also noted. At first the number of polymorphonuclear leukocytes in the blood and bone marrow and of lymphocytes in the blood was greatly reduced, but a marked granulocytosis occurred 12 hr after the injection. This was characterized by an increase in the mitotic index and in the presence of many young myeloid cells in the bone marrow. After about 72–96 hr, the leukocyte count had returned to almost normal values.

Studies on rabbits receiving daily injections of leukocidin for 30 days (Szmigielski *et al.*, 1967b) again showed an increase in 5'N, alkaline phosphatase, and Na-K-ATPase. The number of 5'N-positive cells was at least twice the number expressing alkaline phosphatase activity. The activity peaked at 15 days, and at 28 days normal levels were returning.

The reaction of rabbits to injections of staphylococcal α-hemolysin (Szmigielski *et al.*, 1973) was different than their response to leukocidin. No decrease in the leukocyte count of the peripheral blood or in the bone marrow was noted. Instead an increase in the leukocytes of peripheral blood occurred 2 hr after the administration of the α-hemolysin. This leukocytosis reached a maximum by 4 hr. Slightly elevated leukocyte levels were still present 96 hr after injection. Of the enzymes monitored, the lysosomal enzymes (acid phosphatase, aryl sulfatase, and β-glucuronidase) showed definite increases in activity. The number of cells demonstrating nonspecific esterase decreased. There was no significant change in the percentage of granulocytes with Na-K-ATPase and 5'N.

Szmigielski *et al.* (1973) further characterized the different effects of staphylococcal leukocidin and α-hemolysin on the rabbit leukocyte system. Studies on the bone marrow of α-hemolysin-treated animals by autoradiographic techniques showed the number of cells incorporating [³H]thymidine or [³H]uridine in the treated rabbits was the same as controls. The mitotic index was slightly increased. They concluded that the granulocytosis in α-hemolysin-treated rabbits was not a result of stimulated cell production but a result of the release of the reserve pool of leukocytes. The increased percentage of immature myeloid cells seen in the marrow resulted from the liberation of mature forms and not granulocyte production. In the leukocidin-treated rabbits, incorporation studies indicated DNA and RNA synthesis. These results plus the increased mitotic index suggest active proliferation of myelocytes in the bone marrow. The original decrease in the leukocyte count was most probably a result of cell death caused by the leukocidin (Zucker-Franklin and Hirsch, 1964), which was followed by the production of new cells.

Kolakowska-Polubiec *et al.* (1970) investigated granulopoiesis in rats that had been subjected to third degree burns on 25–30% of the skin on their back. After the real injury there was no increase in 5'N-positive granulocytes. At 48 hr, five of the eight blood samples showed significant increases. In some animals the percentage of positive granulocytes continued to increase at 120 hr whereas others showed a decrease after 96 hr.

Weimar and Haraguchi (1967) studied enzyme activities of invading cells and connective tissue in the corneal wounds of albino rats. In corneas of control animals, polymorphonuclear leukocytes were occasionally found in the connective tissue stroma. These did not have 5'N. More granulocytes in this area were observed 6–12 hr after wounding. Mononuclear leukocytes were also present at this time. Both cells were predominantly negative for 5'N. At the edge of the wound, an occasional 5'N-positive polymorph was seen. After 24 hr, 5'N-positive leukocytes were seen. There seemed to be a relationship between the number of positive cells, the proximity of these cells to the wound, and the degree of inflammation: the more severe the inflammation, the greater the number of 5'N and leukocytes found nearer the wound. By 96 hr only those cells located near the wound showed 5'N activity. At 168 hr the enzyme was limited to leukocytes at the wound's edge. These positive cells were usually polymorphonuclear leukocytes.

The authors suggest that increased synthesis of this enzyme in the infiltrating cells accounted for their findings. However, activation of preexisting enzyme cannot be determined by the data presented. The increase in 5'N active cells, seen by Kolakowska-Polubiec *et al.* (1970), may have been an expression of a similar cell response to the burns as was seen in the eye wounds.

### 8.3.3.2. Human Studies

In the lymphocytes of approximately two-thirds of the chronic lymphocytic patients, 5'N levels were markedly diminished or not detectable (Marique and Hildebrand, 1973; Lopes *et al.*, 1973a,b). The data presented from our laboratory (Quagliata *et al.*, 1974) clearly demonstrated that there was no correlation between the presence (5'N+) or absence (5'N−) of 5'N and the altered B/T cell ratio found in the disease. A survey of the enzyme activity in the lymphocytes of patients with disorders other than CLL, including cardiopulmonary, metabolic, dermatological, and miscellaneous hematological diseases, found the lymphocytes in these patients to be 5'N+. Normal levels were found in the cells of three patients with leprosy, a disease that has a depressed cellular immune response, diminished PHA reactivity, and high levels of B lymphocytes. These are characteristics similar to the lymphocytes of CLL patients (Quagliata *et al.*, 1974). Two additional findings were made as a result of this survey. In the lymphocytes in two of the five patients with acute lymphocytic leukemia (ALL) 5'N activity was not detected, thereby suggesting heterogeneity in this disorder. Studies on patients with infectious mononucleosis showed a transient decrease of the enzyme activity in the early stages of the disease (Quagliata *et al.*, 1974). Recently, diminished 5'N levels have been reported in agammaglobulinemia.

Using an antibody to liver 5'N which inhibited the human lymphocyte enzyme, LaMantia *et al.* (1974) examined the lymphocytes from normal donors and patients with CLL. In the normal samples, 5'N+ and 5'N− lymphocytes were present. There was a good correlation between the percentage of 5'N+ cells determined by the fluorescent antibody method and the values obtained with histochemical technique (Silber *et al.*, 1975). In lymphycytes of CLL patients with detectable 5'N, mixtures of 5'N+ and 5'N− cells were also observed. In the lymphocytes of patients with undetectable 5'N activity, no immunoreactive enzyme was found. It was concluded that undetectable 5'N activity was a result of the absence of immunoreactive enzyme protein on the surface of these lymphocytes. An alternative interpretation of these results that the site of enzymatic activity and immunoreactive protein may be blocked by an inactivating protein is unlikely since activity does not become detectable after homogenization in the presence or absence of the detergent Triton X-100.

At least three explanations can be offered for the high incidence of 5'N negativity in CLL: (a) the negative subpopulation may be more likely to proliferate, or (b) rare 5'N-negative normal subjects may exist, constituting a population more likely to develop CLL, or (c) the activity is lost in the course of leukemogenesis. The possibility that environmental factors may be responsible for the loss of 5'N activity in the majority of CLL cells must also be considered, particularly since profound fluctuations in this activity have recently been reported in macrophages in responses to exogenous stimulation (Karnovsky *et al.*, 1975). Further clinical and experimental studies are required to decide which if any of these hypotheses may account for the heterogeneity of 5'N in CLL. The studies reported herein describe another marker for the increasingly complex pattern of lymphocyte subpopulations.

Rosner *et al.* (1965) studied enzyme levels in the leukocytes of patients with Down's syndrome. In the cells of 12 trisomic patients, elevated levels were seen in leukocyte alkaline phosphatase, acid phosphatase, and 5'N. The erythrocyte glucose-6-phosphate dehydrogenase was also increased when compared to normal control leukocytes. In the leukocytes of patients with translocations, all enzyme activities had normal levels. The authors concluded that these results are an expression of a "derangement of regulating and modifying gene complexes." Benson (1967) studied the rate of protein and RNA synthesis in the leukocytes of trisomic Down's patients by autoradiography. The rate of incorporation of [$^{14}$C]orotic acid and [$^{3}$H]uridine by leukocytes of Down's patients was greater than the incorporation rate in normal cells. He proposed that this increase in synthesis may be responsible for the increase in enzymatic activities observed by Rosner *et al.* (1965).

### 8.3.4. Function of 5'N in Leukocytes

The 5'N activity in leukocytes may be directly related to cellular synthetic processes. High levels are found in the germinal centers of tonsils, lymph nodes, and spleens (Gomori, 1959b; Allan and Crumpton, 1972; Braunstein *et al.*, 1958; Kaiserling and Caesar, 1969; Muller-Hermelink *et al.*, 1974). These are areas of active lymphopoiesis with a high mitotic index. Szmigielski *et al.* (1966a,b, 1968, 1973) reported a marked increase in 5′N+ leukocytes of rabbits treated with leukocidin which was associated with an increased mitotic index (1973), with active RNA and DNA synthesis occurring. Studies by Rosner *et al.* (1965) and Benson (1967) suggest a correlation between the elevated enzyme activities of trisomic Down's leukocytes and increased protein synthesis. In synchronized mouse leukemic cells, 5′N activity increases in the S phase of the cycle. Weimar and Haraguchi (1967) noted either activation or production of 5′N in leukocytes, concurring with the production of new cytoplasm and changes in the leukocyte nucleus.

A role for 5′N in nucleoside uptake has been demonstrated by Fleit *et al.* (1975). Lymphocytes containing 5′N from normal donors and CLL patients and those demonstrating no enzyme activity were examined for their ability to take up adenosine presented as the nucleoside, the 5′-nucleotide. When 5′N+ and 5′N− lymphocytes were incubated with [$^3$H]AMP, the uptake of labeled adenosine was four times greater in 5′N+ lymphocytes. With [$^{32}$P]AMP in the medium, the 5′N+ cells also showed a fourfold increase in uptake. However, 5′N+ and 5′N− lymphocytes were equally able to transport $^{32}$Pi or adenosine. When the cells were incubated with [$^3$H]AMP or [$^{32}$P]AMP in the presence of 10% autologous serum as an exogenous source of 5′N, the uptake of [$^3$H]adenosine or $^{32}$Pi by 5′N− and 5′N+ lymphocytes was the same. These experiments showed that the ectoenzyme would cleave the nucleotide to which cells are relatively impermeable and allow the uptake of the nucleoside and Pi. The absence of nucleotides and the presence of 5′N in plasma make it doubtful whether these *in vitro* experiments pertain to an *in vivo* situation.

An inverse relationship between 5′N activity and protein synthesis has been reported. Fritzson (1967) studied the cyclic variations in 5′N activity and rat liver regeneration. The 5′N levels decreased at the initiation of growth of new rat liver. The enzyme activity increased as protein synthesis ceased. He concluded that the 5′N may act as a controlling factor in liver regenesis by interfering with protein synthesis in some manner.

## 8.4. Summary and Conclusions

The enzyme 5′N which cleaves the phosphate group of the 5′-ribonucleotides and 5′-deoxyribonucleotides has been described in many tissues. The enzymes isolated from different sources show differences in affinity for various 5′-nucleotide substrates. The leukocyte enzyme is usually measured at pH 7.0–7.5 and requires divalent cations, usually

$Mg^{2+}$ or $Mn^{2+}$. Like 5'N obtained from other sources, the leukocyte enzyme is stimulated by low concentrations of detergents. Studies on purified enzyme suggest 5'N exists as a large molecule (130,000–140,000 molecular weight) which is composed of two smaller enzymatically active glycoproteins (70,000–85,000).

The leukocytes of many animals have 5'N activity. Studies by DePierre and Karnovsky (1974) have shown that not all the different white blood cells in a given species possess the enzyme. The heterogeneity of 5'N in human lymphocytes has been demonstrated. The percentage of lymphocytes containing the enzyme varies among different donors but is constant for any one donor (Silber et al., 1975). Lymphocytes from about two-thirds of the patients with CLL have diminished or absent 5'N activity. A transient decrease in 5'N is found early in the course of infectious mononucleosis. There was no relationship established between the level of enzymatic activity in lymphocytes from peripheral blood and the B/T cell ratio (Quagliata et al., 1974). However, studies on lymphocytes in spleen, lymph nodes, and tonsil tissue have reported that 5'N is limited to the follicle and germinal center areas of B lymphocytes. The conclusion from these studies was that 5'N is limited to B cells. Reports from two laboratories (Allen and Crumpton, 1972; Quagliata et al., 1974) demonstrate this enzyme in T lymphocytes from thymus, although the activity in these cells was generally lower than lymphocytes in peripheral blood and tonsil. Possible explanations for these findings have been discussed.

The presence of 5'N in human granulocytes has been reported by two laboratories (Gough and Elves, 1967; Szmigielski et al., 1967a). A third (Strauss and Burrows, 1975) failed to detect the enzyme in the plasma membranes.

The enzyme has been described in the plasma membranes of leukocytes from man and animals. This enzyme was also detected in other subcellular fractions (Warley and Cook, 1973; Demus, 1973). Demus (1973) suggests that the presence of 5'N in these other fractions was a result of contamination by plasma membranes. The possibility that the enzyme is located in other cellular organelles has not been ruled out. Several studies have presented evidence that in guinea pig granulocytes and human lymphocytes this enzyme is localized to the plasma membrane with the active site facing the environment.

The localization of 5'N may determine the function of the enzyme in the cells. The action of the membrane-bound 5'N of human lymphocytes is necessary for the uptake of adenosine from AMP in the external medium (Fleit et al., 1975). The observed high enzymatic activities of the lymphocytes on areas known for active lymphopoiesis and in systems in which leukopoiesis was induced have suggested a relationship between 5'N and cellular synthetic processes.

ACKNOWLEDGMENT

This work was supported by U.S. Public Health Service Grant CA-11655.

# References

Ahmed, Z., and Reis, J. L., 1958, The activation and inhibition of 5'-nucleotidase, *Biochem. J.* **69**:386.

Allan, D., and Crumpton, M.J., 1970, Preparation and characterization of the plasma membrane of pig lymphocytes, *Biochem. J.* **120**:133.

Allan, D., and Crumpton, M. J., 1971, Solubilization of pig lymphocyte plasma membrane and fractionation of some of the components, *Biochem. J.* **123**:967.

Allan, D., and Crumpton, M. J., 1972, Isolation and composition of human thymocyte plasma membrane, *Biochim. Biophys. Acta* **274**:22.

Bainton, D. F., and Farquhar, M. G., 1968a, Differences in enzyme content of azurophil and specific granules of polymorphonuclear leukocytes. I. Histochemical staining of bone marrow smear, *J. Cell Biol.* **39**:286.

Bainton, D. F., and Farquhar, M. G., 1968b, Differences on enzyme content of azurophil and specific granules of polymorphonuclear leukocytes. II. Cytochemistry and electron microscopy of bone marrow cells, *J. Cell Biol.* **39**:299.

Belfield, A., and Goldberg, D. M., 1968, Inhibition of the nucleotidase effect of alkaline phosphatase by β-glycerophosphate, *Nature (London)* **219**:73.

Benson, P. F., 1967, Protein and RNA synthesis in trisomic Down's syndrome leukocytes, *Nature (London)* **215**:1290.

Bosmann, H. B., 1972, Half-lives of enzyme activities in an L51784 mouse leukemic cell, *J. Cell Sci.* **10**:153.

Braunstein, H., Freiman, D. G., and Gall, E. R., 1958, A histochemical study of the enzymatic activity of lymph nodes. I. The normal and hyperplastic lymph node, *Cancer* **11**:829.

Braunstein, H., Freiman, D. F., and Gall, E. R., 1962, A histochemical study of the enzymatic activity of lymph nodes. III. Granulomatous and primary neoplastic conditions of lymphoid tissue, *Cancer* **15**:139.

Cohn, Z. A., and Hirsch, J. C., 1960a, The isolation and properties of the specific cytoplasmic granules of rabbit polymorphonuclear leukocytes, *J. Exp. Med.* **112**:983.

Cohn, Z. A., and Hirsch, J. G., 1960b, The influence of phagocytosis on the intercellular distribution of granule-associated components of polymorphonuclear leukocytes, *J. Exp. Med.* **112**:1015.

Demus, H., 1973, Subcellular fractionation of human lymphocytes: Isolation of two plasma components of the various lymphocytic organelles, *Biochim. Biophys. Acta* **291**:93.

DePierre, J. W., and Karnovsky, M. L., 1972, Ectoenzyme of granulocytes:5'-nucleotidase, *Science* **183**: 1096.

DePierre, J., and Karnovsky, M. L., 1974a, Ectoenzymes of the guinea pig poly-morphonuclear leukocyte. II. Properties and suitability as markers for the plasma membrane, *J. Biol. Chem.* **249**:7121.

DePierre, J. W., and Karnovsky, M. L., 1974b, Ectoenzymes of the guinea pig polymorphonuclear leukocyte. I. Evidence for an ecto-adenosine monophos-phatase,-adenosine triphosphatase and -*p*-nitropehnyl phosphatase, *J. Biol. Chem.* **249**:7111.

Drummond, G. I., and Yamamoto, M., 1971, Nucleotide phosphomonesterases, *in The Enzyme*, Vol. 4 (P. D. Boyer, ed), pp. 337–354, Academic Press, New York.

Evans, W. H., and Gurd, J. W., 1973, Properties of a 5'-nucleotidase purified from mouse liver plasma membranes, *Biochem. J.* **133**:189.

Ferber, E., Kesch, K., Wallach, D. F. H. and Imm, W., 1972, Isolation and characterization of lymphocyte plasma membranes, *Biochim. Biophys. Acta* **266**:494.

Fiske, C. H., and SubbRow, Y., 1925. The colorimetric determination of phos-phorous, *J. Biol. Chem.* **66**:375.

Fleit, H., Conklyn, M., Stebbins, R. D., and Silber, R., 1975, Function of 5'-nucleotidase in the uptake of adenosine from AMP by human lymphocytes, *J. Biol. Chem.* **250**:8889.

Follette, J. H., Valentine, W. N., and Reynolds, J., 1959, A comparison of human leukocyte phosphotase activity toward sodium-β-glycerophosphate, adeno-sine 5'-phosphate and glucose 6-phosphate, *Blood* **14**:415.

Fritzson, P., 1967, Dephosphorylation of pyrimidine nucleotides in the soluble fraction of homogenates from normal and regenerating rat liver, *Eur. J. Biochem.* **1**:12.

Gomori, G., 1.49a, Histochemical specificity of phosphatases, *Proc. Soc. Exp. Biol. Med.* **70**:7.

Gomori, G., 1949b, Further studies on the histochemical specificity of phospha-tase, *Proc. Soc. Exp. Biol. Med.* **72**:449.

Gough, J., and Elves, M. W., 1967, Studies of lymphocytes and their derivative cells *in vitro*. II. Enzyme cytochemistry, *Acta Hematol.* **37**:42.

Hardonk, M. J., 1968, 5'-Nucleotidase. I. Distribution of 5'-nucleotidase in tissues of rat and mouse, *Histochemie* **12**:1.

Hardonk, M. J., and de Boer, H. G. A., 1968, 5'-Nucleotidase. III. Determinations of 5'-nucleotidase isoenzymes in tissues of rat and mouse, *Histochemie* **12**:29.

Hill, P. G., and Sammons, H., 1971, the pH optimum of human 5'-nucleotidases, *Enzyme* **12**:201

Hirsch, J., and Cohn, Z. A., 1960, Degranulation of polymorphonuclear leuko-cytes following phagocytosis of micro-organisms, *J. Exp. Med.* **112**:1005.

Ipata, P. L., 1968, Sheep brain 5'-nucleotidase. Some enzymic properties and allosteric inhibition by nucleoside triphosphates, *Biochemistry* **7**:507.

Kaiserling, E., and Caesar, R., 1969, Elektronenmikroskopischler Nachweis der 5'-Nucleotidase im Keimzentrum de menschichen Tonsille, *Z. Zellforsh.* **95**:202 (Abstract).

Karnovsky, M. L., Lazdino, J., Drath, D., and Harper, A., 1975, Biochemical characteristics of activated macrophages, *Ann. N.Y. Acad. Sci.* **256**:266.

Kolakowska-Polubiec, K., Litwin, J., Nasilowski, W., Slomkowski, M., and Zupan-
    ska, B., 1970, 5'-Ribonucleotide phosphohydrolase activity in peripheral
    blood granulocytes of rats after burns, *Pol. Med. J.* **9**:110.
Ladoulis, C. T., Misra, D. N., Estes, L. W., and Gill, T. J., 1974, Lymphocyte
    plasma membranes. I. Thymic and splenic membranes from inbred rats,
    *Biochim. Biophys. Acta* **356**:27.
LaMantia, K., Conklyn, M., Quagliata, F., and Silber, R., 1974, Immunologic
    studies of 5'-nucleotidase in normal and chronic lymphocytic leukemia lym-
    phocytes, *Blood* **46**:1042 (Abstract).
Lopes, J., Nachbar, M., Zucker-Franklin, D., and Silber, R., 1973a, Lymphocyte
    plasma membranes: Analyses of proteins and glycoproteins by SDS-gel elec-
    trophoresis, *Blood* **41**:131.
Lopes, J., Zucker-Franklin, D., and Silber, R., 1973b, Heterogeneity of 5'-nucleoti-
    dase activity in lymphocytes in chronic lyphocytic leukemia, *J. Clin. Invest.*
    **52**:1297.
Marique, D., and Hildebrand, J., 1973, Evidence for a 5'-nucleotidase in human
    leukemic leukocytes, *Clin. Chim. Acta* **45**:93.
Misra, D. N., Gill, T., and Estes, L. W., 1974, Lymphocyte plasma membranes. II.
    Cytochemical localization of 5'-nucleotidase in rat lymphocytes, *Biochim.
    Biophys. Acta* **352**:455.
Mitchell, R., and Hawthorne, J. N., 1965, The site of dephosphoenositide synthe-
    sis in rat liver, *Biochem. Biophys. Res. Commun.* **21**:333.
Muller-Hermelink, H. K., 1974, Characterization of the B-cell and T-cell regions
    of human lymphatic tissue through enzyme histochemical demonstration of
    ATPase and 5'-nucleotidase activities, *Virchows Arch. Cell Pathol.* **16**:371.
Muller-Hermelink, H. K., Heuserman, U., and Slutte, H. J., 1974, Enzyme
    histochemical observation on the localizations and structure of T-cell and B-
    cell regions in the human spleen, *Cell Tiss. Res.* **154**:167.
Nakamura, S., 1976, Effect of sodium deoxycholate on 5'-nucleotidase, *Biochim.
    Biophys. Acta* **426**:339.
Oliver, J. M., Ukena, T. E., and Berlin, R. D., 1974, Effects of phagocytosis and
    colchicine on the distribution of lectin-binding sites on cell surfaces, *Proc. Nat.
    Acad. Sci. U.S.A.* **71**:394.
Paglia, D. E., and Valentine, W. N., 1975, Characteristics of a pyrimidine-specific
    5'-nucleotidase in human erythrocytes, *J. Biol. Chem.* **250**:7973.
Pearse, A. G. E., 1968, *in Histochemistry, Theoretical and Applied,* pp. 475–546,
    William & Willin, Boston, Massachusetts.
Pearse, A. G. E., and Reis, J. L., 1952, The histochemical demonstration of a
    specific phosphatase 5'-nucleotidase, *Biochem. J.* **50**:534.
Quagliata, F., Faig, D., Conklyn, M., and Silber, R., 1974, Studies on the lympho-
    cyte 5'-nucleotidase in chronic lymphocytic leukemia, infectious mononucleo-
    sis, normal subpopulations and phytohemagglutin stimulated cells, *Cancer
    Res.* **34**:3197.
Reis, J., 1937, Uber die aktivitat der 5'-nukleoticle in den tierischen und menschel-
    ichen Geweben, *Enzyme* **2**:183 (Abstract).
Reis, J., 1939, La nucleotidase et sa relation avec la desamenation des nucleotides
    dano le cour et dano le muscle, *Bull. Soc. Chim. Biol.* **16**:385.

Reis, J. L., 1951, The specificity of phosphormonesterases in human tissues, *Biochem. J.* **48**:548.

Rosner, F., Ony, B., Paine, R., and Mahanand, D., 1965, Biochemical differentiation of trisomic Down's syndrome from that due to translocation, *N. Engl. J. Med.* **273**:1356.

Silber, R., Conklyn, M., Grusky, G., and Zucker-Franklin, D., 1975, Human lymphocytes: 5'-Nucleotidase-positive and-negative subpopulations. *J. Clin. Invest.* **56**:1324.

Strauss, R., and Burrows, S., 1975, Letter to the Editor, *Blood* **46**:655.

Swendsied, M., Wright, P. D., and Bethell, F. H., 1952, Variations in nucleotidase activity of leukocytes. Studies with leukemic patients, *J. Lab. Clin. Med.* **40**:515.

Szmigielski, S., 1965, 5'-Nucleotidase activity in human blood granulocytes during acute infections, *Folia Hematol.* **84**:402.

Szmigielski, S., Jeljaszewicz, J., and Wilczynski, J., 1966a, 5'-Nucleotidase activity in rabbit leukocytes during experimental infections, *Pathol. Microbiol.* **29**:186.

Szmigielski, S., Jeljaszewicz, J., Wilczynski, J., and Korbecki, M., 1966b, Reaction of rabbit leukocytes to staphylococcal (Panton–Valentine) leukocidine *in vitro*, *J. Pathol. Bacteriol.* **91**:599.

Szmigielski, S., Kolakowska-Polubiec, K., Litwin, J., Slomkowski, M., and Zupanska, B., 1967a, Histochemical studies on 5'-nucleotidase in blood and bone marrow cells, *Pol. Med. J.* **6**:631.

Szmigielski, S., Jeljaszewicz, J., and Zak, C., 1967b, Reaction of rabbit leukocytes to staphylococcal alpha hemolysin *in vitro*, *J. Infect. Dis.* **117**:209.

Szmigielski, S., Jeljaszewicz, J., and Zak, C., 1968, Leukocyte system of rabbits receiving repeated injections of staphylococcal leukocidin, *Pathol. Microbiol.* **31**:328.

Szmigielski, S., Kwarecki, K., Jeljaszewicz, J. L., Mollby, R., and Wadstiom, T., 1973, Alpha-toxin and leucocidin effects on granulopoiesis, *Microbiol. Immunol.* **1**:202.

Trubowitz, S., Fellman, D., Morgenetern, S., and Wand, V. M., 1961, The isolation, purification, and some properties of the alkaline phosphatase of human leucocytes, *Biochem. J.* **80**:369.

Wachstein, M., and Meisel, E., 1957, Histochemistry of hepatic phosphatases at a physiological pH, *Am. J. Clin. Pathol.* **27**:13.

Warley, A., and Cook, G. M. W., 1973, The isolation and characterization of plasma membranes from normal and leukemic cells of mice, *Biochim. Biophys. Acta* **323**:55.

Weimar, V. L., and Haraguchi, K. H., 1967, The lag phase of wound repair: A comparison of leukocytic and cornial connective tissue enzyme activities, *Exp. Eye Res.* **6**:283.

Widnell, C. C., 1974, Purification of rat liver 5'-nucleotidase as a complex with sphingomyelin, *in Methods in Enzymology*, Vol. 32 (Fleischer Sand Packer, ed.), pp. 368–374, Academic Press, New York.

Zucker-Franklin, D., and Hirsch, J. G., 1964, Electron microscope studies on the degranulation of rabbit peritoneal leukocytes during phagocytosis, *J. Exp. Med.* **120**:569.

# 9

# Metabolism and Functions of Monocytes and Macrophages

## Martin J. Cline and David W. Golde

Mononuclear phagocytes comprise a cell line that includes primitive forms in the bone marrow (monoblasts and promonocytes), intermediate cells in the blood (monocytes), and mature forms in the tissues (macrophages). Tissue macrophages are heterogeneous and include alveolar macrophages, Kupffer's cells, the macrophages of the splenic sinusoids, and a variety of other forms. The concept of a continuum of cells from bone marrow precursors through the monocyte to the tissue macrophages is important to the understanding of the function and metabolism of these cells. Mononuclear phagocytes at different levels of maturation have distinctive morphologic, functional, and metabolic characteristics.

## 9.1. Proliferation and Maturation

Mononuclear phagocytes probably share a common progenitor cell with the granulocytic series as suggested by cytochemical studies (Leder, 1967), by mixed cellular proliferation in certain types of leukemia (Brandt

MARTIN J. CLINE and DAVID W. GOLDE • Department of Medicine, University of California School of Medicine, Los Angeles, California 90024.

*et al.*, 1974), and by observations of proliferation of bone marrow cells in tissue cultures (Bradley and Metcalf, 1966; Ichikawa *et al.*, 1966).

### 9.1.1. Monoblast

Because of their rarity and the absence of distinctive cytological features, the youngest monocyte precursors are not identifiable in normal human bone marrow but have been observed in cultures of mouse bone marrow (Goud *et al.*, 1975). Blast cells ("monoblasts") presumed to be the progenitors of differentiated mononuclear phagocytes are seen with frequency only in the variants of monocytic leukemia. These cells show little motility, adhesiveness to glass, or phagocytic activity. When these undifferentiated blast cells mature and develop a complex Golgi apparatus and a definite granule population, they are identifiable and are designated promonocytes.

### 9.1.2. Promonocyte

The promonocyte has a high nucleus-to-cytoplasm ratio, a basophilic cytoplasm, some peroxidase activity, and DNA synthetic activity. The cell is capable of endocytosis but generally shows little phagocytosis. With cellular maturation, the activity of certain hydrolases increases, peroxidase activity diminishes, and phagocytic ability increases (Cline, 1975; Nichols *et al.*, 1971; van Furth *et al.*, 1970, 1972).

### 9.1.3. Blood Monocyte

By light microscopy, Wright-stained human monocytes appear as large cells (10–18 $\mu$m in diameter) with grayish-blue cytoplasm frequently containing small numbers of faint, azurophilic granules. Monocytes are generally smaller than promonocytes. Their centrally located nucleus is usually indented or horseshoe-shaped and has a fine, lacy chromatin structure. The living monocyte observed by phase microscopy is slowly motile by means of blunt pseudopodia.

The monocyte is usually easily distinguished from other types of circulating leukocytes by its ultrastructural characteristics (Nichols *et al.*, 1971; Nichols and Bainton, 1973); however, by light microscopy there are some cells that appear to be intermediate in structure between monocytes and large lymphocytes (Horwitz *et al.*, 1970). To distinguish monocytes from such cells one must apply functional criteria, such as phagocytic ability, and the presence of certain enzymatic activities, such as $\alpha$-naphthyl butyrase (Leder, 1967).

### 9.1.4. Tissue Macrophages

Tissue macrophages (synonym: histiocytes) are a later stage of maturation of the monocyte. They are abundant in the alveolar spaces, in the pleural and peritoneal spaces, and in parenchymal organs such as the liver and spleen, and are found in lesser numbers in lymph nodes. Human macrophages are large cells measuring 20–80 $\mu$m in diameter. They contain one or more large vesicular nuclei, often with prominent nucleoli, cytoplasmic granules, and numerous mitochondria, lysosomes, and inclusions (Cline, 1975).

The living cells are slowly motile and are constantly pushing out giant pseudopods many cell diameters in length. This cell movement appears to depend on the complex of microfilaments found in the cell cytoplasm (Allison *et al.*, 1971). Immature macrophages are capable of DNA synthesis and cell division. Ultimately, the immature cell gives rise to a mature, nondividing macrophage. The immature cell has loose nuclear chromatin and basophilic cytoplasm; the mature macrophage has a condensed nuclear chromatin and cytoplasm that stains pink or light red with Romanovsky stains.

Macrophages may form multinucleate giant cells, probably by the process of cell fusion. The maturation of these cells results in the typical giant cells seen in chronic granulomatous reactions. These giant cells are extremely rich in granules, hydrolytic enzymes, and mitochondria.

## 9.2. Kinetics

The studies of Meuret and his colleagues (Meuret, 1974; Meuret and Fliedner, 1974; Meuret *et al.*, 1974a,b, 1975a,b) provide the following information on monocyte kinetics in man: (a) In healthy subjects monocyte counts in the blood oscillate with a cycle frequency of 3–6 days. (b) The total blood monocyte pool includes a circulating pool and a marginated pool. The marginated pool is about three times the size of the circulating pool. (c) Monocytes leave the blood exponentially with a $T\frac{1}{2}$ of 8.4 hr. (d) The $T\frac{1}{2}$ may be prolonged in patients with monocytosis and shortened in patients with acute infection or splenomegaly. (e) Normal monocyte turnover rate averages $7 \times 10^6$ cells/hr/kg of body weight. (f) The promonocyte pool size is about $6 \times 10^8$ cells/kg of body weight. Cells in this pool have a DNA synthesis time of about 10 hr. Considerably more information is available on granulocyte kinetics in normal man (Golde and Cline, 1977). In contrast to these observations in normal man, studies of monocyte kinetics in leukemia are rare (Killman *et al.*, 1962; Osgood *et al.*, 1952).

The relative rapidity with which total labeling of monocytes occurs with the continuous infusion of tritiated thymidine suggests that there is not significant reentry of monocytes into the bloodstream once they have left the circulation. Monocytes enter the tissues to mature to macrophages. For example, the major source of mononuclear phagocytes accumulating at inflammatory foci is the monocyte precursors of the bone marrow (Horwitz, 1972; Lubaroff and Waksman, 1968; Schmalzl et al., 1969; Spector and Willoughby, 1968; Virolainen, 1968). These inflammatory mononuclear cells arise from rapidly proliferating bone marrow cells and reach the inflammatory site by the bloodstream. Under noninflammatory conditions tissue macrophages may also arise from endogenous replicating cells as well as from marrow precursors (Bowden et al., 1969; Golde et al., 1974; Weiden et al., 1975; Widmann and Fahimi, 1975).

A variety of factors influence the numbers of circulating monocytes. Many disease states, including sarcoidosis, tuberculosis, and Hodgkin's disease, may be associated with blood monocytosis. Administration of endotoxin results in a monocytopenia followed by a recovery phase that is slow and incomplete relative to the granulocyte response. Injection of antibody-coated erythrocytes produces a prompt fall in circulating monocytes, persisting at least 3–6 hr (Jandly and Tomlinson, 1958). Glucocorticoids may induce a monocytopenia, probably by interfering with the release of monocytes from the bone marrow (Thompson and Van Furth, 1973). In cyclic neutropenia, monocyte kinetics also vary cyclically (Meuret and Fliedner, 1974).

Whole body irradiation produces a sharp fall in the number of circulating monocytes and of newly formed macrophages because the dividing progenitor cells in the bone marrow are radiosensitive (Hulse, 1959; Volkman and Collins, 1968).

## 9.3. Metabolism

The metabolism and enzymatic activities of mononuclear phagocytes change profoundly with cell maturation, with changes in cellular environment, and with various cellular activities (Cline, 1975; Cohn, 1968). The principal energy source for the human monocyte and probably for most tissue macrophages is glycolysis, even under aerobic conditions (Frei et al., 1961; Oren et al., 1963), with a relatively small amount of the total glucose being metabolized via the hexose monophosphate shunt (West et al., 1968). In contrast to other tissue macrophages, the metabolism of the resting (nonphagocytic) human alveolar macrophage appears to be primarily aerobic (Cline, 1975; Cohen and Cline, 1971). The morphological correlate of this aerobic metabolism is that the alveolar macrophage has abundant mitochondria.

Macrophages have an active lipid metabolism, and phospholipid synthesis is increased during phagocytosis (Elsbach, 1967, 1968; Karnovsky, 1962; Oren et al., 1963; Werb and Cohn, 1971). The more mature cells of the series have abundant rough endoplasmic reticulum and a high rate of protein synthesis (Cohn, 1968; Cline, 1975; Stecher and Thorbecke, 1967). Much of this synthetic activity is directed toward the production of lysosomal enzymes (Cohn and Benson, 1965a,b).

A characteristic feature of mononuclear phagocytes is their prominent lysosomal granules. The enzymes of these granules are made in the endoplasmic reticulum and packaged in the Golgi apparatus to form the primary lysosome (Cohn, 1968; Nichols et al., 1971). These primary lysosomes may then fuse with phagocytic vacuoles or pinocytic vesicles, resulting in the production of structures called secondary lysosomes. A large number of hydrolytic enzymes have been localized within the lysosomal cell fraction, including acid phosphatase, lysozyme, $\beta$-glucuronidase, $\beta$-galactosidase, BPN-hydrolase, esterases, aryl sulfatase, myeloperoxidase (in young cells), elastase, and probably hyaluronidase (Cline, 1975; Cohn, 1968). These enzymes probably have a major role in digestion of phagocytized organic materials, including microorganisms. Some lysosomal enzymes may be secreted by the macrophage (Gordon et al., 1974; Werb and Gordon, 1975) or released on endocytosis (Ackerman and Beebe, 1974). The number and contents of the lysosomes vary with cellular maturation and with activation by cellular immune processes (Mackaness, 1970).

The transformation from monoblast to mature macrophage is associated with changes in cellular composition and metabolism. With maturation, the number of cytoplasmic lysosomes and mitochondria increases, and the activity level of associated lysosomal and mitochondrial enzymes changes correspondingly. This increase in enzyme activity results from the increased synthesis of enzymes accompanying cellular differentiation (Cohn and Benson, 1965b; Cohn et al., 1966). Cytoplasmic organelles, thought to be involved in protein synthesis, are abundant in all phases of monocyte differentiation but are particularly numerous in giant cells. The Golgi apparatus, which is small in monocytes, increases in size and complexity with cell differentiation. Glycolysis and not respiration provides the energy necessary for the phagocytic activity of mammalian monocytes (Cline and Lehrer, 1968). As human monocytes differentiate into macrophages in vitro, phagocytosis is still dependent on glycolytic mechanisms, although the mature macrophage derives its energy from both glycolytic and aerobic pathways. Macrophages, with the exception of the alveolar macrophage, are effective phagocytes even under anaerobic conditions. This characteristic must be advantageous to cells that often function at sites remote from oxygenated blood. Human alveolar macrophages are, in contrast, critically dependent on a $P_{O_2}$ of greater than 25 mm Hg for phagocytosis and energy production (Cohen and Cline, 1971). Monocytes increase their oxygen consumption and the fraction of glucose metabolized via the HMP shunt during phagocytosis and probably generate $H_2O_2$ and superoxide.

It is clear that differentiation to mature macrophages and the accompanying increase in specific activity of certain lysosomal enzymes are dependent on intact protein synthesis. When macrophages are cultivated *in vitro* under circumstances in which pinocytic activity is reduced, the numerous secondary lysosomes gradually disappear from the cytoplasm (Cohn, 1968). This influence of *in vitro* environmental factors on the cellular level of lysosomal enzymes may reflect the situation in the intact animal in which the metabolic and functional status of the macrophages is adaptable. This phenomenon is most clearly demonstrated in the macrophage "activated" by infection with an intracellular parasite such as *Mycobacterium tuberculosis*. Such mononuclear phagocytes are larger, spread more readily on a surface, and have increased metabolic and microbicidal activity. Activation may be mediated by products of sensitized lymphoid cells (Mackaness, 1970).

## 9.4. Functions

There are five major areas of mononuclear phagocyte function: (a) defense against microorganisms; (b) removal of dead or damaged cells, cell debris, and inorganic materials; (c) cooperative and effector functions in immune responses; (d) regulatory interactions in hematopoiesis; and (e) synthesis of biologically active compounds in addition to those involved in the foregoing regulatory processes. These cells may also play a role in wound repair and remodeling of embryonic tissues. Many of these functions are dependent on the active endocytic activity of macrophages and their surface receptors for the Fc portion of certain subclasses of IgG molecules and complement components (Allison *et al.*, 1971; Arend and Mannik, 1973; Cline, 1975; Rabinovitch *et al.*, 1975; Rosse *et al.*, 1975).

## 9.5. Defense against Microorganisms

Monocytes and macrophages have an important role in the defense against a variety of infectious organisms (Territo and Cline, 1975, 1977).

They are the principal cells involved in killing intracellular parasites, including *Mycobacterium* (Dannenberg, 1975), *Listeria*, and *Toxoplasma* species (Remington *et al.*, 1972; Anderson and Remington, 1974), as well as other fungi, bacteria, and protozoa (Behin *et al.*, 1974; Cline, 1975; Mackaness, 1970; Territo and Cline, 1975). Macrophages participate with immunocompetent cells in the defense against viral illness and may directly kill virus and virus-infected cells (Stott *et al.*, 1975). They have been demonstrated to produce interferon and to enhance lymphocyte production of interferon (Epstein *et al.*, 1971; Silverstein, 1975). Viruses in turn may interfere with normal macrophage function (Twomey *et al.*, 1974).

Mononuclear phagocytes must travel to and accumulate at an infective focus, phagocytize, and eventually kill the invading organism. Cell movement probably requires the complex of microtubules and microfilaments and actin- and myosinlike proteins found in the macrophage (Stossel and Hartwig, 1975). Significantly less is known about the chemotaxis of mononuclear phagocytes than of granulocytes. The activated fifth component of complement is chemotactic for monocytes (Snyderman *et al.*, 1971; Dannenberg, 1975), as are factors released by mitogen- and antigen-stimulated lymphocytes (Boetcher and Meltzer, 1975; Boumsell and Meltzer, 1976). Lymphocyte products may be important in the accumulation of monocytes at sites of immunologically mediated inflammation. A number of other specific and nonspecific factors are involved in mononuclear phagocyte chemotaxis, and macrophages respond differently from monocytes in certain of the chemotactic assays (Boumsell and Meltzer, 1977). Increased chemotactic activity has been described in activated macrophages from BCG-infected mice (Meltzer *et al.*, 1975a).

Once macrophages are chemotactically attracted to an inflammatory focus, they may accumulate under the influence of another lymphocyte-derived factor, migration-inhibitory factor (MIF) (Dannenberg, 1975; Kostiala and McGregor, 1975). MIF may be the same molecule that activates macrophages (macrophage-activating factor, MAF) and is probably one of the inducers of the complex series of metabolic changes that result in the activated state (David, 1975). These macrophage-directed "lymphokines" play an important role in macrophage attraction, accumulation, and "activation."

The precise mechanisms by which mononuclear phagocytes kill ingested microorganisms have not been clearly defined (Lehrer, 1975; Cline, 1975). Monocytes and macrophages are probably similar to granulocytes in that microbicidal mechanisms probably involve both oxygen-dependent and -independent functions (Klebanoff, 1971). The activated macrophage has been shown to kill some microorganisms more efficiently than the "resting" cell. Monocytes from patients with chronic granulomatous disease (CGD) manifest defective bactericidal and fungicidal capacity (Lehrer, 1975). Since the defect in CGD is related to impaired $H_2O_2$ and $O_2^-$ generation, it is likely that mononuclear phagocytes share this microbicidal mechanism with granulocytes.

Myeloperoxidase is present in human monocytes but not in macrophages. This enzyme interacts with $H_2O_2$ in one microbicidal system. In the genetic deficiency of myeloperoxidase, monocytes have impaired fungicidal capacity but macrophage killing is normal (Lehrer and Cline, 1969). Monocytes from patients with myeloperoxidase deficiency or CGD have impaired ability to kill *Candida albicans*. The failure of iodination of microorganisms in CGD and myeloperoxidase-deficient monocytes is consistent with the supposition that iodination is catalyzed by a myeloperoxidase- and $H_2O_2$-linked mechanism in the monocyte as it is in the granulocyte (Lehrer and Cline, 1969).

Myeloperoxidase-independent mechanisms also exist in monocytes and macrophages (Lehrer, 1975). Cationic proteins are probably an important microbicidal component, and many other as yet unidentified mechanisms may be operative in killing by cells of the mononuclear phagocyte system.

## 9.6. Removal of Damaged Cells and Inorganic Materials

Mononuclear phagocytes function in the removal of damaged or dying cells. The macrophage seems able to recognize alterations in the erythrocyte surface caused by antibody, physical or chemical injury, or the aging process (Kay, 1975). Old erythrocytes are phagocytized and their hemoglobin catabolized (Gemsa *et al.*, 1973, 1974, 1975). Splenic macrophages remove nuclear remnants and precipitated hemoglobin from circulating red cells ("pitting"). They also ingest immunologically injured white cells and platelets. Alveolar macrophages have a special function in clearing particulate material from inspired air (Golde, 1976).

Macrophages also localize various inorganic materials within tissues. Beryllium, zirconium, and silica cause granulomatous tissue reactions, and silica is known to be highly toxic to macrophages. These substances may produce important clinical diseases.

Because of the macrophage's "housekeeping" role, it participates in several human disorders. For example, Gaucher's disease is due to a deficiency of the enzyme, glucocerebrosidase. Lipid-laden macrophages accumulate in spleen, bone marrow, and other organs because these enzyme-deficient cells cannot handle the large amount of cerebroside from ingested cell membranes. "Storage cells" morphologically similar to those seen in Gaucher's disease and Niemann–Pick disease can occur in a variety of hematologic disorders such as chronic myelocytic leukemia. They are thought to result from an overloading of the normal macrophage's digestive capacity because of the high turnover of hematopoietic elements.

## 9.7. Cooperative Functions in Immune Responses

Mononuclear phagocytes have a crucial role in both cell-mediated and humoral immunity (Mackaness, 1970; Unanue and Cerottini, 1970; Cline, 1975). They operate in the afferent limb of the immune response in antigen handling, and in the efferent limb as effector cells.

Monocytes and macrophages are the primary cells involved in processing certain antigens. They collect, catabolize, and eliminate certain potentially immunogenic materials and retain other immunogenic molecules. The mononuclear phagocytes then can selectively present antigen to immunocompetent lymphoid cells and can thereby regulate the initial immunologic response to antigen (Unanue and Cerottini, 1970). Ultimately, lymphoid cells are responsible for the specificity of this response.

Once antigen is taken up by macrophages, partial degradation occurs in phagolysosomes, and a small fraction may be retained in its native state and can be stored for long periods of time (Unanue and Cerottini, 1970). It is not known with certainty how the mononuclear phagocyte presents antigen or immune information to the lymphocyte, although RNA-associated antigen has been demonstrated. Close contact between the mononuclear phagocyte and lymphocyte is apparently important in the transfer of immunologic information (Lipsky and Rosenthal, 1975a).

Mononuclear phagocytes interact with lymphocytes in many ways (Cline, 1975; Dannenberg, 1975; David, 1975; Greineder and Rosenthal, 1975a,b; Wahl et al., 1975b). Some subclasses of lymphocytes show little response to certain categories of antigen or mitogen in the complete absence of macrophages. Consequently, mononuclear phagocytes are believed important for activation and blast transformation of these lymphocytes. Macrophages and subclasses of T lymphocytes must interact with certain types of antigen before a maximal B-lymphocyte response comprising proliferation and secretion of humoral antibody is expressed. Similarly, optimal T-lymphocyte proliferative response to mitogen and the generation of helper T cells require macrophage membrane interactions (Greineder and Rosenthal, 1975a,b; Erb and Feldmann, 1975). Macrophage–T-cell interaction requires cells that are genetically identical or very similar (Erb and Feldmann, 1975; Lipsky and Rosenthal, 1975b).

In the presence of an antigen such as PPD, T lymphocytes form clusters around macrophages, forming an "immunologic island" (Cline and Swett, 1968; Nielsen *et al.*, 1974).

Another aspect of the macrophage–lymphocyte interaction is that lymphocytes undergoing blast transformation release a variety of bioactive humoral substances (lymphokines) that affect macrophage function. They may also produce specific high-affinity antibodies (cytophilic antibodies) that can bind to, "arm," and direct the effector function of monocytes (Mitchell *et al.*, 1973; Pels and Den Otter, 1974). In short, it can be said that lymphoid cells may activate and direct macrophages and that macrophages may activate and direct lymphocytes.

## 9.8. Cell-Mediated Cytotoxicity and Antitumor Immunity

The role of monocytes and macrophages in the control of neoplasia and in tumor cell destruction is an area of great interest (Fink, 1977). The mononuclear phagocytes may act as effector ("killer") cells in various cytotoxic reactions. One form of specific cytotoxicity is referred to as antibody-dependent, cell-mediated cytotoxicity (ADCC). The ADCC mechanism depends on the coating of target cells with specific antibody and subsequent identification and destruction by effector cells. Although the "null" lymphocyte may be the most important effector cell in human peripheral blood (Brier *et al.*, 1975), mononuclear phagocytes, as well as granulocytes, can function in ADCC (Greenberg *et al.*, 1973; Holm and Hammarström, 1973; Gale and Zighelboim, 1975). Effector cell recognition of antibody-coated target cells depends on cell surface receptors for subclasses of IgG antibody.

Monocytes and macrophages also participate in specific cytotoxic reactions mediated by humoral antibody (cytophilic antibody) that attaches first to the effector cell. This high-affinity cytophilic antibody is an immunoglobulin produced by lymphocytes which binds to macrophages and directs its cytotoxic activity against a specific target (Mitchell *et al.*, 1973; Pels and Den Otter, 1974). This type of antitumor cell activity is specific, is mediated by humoral antibody, and is effective in initiating macrophage cytotoxicity against neoplastic cells. A third form of "specific" stimulation of macrophage tumoricidal mechanisms is mediated by a nonimmunoglobulin humoral factor derived from immune lymphocytes. This material is referred to as specific macrophage-activating factor (SMAF) and appears to act in a manner similar to cytophilic antibody (Pels and Den Otter, 1974; Evans *et al.*, 1972).

An observation of central importance regarding antitumor immunity was the finding that nonspecifically activated macrophages could also kill syngeneic tumor cells (Fink, 1977; Hibbs *et al.*, 1972; Evans, 1975). This phenomenon has been demonstrated both *in vitro* and *in vivo* (Fidler, 1974; Norsbury and Fidler, 1975). Surprisingly, the nonspecifically activated macrophages are capable of distinguishing normal from "neoplastic" or "transformed" target cells and show selective cytotoxicity against the malignant cells (Hibbs, 1974a,b; Piessens *et al.*, 1975; Meltzer *et al.*, 1975b; Droller and Remington, 1975). Human peripheral blood monocytes are also capable of killing neoplastic cells (Holtermann *et al.*, 1974). Nonspecific macrophage activation occurs with intracellular parasitosis, such as *Toxoplasma* or tuberculosis infection, and in response to certain other biological materials, such as phytohemagglutinin, endotoxin, pyran copolymer, and glucan (Fink, 1977). Nonspecific macrophage activation may be mediated by a variety of lymphocyte products (lymphokines), one of which is called macrophage-activating factor (MAF) (David, 1975; Fidler, 1975). Macrophage-activating factor is believed to be the same molecule as the migration-inhibition factor (MIF); i.e., it is the same lymphocyte product assayed by different experimental systems. This factor(s) is released by lymphocytes undergoing a blastogenic response to plant mitogens or to antigen (David, 1975). Macrophage-activating factor is thought to operate via a fucose-containing macrophage surface receptor mechanism (Remold, 1973), since activation can be blocked by L-fucose or fucosidase. A surface membrane esterase may also regulate the response to MAF (David, 1975).

A precise characterization of the activated macrophage is not currently available, but some of its properties are known (David, 1975). The activated cell has a large size, increased adhesiveness to glass, and increased spreading on glass. It has a greater number of lysosome particles than the unactivated cell, but certain of its enzyme activities are decreased whereas others are increased. Collagenase is released in large quantities from activated macrophages (Wahl *et al.*, 1975a). The activated cells have increased chemotactic activity, augmented microbicidal capacity, and enhanced cytotoxicity for syngeneic tumor cells. Table I lists some of the reported characteristics of the activated macrophage.

The mechanisms by which activated macrophages kill tumor cells are not well understood. Killing requires an intact cell membrane and energy production, but is independent of DNA, RNA, or protein synthesis. Cytotoxicity does not depend on phagocytosis; however, close cell–cell contact appears necessary. Transfer of lysosomal material may be important in the killing process (Hibbs, 1974a).

There is now a substantial literature dealing with the activated macro-

**Table I.**   Characteristics of the Activated Macrophage

Increased adherence and spreading on glass
Increased cell size
Increased ruffled membrane movement
Augmented microbicidal activity *(Listeria)*
More effective allogeneic cytotoxicity
Enhanced syngeneic tumor cell cytotoxicity
Increased glucose oxidation via hexose monophosphate shunt
Increased lactic dehydrogenase activity
Greater number of lysosomes
Release of collagenase
Augmented incorporation of glucosamine
Increased DNA synthesis
Increased chemotactic activity
Increased membrane adenylate cyclase
Decrease in lysosomal enzymes, acid phosphatase, cathepsin D, and $\beta$-glucuronidase

phage and its antitumor cell activity. Some of this work has been supported by studies of macrophages isolated directly from animal and human neoplasms (Eccles and Alexander, 1974; Evans, 1973; Wood and Gillespie, 1975). The number of macrophages present in tumor tissue has been inversely correlated with growth and metastatic potential. Macrophages recovered from experimental tumors also have been shown capable of cytotoxic reactions against the tumor cells of the neoplasm from which they were isolated.

Nonspecific mononuclear phagocyte activation *in vivo* may be of potential therapeutic importance. Many investigators believe that immunotherapy with BCG, *Corynebacterium parvum,* and other biologic materials is dependent on macrophage activation. Conversely, they believe monocyte–macrophage dysfunction may permit or facilitate tumor growth. For example, defects in monocyte chemotaxis have been reported in approximately 50% of patients with various types of cancer (Boetcher and Leonard, 1974). Recently, a humoral substance elaborated by tumor cells has been described which is said to interfere with monocyte chemotaxis (Snyderman and Pike, 1976).

## 9.9. Control of Granulopoiesis

Monocytes and macrophages may have a regulatory role in granulopoiesis related to their elaboration of a humoral "granulopoietin." The formation of granulocyte and monocyte colonies in semisolid gel culture is dependent on the presence of stimulating substances collectively called colony-stimulating activity (CSA) (Golde and Cline, 1974). Although there is considerable biochemical heterogeneity associated with this activity, the best characterized material is a glycoprotein having many of the properties of a hormone (Metcalf and Moore, 1971). In mouse systems there are a number of tissue sources of CSA (Sheridan and Stanley, 1971). In man, however, the main sources of CSA appear to be the circulating monocyte and tissue macrophage (Chervenick and LoBuglio, 1972; Golde and Cline, 1972; Golde et al., 1972). Because monocytes and granulocytes probably originate from a common stem cell, the production of stimulatory material may be viewed in terms of a positive humoral feedback system. Thus, monocytes and tissue macrophages may regulate the production of granulocytes as well as their own production (Golde and Cline, 1974). Monocyte CSA elaboration can be increased by endotoxin and certain nucleotides (Ruscetti and Chervenick, 1974). Endotoxin appears to have an important role in granulopoiesis and the production of CSA (Quesenberry et al., 1972; Golde and Cline, 1975).

The role of monocytes and macrophages in the regulation of granulopoiesis is uncertain and undoubtedly will become clearer when the physiologic importance of CSA is defined. At present, there is only indirect evidence that CSA is a physiologic regulator of granulopoiesis in vivo (Golde and Cline, 1974).

## 9.10. Mononuclear Phagocyte Dysfunction Syndromes

Relatively little is known about the dysfunction syndromes of monocytes and macrophages as compared to the well-cataloged disorders of granulocyte function (Cline and Golde, 1977). Defects in monocyte chemotaxis are reported in some patients with cancer (Boetcher and Leonard, 1974) and in patients and animals with the Chediak–Higashi syndrome (Gallin et al., 1975). Of particular clinical importance is the finding that monocyte accumulation in skin windows is markedly impaired by corticosteroids in man (Dale et al., 1974). Glucocorticoids may also reduce monocyte killing of certain bacteria and fungi (Rinehardt et al., 1975).

Monocytes from patients with chronic granulomatous disease (CGD) have defective bactericidal and fungicidal capacity (Lehrer, 1975). In the rare genetic deficiency of myeloperoxidase, the monocytes have defective fungicidal capacity, but macrophage killing is normal (Lehrer and Cline, 1969).

A defect in monocyte microbicidal function has been demonstrated in acute myelomonocytic leukemia and in some patients with lymphoma (Cline, 1973). Some viral infections may be associated with monocyte dysfunction (Kleinerman et al., 1975; Twomey et al., 1974), and a genetic deficiency of the second component of complement has been related to failure of monocyte complement synthesis (Einstein *et al.*, 1975).

Certain substances, such as silica, are toxic to mononuclear phagocytes (Allison *et al.*, 1968), but a clear description of silica-related human mononuclear phagocyte dysfunction syndromes is not available. Recently, an acquired defect of human alveolar macrophage function has been delineated in pulmonary alveolar proteinosis (Golde *et al.*, 1976). In this disease there is an extraordinary incidence of *Nocardia* and fungal infection. Macrophages retrieved by bronchopulmonary lavage from patients with alveolar proteinosis demonstrate impaired adherence to glass, decreased chemotaxis, and reduced fungal killing. The circulating monocytes in this disorder are normal. The defect in lung macrophage function is believed due to the ingestion of lipoproteinaceous material in the alveoli- and consequent depletion of lysosomes.

Many other diseases are thought to involve dysfunction of the mononuclear phagocytes. Situations in which there is failure to contain intracellular parasitosis, such as disseminated tuberculosis and disseminated fungal disease, may be due to monocyte–macrophage defects. Defects have also been postulated in Hodgkin's disease and lepromatous leprosy.

## 9.11. Malignant Mononuclear Phagocytes

Proliferative disorders of monocytes and macrophages have been difficult to categorize, and a cumbersome nomenclature has added to the confusion (Cline and Golde, 1973, 1977). Certain diseases associated with large accumulations of macrophages are clearly not neoplastic. Examples would include the "storage diseases" such as Gaucher's and Niemann–Pick disease in which the underlying disorder relates to the accumulation of complex lipid due to a specific enzyme deficiency (Brady, 1972). One form of sea-blue histiocytosis, a storage disease, results from a partial deficiency of sphingomyelinase (Golde *et al.*, 1975). Certain apparently nonmalignant diseases of unknown etiology are characterized by destructive accumulations of mononuclear phagocytes. A catalog of such diseases would encompass Wegener's granulomatosis, sarcoidosis, multicentric reticulohistiocytosis, Hand–Schüller–Christian disease, and eosinophilic granuloma of bone (Golde, 1975; Territo and Cline, 1977). The latter two disorders and Letterer–Siwe disease are often considered together under the title histiocytosis X, but there seems little reason for doing so (Lieberman *et al.*, 1969; Vogel and Vogel, 1972; Cline and Golde, 1973).

The acute monocytic and myelomonocytic leukemias are types of acute leukemia in which there is a proliferation of hematopoietic cells with sufficient differentiation to exhibit characteristics identifiable as belonging to cells of the mononuclear phagocyte line (Kass and Schnitzer, 1973). There may be a variable admixture of granulocytic elements in monocytic leukemia; historically the term "Naegli type" has been applied to the myelomonocytic leukemia, and "Schilling type" to the form in which there is a pure monocytic proliferation. Since it is likely that normal monocytes and granulocytes share a common progenitor, it is not surprising to find variability in the spectrum of differentiation in myelomonocytic leukemia (Metcalf and Moore, 1971; Brandt *et al.*, 1974). Acute monocytic leukemia cells exhibit morphologic and functional maturation ranging from blast cells to phagocytic cells with the characteristics of macrophages (Bainton, 1975; Schiffer *et al.*, 1975; Lichtman and Weed, 1972). The cells of acute monocytic leukemia usually contain the nonspecific esterase characteristic of monocytes and macrophages (Kass and Schnitzer, 1973). These cells adhere well to glass, may be highly phagocytic, and elaborate substantial quantities of colony-stimulating activity (Golde *et al.*, 1974). Clinically the disease is similar to acute granulocytic leukemia, but tissue infiltration is more common and there may be high levels of serum lysosome and marked lysozymuria.

A chronic form of myelomonocytic leukemia has been delineated that is characterized by anemia, peripheral monocytosis, and immature myelocytic cells in the bone marrow (Miescher and Faquet, 1974; Geary *et al.*, 1975). The clinical course is usually protracted and the role of chemotherapy is uncertain. Chronic erythromonocytic leukemia may be a variant of this disorder (Broun, 1969; Shaw *et al.*, 1973).

Histiocytic lymphoma or reticulum cell sarcoma has classically been considered as a neoplastic proliferation of mononuclear phagocytes. However, recent studies suggest that many of the previously described histiocytic lymphomas are in fact large cell ("immunoblast") lymphocytic malignancies (Lukes and Collins, 1974; Taylor, 1974). Nevertheless, histiocytic neoplasms of lymphoid organs do occur where the proliferating cells appear to be of the monocyte–macrophage line (Rappaport, 1966).

The malignant histiocytoses include Letterer–Siwe disease in children and histiocytic medullary reticulosis in adults (Cline and Golde, 1973; Golde, 1975). These disorders are fairly well-defined clinical entities characterized by the proliferation of moderately differentiated mononuclear cells in lymph nodes, bone marrow, and spleen. Erythrophagocytosis and thrombophagocytosis are common in histiocytic medullary reticulosis and may lead to severe peripheral cytopenias. Hemophagocytic reticulosis is a poorly understood but similar disorder seen in children (Fullerton *et al.*, 1975; Blennow *et al.*, 1974).

Hairy cell leukemia, or "leukemic reticuloendotheliosis," has been classified by some investigators as a monocytic disorder (King *et al.*, 1975; Jaffe *et al.*, 1974). Although in certain instances these "hairy cells" exhibit some of the attributes of mononuclear phagocytes, we believe the weight of evidence suggests that this syndrome usually is a lymphocytic malignancy of the B-cell type (Catovsky *et al.*, 1974; Haak *et al.*, 1974; Golde *et al.*, 1977, Katayama *et al.*, 1972).

## 9.12. Summary

The mononuclear phagocyte cell line has several morphologically defined cell types at different levels of maturation. Each of these has a characteristic composition, function, and metabolism. Mononuclear phagocytes interact with many other cells and in particular with lymphocytes. Disorders of mononuclear phagocyte function and differentiation have been identified.

## References

Ackerman, N. R., and Beebe, J. R., 1974, Release of lysosomal enzymes by alveolar mononuclear cells, *Nature (London)* **247**:475.

Allison, A. C., Harington, J. S., and Birbeck, M., 1968, An examination of the cytotoxic effects of silica on macrophages, *J. Exp. Med.* **124**:141.

Allison, A. C., Davies, P., and De Petris, S., 1971, Role of contractile microfilaments in macrophage movement and endocytosis, *Nature New Biol.* **232**:153.

Anderson, S. E., and Remington, J. S., 1974, Effect of normal and activated human macrophages on *Toxoplasma gondii*, *J. Exp. Med.* **139**:1154.

Arend, W. P., and Mannik, M., 1973, The macrophage receptor for IgG: Number and affinity of binding sites, *J. Immunol.* **110**:1455.

Bainton, D. F., 1975, Ultrastructure and cytochemistry of monocytic leukemia, *in Mononuclear Phagocytes in Immunity, Infection, and Pathology* (R. Van Furth, ed), pp. 83–93, Blackwell, Oxford.

Behin, R., Mauel, J., Biroum-Noerjasin, N., and Rowe, D. S., 1974, Mechanisms of protective immunity in experimental cutaneous leishmaniasis of the guinea pig. II. Selective destruction of different *Leishmania* species in activated guinea pig and mouse macrophages, *Clin. Exp. Immunol.* **20**:351.

Blennow, G., Berg, B., Brandt, L., Messeter, L., Löw, B., and Söderström, N., 1974, Haemophagocytic reticulosis. A state of chimerism? *Arch. Dis. Child.* **49**:960.

Boetcher, D. A., and Leonard, E. J., 1974, Abnormal monocyte chemotactic response in cancer patients, *J. Nat. Cancer Inst.* **52**:1091.

Boetcher, D. A., and Meltzer, M. S., 1975, Brief communication: Mouse mononuclear cell chemotaxis: Description of system, *J. Nat. Cancer Inst.* **54**:795.

Boumsell, L., and Meltzer, M. S., 1976, Mouse mononuclear cell chemotaxis. I. Differential response of monocytes and marcophages, *J. Immunol.* **115**:1746.

Bowden, D. H., Adamson, I. Y. R., Grantham, W. G., and Wyatt, J. P., 1969, Origin of the lung macrophage, *Arch. Pathol.* **88**;540.

Bradley, T. R., and Metcalf, D., 1966, The growth of mouse bone marrow cells *in vitro, Aust. J. Exp. Biol. Med. Sci.* **44**:287.

Brady, R. O., 1972, Biochemical and metabolic basis of familial sphingolipidoses, *Semin. Hematol.* **9**:273.

Brandt, L., Levan, G., Mitelman, F., Olsson, I., and Sjögren, U., 1974, Trisomy G-21 in adult myelomonocytic leukaemia. An abnormality common to granulocytic and monocytic cells, *Scand. J. Haematol.* **12**:117.

Brier, A. M., Chess, L., and Schlossman, S. F., 1975, Human antibody-dependent cellular cytotoxicity. Isolation and identification of a subpopulation of peripheral blood lymphocytes which kill antibody-coated autologous target cells, *J. Clin. Invest.* **56**:1580.

Broun, G. O., Jr., 1969, Chronic erythromonocytic leukemia, *Am. J. Med.* **47**:785.

Catovsky, D., Pettit, J. E., Galetto, J., Okos, A., and Galton, D., 1974, The B-lymphocyte nature of the hairy cell of leukaemic reticuloendotheliosis, *Br. J. Haematol.* **26**:29.

Chervenick, P. A., and LoBuglio, A. F., 1972, Human blood monocytes: Stimulators of granulocyte and mononuclear colony formation *in vitro, Science* **178**:164.

Cline, M. J., 1973, Defective mononuclear phagocyte function in patients with myelomonocytic leukemia and in some patients with lymphoma, *J. Clin. Invest.* **52**:2185.

Cline, M. J., 1975, *The White Cell,* Harvard University Press, Cambridge, Massachusetts.

Cline, M. J., and Golde, D. W., 1973, A review and reevaluation of the histiocytic disorders, *Am. J. Med.* **55**:49.

Cline, M. J., and Golde, D. W., 1977, Granulocytes and monocytes: Function and functional disorders, *in Recent Advances in Haematology* (A. V. Hoffbrand, ed.), Churchill Livingstone, London, in press.

Cline, M. J., and Lehrer, R. I., 1968, Phagocytosis by human monocytes, *Blood* **32**:423.

Cohen, A. B., and Cline, M. J., 1971, The human alveolar macrophage: Isolation, cultivation *in vitro,* and studies of morphologic and functional characteristics, *J. Clin. Invest.* **50**:1390.

Cohn, Z. A., 1968, The structure and function of monocytes and macrophages, *Adv. Immunol.* **9**:163.

Cohn, Z. A., and Benson, B. A., 1965a, The differentiation of mononuclear phagocytes: Morphology, cytochemistry, and biochemistry, *J. Exp. Med.* **121**:153.

Cohn, Z. A., and Benson, B. A., 1965b, The *in vitro* differentiation of mononuclear phagocytes. I. The influence of inhibitors and the results of autoradiography, *J. Exp. Med.* **121**:279.

Cohn, Z. A., Fedorko, M. D., and Hirsch, J. G., 1966, The *in vitro* differentiation of mononuclear phagocytes. V. The formation of macrophage lysosomes, *J. Exp. Med.* **123**:757.

Dale, D. C., Fauci, A. S., and Wolff, S. M., 1974, Alternate-day prednisone. Leukocyte kinetics and susceptibility to infections, *N. Engl. J. Med.* **291**:1154.

Dannenberg, A. M., 1975, Macrophages in inflammation and infection, *N. Engl. J. Med.* **293**:489.

David, J. R., 1975, Macrophage activation by lymphocyte mediators, *Fed. Proc.* **34**:1730.

Droller, M. J., and Remington, J. S., 1975, A role for the macrophage in *in vitro* and *in vitro* resistance to murine bladder tumor cell growth, *Cancer Res.* **35**:49.

Eccles, S. A., and Alexander, P., 1974, Macrophage content of tumours in relation to metastatic spread and host immune reaction, *Nature (London)* **250**:667.

Einstein, L. P., Alper, C. A., Bloch, K. J., Herrin, J. T., Rosen, F. S., David, J. R., and Colten, H. R., 1975, Biosynthetic defect in monocytes from human beings with genetic deficiency of the second component of complement, *N. Engl. J. Med.* **292**:1169.

Elsbach, P., 1967, Metabolism of lysophosphatidyl ethanolamine and lysophosphatidyl choline by homogenates of rabbit polymorphonuclear leukocytes and alveolar macrophages, *J. Lipid Res.* **8**:359.

Elsbach, P., 1968, Increased synthesis of phospholipid during phagocytosis, *J. Clin. Invest.* **47**:2217.

Epstein, L. B., Cline, M. J., and Merigan, T. C., 1971, The interaction of human macrophages and lymphocytes in the PHA-stimulated production of interferon, *J. Clin. Invest.* **50**:744.

Erb, P., and Feldmann, M., 1975, The role of macrophages in the generation of T-helper cells. II. The genetic control of the macrophage T-cell interaction for helper cell induction with soluble antigens, *J. Exp. Med.* **142**:460.

Evans, R., 1973, Macrophages and the tumour-bearing host, *Br. J. Cancer* **28**:19.

Evans, R., 1975, Macrophage cytotoxicity, in *Mononuclear Phagocytes in Immunity, Infection, and Pathology* (R. Van Furth, ed.), pp. 827–844, Blackwell, Oxford.

Evans, R., Grant, C. K., Cox, H., Steele, K., and Alexander, P., 1972, Thymus-derived lymphocytes produce an immunologically specific macrophage-arming factor, *J. Exp. Med.* **136**:1318.

Fidler, I. J., 1974, Inhibition of pulmonary metastasis by intravenous injection of specifically activated macrophages, *Cancer Res.* **34**:1074.

Fidler, I. J., 1975, Activation *in vitro* of mouse macrophages by syngeneic, allogeneic, or xenogeneic lymphocyte supernatants, *J. Nat. Cancer Inst.* **55**:1159.

Fink, M. A. (ed.), 1977, *The Macrophage in Neoplasia,* Academic Press, New York, in press.

Frei, J., Borel, C., Horvath, G., Cullity, B., and Vannotti, A., 1961, Enzymatic studies in the different types of normal and leukemic human white cells, *Blood* **18**:317.

Fullerton, P., Ekert, H., Hosking, C., and Tauro, G. P., 1975, Hemophagocytic reticulosis. A case report with investigations of immune and white cell function, *Cancer* **36**:441.

Gale, R. P., and Zighelboim, J., 1975, Polymorphonuclear leukocytes in antibody-dependent cellular cytotoxicity, *J. Immunol.* **114**:1047.

Gallin, J. I., Klimerman, J. A., Padgett, G. A., and Wolff, S. M., 1975, Defective mononuclear leukocyte chemotaxis in the Chediak–Higashi syndrome of humans, mink, and cattle, *Blood* **45**:863.

Geary, C. G., Catovsky, D., Wiltshaw, E., Milner, G. R., Scholes, M. C., Van Noorden, S., Wadsworth, L. D., Muldal, S., MacIver, J. E., and Galton, D. A. G., 1975, Chronic myelomonocytic leukaemia, *Br. J. Haematol.* **30**:289.

Gemsa, D., Woo, C. H., Fudenberg, H. H., and Schmid, R., 1973, Erythrocyte
    catabolism by macrophages *in vitro*. The effect of hydrocortisone on erythro-
    phagocytosis and on the induction of heme oxygenase, *J. Clin. Invest.*
    **52**:812.
Gemsa, D., Woo, C. H., Fudenberg, H. H., and Schmid, R., 1974, Stimulation of
    heme oxygenase in macrophages and liver by endotoxin, *J. Clin. Invest.*
    **53**:647.
Gemsa, D., Woo, C. H., Webb, D., Fudenberg, H. H., and Schmid, R., 1975,
    Erythrophagocytosis by macrophages: Suppression of heme oxygenase by
    cyclic AMP, *Cell. Immunol.* **15**:21.
Golde, D. W., 1975, Disorders of mononuclear phagocyte proliferation, matura-
    tion and function, *Clin. Haematol.* **4**:705.
Golde, D. W., 1976, Human pulmonary macrophages in disease and neoplasia, *in*
    *Role of Macrophages in Neoplasia (Wood's Hole Symposium)* (M. Fink, ed.), Aca-
    demic Press, New York.
Golde, D. W., and Cline, M. J., 1972, Identification of the colony-stimulating cell in
    human peripheral blood, *J. Clin. Invest.* **51**:2981.
Golde, D. W., and Cline, M. J., 1974, Regulation of granulopoiesis, *N. Engl. J. Med.*
    **291**:1388.
Golde, D. W., and Cline, M. J., 1975, Endotoxin-induced release of colony-
    stimulating activity in man, *Proc. Soc. Exp. Biol. Med.* **149**:845.
Golde, D. W., and Cline, M. J., 1977, Production, distribution, and fate of
    granulocytes, *in Hematology* (W. J. Williams, E. Beutler, A. J. Erslev, and R. W.
    Rundles, eds.), McGraw-Hill, New York, in press.
Golde, D. W., Finley, T. N., and Cline, M. J., 1972, Production of colony-
    stimulating factor by human macrophages, *Lancet* **ii**:1397.
Golde, D. W., Rothman, B., and Cline, M. J., 1974, Production of colony-stimulat-
    ing factor by malignant leukocytes, *Blood* **43**:749.
Golde, D. W., Schneider, E. L., Bainton, D. F., Penchev, P. G., Brady, R. O.,
    Epstein, C. J., and Cline, M. J., 1975, Pathogenesis of one variant of sea-blue
    histiocytosis, *Lab. Invest.* **33**:371.
Golde, D. W., Territo, M. C., Finley, T. N., and Cline, M. J., 1976, Defective lung
    macrophages in pulmonary alveolar proteinosis, *Ann. Intern. Med.* **85**:304.
Gordon, S., Todd, J., and Cohn, Z. A., 1974, *In vitro* synthesis and secretion of
    lysozyme by mononuclear phagocytes, *J. Exp. Med.* **139**:1228.
Goud, T. J. L. M., Chotte, C., and van Furth, R., 1975, Identification and
    characterization of the monoblast in mononuclear phagocyte colonies grown
    *in vitro, J. Exp. Med.* **142**:1180.
Greenberg, A. H., Shen, L., and Roitt, I. M., 1973, Characterization of the
    antibody-dependent cytotoxic cell. A nonphagocytic monocyte? *Clin. Exp.*
    *Immunol.* **15**:251.
Greineder, D. K., and Rosenthal, A. S., 1975a, Macrophage activation of alloge-
    neic lymphocyte proliferation in the guinea pig mixed leukocyte culture, *J.*
    *Immunol.* **114**:1541.
Greineder, D. K., and Rosenthal, A. S., 1975b, The requirement for macrophage–
    lymphocyte interaction in T-lymphocyte proliferation induced by generation
    of aldehydes on cell membranes, *J. Immunol.* **115**:932.
Haak, H. L., De Man, J. C. H., Hijmans, W., Knapp, W., and Speck, B., 1974,

Further evidence for the lymphocytic nature of leukaemic reticuloendotheliosis (hairy-cell leukaemia), *Br. J. Haematol.* **27**:31.

Hibbs, J. B., Jr., 1974a, Discrimination between neoplastic and nonneoplastic cells *in vitro* by activated macrophages, *J. Nat. Cancer Inst.* **53**:1487.

Hibbs, J. B., Jr., 1974b, Heterocytolysis by macrophages activated by bacillus Calmette–Guérin: Lysosome exocytosis into tumor cells, *Science* **184**:468.

Hibbs, J. B., Jr., Lambert, L. H., Jr., and Remington, J. S., 1972, Control carcinogenesis: A possible role for the activated macrophage, *Science* **177**:998.

Holm, G., and Hammarström, S., 1973, Haemolytic activity of human blood monocytes. Lysis of human erythrocytes treated with anti-A serum, *Clin. Exp. Immunol.* **13**:29.

Holtermann, O. A., Djerassi, I., Lisafeld, B. A., Elias, E. G., Papermaster, B. W., and Klein, E., 1974, *In vitro* destruction of tumor cells by human monocytes, *Proc. Soc. Exp. Biol. Med.* **147**:456.

Horwitz, D. A., 1972, The development of macrophages from large mononuclear cells in the blood of patients with inflammatory disease, *J. Clin. Invest.* **51**:760.

Horwitz, D. A., Stastny, P., and Ziff, M., 1970, Circulating deoxyribonucleic acid-synthesizing mononuclear leukocytes. I. Increased numbers of proliferating mononuclear leukocytes in inflammatory diseases, *J. Lab. Clin. Med.* **76**:891.

Hulse, E. V., 1959, The total white cell count of the blood as an indicator of acute radiation damage and its value during the first few hours after exposure, *J. Clin. Pathol.* **13**:37.

Ichikawa, Y., Pluznik, D. H., and Sachs, L., 1966, *In vitro* control of the development of macrophage and granulocyte colonies, *Proc. Nat. Acad. Sci. U.S.A.* **56**:488.

Jaffe, E. S., Shevach, E. M., Frank, M. M., and Green, I., 1974, Leukemic reticuloendotheliosis: Presence of a receptor for cytophilic antibody, *Am. J. Med.* **57**:108.

Jandl, J. H., and Tomlinson, A. S., 1958, The destruction of red cells by antibodies in man. II. Pyrogenic, leukocytic, and dermal response to immune hemolysis, *J. Clin. Invest.* **37**:1202.

Karnovsky, M. L., 1962, The physiological basis of phagocytosis, *Physiol. Rev.* **42**:143.

Kass, L., and Schnitzer, B., 1973, *Monocytes, Monocytosis and Monocytic Leukemia*, Charles C. Thomas, Springfield, Illinois.

Katayama, I., Li, C. Y., and Yam, L. T., 1972, Histochemical study of acid phosphatase isoenzyme in leukemic reticuloendotheliosis, *Cancer* **29**:157.

Kay, M. M. B., 1975, Mechanism of removal of senescent cells by human macrophages *in situ*, *Proc. Nat. Acad. Sci. U.S.A.* **72**:3521.

Killman, S.-A., Cronkite, E. P., Bond, V. P., and Fliedner, T. M., 1962, Proliferation of human leukemic cell studies with tritiated thymidine *in vivo*, in *Proceedings of the VIII Congress of the European Society of Hematology*, p. 63, Karger, Basel.

King, G. W., Hurtubise, P. E., Sagone, A. L., Jr., LoBuglio, A. F., and Metz, E. N., 1975, Leukemic reticuloendotheliosis. A study of the origin of the malignant cell, *Am. J. Med.* **59**:411.

Klebanoff, S. J., 1971, Intraleukocytic microbicidal defects. *Ann. Rev. Med.* **22**:39.

Kleinerman, E. S., Snyderman, R., and Daniels, C. A., 1975, Depressed monocyte chemotaxis during acute influenza infection, *Lancet* **ii**:1063.

Kostiala, A. A. I., and McGregor, D. D., 1975, The mediator of cellular immunity. IX. The relationship between cellular hypersensitivity and acquired cellular resistance in rats infected with *Listeria monocytogenes, J. Exp. Med.* **141**:1249.

Leder, L. D., 1967, The origin of blood monocytes and macrophages, *Blut* **16**:86.

Lehrer, R. I., 1975, The fungicidal mechanisms of human monocytes. I. Evidence for myeloperoxidase-linked and myeloperoxidase-independent candidacidal mechanisms, *J. Clin. Invest.* **55**:338.

Lehrer, R. I., and Cline, M. J., 1969, Leukocyte myeloperoxidase deficiency and disseminated candidiasis: The role of myeloperoxidase in resistance to Candida infection, *J. Clin. Invest.* **48**:1478.

Lichtman, M. A., and Weed, R. I., 1972, Peripheral cytoplasmic characteristics of leukocytes in monocytic leukemia: Relationship to clinical manifestations, *Blood* **40**:52.

Lieberman, P. H., Jones, C. R., Dargeon, H. W. K., and Begg, C. F., 1969, A reappraisal of eosinophilic granuloma of bone, Hand–Schüller–Christian syndrome and Letterer–Siwe syndrome, *Medicine* **48**:375.

Lipsky, P. E., and Rosenthal, A. S., 1975a, Macrophage–lymphocyte interaction. II. Antigen-mediated physical interactions between immune guinea pig lymph node lymphocytes and syngeneic macrophages, *J. Exp. Med.* **141**:138.

Lipsky, P. E., and Rosenthal, A. S., 1975b, Macrophage–lymphocyte interaction: Antigen-independent binding of guinea pig lymph node lymphocytes by macrophages, *J. Immunol.* **115**:440.

Lubaroff, D. M., and Waksman, B. H., 1968, Bone marrow as source of cells in reactions of cellular hypersensitivity. I. Passive transfer of tuberculin sensitivity in syngeneic systems, *J. Exp. Med.* **128**:1437.

Lukes, R. J., and Collins, R. D., 1974, Immunologic characterization of human malignant lymphomas, *Cancer* **34**:1488.

Mackaness, G. B., 1970, The monocyte in cellular immunity, *Semin. Hematol.* **7**:172.

Meltzer, M. S., Jones, E. E., and Boetcher, D. A., 1975a, Increased chemotactic responses of macrophages from BCG-infected mice, *Cell. Immunol.* **17**:268.

Meltzer, M. S., Tucker, R. W., Sanford, K. K., and Leonard, E. J., 1975b, Interaction of BCG-activated macrophages with neoplastic and nonneoplastic cell lines *in vitro:* Quantitation of the cytotoxic reaction by release of tritiated thymidine from prelabeled target cells, *J. Nat. Cancer Inst.* **54**:1177.

Metcalf, D., and Moore, M. A. S., 1971, Haemopoietic cells, in *Frontiers in Biology* (A. Neuberger and E. L. Tatum, eds.), pp. 468–478, North-Holland Publ., Amsterdam.

Meuret, G., 1974, Human monocytopoiesis, *Exp. Hematol.* **2**:238.

Meuret, G., and Fliedner, T. M., 1974, Neutrophil and monocyte kinetics in a case of cyclic neutropenia, *Blood* **43**:565.

Meuret, G., Bremer, C., Bammert, J., and Ewen, J., 1974a, Oscillation of blood monocyte counts in healthy individuals, *Cell Tissue Kinet.* **7**:223.

Meuret, G., Bammert, J., and Hoffmann, G., 1974b, Kinetics of human monocytopoiesis, *Blood* **44**:801.

Meuret, G., Batara, E., and Furste, H. O., 1975a, Monocytopoiesis in normal man:

Pool size, proliferation activity and DNA synthesis time of promonocytes, *Acta Haematol.* **54**:261.

Meuret, G., Detel, U., Kilz, H. P., Senn, H. J., and van Lessen, H., 1975b, Human monocytopoiesis in acute and chronic inflammation, *Acta Haematol.* **54**:328.

Miescher, P. A., and Farquet, J. J., 1974, Chronic myelomonocytic leukemia in adults, *Semin. Hematol.* **11**:129.

Mitchell, M. S., Mokyr, M. B., Aspnes, G. T., and McIntosh, S., 1973, Cytophilic antibodies in man, *Ann. Intern. Med.* **79**:333.

Nichols, B. A., and Bainton, D. F., 1973, Differentiation of human monocytes in bone marrow and blood. Sequential formation of two granule populations, *Lab. Invest.* **29**:27.

Nichols, B. A., Bainton, D. F., and Farquhar, M. G., 1971, Differentiation of monocytes. Origin, nature and fate of their azurophil granules, *J. Cell Biol.* **50**:498.

Nielsen, M. H., Jensen, H., Braendstrup, O., and Werdelin, O., 1974, Macrophage–lymphocyte clusters in the immune response to soluble protein antigen *in vitro*. II. Ultrastructure of clusters formed during the early response, *J. Exp. Med.* **140**:1260.

Norbury, K. C., and Fidler, I. J., 1975, *In vitro* tumor cell destruction by syngeneic mouse macrophages: Methods for assaying cytotoxicity, *J. Immunol. Methods* **7**:109.

Oren, R., Franham, A. E., Saito, K., Milofsky, E., and Karnovsky, M. L., 1963, Metabolic patterns in three types of phagocytizing cells, *J. Cell Biol.* **17**:487.

Osgood, E. E., Tive , H., Davison, K. V., Seaman, A. J., and Li, J. G., 1952, The relative rates of formation of new leukocytes in patients with acute and chronic leukemias. Measured by the uptake of radioactive phosphorus in the isolated desoxyribosenucleic acid, *Cancer* **5**:331.

Pels, E., and Den Otter, W., 1974, The role of a cytophilic factor from challenged immune peritoneal lymphocytes in specific macrophage cytotoxicity, *Cancer Res.* **34**:3089.

Piessens, W. F., Churchill, W. H., Jr., and David, J. R., 1975, Macrophages activated *in vitro* with lymphocyte mediators kill neoplastic but not normal cells, *J. Immunol.* **114**:293.

Quesenberry, P., Morley, A., Stohlman, F., Jr., Rickard, K., Howard, D., and Smith, M., 1972, Effect of endotoxin on granulopoiesis and colony-stimulating factor, *N. Engl. J. Med.* **286**:227.

Rabinovitch, M., Manejias, R. E., and Nussenzweig, V., 1975, Selective phagocytic paralysis induced by immobilized immune complexes, *J. Exp. Med.* **142**:827.

Rappaport, H., 1966, Tumors of the hematopoietic system, *Atlas of Tumor Pathology*, Sec. III, Fasc. 8, Washington, D.C., Armed Forces Institute of Pathology.

Remington, J. S., Krahenbuhl, J. L., and Mendenhall, J. W., 1972, A role for activated macrophages in resistance to infection with *Toxoplasma*, *Infect. Immunol.* **6**:829.

Remold, H. G., 1973, Requirement for α-L-fucose on the macrophage membrane receptor for MIF, *J. Exp. Med.* **138**:1065.

Rinehart, J. J., Sagone, A. L., Balcerzak, S. P., Ackerman, G. A., and LoBuglio, A. F., 1975, Effects of corticosteroid therapy on human monocyte function, *N. Engl. J. Med.* **292**:236.

Rosse, W. F., de Boisfleury, A., and Bessis, M., 1975, The interaction of phagocytic cells and red cells modified by immune reactions. Comparison of antibody and complement-coated red cells, *Blood Cells* **1**:345.

Ruscetti, F. W., and Chervenick, P. A., 1974, Release of colony-stimulating factor from monocytes by endotoxin and polyinosinic-polycytidylic acid, *J. Lab. Clin. Med.* **83**:64.

Schiffer, C. A., Sanel, F. T., Stechmiller, B. K., and Wiernik, P. H., 1975, Functional and morphologic characteristics of the leukemic cells of a patient with acute monocytic leukemia: Correlation with clinical features, *Blood* **46**:17.

Schmalzl, F., Huber, H., Asamer, H., Abbrederis, K., and Braunsteiner, H., 1969, Cytochemical and immunohistologic investigations on the source and the functional changes of mononuclear cells in skin window exudates, *Blood* **34**:129.

Shaw, M. T., Bottomley, S. S., Bottomley, R. H., and Hussein, K. K., 1973, The relationship of erythromonocytic leukemia to other myeloproliferative disorders, *Am. J. Med.* **55**:542.

Sheridan, J. W., and Stanley, E. R., 1971, Tissue sources of bone marrow colony stimulating factor, *J. Cell. Physiol.* **78**:451.

Silverstein, S. C., 1975, The role of mononuclear phagocytes in viral immunity, *in Mononuclear Phagocytes in Immunity, Infection, and Pathology* (R. Van Furth, ed.), Chap. 36, Blackwell, Oxford.

Snyderman, R., and Pike, M. C., 1976, An inhibitor of macrophage chemotaxis produced by neoplasms, *Science* **192**:370.

Snyderman, R., Shin, H. S., and Hausman, M. S., 1971, Chemotactic factor of mononuclear leukocytes, *Proc. Soc. Exp. Biol. Med.* **138**:387.

Spector, W. G., and Willoughby, D. A., 1968, The origin of mononuclear cells in chronic inflammation and tuberculin reactions in the rat, *J. Pathol. Bacteriol.* **96**:389.

Stecher, V. J., and Thorbecke, G. J., 1967, Sites of synthesis of serum proteins: I. Serum proteins produced by macrophages *in vitro*, *J. Immunol.* **99**:643.

Stossel, T. P., and Hartwig, J. H., 1975, Interactions between actin, myosin, and an actin-binding protein from rabbit alveolar macrophages, *J. Biol. Chem.* **250**:5706.

Stott, E. J., Probert, M., and Thomas, L. H., 1975, Cytotoxicity of alveolar macrophages for virus-infected cells, *Nature (London)* **255**:710.

Taylor, C. R., 1974, The nature of Reed–Sternberg cells and other malignant "reticulum" cells, *Lancet* **ii**:802.

Territo, M. C., and Cline, M. J., 1975, Mononuclear phagocyte proliferation, maturation and function, *Clin. Haematol.* **4**:685.

Territo, M. C., and Cline, M. J., 1976, Macrophages and their disorders in man, *in Immunobiology of the Macrophage* (D. S. Nelson, ed.), p. 594, Academic Press, New York.

Thompson, J., and Van Furth, R., 1973, The effect of glucocorticosteroids on the proliferation and kinetics of promonocytes and monocytes of the bone marrow, *J. Exp. Med.* **137**:10.

Twomey, J. J., Gyorkey, F., and Norris, S. M., 1974, The monocyte disorder with herpes zoster, *J. Lab. Clin. Med.* **83**:768.

Unanue, E. R., and Cerottini, J. C., 1970, The function of macrophages in the immune response, *Semin, Hematol.* **7**:225.

van Furth, R., Hirsch, J. G., and Fedorko, M. E., 1970, Morphology and peroxidase cytochemistry of mouse promonocyte, monocyte, and macrophages, *J. Exp. Med.* **132**:794.

van Furth, R., Cohn, Z. A., Hirsch, J. G., Humphrey, J. H., Spector, W. G., and Langevoort, H. L., 1972, The mononuclear phagocyte system: A new classification of macrophages, monocytes, and their precursor cells, *Bull. WHO* **46**:845.

Virolainen, M., 1968, Hematopoietic origin of macrophages as studied by chromosome markets in mice, *J. Exp. Med.* **127**:943.

Vogel, J. M., and Vogel, P., 1972, Idiopathic histiocytosis: A discussion of eosinophilic granuloma, the Hand–Schüller–Christian syndrome, and the Letterer–Siwe syndrome, *Semin. Hematol.* **9**:349.

Volkman, A., and Collins, F. M., 1968, Recovery of delayed-type hypersensitivity in mice following suppressive doses of X-radiation, *J. Immunol.* **101**:846.

Wahl, L. M., Wahl, S. M., Mergenhagen, S. E., and Martin, G. R., 1975a, Collagenase production by lymphokine-activated macrophages, *Science* **24**:261.

Wahl, S. M., Wilton, J. M., Rosenstreich, D. L., and Oppenheim, J. J., 1975b, The role of macrophages in the production of lymphokines by T and B lymphocytes, *J. Immunol.* **114**:1296.

Weiden, P. L., Storb, R., and Tsoi, M., 1975, Marrow origin of canine alveolar macrophages, *J. Reticuloendothel. Soc.* **17**:342.

Werb, Z., and Cohn, Z. A., 1971, Cholesterol metabolism in the macrophage. I. The regulation of cholesterol exchange, *J. Exp. Med.* **134**:1545.

Werb, Z., and Gordon, S., 1975, Elastase secretion by stimulated macrophages. Characterization and regulation, *J. Exp. Med.* **142**:361.

West, J., Morton, D. J., Esmann, V., and Stjernholm, R. L., 1968, Carbohydrate metabolism in leukocytes. VIII. Metabolic activities of the macrophage, *Arch. Biochem. Biophys.* **124**:85.

Widmann, J.-J., and Fahimi, H. D., 1975, Proliferation of mononuclear phagocytes (Kupffer cells) and endothelial cells in regenerating rat liver, *Am. J. Pathol.* **80**:349.

Wood, G. W., and Gillespie, G. Y., 1975, Studies on the role of macrophages in regulation of growth and metastasis of murine chemically induced fibrosarcomas, *Int. J. Cancer* **16**:1022.

# The Production of Immunoglobulins by Mouse Myeloma Cells

## W. Cieplinski and M. D. Scharff

## 10.1. Introduction

When a foreign substance is introduced into the body, the organism responds by synthesizing relatively large amounts of immunoglobulins which will react specifically with the immunogen. Originally, this was thought to involve a relatively straightforward series of events in which antigens were processed by phagocytic cells, plasma cell precursors representing selected clones were activated by specific antigens, and then cell proliferation and differentiation led to the production of specific antibodies. However, within this model it was not clear how recognition of self, tolerance, and the availability of precursor cells ready to make every possible antibody was achieved. Although these and other difficult questions have still not been resolved, it has become clear that between the initial introduction of antigen and the activation of the plasma cell to produce antibodies, the body carries out a highly complex series of events involving a multiplicity of signals mediated through soluble factors and the direct and indirect interactions of multiple cell types. Subpopulations of thymus (T) derived and bone marrow (or in the bird, bursa of Fabricius) (B) derived lymphocytes interact with macrophages and with each

W. CIEPLINSKI and M. D. SCHARFF • Department of Cell Biology, Albert Einstein College of Medicine, Bronx, New York 10461.

other to produce negative (suppressive) or positive (collaborative) responses. Genes are activated. Some cells are stimulated to replicate and differentiate whereas others are prevented from responding. All this requires what Jerne (1974) has called a "network of information" and is so complex that the details are only just beginning to be discussed.

On the other hand, significant progress has been made in understanding the biochemical and molecular events which constitute the final steps in the process and lead to the synthesis and secretion of large amounts of antibody by the plasma cell. These insights have in large part resulted from the realization that the neoplasm, multiple myeloma, represents the amplification of a single clone of antibody-forming cells all making large amounts of a single homogenous immunoglobulin or antibody. Many myeloma tumors representing most of the classes and subclasses of immunoglobulin have been induced in mice. These tumors can be adapted to grow continuously in culture, cloned, and studied both genetically and biochemically. Such studies have provided a rather detailed description of the synthesis, assembly, and secretion of immunoglobulins, and there have been extensive reviews (Potter, 1972; Franklin and Frangione, 1975) of this subject. In this chapter, we will therefore concentrate on the information obtained in several laboratories, including our own, on the production of immunoglobulin by mouse myeloma cells and discuss the potential implications of these findings to the understanding of multiple myeloma in man.

## 10.2. Plasma Cell Tumors and Cell Lines

As Potter (1967) has described in detail in his definitive review on mouse myelomas, spontaneous plasmacytomas are relatively rare in this species. However, this became a useful experimental system when Merwin and Algire (1959) found that myelomas could be consistently induced by implanting Millipore chambers in the peritoneal cavity. Subsequently, other irritants such as Lucite disks and various mineral oils which produce an inflammatory response and granulomas within the peritoneal cavity were also found to be effective (Lieberman et al., 1961; Potter and Boyce, 1962; Merwin and Redman, 1963). Subsequent studies showed that susceptibility to plasmacytomas is genetically controlled and that only BALB/c and NZB inbred mouse strains are readily susceptible. Humoral factors also play a role since the frequency of tumors is higher in males or testosterone-treated females than in normal females (Takakura et al., 1967; Hollander et al., 1968). A variety of viruses have been found associated with mouse myeloma tumors. However, Potter and his colleagues (1973) have recently shown that the Abelson murine leukemia virus can induce murine plasmacytomas.

One of the crucial benefits of mouse myelomas as an experimental system is that they can be readily transplanted from one animal to another and thus provide a continuous and virtually unlimited source of a particular homogeneous immunoglobulin and of the cells producing that particular myeloma protein. The tumor cells can also be frozen away and, when needed, defrosted and reinjected into recipient animals. All these characteristics have allowed investigators to obtain important information on the structure of immunoglobulins (Weigert *et al.*, 1970; McKean *et al.*, 1972; Hood *et al.*, 1975), the kinetics of malignant cell proliferation, the induction of malignancy, and the effect of chemotherapeutic agents (Potter, 1972; Bergsagel *et al.*, 1975).

The ability to conduct biochemical experiments has been greatly facilitated by the adaptation of mouse myeloma cells to suspension cell culture. This was accomplished by dissociating tumors into a single cell suspension and then growing the cells in tissue culture medium (Pottengill and Sorensen, 1967; Horibata and Harris, 1970; Laskov and Scharff, 1970). In most cases, the cells began to die after a short time in culture, but could ultimately be adapted to continuous culture by repeated passage between animals and tissue culture (Laskov and Scharff, 1970). Once fully adapted to culture, most of the cell lines are easy to maintain *in vitro*, divide every 14–24 hr, continue to synthesize and secrete large amounts of the same immunoglobulin as the parent tumor, can be reinjected in mice to form tumors, and can be stored in the frozen state.

Cell lines producing all the major classes and subclasses of mouse immunoglobulin are now available. In order to study these cells using genetic tools similar to those which have been so useful in studying microorganisms, it was necessary to clone the cultured mouse myeloma cells so as to look for cells which had undergone mutations at various steps in the synthesis, assembly, glycosylation, and secretion of immunoglobulin. One very useful approach was described by Coffino *et al.* (1972) who showed that the myeloma cells could be cloned in soft agar with a high efficiency.

Variant or mutant clones were identified by overlaying the clones while they were still small with agar containing antiserum directed against one or both of the immunoglobulin polypeptide chains. For example, if antibody directed against a particular heavy chain was used, parental clones synthesizing and secreting molecules containing heavy chains were surrounded and obscured by an immunologic precipitate. Clones not surrounded by precipitate had either lost the ability to synthesize heavy chains, were blocked in the assembly and secretion of the heavy chains, or were secreting heavy chains that had lost the antigenic determinants recognized by the particular antiserum used. Presumptive mutants can be recovered from the agar, grown to mass culture, and characterized in detail using a variety of biochemical, serological, and genetic techniques.

## 10.3. Types and Frequency of Spontaneous Variants

When cell lines producing the $IgG_{2b}$, $IgG_{2a}$, and $IgG_1$ subclasses and the IgA class of mouse immunoglobulin were examined for clones which differed from the parental heavy- plus light-chain-producing cells, as many as 1–10% of the clones were unstained in the immunoplate assay just described. Even if freshly isolated subclones were studied, 0.5–1% of the clones were not surrounded by an immunologic precipitate. This very high frequency of variants was surprising since it suggested a "mutation rate" much higher than the $10^{-5}$ to $10^{-8}$ per cell per generation which has been observed for most mutations in both animal and bacterial cells. In order to confirm this, Coffino and Scharff (1971) and Baumal et al. (1973) used fluctuation analysis to determine the actual mutation rates in a number of different mouse meyloma cell lines. $IgG_{2b}$ (MPC-11) and $IgG_1$ ($P_3$) producing cells spontaneously lost the ability to produce heavy chains at a rate of $10^{-3}$ per cell per generation. Variants also arose at a high frequency in mouse myeloma tumors (Potter and Kuff, 1964; Baumal and Scharff, 1976) so this seems to be a characteristic of mouse myeloma cells, not just of cells in continuous culture. Nor is this due to an overall genetic instability in these cells, since mutant myeloma cells resistant to 5-bromo-2'-deoxyuridine and 6-thioguanine as well as to four other drugs arise at a frequency of $10^{-6}$ to $10^{-8}$ per cell per generation.

When spontaneously occurring unstained clones were recovered from the agar, recloned, grown to mass culture, and studied in detail, the missing immunoglobulin polypeptide chain could not be detected by a variety of sensitive immunological and biochemical techniques. Antisera made against both native and denatured immunoglobulin molecules were used so that they would react with hidden or abnormal antigenic determinants and thus increase the chance of detecting mutant proteins or fragments. In a few cases, variants which have lost the ability to produce one or both chains have been examined for the respective messenger RNA by in vitro translation in heterologous cell-free systems or by nucleic acid hybridization. Most of the cases lack detectable messenger RNA (Cowan et al., 1974; Kuehl et al., 1975; Green et al., 1975). However, Cowan et al. (1974) have reported one instance in which the messenger is present but defective.

It appears that most of the spontaneously occurring variants have lost the ability to synthesize one or both immunoglobulin polypeptide chains. At this time it is not known whether the variants have lost a structural or regulatory gene or have a defect in the transcription or nuclear processing of messenger RNA. Because of our uncertainty about the genetic basis or molecular mechanism involved, we have called these "variants" rather than "mutants."

Whatever their origins, it is clear that light-chain-producing ($H^-L^+$ phenotype), heavy-chain-producing ($H^+L^-$) (Morrison and Scharff, 1975), and nonproducing ($H^-L^-$) variants arise spontaneously at a high frequency in mouse myeloma cells. Similar abnormalities are seen in the human multiple myeloma where approximately 20% of cases produce only L chains (Bence-Jones myeloma) and approximately 1% of the cases do not have paraprotein in their serum or urine (Osserman and Takatsuki, 1964). It is important to note that, with one possible exception (Lyons et al., 1975), we are not aware of any cases in which a patient's cells have been shown to be synthesizing intact apparently normal heavy chains in the absence of light chains ($H^+L^-$). Similarly, in some mouse myeloma cell lines such variants have never been seen (Baumal et al., 1973), whereas in others such as $P_3$ and MOPC-315 such variants do arise (Morrison and Scharff, 1975; Bailey et al., 1973). We suspect that when large amounts of heavy chains are produced alone, they become insoluble, accumulate intracellularly, and decrease cell viability. When $P_3$ heavy chain producers were isolated, initially they produced similar amounts of heavy chains as their parent but the culture quickly converted to a mixture of nonproducers and cells that were making approximately one-tenth the amount of heavy chains as the parent. These heavy chain producers could then be cloned out and maintained as stable cultures producing very small amounts of heavy chains (Morrison and Scharff, 1975). This suggests that even $P_3$ heavy-chain producers survive only if they can in some way "modulate" heavy-chain production.

The most interesting types of immunoglobulin variants observed in human disease states are those which produce fragments of heavy chains. Because of their structural characteristics, these heavy-chain variants have led Franklin and Frangione (1975) and others to interesting suggestions about the possible structure and organization of the immunoglobulin genes. Potter and his colleagues have observed similarly deleted heavy chains in a few mouse myeloma tumors (Potter and Kuff, 1964) and more recent structural characterization of some of these (Robinson et al., 1974; Mushinski, 1971) reveals deletions similar to those reported for some human proteins. Similar deletion mutants have been reported by Milstein and his colleagues (Milstein et al., 1975; Cotton et al., 1973) to arise spontaneously from the $P_3$ cell line at a frequency of 3 in 7000 clones screened. They have characterized not only the mutant proteins but also the messenger RNAs from which the mutant proteins are translated. Since Milstein and his colleagues have shown that one of these mutants is an internal deletion whereas another is a premature termination due to the mutation of a codon to UAA which is an ocher termination codon in bacteria, these studies provide support for similar genetic mechanisms in prokaryotes and higher organisms.

## 10.4. Effect of Mutagenizing Agents on Mouse Myeloma Cells

Whereas we have also isolated spontaneous mutants which synthesize heavy chains that differ serologically and chemically from the parental chains (H*L$^+$ phenotype), their frequency is much lower than light-chain-producing (H$^-$L$^+$), heavy-chain-producing (H$^+$L$^-$), and nonproducing (H$^-$L$^-$) variants. In order to obtain more primary sequence mutants and to obtain some insight into their genetic basis, we have exposed mouse meyloma cells to a variety of mutagenizing agents (Baumal *et al.*, 1973). Agents such as nitrosoguanidine and ethyl methane sulfonate, which are usually very effective mutagens in both prokaryotes and animal cells, did not increase the frequency of mutants or variants more than two- to threefold above the already high spontaneous level. In contrast, ICR-191, an acridine half-mustard which causes frameshift mutations in microorganisms, was a very effective mutagen, increasing the frequency of variants 20-fold. At high doses of ICR-191, as many as 6% of the surviving clones differed from the parental cells (Table I). Hobbs (1971) has suggested that

**Table I.** Effect of Mutagens on the Loss of Heavy-Chain Production

| Agent | Mutagen ($\mu$g/ml) | Percent cell survival | Incidence of variants | Percent | $P$ |
|---|---|---|---|---|---|
| ICR 191 | 0 | 100 | 18/2104 | 0.86 | — |
| | 1 | 60 | 56/3635 | 1.54 | 0.016 |
| | 2 | 25 | 110/3404 | 3.24 | <0.001 |
| | 4 | <1 | 15/229 | 6.55 | <0.001 |
| Melphalan | 0 | 100 | 17/3777 | 0.45 | — |
| | 0.2 | 32 | 31/2336 | 1.33 | <0.001 |
| | 0.6 | 16 | 55/2961 | 1.86 | <0.001 |
| | 0.8 | 9 | 31/1298 | 2.39 | <0.001 |

Cells were grown in the presence of various doses of each mutagen for 24 hr, then grown in the absence of the mutagen for an additional 24 hr. The cells were then cloned in soft agar and overlayered with antibody against heavy chains; the total number of clones and percentage of unstained clones were determined: $P$ represents the statistical significance of results determined by the $\chi^2$ test.

melphalan (Alkeran) induces changes in immunoglobulin production by human myeloma cells. We found that melphalan was also an effective mutagen of mouse meyloma cells (Table I) (Preud'homme *et al.*, 1973). Most importantly, almost half the variants induced by both ICR-191 and melphalan were synthesizing heavy chains which differed from the parental chain both serologically and chemically (Birshtein *et al.*, 1974; Preud'homme *et al.*, 1975). These fit the usual criteria of true mutants in that they are stable, are induced by mutagens, and are producing defective gene products. These mutant heavy chains either contained deletions in the C-terminal part of the molecule or appeared to contain the genetic information from two constant region genes probably as the result of recombination or some related process. Some of these heavy-chain mutants had defects in assembly, glycosylation, and secretion and are discussed below.

## 10.5. Relationship to Human Heavy-Chain Disease

Franklin and Frangione (1975) have recently reviewed the types of heavy chain fragments that are sometimes synthesized in lymphoproliferative diseases and in myelomas. Many of the mutagen-induced and spontaneous deletions observed *in vitro* in mouse myelomas closely resemble those which have been described in human heavy-chain disease. One major difference is that all the mutant mouse cells continue to synthesize light chains whereas in some cases of human disease only H-chain fragments are synthesized. However, Dr. Sherrie Morrison (personal communication) has recently shown that if one starts with a mutant with an internal deletion in the heavy chain, one can readily generate secondary variants which have lost the ability to synthesize light chains but continue to synthesize and secrete the heavy-chain fragment. This at least shows that it is possible to obtain abnormalities in immunoglobulin production in mouse myeloma cells which are similar to those observed in humans.

## 10.6. Regulation of Immunoglobulin Synthesis, Assembly, and Secretion

The mouse plasmacytomas have also been used to study some of the more unusual aspects of the genetic control of immunoglobulin synthesis. For example, it is not known whether the generation of antibody diversity has occurred through evolution and is based on a large number of germ line genes or if it is based on changes in the DNA which are generated during the development and differentiation of somatic cells (Williamson, 1976). Secondly, structural studies of myeloma proteins (Hood *et al.*, 1975) and the classical genetic studies summarized by Williamson (1976) have provided indirect evidence that there are many more variable than constant region genes and that each immunoglobulin heavy (and light) chain is the product of at least two different genes (Hood *et al.*, 1975). However, it is still not clear exactly how or when the information from the variable and constant region genes is joined to form a single messenger RNA. Finally, we do not know how each immunoglobulin-producing cell expresses only one of the two alleles it contains for each immunoglobulin class or subclass (Cebra, 1969).

Genetic studies indicate that constant region genes that code for the heavy-chain classes and subclasses are closely linked to the heavy-chain variable region genes. Similarly, the constant and variable region genes that code for λ light chains (or for κ light chains) are closely linked. However, the heavy chain, κ light chain, and λ light chain genes are not linked to each other. The three linkage groups are schematically presented in Fig. 1. Genetic studies also suggest that there is a single constant region gene for each subclass and class of immunoglobulin (Williamson, 1976). Nucleic acid hybridization has confirmed that there is no more than a very few copies of each constant region per haploid genome in the plasma cell (Leder *et al.*, 1975; Bernardini and Tonegawa, 1974). All these findings have led to the suggestion that one of the many available variable region genes is "translocated" to a constant region gene and that the joining of variable and constant region gene results in the expression of that particular heavy or light chain. Recently, using nucleic acid hybridization, Tonegawa *et al.* (1976) have obtained evidence that suggests that the variable and constant region genes are separate in the germ cell and in nonimmunoglobulin-producing cells but are closely associated in the differentiated myeloma cell. A variety of molecular mechanisms have been proposed for these changes in DNA structure, but it is not known which, if any, of these mechanisms is correct.

Whatever the molecular mechanism, the evidence currently available

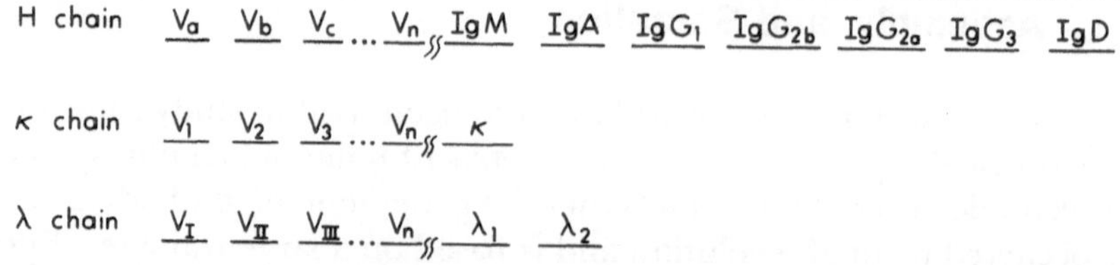

**Fig. 1.** Schematic representation of the organization of the immunoglobulin genes.

suggests that initially the variable and constant region genes are genetically linked but not contiguous. During embryogenesis or differentiation of the immune system, it is thought that different combinations of variable (V) and constant (C) regions are joined and the synthesis of small amounts of a given immunoglobulin begins. This immunoglobulin, probably IgM, serves as a surface receptor and when it interacts with a specific antigen, the precursor cell undergoes replication and differentiation to form a mature plasma cell which has switched from making IgM to IgG (Cooper et al., 1976; Ander et al., 1976). The mature plasma cell synthesizes approximately one million heavy chains per cell each minute and slightly more light chains, has a large amount of well-organized endoplasmic reticulum, and a large Golgi apparatus.

In order to examine the genetic mechanisms involved in these processes, a variety of hybrids have been formed between nonimmunoglobulin- and immunoglobulin-producing cells (Periman, 1970; Coffino et al., 1971) and between immunoglobulin-producing cells from the same and different species (Margulies et al., 1976b). The hybrids between fibroblasts and immunoglobulin-producing cells either have lost the ability to produce immunoglobulin or in one case produce very small amounts of antibody. This would suggest that one or more of the traits needed for immunoglobulin production is repressed, but as Davis and Adelberg (1973) have emphasized, such a conclusion can be made with assurance only if reexpression can be achieved. If not, extinction may be due merely to gene loss or other more complex mechanisms. Furthermore, the studies of numerous intraspecific or interspecific hybrids between immunoglobulin-producing cells suggest that the expression of particular heavy and light chain genes is under "cis-dominant" control: i.e., expression does not require soluble activators or repressors that are synthesized on one chromosome and act on another.

In two recent detailed studies with mouse myeloma cells making different classes and subclasses of immunoglobulins, Kohler and Milstein (1975) and Margulies et al. (1976a) have shown that not only are both parental immunoglobulins produced, but that the hybrids do not express classes or subclasses other than those made by the parents. They were also unable to detect any immunoglobulin polypeptide chains with a different isoelectric focusing pattern than those of the parental heavy and light chain. This means that there is not significant reassortment of the variable and constant regions of the parental chains, again suggesting that the joining of constant and variable region information occurs in the nucleus.

The continued synthesis of the parental immunoglobulin and the lack of synthesis of new chains both suggest that soluble repressors or activators are not involved in the regulation of immunoglobulin synthesis. This is perhaps most easily understood by considering the fusion of an

IgM-producing myeloma (Margulies *et al.*, 1976a) or normal plasma cell (Kohler and Milstein, 1975) with an IgG$_1$-producing myeloma. The resulting hybrid is of particular interest because, as already mentioned, many investigators believe that the normal antibody-forming cell switches from IgM to IgG production during antigen-induced differentiation. The hybrids continue to produce both IgM and IgG$_1$. No IgA, IgG$_{2a}$, or IgG$_{2b}$ is synthesized in detectable amounts. If the normal IgM to IgG switch was caused by the production of activator of IgG$_1$, then this activator should be present in the IgG producer and might be expected to turn on an additional IgG heavy chain in the IgM producer. If the disappearance of IgM production which appears to occur in normal cells during differentiation was due to the production of a trans-acting soluble repressor of IgM, then the synthesis of IgM might be expected to be repressed in the hybrid. Although there are alternatives, cis-dominant control provides the simplest explanation for the continued synthesis of only the parental IgM and IgG$_1$ in the hybrid. The IgM to IgG switch in normal cells could be achieved by translocation of the variable region from the IgM to IgG constant region, but whether this is true or how it is accomplished is still not known.

The coordinated amplification of heavy and light chain expression presents another interesting problem in regulation. As already mentioned, the heavy and light chain genes are not linked and are presumed to be on different chromosomes. Since there does not appear to be any amplification of the immunoglobulin genes (Bernardini and Tonegawa, 1974; Leder *et al.*, 1975) and the immunoglobulin messenger is translated at approximately the same rate as other cell proteins (Scharff and Laskov, 1970), the relatively large amounts of immunoglobulin synthesized must be due to increases in the rate of transcription of immunoglobulin messenger, differences in the processing or stability of the immunoglobulin messenger, or some combination of these. Whatever the mechanism, there appears to be coordinated regulation of heavy- and light-chain production. Such coordination could result from an interdependence between the synthesis of the individual chains. However, as already described in a preceding section, we and others (Scharff *et al.*, 1975; Milstein *et al.*, 1975) have been able to isolate variants which have lost the ability to synthesize heavy chains, light chains, or both immunoglobulin polypeptide chains. The presence of such mutants proves that the synthesis of either chain does not require the continued synthesis of the other one.

It would also be interesting to determine whether the presence of other immunoglobulin-specific traits is dependent on the continued synthesis of immunoglobulin. A large number of studies carried out in many laboratories have shown that immunoglobulin, like other secreted proteins, is synthesized on the membrane-associated polyribosomes which make up the rough endoplasmic reticulum (Harrison *et al.*, 1974; Pryme *et al.*, 1973). Light and heavy chain messenger has been found associated with membrane-associated polyribosomes containing 6–8 and 16–20 ribosomes, respectively (Pryme *et al.*, 1973). Although immunoglobulin messenger has in some reports been found associated with free polyribosome, in general the amounts of such messenger are smaller (Lisowska-Bernstein *et al.*, 1970) than that on the rough endoplasmic reticulum. Most recent studies show that immunoglobulins are made throughout the cell cycle in mouse myeloma cells (Liberti and Baglioni, 1973), but Abraham *et al.* (1973) have reported that larger amounts of immunoglobulin are made in G1 than in S and G2 and that 28% of the cells' ribosomes are membrane associated in G1 whereas 18–20% are membrane associated in S and G2. Finally, in the few cell lines examined, the percentage of membrane-associated polyribosomes seems to be proportional to the amount of immunoglobulin being produced by that particular cell line. All these observations and others have led to the belief that most of the membrane-associated polyribosomes in mouse myeloma cells are synthesizing immunoglobulins. It therefore seemed reasonable to assume that variants which had lost the ability to synthesize heavy and light chains would also lose most of their rough endoplasmic reticulum. However, this is not true since we have now examined nonproducing variants, all of which contain almost as many fully active membrane-associated polyribosomes as the parental heavy- plus light-chain-producing cells (Cieplinski and Scharff, in preparation). Thus, although there is a coordination between immunoglobulin production and the formation of the rough endoplasmic reticulum, the continued presence of large numbers of membrane-associated polyribosomes is not dependent on the continued synthesis of immunoglobulin.

## 10.7. Posttranscriptional Events in the Production of Immunoglobulin

Following their synthesis on membrane-associated polyribosomes, the immunoglobulin polypeptide chains are inserted into the cisternae of the endoplasmic reticulum, assembled into a covalently linked four-chain structure, glycosylated, and secreted from the cell. These processes are summarized schematically in Fig. 2. The molecular mechanism responsible for the selective segregation of immunoglobulin (and other secreted protein in other cell types) within the cisternae has been the subject of

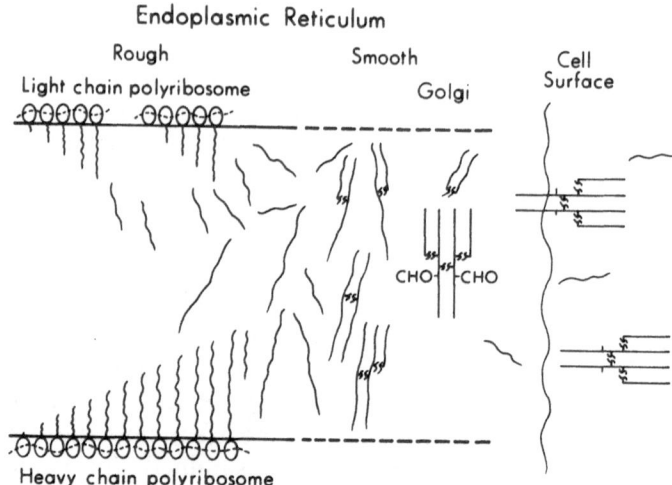

**Fig. 2.** Schematic representation of cellular events in the synthesis, assembly, glycosylation, and secretion of immunoglobulins.

considerable controversy (Rothman, 1975). For example, it has been suggested that since most secreted proteins are glycosylated, the carbohydrate plays an important role in this process. However, the light chains synthesized by some myelomas are not glycosylated and are secreted normally (Melchers, 1971). Using mutants with defects in glycosylation, Weitzman and Scharff (1976) have shown that, at least in these mutants, the carbohydrate is not required for insertion into the cisternae, assembly, or secretion. A number of workers, but especially Blobel and his colleagues (Scheele *et al.,* 1975), have suggested that a short amino acid sequence on the N-terminal part of the molecule, which is present on a newly synthesized polypeptide chain but rapidly removed after synthesis, is required for segregation of secreted proteins into cisternae of the endoplasmic reticulum.

Once the newly synthesized heavy and light chains have been released from the ribosome into the endoplasmic reticulum, they become associated and are held together by both noncovalent bonds and covalent disulfide bonds. Different classes and subclasses assemble primarily through one or the other of the two pathways depicted in Fig. 2—either first joining heavy and light chains to form HL half-molecules and then forming disulfide bonds between two heavy chains for producing the $H_2L_2$ molecule, or first forming the inter-H chain disulfide bond and then attaching the two L chains. Since the pathway of assembly is determined by the heavy chain class or subclass, amino acid sequences in the heavy chain must determine which pathway is preferred (Baumal *et al.*, 1971). The time required to assemble an $H_2L_2$ molecule from heavy and light chains varies from myeloma to myeloma and is quite heterogeneous in normal cells, but requires between 5 and 20 min in most cases.

Glycosylation of the heavy chain, and in some tumors the light chains, appears to start in the rough endoplasmic reticulum but to be largely carried out by glycosyl transferases located in the Golgi apparatus. There is some evidence that the final carbohydrate residues are added close to or at the time of secretion (Melchers and Knopf, 1967). The kinetics of secretion are relatively the same in all mouse myelomas studied so far, except in mutants with blocks in assembly where secretion is often very delayed or inhibited completely. However, the kinetics of secretion in normal lymph node cells appears to be more rapid and orderly than in myeloma cells (Fig. 3). This is the only major difference we have observed in the production of immunoglobulin by normal and malignant cells.

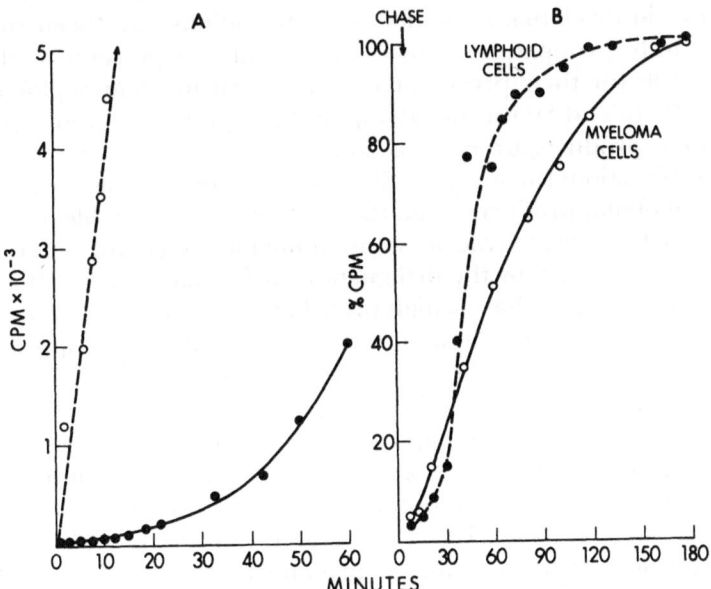

**Fig. 3.** Secretion of immunoglobulins by mouse myeloma and normal immunoglobulin-producing cells. (A) Myeloma cells were incubated with radioactive amino acids and the intracellular and secreted proteins were examined and showed a lag between synthesis and secretion. (B) Both normal (●---●) and malignant (○---○) cells were incubated with radioactive amino acids for 10 min, then incorporation was stopped but protein synthesis allowed to continue. The figure shows the kinetics of secretion of the immunoglobulins made during the first 10-min period. (From Baumal and Scharff, 1973.)

## 10.8. Conclusions

Based even on the limited review presented herein, it is clear that studies on mouse myeloma tumors and cell lines have provided a number of interesting insights into the genetic controls and molecular mechanisms involved in the production of immunoglobulins by plasma cells. Although human multiple myeloma and the solid plasmacytomas of the mouse differ pathologically, they do have some pathophysiological features in common. Studies using cells from human lymphoproliferative disorders and human myelomas suggest that most of the findings described for mouse myelomas in the preceding sections will be confirmed with human cells.

One of the most intriguing aspects of the mouse studies is that they provide a possible explanation for the abnormalities in immunoglobulin production seen in human myeloma. The high frequency of light-chain (Bence-Jones)-producing and the occasional detection of nonproducing human myelomas have always been perplexing as has the production of fragments of heavy chains in some types of lymphoproliferative diseases as well as in myeloma. A number of explanations have been suggested. These can be grouped as follows: (a) A significant percentage of normal plasma cells (or their precursors) are aberrant in immunoglobulin production (Lam and Stevenson, 1973) but their presence is only recognized when their products are produced in large amounts as a result of malignant proliferation; (b) only a small number of normal cells are aberrant in immunoglobulin production but these are highly susceptible to malignant transformation; (c) aberrancies in immunoglobulin production or genetic instability are caused by the malignant transformation; and (d) normal B cells or their progeny have a high probability of undergoing a mutation in immunoglobulin production. Since normal B cells divide approximately 10 times and then die, they are unlikely to undergo such a mutation, whereas malignant cells continue to proliferate and therefore have an increased chance of mutating, overgrowing their parental cell type, and expressing the mutation. We would like to suggest that all myelomas or malignancies producing immunoglobulin start out synthesizing normal heavy and light chains. The high mutation rate we have observed in the mouse myeloma cells could then explain the high frequency of light-chain and lower frequency of nonproducing myelomas in human disease.

ACKNOWLEDGMENTS

The work reported from our laboratory was supported by grants from the National Institutes of Health (NIH AI 10702, NIH AI S231) and the National Science Foundation (NSF PCM7S-13609).

# References

Abraham, K. A., Pryme, I. F., Abro, A., and Dowben, R. M., 1973, Polysomes in various phases of the cell cycle in synchronized plasmacytoma cells, *Exp. Cell Res.* **82**:95.

Anderson, J., Coutinho, A., Melchers, F., and Watanabe, T., 1976, Growth and maturation of lymphocytes in culture, in "The Origins of Lymphocyte Diversity," *Cold Spring Harbor Symp. Quant. Biol.* **XLI** (in press).

Bailey, L. K., Hannestad, K., and Eisen, H. N., 1973, Aberrant immunoglobulin production in stable mouse myeloma tumor variants, *Fed. Proc.* **32**:1013.

Baumal, R., and Scharff, M. D., 1973, Synthesis, assembly and secretion of mouse immunoglobulin, *Transplant. Rev.* **14**:163.

Baumal, R., and Scharff, M. D., 1976, Immunoglobulin biosynthesis by the MOPC 173 mouse myeloma tumor and variant spleen clones, *J. Immunol.* **116**:65.

Baumal, R., Potter, M., and Scharff, M. D., 1971, Synthesis, assembly and secretion of gammaglobulin by mouse myeloma cells, *J. Exp. Med.* **134**:1316.

Baumal, R., Birshtein, B. K., Coffino, P., and Scharff, M. D., 1973, Mutations in immunoglobulin-producing mouse myeloma cells, *Science* **182**:164.

Bergsagel, D. E., Ogawa, M., and Librach, S. L., 1975, Mouse myeloma, *Arch. Intern. Med.* **135**:109.

Bernardini, A., and Tonegawa, S., 1974, Hybridization studies with an antibody heavy chain mRNA, *FEBS Lett.* **41**:73.

Birshtein, B. K., Preud'homme, J.-L., and Scharff, M. D., 1974, Variants of mouse myeloma cells that produce short immunoglobulin heavy chains, *Proc. Nat. Acad. Sci. U.S.A.* **71**:3478.

Cebra, J. J., 1969, Immunoglobulins and immunocytes, *Bacteriol. Rev.* **33**:159.

Coffino, P., and Scharff, M. D., 1971, Rate of somatic mutation in immunoglobulin production by mouse myeloma cells, *Proc. Nat. Acad. Sci. U.S.A.* **68**:219.

Coffino, P., Knowles, B., Nathenson, S., and Scharff, M. D., 1971, Suppression of immunoglobulin synthesis by cellular hybridization, *Nature New Biol.* **231**:87.

Coffino, P., Baumal, R., Laskov, R., and Scharff, M. D., 1972, Cloning of mouse myeloma cells and detection of rare variants, *J. Cell. Physiol.* **79**:429.

Cooper, M. D., Kearney, J. F., Lydyard, P. M., Grossi, C. E., and Lawton, A. R., 1976, Comparative analysis of B-cell generation in mouse, man and chicken, in "Origins of Lymphocyte Diversity," *Cold Spring Harbor Symp. Quant. Biol.* **XLI** (in press).

Cotton, R. G. H., Secher, D. S., and Milstein, C., 1973, Somatic mutation and the origin of antibody diversity. Clonal variability of the immunoglobulin produced by MOPC 21 cells in culture, *Eur. J. Immunol.* **3**:135.

Cowan, N. J., Secher, D. S., and Milstein, C., 1974, Intracellular immunoglobulin chain synthesis in nonsecreting variants of a mouse myeloma: Detection of inactive light chain messenger RNA, *J. Mol. Biol.* **90**:691.

Davis, F. M., and Adelberg, E. A., 1973, Use of somatic cell hybrids for analysis of the differentiated state, *Bacteriol. Rev.* **37**:197.

Franklin, E. C., and Frangione, B., 1975, Structural variants of human and murine immunoglobulins, *in Contemporary Topics in Molecular Immunology*, Vol. 4 (F. P. Inman and W. J. Mandy, eds.), Plenum Press, New York.

Green, M., Graves, P. N., Zehavi-Willner, T., McInnes, J., and Pestka, S., 1975, Cell-free translation of immunoglobulin messenger RNA from MOPC 315 plasmacytoma and MOPC 315 NR, a variant synthesizing only light chain, *Proc. Nat. Acad. Sci. U.S.A.* **72**:224.

Harrison, T. M., Brownlee, G. G., and Milstein, C., 1974, Studies on polysome-membrane interactions in mouse myeloma cells, *Eur. J. Biochem.* **47**:613.

Hobbs, J. R., 1971, Immunocytoma o'mice an' men, *Br. Med. J.* **2**:67.

Hollander, V. P., Takakura, K., and Yamada, H., 1968, Endocrine factors in the pathogenesis of plasma cell tumors, *Recent Prog. Horm. Res.* **24**:81.

Hood, L., Campbell, J. H., and Elgin, S. C. R., 1975, The organization, expression, and evolution of antibody genes and other multigene families, *Annu. Rev. Genet.* **9**:305.

Horibata, K., and Harris, A. W., 1970, Mouse myelomas and lymphomas in culture, *Exp. Cell Res.* **60**:61.

Jerne, N. K., 1974, Towards a network theory of the immune system, *Ann. Immunol. (Inst. Pasteur)* **125C**:373.

Kohler, G., and Milstein, C., 1975, Continuous cultures of fused cells secreting antibody of predefined specificity, *Nature (London)* **256**:495.

Kuehl, W. M., Kaplan, B. A., Scharff, M. D., Nav, M., Honjo, T., and Leder, P., 1975, Characterization of light chain and light chain constant region fragment mRNAs in MPC 11 mouse myeloma cells and variants, *Cell* **5**:139.

Lam, C., and Stevenson, G., 1973, Detection in normal plasma of immunoglobulin resembling the protein of γ-chain disease, *Nature (London)* **246**:419.

Laskov, R., and Scharff, M. D., 1970, Synthesis, assembly, and secretion of gammaglobulin by mouse myeloma cells. I. Adaptation of the Merwin plasma cell tumor 11 to culture, cloning and characterization of gammaglobulin synthesis, *J. Exp. Med.* **131**:515.

Leder, P., Honjo, T., Packman, S., Swan, D., Nav, M., and Norman, B., 1975, The organization and diversity of immunoglobulin K and γ genes, *in Molecular Approaches to Immunology* (E. E. Smith and D. S. Ribbons, eds.), p. 173, Academic Press, New York.

Liberti, P., and Baglioni, C., 1973, Synthesis of immunoglobulin and nuclear protein in synchronized mouse myeloma cells, *J. Cell. Physiol.* **82**:113.

Lieberman, R., Mantel, N., and Humphrey, W. Jr., 1961, Ascites production in 17 mice strains, *Proc. Soc. Exp. Biol. Med.* **107**:163.

Lisowska-Bernstein, B., Lamm, M. E., and Vassali, P., 1970, Synthesis of immuno-globulin heavy and light chains by the free ribosomes of a mouse plasma cell tumor, *Proc. Nat. Acad. Sci. U.S.A.* **66**:425.

Lyons, R. M., Chaplin, H., and Tillack, T. W., 1975, Gamma-heavy chain disease: Rapid sustained response to cyclophosphamide and prednisone, *Blood* **46**:1.

Margulies, D. H., Kuehl, W. M., and Scharff, M. D., 1976, Somatic cell hybridization of mouse myeloma cells, *Cell* **8**:405.

Margulies, D. H., Cieplinski, W., Dharmgrongartama, B., Gefter, M. L., Morrison, S. L., Kelley, T., and Scharff, M. D., 1976b, Regulation of immunoglobulin expression in mouse myeloma cells, in "Origins of Lymphocyte Diversity," *Cold Spring Harbor Symp. Quant. Biol.* **XLI** (in press).

McKean, D. J., Potter, M., and Hood, L., 1972, Amino acid sequence comparison of three new Balb/C mouse kappa chains, *Fed. Proc.* **31**:772 (Abstract).

Melchers, F., 1971, The secretion of a Bence-Jones type light chain from a mouse plasmacytoma, *Eur. J. Immunol.* **1**:330.

Melchers, F., and Knopf, P. M., 1967, Biosynthesis of the carbohydrate portion of immunoglobulin chains: Possible relation to secretions, in "Antibodies," *Cold Spring Harbor Symp. Quant. Biol.,* p. 255.

Merwin, R. M., and Algire, G. H., 1959, Induction of plasma cell neoplasms and fibrosarcomas in BALB/c mice carrying diffusion chambers, *Proc. Soc. Exp. Biol. Med.* **101**:437.

Merwin, R. M., and Redman, L. W., 1963, Induction of plasma cell tumors and sarcomas in mice by diffusion chambers placed in the peritoneal cavity, *J. Nat. Cancer Inst.* **31**:998.

Milstein, C., Adetugbo, K., Brownlee, G. G., Cowan, N. J., Proudfoot, N. J., Rabbitts, T. H., and Secher, D. S., 1975, Immunoglobulin genes in a mouse myeloma and in mutant clones, in *Molecular Approaches to Immunology* (E. E. Smith and D. W. Ribbons, eds.), p. 131, Academic Press, New York.

Morrison, S. L., and Scharff, M. D., 1975, Heavy chain-producing variants of a mouse myeloma cell line, *J. Immunol.* **114**:655.

Mushinski, J. F., 1971, γA half molecules: Defective heavy chain mutants in mouse myeloma proteins, *J. Immunol.* **106**:41.

Osserman, E. F., and Takatsuki, K., 1964, Considerations regarding the pathogenesis of the plasmacytic dyserasias, *Scand. J. Haematol.* **4** (Suppl.):28.

Periman, P., 1970, IgG synthesis in hybrid cells from an antibody-producing mouse myeloma and an L cell substrain, *Nature (London)* **228**:1086.

Preud'homme, J.-L., Buxbam, J., and Scharff, M. D., 1973, Mutagenesis of mouse myeloma cells with "Melphalan," *Nature (London)* **245**:320.

Preud'homme, J.-L., Birshtein, B. K., and Scharff, M. D., 1975, Variants of mouse myeloma cells that produce short immunoglobulin heavy chains, *Proc. Nat. Acad. Sci. U.S.A.* **72**:1427.

Pottengill, G. S., and Sorensen, G. D., 1967, Murine myeloma cells in suspension culture, *Exp. Cell Res.* **47**:608.

Potter, M., 1967, The plasma cell tumors and myeloma proteins of mice, in *Methods in Cancer Research* (H. Busch, ed.), Vol. II, p. 105, Academic Press, New York.

Potter, M., 1972, Immunoglobulin-producing tumors and myeloma proteins of mice, *Physiol. Rev.* **52**:631.

Potter, M., and Boyce, C., 1962, Induction of plasma cell neoplasms in strain BALB/c mice with mineral oil and mineral oil adjuvants, *Nature (London)* **193**:1086.

Potter, M., and Kuff, E. L., 1964, Disorders in the differentiation of protein secretion in neoplastic plasma cells, *J. Mol. Biol.* **9**:537.

Potter, M., Sklar, M. D., and Rowe, W. P., 1973, Rapid viral induction of plasmacytomas in pristane-primed BALB/c mice, *Science* **182**:592.

Pryme, I. F., Garantun-Tjeldsto, O., Birekbichler, P. J., Weltman, J. K., and Dowben, R. M., 1973, Synthesis of immunoglobulins by membrane-bound polysomes and free polysomes from plasmacytoma cells, *Eur. J. Biochem.* **33**:374.

Robinson, E. A., Smith, D. F., and Appella, E., 1974, Chemical characterization of a mouse immunoglobulin A heavy chain with a 100 residue deletion, *J. Biol. Chem.* **249**:6605.

Rothman, S. S., 1975, Protein transport by the pancreas, *Science* **190**:747.

Scharff, M. D., and Laskov, R., 1970, Synthesis and assembly of immunoglobulin polypeptide chains, *Prog. Allergy* **14**:37.

Scharff, M. D., Birshtein, B. K., Dharmgrongartama, B., Frank, L., Kelly, T., Kuehl, W. M., Margulies, D. H., Morrison, S. L., Preud'homme, J.-L., and Weitzman, S., 1975, The use of mutant myeloma cells to explore the production of immunoglobulins, *in Molecular Approaches to Immunology* (E. E. Smith and D. M. Ribbons, eds.), p. 109, Academic Press, New York.

Scheele, G. A., Dobberstein, B., Devillers-Thiery, A., and Blobel, G., 1975, *In vitro* translation of cell fractions from dog pancreas, *J. Cell Biol.* **67**:385a.

Takakura, K., Yamada, H., Weber, A. H., and Hollander, V. P., 1967, Studies on the pathogenesis of plasma cell tumors, effect of sex hormones on the development of plasma cell tumors, *Cancer Res.* **27**:932.

Tonegawa, S., Hozumi, N., Matthyssens, G., and Schuller, R., 1976, Somatic changes in content and context of immunoglobulin genes, in "Origin of Lymphocyte Diversity," *Cold Spring Harbor Symp. Quant. Biol.* **XLI** (in press).

Weigert, M., Cesari, M., Yonkovich, S. J., and Cohn, M., 1970, Variability in the lambda light chain sequences of mouse antibody, *Nature (London)* **228**:1045.

Weitzman, S., and Scharff, M. D., 1976, Mouse myeloma mutants blocked in the assembly, glycosylation, and secretion of immunoglobulin, *J. Mol. Biol.* **102**:237.

Williamson, A. R., 1976, The biological origin of antibody diversity, *Annu. Rev. Biochem.* **45**:467.

# 11

# The Origin of RNA Tumor Viruses and Their Relation to Human Leukemia

## Robert C. Gallo and David H. Gillespie

## 11.1. Origin of RNA Tumor Viruses

Type C RNA viruses (RNA tumor viruses, oncornaviruses, leukemia–sarcoma viruses, retraviruses) have been isolated from many species. In several species the viruses have been associated with leukemia, and sometimes the disease has been reproduced when the virus was inoculated into animals. In a few species the evidence seems to be conclusive that these viruses are a contributing factor in the etiology of the naturally occurring leukemia. This appears to be the case in chickens, cats, gibbons, cows, and some wild-type mice. There are three major problems in proving that type C viruses cause leukemia in some animal systems: (a) a long latent period for effect; (b) the fact that susceptibility appears to vary enormously among different members of a species; and (c) many type C viruses apparently are not leukemogenic.

Type C viruses are a distinct class of viruses present among many vertebrates and share common morphology, composition, and life cycle. They are spherical particles approximately 1000 Å in diameter, contain-

ROBERT C. GALLO and DAVID H. GILLESPIE  •  Laboratory of Tumor Cell Biology, National Cancer Institute, Bethesda, Maryland 20014.

ing a centrally placed, electron-dense core surrounded by a unit membrane. In our view, the *sine qua nons* of type C viruses are (a) condensation of the virus core beneath the cell surface with subsequent budding of the virus from the cell membrane; and (b) the essential components of the RNA → DNA mode of replication of these viruses, including a high molecular weight, single-stranded genome of RNA associated with a DNA polymerase (reverse transcriptase). However, although these features, as well as biological activity, are deemed necessary to conclude that a particle in question is type C and a virus, we emphasize that in our view there is a continuum of particles ranging from immature or defective particles which may even remain in the cytoplasm, to the fully mature, replicating type C virus.

The mode of replication of these viruses is now fairly well understood (see Tooze, 1973). The infectious cycle involves virus adhering to the cell membrane, penetration and uncoating, synthesis of complementary DNA copies of the viral RNA (synthesis of the provirus), formation of a double-stranded DNA provirus, integration of the provirus into the host cell DNA, expression of the proviral DNA (i.e., synthesis and processing of viral RNA mediated presumably by cellular RNA polymerases), synthesis of viral proteins, assembly of the particle, budding, and release. When a cell is not permissive to infection by type C RNA viruses, the block may be at any one of these levels.

Type C viruses can be transmitted from animal to animal (infectious horizontal) or from mother to offspring, e.g., via milk or across the placenta (congenital infection), or genetically in the germ line (vertical) from parent to progeny along with other cellular genes.

In this chapter we will consider in more detail ideas and data relevant to the origin of type C viruses, the development of oncogenic viruses, interspecies transmission of type C viruses, their identification and isolation from primates, the evidence for the presence of type C viral information in humans, and the implications to human leukemia.

### 11.1.1. RNA-Containing Viruses Coded by Genes of Normal Cells

Huebner and Todaro (1969), Bentvelzen *et al.* (1970), and Temin (1971) have proposed that the RNA genomes of RNA "tumor" viruses originate by the "escape" and subsequent autonomous replication of particular cell genes, called "virogenes" (Huebner and Todaro, 1969), found in normal cells. These ideas are well supported by experimental evidence in several species. The evidence applies most directly to a group of viruses that are indistinguishable from oncogenic RNA-containing viruses by morphological, biophysical, and biochemical criteria, but in general they do not cause cancer as far as anyone knows. Some of these are type A particles and others are type B and type C viruses. Similar viruses that do cause cancer will be called "type C RNA tumor viruses" or just "RNA tumor viruses." The prevailing opinion is that RNA tumor viruses that cause sarcomas and/or leukemias are derived from the nononcogenic type C RNA viruses by genetic modification of the latter (see later).

The evidence that the genomes of type C RNA viruses originate from virogenes of normal cells is of four types. First, type A, type B, and type C RNA viruses have been detected by electron microscopy in some tissues of apparently normal animals. All these viruses are 1000-Å-diameter, membrane-bound particles having an inner structure (the "core" or "nucleoid"), also membrane-bound and containing the virus RNA (for reviews see Tooze, 1973; Gillespie et al., 1975b). Type A RNA virus particles, characterized by a doughnut-shaped, centrally located core, have been seen in early embryos of normal mice (Calarco and Szollosi, 1973). Type B RNA virus particles, characterized by an eccentric, electron-dense core, have been detected in mammary glands of normal mice (East et al., 1975). Type C RNA virus particles characterized by a centrally located, electron-dense core, have been visualized in placenta of several primates (Kalter et al., 1973a,b; Schidlovsky and Ahmed, 1973; Jensen, personal communication). They are especially numerous in baboon placentas and are also found in other tissues of this animal (Kalter et al., 1973a). On the other hand, this is, of course, not substantial proof since a normal animal may harbor an acquired virus.

Second, type A, type B, and type C RNA viruses are produced after culturing cells from tissues of normal animals (Lieber et al., 1973). The production of type C RNA viruses in some systems can be markedly enhanced by pretreating the cells with halogenated pyrimidine deoxyribonucleosides that replace natural nucleosides during DNA or RNA synthesis and are mutagenic, for example with iododeoxyuridine (IdU) (Lowy et al., 1971; Aaronson et al., 1971). It can also be slightly enhanced with cyclohexemide, an inhibitor of protein synthesis (Aaronson and Dunn, 1974). The IdU induction is sometimes augmented by adding steroid hormones, for example dexamethasone (Paran et al., 1973), or by cyclic AMP (Tihon and Green, 1973), and can be inhibited by antagonists of nucleic acid metabolism, for example 3'-deoxyadenosine (cordycepin) (Wu et al., 1972) or actinomycin D (Gallo, Ben Horin, and Wu, unpublished results). The augmentors and inhibitors of IdU induction of type C RNA virus production are active at particular times of the IdU induction process. Type C RNA viruses have been induced from chickens, cats, guinea pigs, mice, rats, and baboons, among other animals. These viruses usually replicate in some normal cells but have not been shown to be tumorigenic. Ordinarily, the viruses induced from normal cells grow poorly in cells from the animal that yielded them. They grow better in cells from other animals or in cells from different strains of the same animal (Levy, 1973). These growth patterns denote the "tropism" of virus (see later).

Third, the RNA of viruses or, alternatively, the DNA copies of the RNA of viruses (cDNA) induced from or produced by normal cells in culture have nucleotide sequences that are indistinguishable from sequences in DNA from any tissue of any member of the animal species that produced the virus (Neiman, 1973a,b; Gillespie and Gallo, 1975; Nayak et al., 1974; Gillespie et al., 1973; Benveniste and Todaro, 1974a–c). To measure this, radioactive RNA or cDNA from a particular virus is hybridized to DNA from virus-producing cells or to DNA from tissues of apparently normal uninfected animals. In the case of a type C RNA virus produced by cells of a normal baboon, as much of the viral RNA or cDNA hybridizes to DNA from normal baboon tissues as it does to DNA from cells deliberately infected by the baboon virus, e.g., infected bat, mink, dog, or human cells (Benveniste and Todaro, 1974a–c, 1976; Wong-Staal et al., 1976). The quality of a hybrid, i.e., how "perfect" the match between two nucleic acids, can be estimated by determining the hybrid thermal stability. The thermal stability of hybrids formed with DNA from all of these sources is about the same. In contrast, very little of the RNA or cDNA from the baboon virus hybridizes to DNA from uninfected human cells, and there is no detectable hybridization to DNA from uninfected bat, mink, or dog cells. The same type of molecular hybridization experiment has been done with type C RNA viruses induced from chickens (Neiman, 1973a), cats (Neiman, 1973b; Gillespie et al., 1973), guinea pigs (Nayak et al., 1974), rats (Benveniste and Todaro, 1974a–c), and mice (Callahan et al., 1974, 1975; Benveniste and Todaro, 1975). Thus, DNA of these normal animals contains nucleotide sequences that can be packaged into infectious, type C RNA virus particles after IdU induction and the virus can transfer these sequences to the DNA of a new host cell. Since there is apparently at least one complete copy of the viral genome in the DNA of every cell of every tissue of the normal animal, these results provide the strongest evidence that these viral genes are indeed endogenous, genetically transmitted elements.

Fourth, the DNA of "normal" chicken or mouse cells when introduced into cells of a new species can cause production of virus characteristic of the donor cell species (Cooper and Temin, 1974; Scolnick and Bumgarner, 1975). Although the transmitted viruses were classified as xenotropic, they have not been shown to be true endogenous viruses that were transfected with the normal cell DNA. In fact, Cooper and Temin (1974) point out that the true endogenous virus genes may *not* be infectious in their system.

RNA-containing viruses obtained from normal cells are called

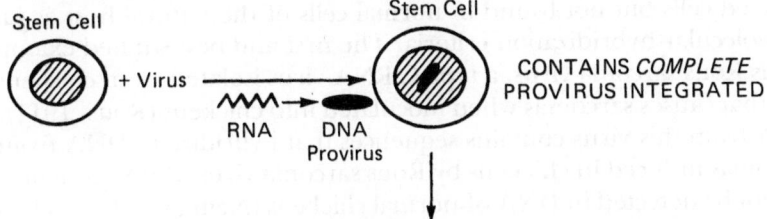

Stem Cell is TRANSFORMED. Virus is Rare Because
Repressors Prevent Expression. Provirus is Difficult to
Detect Because Available Probes are Very Inappropriate.

**Fig. 1.** Classical scheme for infection and transformation of a cell by an RNA tumor virus (leukemic cells intrinsically abnormal). The infected cell in this case is a stem cell. Viral RNA is transcribed to DNA via reverse transcriptase. The newly synthesized DNA provirus is completely integrated into the cellular chromosomal DNA. The provirus carries genes for leukemogenesis. When expressed the cells are transformed to leukemic cells. All daughter cells (derived from one transformed original cell) contain at least one complete provirus. Virus could rarely be seen because provirus is rarely *completely* expressed, but partial expression is sufficient for transformation. However, in this model the provirus should be easily identified. Since this is not the case in every human leukemia, then the model must be incorrect or else all the available probes and virus isolates today are not applicable (wrong viruses and not even modest homology between available animal viruses and human candidate viruses and a putative very specific human acquired virus).

"endogenous," "xenotropic" (Levy, 1973), or "class 1" (Gillespie and Gallo, 1975) viruses. The term "endogenous virus" signifies that the virus was a resident of normal cells and implies that the animal carried genes coding for it in its DNA. The term "xenotropic virus" signifies that the virus grows better in cells from some other species than in cells from the same species that yielded the virus. Most endogenous type C RNA viruses are xenotropic. The term "class 1 virus" denotes a virus whose RNA genome or DNA copies of it hybridize equally to DNA from normal or virus-infected cells (see earlier). All endogenous viruses must be class 1, by the implied definition of the word "endogenous" (for a listing of endogenous viruses, see Gillespie *et al.*, 1975b; Gallo and Todaro, 1976).

It may appear that having three terms to describe one type of virus is redundant. However, each terminology is based on a different property of the viruses (Gillespie and Gallo, 1975) and has a particular use in describing the oncogenic RNA viruses, as opposed to the nononcogenic RNA viruses already described.

### 11.1.2. Type C RNA-Containing Viruses Not Coded by Genes of Normal Cells

RNA or cDNA from some type C RNA viruses, in particular those that cause sarcomas and leukemias, contain sequences found in virus-infected cells but not found in normal cells of the natural host as judged by molecular hybridization criteria. The first and best studied example of this is Rous sarcoma virus, a type C RNA virus isolated from chickens and one that causes sarcomas when inoculated into chickens (Rous, 1911). The RNA from this virus contains sequences that hybridize to DNA from web sarcomas induced in chickens by Rous sarcoma virus, RNA sequences that cannot be detected in DNA of normal chickens (Neiman, 1972). The RNA or cDNA of Rauscher leukemia virus, a type C RNA virus isolated from mice and one that causes leukemia in mice (Rauscher, 1962), contains sequences that hybridize to DNA from cells infected by the virus or in blood cells of leukemic mice that are missing in DNA of normal mice (Gillespie *et al.*, 1973,1975c). The RNAs of feline sarcoma–leukemia and leukemia viruses isolated from cats (Snyder and Theilen, 1969) and capable of causing tumors in a wide variety of animals, contain few sequences in common with DNA from normal cats (Gillespie *et al.*, 1973). Finally, RNA from simian sarcoma–leukemia virus, a virus isolated from woolly monkeys and capable of causing tumors in marmosets (Theilen *et al.*, 1971; Wolfe *et al.*, 1971), and RNA from gibbon ape leukemia virus, a virus family isolated from several gibbon apes (De Pauli *et al.*, 1973; Kawakami *et al.*, 1972) and which can cause leukemia in this species, contain no sequences that hybridize to DNA from primates. However, the RNA or cDNA from these viruses hybridizes to DNA from cells infected by them (Benveniste *et al.*, 1974a,b; Wong-Staal *et al.*, 1975; Scolnick *et al.*, 1974; Gillespie *et al.*, 1975b).

These viruses have been called "exogenous," "ecotropic," or "class 2" viruses. The term "exogenous" has little meaning except that it is the opposite of "endogenous" and therefore implies that the genomes of exogenous viruses are *not* coded by DNA of normal cells, at least not *en toto*. "Ecotropic" viruses replicate relatively well in cells from their natural host, ordinarily better than in cells from another species. "Class 2" virus indicates that the virus contains RNA sequences missing in DNA of normal cells as measured by molecular hybridization. Specifically, class 2 viruses are those containing RNA sequences that hybridize to DNA from cells producing the virus, and at least some of these RNA sequences do not hybridize to DNA from normal cells. Often class 2 viruses also contain RNA sequences that hybridize to DNA from both normal and virus-producing cells (see later).

Beside containing RNA sequences not found in DNA from normal cells, class 2 viruses have other properties that distinguish them from class 1 viruses. Class 2 viruses are generally isolated from tumor tissues, although sometimes they can be isolated from an infected "carrier" animal (Wolfe *et al.*, 1971). Viruses that cause leukemias when inoculated into animals have been isolated from both sarcomatous and leukemic tissues. Viruses that cause sarcomas have been isolated from sarcomatous tissue and by repeated passage of a leukemogenic virus through animals or cultured cells. All class 2 type C RNA viruses studied to date are oncogenic, whereas most class 1 viruses are not known to be.

*Although class 2 viruses contain RNA sequences that are not found in DNA from normal cells, it appears that virtually all their RNA sequences were derived from normal cells.* Between 60 and 80% of the sequences in RNA from Rauscher mouse leukemia virus can be hybridized to DNA from cells producing Rauscher leukemia virus when formation of viral RNA–cell DNA hybrids resistant to RNAse-A treatment at 37°C in 0.3 M NaCl is measured, whereas only 15–20% of the same RNA forms complexes of comparable RNAse stability with DNA from normal mouse cells (Gillespie *et al.*, 1973,1975c). However, when one assays complexes that bind nitrocellulose (Gillespie *et al.*, 1975c) or those that are resistant to RNAse-A at 25°C in 1 M NaCl (unpublished results with F. Wong-Staal), 60–70% of the RNA is found to interact specifically with DNA sequences from normal mice. The thermal stability of hybrids formed with DNA of normal mice and involving the 20% of RNA from Rauscher leukemia virus resistant to RNAse-A at 37°C is some 5° lower than that of hybrids formed with DNA from virus-producing cells. The results with RNA of this virus indicate that few sequences exist in DNA of normal mice that are *identical* to those in the Rauscher leukemia virus genome but that sequences *related* in a specific fashion to a major fraction of the virus RNA are present. Similar results have been obtained with RNA from simian sarcoma–leukemia virus, where sequences related to 50% of the virus RNA have been detected in DNA of normal mice (Wong-Staal *et al.*, 1975), the animal that may have been the original source of this virus (Lieber *et al.*, 1975). RNA from Rous sarcoma virus contains sarcomagenic sequences (Lai *et al.*, 1973; Duesberg and Vogt, 1970) related but not identical to sequences in DNA of normal chickens. Thus, in these cases it appears that the sequences in class 2 viruses not found per se in genes of normal animals were somehow derived from them. Either the viral RNA sequences originated in genes of normal cells then evolved away or they originated elsewhere and through recombination have become more hostlike. In the cases of some class 2 viruses there is evidence for the latter, especially following laboratory manipulation (Scolnick *et al.*, 1973; Scolnick and Parks, 1974; Haywood and Hanafusa, 1975; Weiss, 1973; Altaner and Temin, 1970); in every case so far studied there is evidence for the former.

### 11.1.3. Class 2 Viruses Arise from Class 1 Viruses

Clearly, the simplest explanation of the observations summarized in the preceding two sections is that cell genes give rise directly to the RNA genomes of class 1 nononcogenic viruses, which in turn can be genetically modified, giving rise to tumorigenic class 2 viruses (Temin, 1971; Gillespie and Gallo, 1975; Gillespie *et al.*, 1973). Other than the close homology of class 1 virus genomes and the distant relatedness of class 2 virus genomes to normal cell genes, the most compelling evidence that class 2 viruses arise from modifications of class 1 viruses concerns their interrelationships. Class 1 and 2 viruses from mice have RNA genomes with related nucleotide sequences (Benveniste and Todaro, 1973; Miller *et al.*, 1974; East *et al.*, 1975; Callahan *et al.*, 1974,1975) and the same is true for class 1 and 2 viruses from chickens (Neiman *et al.*, 1974; Kang and Temin, 1973). The interrelatedness is measured by hybridizing cDNA from one virus to RNA from another. If one uses the relatedness of mouse viruses to DNA of normal mice and the interrelatedness among mouse viruses to construct genetic linkage maps, the maps are consistent with the cell gene → class 1 virus → class 2 virus scheme (Gillespie and Gallo, 1975; Gillespie *et al.*, 1975a).

Class 1 (RD-114) and class 2 viruses (FeLV, FeSV) from cats are not detectably related (Benveniste and Todaro, 1973; Miller *et al.*, 1974; East *et al.*, 1975), but there is evidence that both classes of virus entered cats from other animals (Benveniste and Todaro, 1974a,b; and see later). Similarly, class 1 and 2 viruses from primates are not interrelated and again there is evidence that the class 2 primate viruses came from another animal (Benveniste *et al.*, 1974a,b; Wong-Staal *et al.*, 1975; and see later).

In terms of the ability of type C RNA viruses to cause tumors, available molecular hybridization results are consistent with the essence of Temin's protovirus theory (1971). Temin proposed that RNA viruses become tumorigenic only after genetic modification of "protoviruses." Temin proposed that protoviruses contain an RNA genome that originates directly from cell DNA sequences and that the genetic modifications causing the nononcogenic protovirus to acquire tumorigenic potential involve reverse transcription and/or recombination with cell DNA.

No reports indicate that type A RNA viruslike particles have oncogenic potential, and the relatedness between their RNA genome and cell DNA sequences is unknown. The type B RNA virus, mouse mammary tumor virus, is suspected of causing mammary tumors in mice. The genome of this virus is closely related to genes in normal mice (Varmus *et al.*, 1972; Gillespie and Gallo, 1975), though one report suggests small differences in nucleotide sequence (Gillespie and Gallo, 1975). Specifically, though all the cDNA (Varmus *et al.*, 1972) or RNA (Gillespie and Gallo, 1975) from mouse mammary tumor virus hybridizes to cell DNA, the thermal stability of the viral RNA–cell DNA hybrid is lower than would be expected if the cell DNA contained sequences identical to those in the virus (Gillespie and Gallo, 1975).

## 11.1.4. Type C RNA Viruses Are Transmitted among Hosts of Different Species in the Wild

Whether from class 1 or class 2 viruses, the RNA or cDNA from type C RNA viruses usually hybridizes better to DNA from the animal that originated the virus (usually its natural host) than to DNA from other animals and, among other animals, hybridizes more fully to DNA from animals more closely related phylogenetically to the progenitor or natural host of the virus. This is true for class 1 and class 2 chicken viruses (Baluda and Nayak, 1970; Neiman, 1972,1973a; Baluda and Drohan, 1972), class 1 and class 2 mouse viruses (Gillespie and Gallo, 1975; Gillespie et al., 1973,1975c), a class 1 virus from baboons (Benveniste and Todaro, 1974a,b,1976; Wong-Staal et al., 1976), a class 1 virus from guinea pigs (Nayak et al., 1974), and a class 1 virus from rats (Scolnick et al., 1973). This type of result indicates that the cell DNA sequences involved in the viral RNA–DNA hybrids are evolutionarily selected, cellular, genomic components. The confidence in this interpretation varies directly with the number of different animals tested. In the cases of type C RNA viruses from chickens, mice, and baboons the number is large and one can conclude that the viral or viral-related DNA sequences in these animals have existed in the evolutionary lines that led to them for some 100 million years or more.

The exceptions to this phylogenetic pattern are interesting and indicate interspecies transmission of some type C RNA viruses. Among DNA preparations from many animals tested, the cDNA from the RD-114/CCC group of class 1 feline viruses hybridizes more than expected to DNA from normal baboons (Benveniste and Todaro, 1974a); cDNA and RNA from simian sarcoma–leukemia virus and gibbon ape leukemia virus do not hybridize to DNA fron normal primates but do hybridize to DNA from normal mice or rats (Benveniste et al., 1974a,b; Wong-Staal et al., 1975); and cDNA from feline leukemia virus or pig type C RNA virus hybridizes more than expected to DNA from rats or mice, respectively (Benveniste and Todaro, 1974a,b). The results suggest that the RD-114/ CCC virus originated in baboons and was transferred to cats, that simian sarcoma–leukemia virus and gibbon ape leukemia virus originated in mice or rats and was transferred to primates. In some instances, these results are substantiated by direct comparisons of the respective viruses by biological tests, protein antigenic tests, and tests of nucleic acid relatedness by molecular hybridization. For instance, the RD-114 virus of cats is unusually related by these three approaches to the baboon endogenous virus, and the infectious primate viruses (woolly monkey simian sarcoma virus and gibbon ape leukemia virus) are unusually related to certain viruses of rodents (Benveniste and Todaro, 1973).

All these interspecies transfers probably occurred within the past 15 million years. In at least one case, the transfer of the baboon virus (or a related ancestral virus) to an ancestor of domestic and a few other cat species, the results strongly suggest that the virus inserted DNA sequences into the cat germ line. Thus, RD-114/CCC is now an endogenous, xenotropic class 1 virus of cats even though at one time in the evolutionary past it was not. In another case, the mouse or rat → primate transfer of simian sarcoma–leukemia virus and/or gibbon ape leukemia virus, the virus(es) certainly did not insert DNA sequences into the germ line of any individual primates tested. In the two remaining cases it has been claimed that viruslike sequences were transferred into the germ line of cats and pigs (Benveniste and Todaro, 1975,1976), but the data are also consistent with an infection restricted to somatic cells and a gradual convergence of virus sequences with host genes by recombination.

Whatever details prove correct, the fact of interspecies transfer of type C RNA viruses seems to us to be well supported, and there is no reason to exclude man or any other species as a potential recipient host.

Before considering the problem of type C RNA viruses in man, it is useful to discuss the details of the history and characteristics of the known primate type C viruses because first, they are the first type C viruses to be isolated from close relatives of man; second, several are oncogenic; third, they provide the closest models to man of viral-induced neoplasias; and fourth, they have provided the most useful probes for detecting type C viral information in humans, i.e., viruses like these could be present in the human population.

## 11.1.5. Primate Type C RNA Tumor Viruses

As we have mentioned, type C viruses have been isolated from primates in recent years, and they consist of members of both major virus classes. The first isolate came from woolly monkey, a household pet of a woman in California. The monkey developed a spontaneous fibrosarcoma of the neck. The virus was identified by Gordon Theilen and his associates (Theilen *et al.*, 1971), and it was isolated subsequently by Wolfe and Deinhardt in collaboration with Theilen and Kawakami from tumors of marmoset monkeys after they were inoculated with extracts from the woolly monkey tumor (Wolfe *et al.*, 1971). This virus has become known as the woolly monkey virus, the simian sarcoma–leukemia virus, or the simian sarcoma virus–simian sarcoma-associated virus (SSV-SSAV). It consists of a virus which transforms fibroblasts *in vitro* (the sarcoma component) and a helper virus for replication (the leukemia virus or associated virus component). There is still *only one isolate* of this virus from a woolly monkey. At about the same time, type C viruses were isolated from gibbon apes with different types of hematopoietic neoplasms, including both myelogenous and lymphoid leukemias (Kawakami et al., 1972). It may be important to note that some of these isolates came from a colony of gibbons inoculated directly or indirectly with human blood from people with malaria (De Pauli et al., 1973). In a colony of 195 apes in Thailand, 103 animals were injected with the human blood. Neoplasms developed in 10 animals, all from the inoculated group. Virus was isolated from some of these animals. Other isolates came from gibbons in a San Francisco zoo that developed spontaneous leukemia. More recently, three isolates of the gibbon ape leukemia virus (GaLV) were obtained from extracts of "normal" gibbon brains. Two of these gibbons had been inoculated with extracts of brains from humans with kuru (Todaro et al., 1975). The third animal was a cagemate of the other two. Finally, we recently isolated a GaLV from a gibbon ape called "Hugo" kept at Hall's Island near Bermuda. This animal spontaneously developed lymphoid leukemia and virus was isolated (GaLV-H) from several tissues. An extremely high virus titer was found in the plasma, saliva, and several tissues.

Kawakami has clearly shown that the gibbon ape leukemia virus moves horizontally among contacts, and that only some animals are susceptible to the development of leukemia, possibly dependent on the immune response of the animal (Kawakami et al., 1973). It is clear that gibbons are extremely susceptible to this virus, and we think the transmission is probably from the saliva.

Analyses of these viruses then proceeded in several laboratories, and several important observations soon emerged. (1) It was quickly determined that both the GaLV and SSV-SSAV are not endogenous to primates (Scolnick et al., 1974; Benveniste et al., 1974a,b; Wong-Staal et al., 1975). Instead they are typical class 2 infectious viruses. (2) Both SSV-SSAV and the various GaLV form members of a very closely related group (for a recent summary, see Gallo and Todaro, 1976). Based on biological, immunological, and biochemical assays, this group of infectious type C viruses has been shown to consist of several members of a highly related group. They consist of at least four distinct subgroups (see Table I). The close relatedness of members of this group indicates that they have a common origin. This is surprising in view of the rapid rate of divergence of viral genes in general (Gallo et al., 1973; Benveniste and Todaro, 1976) and the ecological and phylogenetic differences of the host animals of the GaLV and SSV-SSAV virus family, i.e., gibbons are Old World apes and woolly monkeys are New World monkeys. The extreme susceptibility of gibbons to GaLV suggests that the virus entered these animals relatively recently, and indicates to us that this transmission may have been influenced by man removing these animals from their natural habitat.

**Table I.** Infectious (Class 2) Primate Type C Viruses

| Proposed subgroup[a] | Isolate | Source of isolate | Mode of transmission | Reference |
|---|---|---|---|---|
| A | SSV-SSAV | Woolly monkey fibrosarcoma | Horizontal | Wolfe et al., 1971 |
| B | GALV-1 | Gibbon ape leukemia | Horizontal | Kawakami et al., 1972, 1973 |
| C | GALV-SEATO | Gibbon ape leukemia | Horizontal | Kawakami et al., 1972, 1973 |
| D | GBr-1 GBr-2 GBr-3 | Gibbon brains | Horizontal | Todaro et al., 1975 |
| E | GALV-H | Gibbon leukemia | Horizontal | Gallo et al., submitted for publication |

[a] See Gallo and Todaro (1976).

It is interesting to speculate about the origin of this group. Early results suggested that these viruses were more unusually related to some of the type C viruses of mice. This prompted us to look for nucleic acid sequences in the DNA from mice related to the viral genes SSV-SSAV and GaLV. Such sequences were found and interpreted as suggestive that the origin of the infectious primate type C virus group might be from a mouse virus (Wong-Staal *et al.*, 1975). Independently, an Asian mouse type C virus was isolated by Lieber *et al.* (1975) and found to be particularly closely related to the infectious primate virus group. As will be described fully in the following section, there is evidence to suggest that viruses of the SSV-SSAV–GaLV group may have also entered the human population.

Endogenous (class 1) type C viruses have been isolated from only one primate, the baboon, despite numerous attempts with many primates, especially man. In baboons there are now several isolates from many tissues and from different species of baboons. The first evidence for these viruses came from electron microscopic visualization of viruslike particles in normal placentas and in leukemic tissues (Kalter *et al.*, 1973a; Lapin, 1973). However, it was only after their successful propagation in tissue culture (i.e., isolation) (Melnick *et al.*, 1973; Benveniste *et al.*, 1974b), particularly by culturing baboon cells with cells from heterologous species, that they could clearly be shown to be true type C virus and to be fully characterized as new viruses. *Thus, unlike any other primate, baboons appear not to have strong control over their endogenous virus, and apparently the virus has been out of control for a long period.*

The baboon virus (BaEV) isolates are closely related to one another in their biological properties, in the relatedness of their antigenic proteins, and in the similarities of the nucleotide sequences of their RNA genomes, but they are distinct from all other type C viruses. They are truly endogenous to baboons, and there are phylogenetically related genes in DNA from other primates (Benveniste and Todaro, 1976; Wong-Staal *et al.*, 1976).

The baboon virus has been of particular interest for at least two reasons. (1) If it were a truly endogenous virus of primates and evolved as the species evolved, it might provide useful molecular probes for determining whether other Old World primates (including man) possess related virogenes and, inferentially, harbor their own endogenous type C virus. Indeed, this was found to be the case (Benveniste and Todaro, 1974c,1976; Wong-Staal *et al.*, 1976). We believe that these viral-related genes serve a useful biological role (Mayer *et al.*, 1974; Gillespie and Gallo, 1975) and that the release of infectious type C virus is usually accidental. It would follow that most primates "tightly" control the expression of their virogenes whereas baboons for some reason cannot. (2) As was noted earlier, the baboon endogenous viruses are easy to isolate and hence may be viewed as out of normal host control. Supporting this is evidence that the baboon virus (or an ancestral precursor) was transmitted into the germ line of the ancestor of the domestic cat some 3 to 10 million years ago in Africa (Benveniste and Todaro, 1974a). This transmitted virus appears to be the precursor of today's endogenous class 1 virus of domestic cats, RD-114. It appears then that this type of virus has been out of control in baboons and cats for an extensive period. These results have major implications to our isolation of a virus highly related to the baboon endogenous virus from a woman with AML (Gallagher and Gallo, 1975; Teich *et al.*, 1975), and to our recent evidence for proviral sequences highly related to sequences of the baboon virus RNA genome in DNA from some people with leukemia (Wong-Staal *et al.*, 1976; and see later).

## 11.2. Type C RNA Viruses in Human Cells

Class 2, type C RNA tumor viruses cause sarcomas and leukemias in a variety of animal model systems. In some (chickens, wild-type mice, cats, cows, and captive gibbons), they may be the major natural cause of leukemia in the species. On this basis, it seems reasonable to see whether the same could be true in humans. On the other hand, chemicals can cause tumors in (apparently) virus-free animals, *so one need not expect that all human sarcomas and leukemias would have a viral etiology, even if evidence for viral involvement can be demonstrated in some cases.* This may be an important qualification to make, for particular viral markers are found in human cells only rarely. Widespread presence of some markers has been reported, but in our experience most viral markers are detectable in only a small fraction of patients examined. As will be discussed later, there are several possibilities which might account for the usual failure to detect evidence for acquired virus even if such virus were responsible for all leukemias.

## 11.2.1. Detection of Type C RNA Virus Components in Tissue of Leukemic Patients

### 11.2.1.1. Reverse Transcriptase; Direct Demonstration

The direct demonstration of reverse transcriptase is defined here as the detection of an enzyme capable of synthesizing DNA copies of RNA and having structural and/or immunological similarity to reverse transcriptase from laboratory RNA tumor viruses. Of blood leukocyte samples from many patients only 10 cases have been reported to contain reverse transcriptase that meets this criteria. The enzyme activity detected in human cells chromatographed on DEAE-cellulose, phosphocellulose, and hydroxyapatite-like viral reverse transcriptase. It had a molecular weight of about 70,000 (Sarngadharan *et al.*, 1972; Gallo *et al.*, 1974) and an aggregate form of molecular weight 140,000 (Mondal *et al.*, 1974). It utilized poly A and heteropolymeric RNA as template for DNA synthesis *in vitro* (Sarngadharan *et al.*, 1972), and the utilization of poly A was inhibited by antisera raised against reverse transcriptase of simian sarcoma virus and gibbon ape leukemia virus (Mondal *et al.*, 1974; Todaro and Gallo, 1973; Gallo *et al.*, 1974). The utilization of RNA templates required a complementary primer (Sarngadharan *et al.*, 1972).

This enzyme activity has been found only in blood leukocytes from patients with acute myelogenous leukemia, of patients tested. In the cases of patients with chronic myelogenous leukemia in chronic or acute phase, patients with chronic lymphocytic leukemia, and patients with acute lymphocytic leukemia the enzyme was not found. A spleen sample from a child with myelofibrosis was reported to contain high levels of viral-related reverse transcriptase. This enzyme was also antigenically closely related to reverse transcriptase of the simian sarcoma virus–gibbon ape leukemia virus group (Steele *et al.*, 1977). This is of particular interest in view of the preleukemic nature of myelofibrosis.

Often an enzyme or enzymes having *some* of the properties of viral reverse transcriptase could be detected in human tumor tissue. Many reports show enzyme activities in extracts of tumor tissue capable of utilizing oligo dT · poly A but not oligo dT · poly dA as primer template for DNA synthesis *in vitro* that is missing or present at low levels in normal "control" tissue. In most cases in which this activity has been found it has not had the biophysical and immunological properties of reverse transcriptase, but behaves more like cell DNA polymerase γ (Gallo *et al.*, 1974). Thus, while the rigid criteria listed herein may create false negative results by being too selective, enzyme activities that have not met these criteria usually have been shown not to be reverse transcriptase. An exception to this may be the enzyme activity purified from the spleen of a patient with chronic lymphocytic leukemia and having biophysical and biochemical properties in common with reverse transcriptases of laboratory viruses (Witkin *et al.*, 1975) but lacking immunological relatedness to them (Spiegelman, personal communication). This type of enzyme has also been found in our laboratory in blood cells from about 35 leukemic patients. Although antisera raised against reverse transcriptases of simian sarcoma–leukemia virus, Rauscher leukemia virus, the feline endogenous virus RD-114, feline leukemia virus, and avian myeloblastosis virus have been tested, only the antisera prepared against the reverse transcriptases of SSV-SSAV and gibbon ape leukemia virus inhibit the DNA polymerase activity from human leukemic cells, and then only occasionally (Gallo *et al.*, 1974; Gallo, Gallagher, and Saxinger, unpublished results). It could be that this polymerase, biochemically a reverse transcriptase but not detectably antigenically related to known viral reverse transcriptase, does nonetheless represent a viral reverse transcriptase, but the appropriate viral immunological reagent has not yet been tested. For instance, it will, of course, be of interest to test those polymerases which are biochemically like viral reverse transcriptase but did not show antigenic relatedness to reverse transcriptase of the simian sarcoma virus–gibbon ape leukemia virus group (or to reverse transcriptase from any other virus tested) with antibodies prepared against reverse transcriptase from baboon endogenous virus. (For recent reviews emphasizing findings of reverse transcriptase in cells see Sarin and Gallo, 1974; Wu and Gallo, 1975. For detailed methods see Sarngadharan *et al.*, 1976.)

### 11.2.1.2. High Molecular Weight RNA; Direct Demonstration

The RNA genome of all type C RNA viruses studied is an aggregate of two "subunit" RNA molecules, each 5000 nucleotides in length. The isolation of such an RNA from human tumors has not been reported.

### 11.2.1.3. Reverse Transcriptase and High Molecular Weight RNA; Simultaneous (Indirect) Demonstration

The synthesis of cDNA on a viral RNA template mediated by endogenous reverse transcriptase results in a complex consisting of a short DNA chain complexed with the much larger template viral RNA. If the DNA is radiolabeled and the template RNA is not, the biophysical properties of the label will be like that of the template. It has been reported that the cytoplasm of human tumor cells generally contains the apparatus for synthesizing DNA on a high molecular weight RNA whereas the cytoplasm of a variety of tissues from normal humans does not (Schlom and Spiegelman, 1971; Baxt *et al.*, 1972; Gallo *et al.*, 1973,1974). This is one marker reported to be almost characteristic of tumor cells, including sarcomas, leukemias, and carcinomas of several types (Spiegelman, 1976). It has never been shown that the assay measures anything but synthesis of cDNA on a viral RNA; however, the assay is indirect and the reaction product has not been analyzed in detail. It is not clear whether this is always a consequence of viral infection or can be due to endogenous virogene expression. (For a more detailed discussion see reviews by Sarin and Gallo, 1974, and Wu and Gallo, 1975.)

### 11.2.1.4. Viral-Related Sequences in RNA from Human Tumor Tissue

This assay has been carried out by hybridizing partial DNA copies of the RNA genome of laboratory RNA tumor viruses to RNA of human cells. Using cDNA from Rauscher (Kufe *et al.*, 1972; Hehlman *et al.*, 1972; Gallo *et al.*, 1974) or Moloney (Larsen *et al.*, 1975; Tavitian *et al.*, 1976) mouse leukemia viruses, some patients with sarcomas or leukemias contain RNA sequences in malignant tissues capable of hybridizing more of the cDNA than can be hybridized by RNA of tissues from normal donors. Similar results have been obtained with cDNA from baboon endogenous virus (Reitz and Gallo, unpublished results) and simian sarcoma virus (Gallo *et al.*, 1974; Tavitian *et al.*, 1976). The amount of cDNA hybridized is usually so low and the cell RNA so complex that the results are quite difficult to interpret in terms of the presence of a particular viral RNA. No purification of the relevant RNA from human tumor tissue has been reported.

### 11.2.1.5. Viral-Related Sequences in cDNA Synthesized by Cytoplasmic Particles of Human Leukemic Tissues

cDNA can be synthesized *in vitro* by a cytoplasmic, particulate fraction from fresh uncultured human leukemic cells (Baxt *et al.*, 1972; Sarngadharan *et al.*, 1972; Gallo *et al.*, 1973,1974). A portion of the sequences in this cDNA hybridizes to RNA from some mammalian RNA tumor viruses. From particles purified by differential centrifugation (100–5000S) about 1–10% of the sequences hybridize to viral RNA. As much as 50–60% of the sequences are viral related if synthesized by cytoplasmic particles subsequently purified by isopycnic fractionation in sucrose gradient (Gallo *et al.*, 1973,1974; Reitz *et al.*, 1976). In the case of the isopycnically purified particles, both the cDNA and viral RNA are relatively pure so one can be confident of examining specific cDNA–RNA hybridization. cDNA synthesized by isopycnically purified cytoplasmic particles in blood leukocytes from patients with myelogenous leukemia shows relatedness to the primate class 1 and 2 viruses, i.e., to baboon endogenous virus (Reitz *et al.*, 1976), simian sarcoma virus (Gallo *et al.*, 1973,1974; Reitz *et al.*, 1976; Mak *et al.*, 1975), and to a class 2 virus of both mouse and rat origin, Kirsten sarcoma–leukemia virus (Gallo et al., 1973,1974; Miller et al., 1974). About half of the cDNA sequences hybridized to RNA from one of these viruses in over 90% of a total of 20 cases examined (for a summary, see Gallo et al., 1974). A smaller fraction (5–20%) of the cDNA routinely hybridized to RNA from mouse viruses. The sequences complementary to the RNA of simian sarcoma virus apparently are not the same as those complementary to the RNA of murine leukemia virus (Tavitian et al., 1976). Particles from none of the patients synthesized cDNA that hybridized significantly to RNA from feline leukemia virus or avian myeloblastosis virus.

### 11.2.1.6. Viruslike Particles in Human Leukemic Cells

All the virus markers described previously are recoverable from small, cytoplasmic particles in leukemic tissues. The buoyant density of the particles capable of synthesizing cDNA with viral sequences (Baxt et al., 1972; Todaro and Gallo, 1973; Gallo et al., 1973) or of synthesizing the simultaneous detection complex (Baxt et al., 1972) (see Section 11.2.1.4) is between 1.18 and 1.2 g/ml. In a few cases of cytoplasmic particles from blood leukocytes of leukemic patients, the particles were shown to be about 1000S and convertible to a 200–500S form ($p$ 1.25 g/ml) after treatment with nonionic detergent (Gallo et al., 1974). Blood leukocytes from normal donors also contain cytoplasmic particles capable of synthesizing small amounts of cDNA in vitro, but this synthesis, at least in part, appears to be DNA directed (Bobrow et al., 1972; Reitz et al., 1974; Gallo et al., 1974).

### 11.2.1.7. Viral Structural Proteins in Human Tumor Cells

There have been some reports describing proteins in human tumor cells that immunologically cross-react with antisera raised against a variety of RNA tumor viruses or against structural proteins (generally p30) purified from them (Strand and August, 1974; Sherr and Todaro, 1974, 1975; Nooter et al., 1975; Mellors and Mellors, 1976; Metzgar et al., 1976). As with other viral markers, the cross-reacting proteins are found only infrequently. The positive results have been criticized (Stephenson and Aaronson, 1976) because the human antigens were not purified. Some studies involving partial purification of proteins from human tumors and quantitative, sensitive radioimmune assays have yielded impressive negative results (Stephenson and Aaronson, 1976). These experiments serve to show that if viral proteins do exist in human tumors, their frequency and/or concentration must be low or their antigenic cross-reactivity is unstable. However, experiments of this sort cannot be used as a basis for dismissing consideration of the viral etiology of human tumors, especially since model systems exist in which cell transformation is not accompanied by expression of viral proteins (Aaronson *et al.*, 1975). Nonetheless, there is no concrete and noncontested evidence for the presence of viral proteins, excepting reverse transcriptase (see Section 11.2.1.1), in human tumor cells, and in our view the presence of a *viral-related* reverse transcriptase has only rarely been documented.

### 11.2.1.8. Viral Sequence in DNA of Human Tumors

*11.2.1.8a. "Extra" Sequences.* The cDNA synthesized by cytoplasmic particles of human tumor tissues contains some sequences (about 1% of the total) that hybridize to nuclear DNA from the same tumor but not to DNA from normal control tissue (Baxt and Spiegelman, 1972; Baxt *et al.*, 1973; Baxt, 1974). In two cases, the control tissue was from an identical twin of the donor of the tumor tissue (blood leukocytes of a leukemic individual) (Baxt *et al.*, 1973). To enrich for the "extra" sequences in the cDNA preparation, sequences that hybridize to DNA from a normal tissue are first removed (Baxt and Spiegelman, 1972). It is the "recycled" residue that contains the "extra" sequences (up to 50% of the total, but as little as none). Of the recycled cDNA sequences, some are viral related (i.e., hybridize to the RNA of a type C animal virus) (Baxt, 1974). There is little published to indicate the regularity of occurrence of extra sequences in tumor tissue, partly because the recycled DNA probe is difficult to prepare in quantity, and the experiments are very difficult. The simplest interpretation of the positive results is that the cells were infected some time after fertilization by a type C virus.

*11.2.1.8b. Proviral DNA Sequences Related to the RNA Genome of Baboon Endogenous Virus in Human Tumor Tissues.* Except·for the small fraction related to RNA of Rauscher leukemia virus, the extra DNA sequences in human tumors just described are not defined as related to any known laboratory RNA tumor virus. Attempts have been made to hybridize viral RNA or cDNA to genomic DNA from human tumors but predominantly negative results have been reported (Gallo *et al.*, 1974). RNA and/or cDNA from simian sarcoma–leukemia virus, gibbon ape leukemia virus, Rauscher mouse leukemia virus, and Kirsten mouse–rat sarcoma–leukemia virus hybridize equally to DNA from human tumor or normal tissues (Benveniste and Todaro, 1974c, 1976; Benveniste *et al.*, 1974a; Scolnick *et al.*, 1974; Gallo *et al.*, 1974; summarized in Gillespie *et al.*, 1975b, and more recently in Gallo *et al.*, 1977). A few high values were obtained with cDNA from baboon endogenous virus (Benveniste and Todaro, 1976), but the authors chose to call them "spurious." All reports that have given negative results involved studies of relatively few tumor samples (10–20 in total).

In contrast are the following recent results from our laboratory. Hybridizations with RNA from baboon endogenous virus labeled to $10^8$ cpm/$\mu$g with $^{125}$I have resulted in the detection of DNA sequences in tissues from *some* leukemic patients (about 10–20%) that are not detectable in the DNA of at least most normal human tissues (Wong-Staal *et al.*, 1976; Reitz *et al.*, 1976). It is particularly difficult to demonstrate the presence of baboon virus-related *extra* (proviral) DNA sequences in human tumor tissues, that is, sequences not found in DNA of normal humans, because normal humans contain sequences in their DNA which are evolutionarily related to the baboon virogene sequences, much in the same way that genes coding for hemoglobin in the two species would be related. The situation with baboon endogenous virus sequences is not quite as difficult as with other structural genes in terms of normal humans containing related sequences because the baboon endogenous virogenes appear to have evolved at about three times the rate of the bulk of single-copy DNA sequences. Thus, 20 times more of the sequences in cDNA from baboon endogenous virus hybridizes to normal baboon than to normal human DNA (Benveniste and Todaro, 1976) and four times more of the sequences in RNA from the same virus show this specificity (Wong-Staal *et al.*, 1976).

The evidence (Wong-Staal *et al.*, 1976) for proviral sequences related to baboon endogenous virus in DNA of human tumor tissues is the following. First, using a fixed cell DNA-to-$^{125}$I-labeled RNA weight ratio ($10^7$:1) and varying the time of hybridization, DNA from spleens or blood leukocytes from some patients with leukemia hybridize about three times more of the sequences in the [$^{125}$I]RNA than were hybridized by DNA of normal human tissues. The hybridization reaction was taken to a condition ($C_0 t = 2 \times 10^4$, with respect to DNA) in which hybridization of the RNA to single-copy DNA sequences was nearly complete. Some of the hybridization of the [$^{125}$I]RNA to DNA from the positive leukemic patients proceeded more slowly than the case of hybridization of the same RNA to DNA from a single-copy standard, suggesting that the presence of some of the proviral sequences was restricted to a particular fraction of cells in the tissues.

Second, when the time of hybridization was held constant and the DNA/RNA ratio was varied, DNA from some leukemic tissues hybridized three times more of the sequences in the [$^{125}$I]RNA than could be hybridized by DNA from normal human tissues, even at the highest DNA/RNA ratio ($>10^8$:1). When the data were subjected to a double reciprocal analysis and extrapolated to an infinite DNA/RNA ratio, DNA from the positive leukemics and normal tissues still showed the threefold differential. Thus, the sequences in the leukemics that hybridized the extra sequences in RNA of baboon endogenous virus were not detectable, even at very low frequency (<0.1–0.01 copies per cell), in DNA from normal humans.

Third, the thermal stability of the hybrids with DNA from tissues of the positive leukemic patients was some 5° higher than that of hybrids involving DNA from normal humans. This suggests a *qualitative* difference between the new proviral sequences in DNA from leukemic cells and the sequences in DNA from normal humans and presumably also in the DNA from leukemic cells that are evolutionarily related to baboon endogenous virogenes.

The fraction of the hybridizable sequences in [$^{125}$I]RNA from baboon endogenous virus reported to hybridize to DNA *from the positive* leukemic patients ranged from 30 to 70% of the RNA compared to 20 to 25% hybridized by DNA from normal tissues (Wong-Staal *et al.,* 1976). However, our unpublished results with N. Miller, M. Reitz, and F. Wong-Staal suggest that DNA from malignant tissues of the *majority* of leukemic patients does not hybridize significantly more of the sequences in RNA from baboon endogenous virus than is hybridized by DNA from a variety of tissues from normal humans. The detection of proviral sequences related to baboon endogenous virus by hybridization with RNA from the virus is a relatively unusual event, occurring in some 10–20% of the patients tested (about 60 patients), as is the case with other viral markers (see earlier). It cannot be predicted whether cDNA from the same virus or related viruses will detect proviral sequences more or less frequently, but we note that using cDNA from baboon endogenous virus it has been documented that DNA from 3 of 36 human tumors tested gave unexpectedly high hybridization values (Benveniste and Todaro, 1976).

*11.2.1.8c. Other Proviral Sequences in DNA of Human Tumor Tissue.* The hybridization of cDNA from Rauscher leukemia virus to DNA from some solid tissues from some patients with leukemia or lymphoma yields positive results in some 10–20% of the patients tested (unpublished results with G. Aulakh, N. Miller, and F. Wong-Staal; also W. Baxt, personal communication). Positive results, involving hybridization of 20–50% of the cDNA sequences compared to less than 10% hybridized by DNA from normal human tissues, were first detected by chromatography of the hybrids on hydroxyapatite (with G. Aulakh). This was subsequently confirmed by monitoring hybrid formation with S1 nuclease (with N. Miller and F. Wong-Staal). Surprisingly, with DNA from blood leukocytes of leukemic patients, complexes that bind hydroxyapatite could be detected, but these were not resistant to S1 nuclease (unpublished results with N. Miller and F. Wong-Staal).

DNA from some humans hybridizes a substantially larger fraction of the sequences in RNA or cDNA from simian sarcoma–leukemia virus (over 50%) than can be hybridized to DNA from tissues of most humans (10–15%), when hybrid formation is monitored by resistance to S1 nuclease (with M. Reitz and F. Wong-Staal, unpublished observations). However, positive results with probes from this virus have been very rare and the number of DNA samples analyzed is too small to estimate the frequency at which these sequences are detected.

In no case has it been adequately documented that the putative proviral sequences are confined to malignant tissues of cancer patients or even to persons with malignancies. There is no reason to anticipate that either correlation will hold, even it it proves that RNA tumor viruses are involved in the etiology of human cancer (see Section 11.2.2).

### 11.2.1.9. Type C Viruses Obtained from Human Cells

Particles *resembling* RNA tumor viruses have been observed by microscopy in a variety of human tumor tissues and in some tissues from apparently normal humans (for reviews, see Gillespie *et al.*, 1975b). Following culturing of human cells the short-term release of morphologically similar particles having a density of about 1.16 g/ml, a reverse transcriptaselike activity, high molecular weight RNA, and capable of synthesizing cDNA with viral-related sequences has also been reported (Mak *et al.*, 1974,1975). The best characterized particles, released by bone marrow cells from leukemic patients, are apparently not infectious.

The release of infectious virus from fresh human tissues has never been reported. The release of infectious particles following a few (Gallagher and Gallo, 1974; Teich *et al.*, 1975; Nooter *et al.*, 1975; Gabelman *et al.*, 1975) or many (Panem *et al.*, 1975) passages in culture of human cells has recently been reported by investigators in several laboratories, although this clearly must be a very rare event. The first case involved blood leukocytes (Gallagher and Gallo, 1974) and later bone marrow cells (Teich *et al.*, 1975) from a patient who had and subsequently died of acute myelogenous leukemia (patient HL23). Cells from 20 other leukemic patients and from numerous cell lines from normal persons or persons with neoplastic disease have failed to release virus in the same laboratory (Gallagher *et al.*, 1975; Gallo, Gallagher, Markham, and Ruscetti, unpublished results). The viruses released from cells of patient HL23 were of two types, one related to simian sarcoma–leukemic virus and a second related to baboon endogenous virus (Teich *et al.*, 1975; Chan *et al.*, 1976; Stephenson *et al.*, 1976; Reitz *et al.*, 1976). The virus was reisolated three times from independently drawn clinical samples (Gallagher *et al.*, 1975; see Gallo, 1976, for a review of the isolations). The fresh spleen of patient

HL23 contained proviral sequences related to the baboon endogenous virus but did not carry detectable amounts of DNA related to simian sarcoma–leukemia virus (Reitz *et al.*, 1976; Wong-Staal *et al.*, 1976). CDNA synthesized by cytoplasmic particles from fresh, uncultured blood leukocytes of patient HL23 contained some sequences related to the genome of baboon endogenous virus and others related to the genome of simian sarcoma virus (Reitz *et al.*, 1976). Finally, the fresh blood leukocytes (uncultured) were shown to contain reverse transcriptase antigenically related to the reverse transcriptase of simian sarcoma virus (Mondal *et al.*, 1974). Thus the patient herself had the genetic capacity to generate nucleotide sequences related to those found in the viruses released by her cultured cells. Interestingly, a known contact of patient HL23 who also had acute myelogenous leukemia also had proviral DNA sequences related to those of baboon endogenous virus (Wong-Staal *et al.*, 1976).

A similar pair of infectious viruses have been released from human embryo cells after many (35–50) passages in culture (Panem *et al.*, 1975). Release by two cell lines has been studied in detail. The cell lines show: (a) no evidence of virus expression for 10–20 passages in culture, (b) intracellular expression of viral proteins during passages 20–35, and (c) spontaneously released infectious virus at later passages. The exact scheduling of events may be different with each cell line. The presence of viral nucleic acid components in the early passage cells has not been reported. In both cases once the cells produce viruses two virus types were released, one related to simian sarcoma virus and a second related to baboon endogenous virus (Prochownik *et al.*, 1977, personal communication; unpublished results with M. Reitz and N. Miller).

The release of infectious viruses from human tumor cells has also been recently reported by other laboratories (Nooter *et al.*, 1975; Gabelman *et al.*, 1975; Balbanova *et al.*, 1975; Vosika *et al.*, 1975). In two cases, the release of virus related to simian sarcoma virus is documented (Nooter *et al.*, 1975; Gabelman *et al.*, 1975). In the same two cases, the possibility of release of a second virus related to baboon endogenous virus was not tested; in the remaining two cases the nature of the viruses is unknown.

## 11.2.2. Natural Antibodies in Humans to Primate Type C Viruses

If type C viruses have entered the human population from congenital infection or from classical horizontal infection, we might anticipate finding one or more natural antibodies in the sera of humans directed against the virus or viruses in question. There admittedly could be situations in which this would not be true; for example, if only a few cells were infected or if there was integration of only partial provirus, one may not necessarily develop antibodies to viral proteins. This may be particularly true if the infection developed *in utero*. We conclude that negative data are not meaningful in deciding whether humans can be infected by RNA tumor viruses but positive results from carefully conducted experiments are. To test for antiviral antibodies in human sera we must have the "right" viral reagents, i.e., those of the appropriate virus(es) or those of viruses closely related to the infecting virus(es). As indicated, the primate type C viruses were isolated relatively recently; the most compelling evidence for specific type C viral components in humans involves components related or identical to those of the primate type C viruses. Though seroepidemiological studies using reagents from primate viruses are only just beginning, there are already interesting results, albeit not without controversy. The reported results, searching for natural antibodies in humans directed against proteins of RNA tumor viruses (all within the last year), fall into two groups: (a) Negative results were obtained with two *purified* primate type C viral proteins, p30 and gp69/71. P30 is the protein which is the major antigenic determinant of a type C virus, an internal structural protein with a molecular weight of about 30,000. Gp69/71 is the major viral envelope protein. It is a glycoprotein of molecular weight 69,000–71,000. The approach utilized immune precipitation of these purified, radiolabeled viral proteins by human sera. The negative results were reported by Stephenson and Aaronson (1976). (b) Positive results were obtained with whole primate type C virus by showing either precipitation of specific proteins (Gp69/71) associated with disrupted, radiolabeled virus by human sera (Snyder *et al.*, 1976; Kurth *et al.*, 1976) or by showing through immune electron microscopy the tagging (by ferritin-conjugated human antibodies) of specific primate type C virus budding from cells which had been deliberately infected with the virus (Aoki *et al.*, 1976). Although these approaches are certainly more crude than those using purified viral proteins and have not established conclusively the nature of the protein involved, they do seem to be the more natural approaches to begin the search for antibodies. From this approach one can proceed to determine the exact protein or proteins involved. The published positive reports have, in general, tended to rule out artifacts arising from calf serum, heterophile antigens, ABO blood group proteins, complement, and Forsmanlike antigens. Moreover, in two of the reports, evidence for specificity to the primate type C viruses was shown (Aoki *et al.*, 1976; Kurth *et al.*, 1977), and the antibodies could be removed by absorption of the sera with the virus in question (Aoki *et al.*, 1976) or with a fraction of the virus containing gp69/71 protein (Snyder *et al.*, 1976). However, more specificity studies and a clear delineation of the protein detected are needed. It should be noted that these antibodies are reported to react with viruses such as the HL23 virus isolated from a woman with AML (Gallagher and Gallo, 1974) and the HEL-12 virus isolated from a human embryo (Panem *et al.*, 1975) or with the HL23 and HEL-12 viruses themselves.

The distribution of the antibodies in the population is of considerable interest. Kurth *et al.* (1977) have reported that 100% of normal individuals contain antibodies to the baboon virus and 49% have antibodies to the simian sarcoma virus–gibbon leukemia virus group. Aoki has also found that a high proportion of normal individuals have antibody to both these primate virus groups (Aoki *et al.*, 1976). Both groups have evidence that people with leukemia have little or no detectable antibody (personal communication of R. Kurth, N. Teich, and R. Weiss, and of T. Aoki). These results may have important etiological implications.

It will be important now (a) to carry out prospective studies especially on high risk individuals; (b) to determine the precise proteins involved directly (data available suggest that it involves viral envelope proteins and possibly p30); (c) to clarify the discrepancy with the negative results reported by Stephenson and Aaronson utilizing purified proteins from the onset. Regarding the latter, Aoki has pointed out that the purification and/or iodination procedure may modify or be responsible for loss of the antigenic determinants, and that the assay may not be sufficiently sensitive and might miss the low levels of antibody in human sera. In any case, it is of great importance to resolve this issue.

## 11.3. Summary and Interpretations

Type C RNA tumor viruses may be endogenous or they may be acquired. Some are known to be major factors in the cause of leukemia in certain species, but many have no known pathogenic effect. This seems particularly true of the endogenous viruses which could be serving some unknown normal function. In instances in which there is strong evidence for their involvement in the etiology of leukemia, the virus is usually of the acquired type (chickens, wild-type mice, cats, cows, and gibbon apes). In a few animals with acquired virus as an etiological factor, virus replication is extensive, and the virus is usually easy to isolate. This had led to the view that if acquired virus is present in man, it too should be easy to isolate, but this is not logical. Acquired viruses may be much more widespread than currently known, but for many reasons it may be difficult or impossible to isolate in many species. It is those few animals with very active virus replication that may be the exceptions, not man.

Isolations of type C viruses from primates were achieved in recent years, and they include members of both virus groups, i.e., acquired and endogenous. The acquired ones have been shown to cause sarcoma, lymphoma, or leukemia. Human tumors including leukemias are, of course, not ordinarily virus productive, but intracytoplasmic, viruslike particles have been frequently identified in leukemic blood or bone marrow cells. These may be defective virus. In *one* case, a woman with AML, *complete* infectious virus (HL23V) was isolated. The virus is highly related to the known subhuman primate type C viruses. Some evidence has strongly indicated that the virus is not a contaminant. This includes repeat isolation of the virus from separate clinical specimens and the detection of nucleic acid sequences in the fresh tissue (spleen) of the patient related to the RNA of HL23 viruses. Recent results have shown the presence of proviral sequences in the DNA of fresh uncultured tissues of several patients with leukemia and some with lymphoma. These results and Spiegelman's extra sequences provide evidence for acquired type C viral information in man.

It is sometimes argued that to be etiologically relevant a virus must be commonly identified. We do not agree with this reasoning. The leukemias may be heterogeneous diseases with more than one cause, even more than one viral etiology. In short, we cannot say that the HL23 virus was the cause of the leukemia in patient HL23 nor that the viral information similar to information contained in HL23 virus found in a fraction of other leukemic patients was causative in them. On the other hand, the failure to obtain similar results in all leukemic patients does not preclude their importance in some. It is also possible that this information is present in all patients, but not detectable because only some cells contain the viral information or the information is partial (see below). In fact some recent seroepidemiological results suggest that viruses related or identical to the HL23 viruses may be widespread in man. If so, other factors may be important in determining their pathogenicity. If the serological results are correct, our molecular hybridization approaches are of insufficient sensitivity to provide an estimate of the distribution of viral nucleic acid sequences in the population.

## 11.4. Deductions Concerning Viral Etiology of Human Leukemia

If, as has been reported, normal humans contain natural antibodies directed against primate type C RNA viruses, we would be forced to conclude that infection of the human population is widespread. After infection the viruses can replicate in the human body to the extent that viral antigen(s) is produced in sufficient quantity to stimulate an immune response. At least one of the virus groups implicated is tumorigenic (sarcomagenic and/or leukemogenic) in subhuman primates, so we must consider that they may be leukemogenic in humans as well. *A priori* we expected that these viruses, or molecular markers identifying their presence, would be concentrated in leukemic cells, e.g., in the blast cells of the peripheral blood of leukemic patients.

Our experience with markers in leukemic blood leukocytes, specifically with viral-related reverse transcriptase, viral-related DNA sequences synthesized by cytoplasmic particles, viral-related cytoplasmic RNA, and proviral DNA sequences (Gallo *et al.*, 1974; Gillespie *et al.*, 1975b) and with release of virus particles (Gallagher *et al.*, 1975) shows clearly *that these markers are rare* and are *not characteristic of leukemic blood cell* samples, and suggest strongly that when they are present it is in *a minority of the blood cell population* (e.g., see Gallo *et al.*, 1974,1977). This vexing conclusion is supported by related work from other laboratories and by the electron microscope work of Seman and Seman (1968), who have reported type C viruslike particles in large numbers in blood cells of leukemic patients but *only* in a very small fraction of the blood cell population.

At this point we do not know whether those viral markers detected in leukemic blood cells are produced by infected blood cells or are taken up by uninfected blood cells via phagocytosis or related processes. It is our working model that the markers are not, *in themselves,* responsible for the "blast phenotype" of the leukemic blood cell population and that the antiviral immune response in humans it not directed against antigens produced by infected blood cells.

To conclude that human cells are infected by a type C RNA virus, that the infection event is important to leukemogenesis, but that leukemic blood blast cells themselves do not contain replicating virus or complete viral information seems paradoxical, but we feel that we must be able to link these events. We present five working hypotheses which we believe are consistent with the available data.

## Hypothesis 1: "Partial Provirus Integration"

In this hypothesis it is proposed that it is the leukemic cells or their precursor cells which are infected by a type C virus, but that a complete DNA provirus is not integrated. Instead only a fragment is integrated, a fragment sufficient to transform the cells but insufficient to lead to regular production of viral proteins. Of course this would not yield whole virus either. Whole virus would be a very rare event, requiring the integration of essentially the whole provirus. The most serious problem

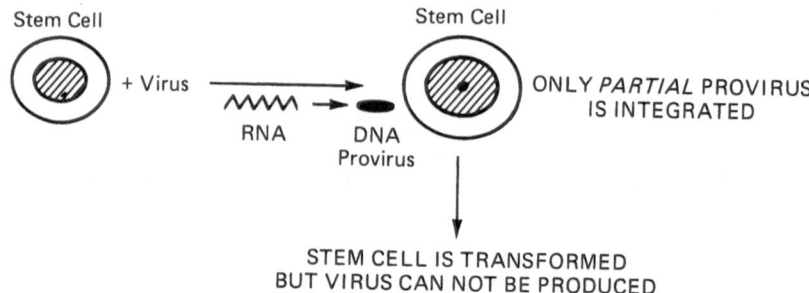

**Fig. 2.** Partial provirus model (leukemic cells intrinsically abnormal) (model 1). In this model, like the first one given, the stem cell is infected by an acquired RNA tumor virus leading to transformation to a leukemic cell. However, in this case only a *partial* DNA provirus is synthesized and/or integrated into the host cell chromosomal DNA. Daughter cells will all be transformed and contain partial provirus. The partial provirus carries sufficient genetic information to transform the cell, but a virus usually cannot be isolated because ordinarily there is insufficient viral information integrated. Viral proteins would be limited and difficult to detect, and provirus would be very difficult to detect.

with this model is that there is no direct proof in animal models that partial proviruses can occur with RNA tumor viruses. However, it is known with DNA tumor viruses and there is evidence consistent with the partial integration model for RNA tumor viruses (Scolnick *et al.*, 1973).

In the context of our ideas on the nature of human leukemic cells, cell transformation caused by partial provirus integration is equatable with differentiation arrest. Whether this occurs by synthesis of a critical viral protein coded by the provirus fragment (Temin, 1971), by "switching on" of endogenous oncogene–virogene sequences (Huebner and Todaro, 1969), by RNA "paraprocessing" (Gillespie and Gallo, 1975), by loss of response to diffusible growth-regulating factors (see below), or by some other mechanism is not resolved. This model is illustrated in Fig. 2.

## Hypothesis 2: "Double Infection"

This model (see Fig. 3) has been presented in detail previously and suggests that if type C RNA viruses contribute to leukemia, there may be two separate infection events (Gillespie and Gallo, 1976). One involves an unknown target cell capable of supporting virus replication (and usually leading to an immune response capable of suppressing that replication) and a second ultimately resulting in the transformation of blood cells. The second infection was compared to a "nonproductive" infection in model systems, involving partial integration of provirus and resulting in cell transformation often without detectable expression of virus markers.

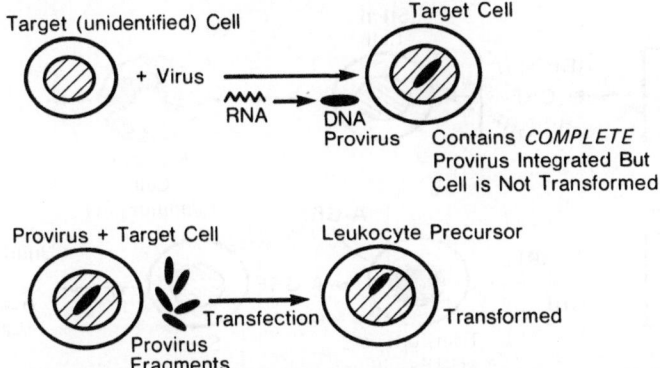

**Fig. 3.** Double infection model (leukemic cells intrinsically abnormal) (model 2). Unlike model 1 (Fig. 2) and the classical scheme (Fig. 1), in this hypothesis the initial cell to be infected is not a leukemic cell progenitor cell. Instead a "double infection" is suggested. In the first step an undesignated target cell is infected by an RNA tumor virus. Complete provirus is integrated but the cell need not be transformed. However, it produces virus which may infect a leukocyte precursor (stem cell), leading to integration (as in model 2) of a partial provirus and transformation of the secondarily infected cell. Any *antiviral* immune response is directed against the virus-producing cell or virus produced by those cells. Any *antitumor* immune response is directed against the secondarily infected, transformed leukocyte precursor. Alternatively, and as depicted here, the secondary event may be by transfection by a DNA fragment derived from the original target cell. The consequences from this point is as for model 2. Complete provirus can be confined to the rare cell (original target cell) of any body tissue. Clonally derived tumor cells will only contain small pieces of provirus.

## Hypothesis 3: "Leukemic Blood Cells Are Intrinsically Normal but a Regulator Cell Is Transformed"

This model (see Fig. 4) proposes that growth and differentiation of leukocytes (particularly granulocytic cells and their precursors) requires factors (proteins) which are produced by other cells (probably hematopoietic). It is the factor-producing cell which is infected. It produces abnormal or insufficient growth (differentiation) regulatory proteins leading to abnormal expansion of the receptor cell compartment. This hypothesis is attractive for several reasons, and there are observations which indicate that leukemic blood cells from at least some patients with AML and CML can be induced *in vitro* to differentiate with appropriate factors (Paran *et al.*, 1970; Gallagher *et al.*, 1975; Gallagher and Gallo, 1977). However, a major difficulty with this hypothesis is the fact that leukemic cells usually show chromosomal abnormalities, indicating they are not intrinsically normal but directly affected by whatever caused the disease.

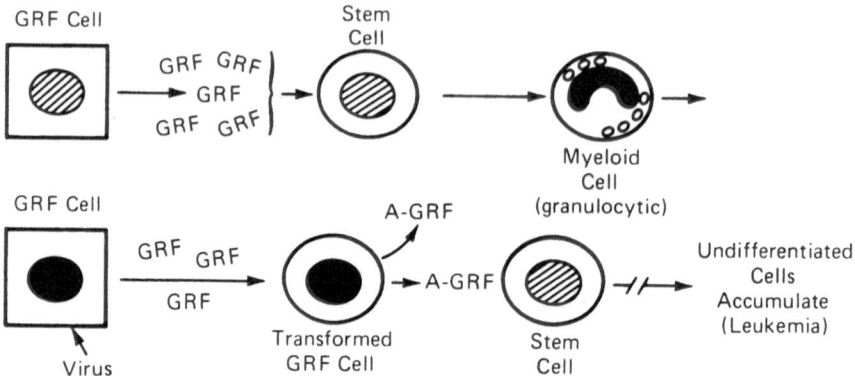

**Fig. 4.** Leukemic cells secondarily affected (but intrinsically normal) (model 3). Similar to model 2, in this hypothesis the original target cell is not a leukemic cell precursor but instead some undesignated cell. However, in this case the target cell is further specified as one which synthesizes and releases one or more growth regulatory factors (GRF). As discussed elsewhere (see Gallo *et al.,* 1977), these are believed to be glycoproteins which may be cell type specific. GRF induce growth and differentiation, e.g., in the granulocytic series they are important for the formation of normal, mature (nondividing) granulocytes. This cell is infected by an RNA tumor virus. Complete provirus is synthesized and integrated into one or more chromosomes of this GRF-producing cell, which leads to either insufficient production of normal GRF, an abnormal GRF (A-GRF), or both. When this occurs, normal differentiation of stem cells cannot occur, e.g., granulocytes are not made. Undifferentiated cells accumulate, thus retaining their capacity to synthesize DNA and divide. The consequence is an expanding pool of blast cells we call leukemia, but as is evident from the preceding, the so-called leukemic cells are intrinsically normal. In keeping with this model is the evidence that mouse and human myelogenous leukemia cells are not autonomous but can be induced to grow and to differentiate *in vitro* under certain conditions. Against the model are the cytogenetic abnormalities in human leukemic leukocytes (unless they are secondary phenomena) and the fact that *special* conditions appear to be required to induce maturation of leukemic myelogenous cells *in vitro.* The model predicts that a rare cell (not the leukemic blood cells) will have complete provirus, that viral proteins will be rarely found, and that the disease is at least theoretically reversible.

## Hypothesis 4: "Loss of Provirus and Differentiation Genes by Chromosomal Rearrangement"

In this model (see Fig. 5) the stem cell, a progenitor of the leukemic cell, is infected by a type C virus. The virus undergoes limited replication, stimulates an immune response, but does *not* necessarily transform the stem cell. The stem cell then contains provirus but can be transformation negative. However, the model predicts that at the site of provirus integration the chromosome is susceptible to breakage. This occurs after an undefined number of divisions of the infected cell. With chromosomal change some or all of the provirus is lost, as well as adjacent cellular genes. Some of these adjacent cellular genes may be important to cell differentia-

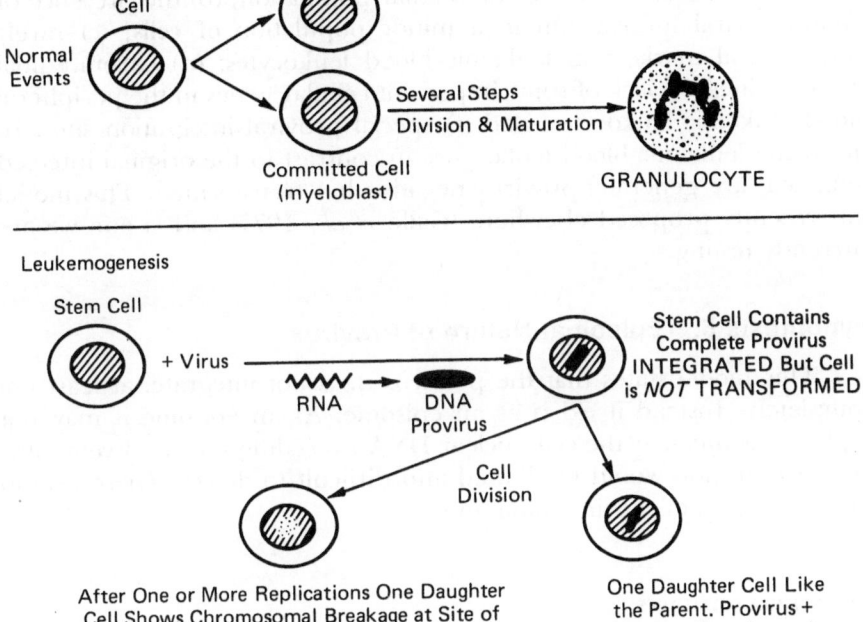

**Fig. 5.** Chromosomal break–provirus loss (model 4). Here we propose that like the classical model (Fig. 1) the leukemic cell precursor, a stem cell, is infected by an RNA tumor virus. Complete DNA provirus is synthesized and complete provirus is integrated into the stem cell chromosomal DNA. Thus, the cell is provirus positive, but unlike the situation depicted in Fig. 1, the stem cell is not transformed. Instead, after one or more cell divisions and because of the integrated provirus, the chromosome is susceptible to breakage, deletion, and translocation. Some of what is lost includes genes for normal cellular differentiation. Some or all of the provirus is also lost. Thus, it is *this* chromosomal change which directly leads to leukemia, not the presence of provirus per se. In this model, provirus is difficult to find, and may never be completely found in leukemic blood leukocytes. Similarly, release of whole virus would be a rare chance event, as would successful virus isolation.

tion. Therefore, some descendants will be blocked in normal maturation and have a proliferative advantage. The deletion is required for cell transformation. The model then predicts: (a) difficulty in finding virus markers in a total hematopoietic cellular population; (b) the presence of complete viral information in a minor population of cells; (c) rarely finding viral markers in leukemic blood leukocytes; (d) chromosomal abnormalities; (e) lack of some important cellular genes in the peripheral blood leukemic leukocytes; and (f) special proviral integration sites. In short, the leukemic blood leukocytes, in contrast to the original infected stem cell, are generally provirus negative but transformed. This model was recently proposed elsewhere (Gallo *et al.,* 1977) and is one we are currently testing.

## Hypothesis 5: "Episomal Nature of Provirus"

This model states that the provirus does not integrate, at least not completely. Instead it exists as an episome. As an episome it may not replicate as much as the cell nuclear DNA preceding mitosis. Eventually, its concentration would be diluted and difficult to detect. There are no clear examples of this in animal models.

ACKNOWLEDGMENTS

We are indebted to a number of colleagues who contributed to this work: especially Dr. Robert Gallagher, Dr. Flossie Wong-Staal, Dr. Marvin Reitz, and Dr. W. Carl Saxinger. We are also grateful for many stimulating discussions with Dr. William Jarrett and Dr. Max Essex which helped formulate some of the ideas in this chapter.

## References

Aaronson, S. A., and Dunn, C. Y., 1974, High-frequency C-type virus induction by inhibitors of protein synthesis, *Science* **183**:422.

Aaronson, S. A., Todaro, G. J., and Scolnick, E. M., 1971, Induction of murine C-type viruses from clonal lines of virus-free BALB/3T3 cells, *Science* **174**:157.

Aaronson, S. A., Stephenson, J. R., Hino, S., and Tronick, S. R., 1975, Differential expression of helper viral structural polypeptides in cells transformed by clonal isolates of woolly monkey sarcoma virus, *J. Virol.* **16**:1117.

Altaner, C., and Temin, H. M., 1970, Carcinogenesis by RNA sarcoma viruses. XII, *Virology* **40**:113.

Aoki, T., Walling, M. J., Bushar, G. S., Liu, M., and Hsu, K. C., 1976, Natural antibodies in sera from healthy humans to antigens on surfaces on type C RNA viruses and cells from primates, *Proc. Nat. Acad. Sci. U.S.A.* **73**:2491.

Balbanova, H., Kotler, M., and Becker, Y., 1975, Transformation of cultured human embryonic fibroblasts by oncornavirus-like particles released from a human carcinoma cell line, *Proc. Nat. Acad. Sci. U.S.A.* **72**:2794.

Baluda, M. A., and Drohan, W. N., 1972, Distribution of deoxyribonucleic acid complementary to the ribonucleic acid of avian myeloblastosis virus in tissues of normal and tumor-bearing chickens, *J. Virol.* **10**:1002.

Baluda, M. A., and Nayak, D. P., 1970, DNA complementary to viral RNA in leukemic cells induced by avian myeloblastosis virus, *Proc. Nat. Acad. Sci. U.S.A.* **66**:329.

Baxt, W., 1974, Sequences present in both human leukemic cell nuclear DNA and Rauscher leukemia virus, *Proc. Nat. Acad. Sci. U.S.A.* **71**:2853.

Baxt, W., and Spiegelman, S., 1972, Nuclear DNA sequences present in human leukemic cells and absent in normal leukocytes, *Proc. Nat. Acad. Sci. U.S.A.* **69**:3737.

Baxt, W., Hohlman, R., and Spiegelman, S., 1972, Human leukemic cells contain reverse transcriptase associated with a high molecular weight virus-related RNA, *Nature New Biol.* **244**:72.

Baxt, W., Yates, J. W., Wallace, H. J., Holland, J. F., and Spiegelman, S., 1973, Leukemia-specific DNA sequences in leukocytes of the leukemic member of identical twins, *Proc. Nat. Acad. Sci. U.S.A.* **70**:2629.

Bentvelzen, P., Daams, J. H., Hagerman, P., and Calafat, J., 1970, Genetic transmission of viruses that incite mammary tumor virus in mice, *Proc. Nat. Acad. Sci. U.S.A.* **67**:377.

Benveniste, R. E., and Todaro, G. J., 1973, Homology between type-C viruses of various species as determined by molecular hybridization, *Proc. Nat. Acad. Sci. U.S.A.* **70**:3316.

Benveniste, R. E., and Todaro, G. J., 1974a, Evolution of C-type viral genes: Inheritance of exogenously acquired genes, *Nature (London)* **252**:456.

Benveniste, R. E., and Todaro, G. J., 1974b, Multiple divergent copies of endogenous C-type virogenes in mammalian cells, *Nature (London)* **252**:170.

Benveniste, R. E., and Todaro, G. J., 1974c, Evolution of type-C viral genes: I. Nucleic acid from baboon type C virus as a measure of divergence among primate species, *Proc. Nat. Acad. Sci. U.S.A.* **71**:4513.

Benveniste, R. E., and Todaro, G. J., 1975, Evolution of type C viral genes: Preservation of ancestral murine type C viral sequences in pig cellular DNA, *Proc. Nat. Acad. Sci. U.S.A.* **72**:4090.

Benveniste, R. E., and Todaro, G. J., 1976, Evolution of type C viral genes: Evidence for an Asian origin of man, *Nature (London)* **261**:101.

Benveniste, R. E., Heinemann, R., Wilson, G. L., Callahan, R., and Todaro, G. J., 1974a, Detection of baboon type C viral sequences in various primate tissues by molecular hybridization, *J. Virol.* **14**:56.

Benveniste, R. E., Lieber, M. M., Livingston, D. M., Sherr, C. J., Todaro, G. J., and Kalter, S. S., 1974b, Infectious C type virus isolated from baboon placenta, *Nature (London)* **248**:17.

Benveniste, R. E., Sherr, C. J., and Todaro, G. J., 1975, Evolution of type C viral genes: Origin of feline leukemia virus, *Science* **190**:886.

Bobrow, S. N., Smith, R. G., Reitz, M. S., and Gallo, R. C., 1972, Stimulated normal human lymphocytes contain a ribonuclease-sensitive DNA polymerase which is distinct from viral RNA-directed DNA polymerase, *Proc. Nat. Acad. Sci. U.S.A.* **69**:3228–3232.

Calarco, P. G., and Szollosi, D., 1973, Intracisternal A particles in ova and preimplantation stages of the mouse, *Nature New Biol.* **243**:91.

Callahan, R., Benveniste, R. E., Lieber, M. M., and Todaro, G. J., 1974, Nucleic acid homology of murine type C viral genes, *J. Virol.* **14**:1394.

Callahan, R., Lieber, M. M., and Todaro, G. J., 1975, Nucleic acid homology of murine xenotropic type C viruses, *J. Virol.* **15**:1378.

Chan, E., Peters, W. P., Sweet, R. W., Ohno, T., Kufe, D. W., Spiegelman, S., Gallo, R. C., and Gallagher, R. E., 1976, Characterization of a virus (HL23V) isolated from cultured acute myelogenous leukemic cells, *Nature (London)* **260**:266.

Cooper, G. M., and Temin, H. M., 1974, Infectious DNA from cells infected with Rous sarcoma virus, reticuloendeliotheliosis virus or Rous-associated virus-o, *Cold Spring Harbor Symp. Quant. Biol.* **39**:1027.

De Pauli, A., Johnsen, D. O., and Noll, W. W., 1973, Granulocytic leukemia in white-handed gibbons, *J. Am. Vet. Med. Assoc.* **963**:624.

Duesberg, P. H., and Vogt, P. K., 1970, Differences between the ribonucleic acids of transforming and nontransforming avian tumor viruses, *Proc. Nat. Acad. Sci. U.S.A.* **67**:1673.

East, J. L., Kneslk, J. E., Chan, J. C., and Dmochowski, L., 1975, Quantitative nucleotide sequence relationships of mammalian RNA tumor viruses, *J. Virol.* **15**:1396.

Gabelman, N., Waxman, S., Smith, W., and Douglas, S. D., 1975, Appearance of C-type virus-like particles after co-cultivation of a human tumor-cell line with rat (XC) cells, *Int. J. Cancer* **16**:355.

Gallagher, R. E., and Gallo, R. C., 1974, Type C RNA tumor virus isolated from cultured human acute myelogenous leukemia cells, *Science* **187**:350.

Gallagher, R. E., and Gallo, R. C., 1977, Continuous production of complete type-C virus by exponentially growing cultured leukocytes from one to sixteen patients with myelogenous leukemia, *in Proceedings of the IInd International Congress on Pathological Physiology, Prague, Czechoslovakia,* in press.

Gallagher, R. E., Salahuddin, S. Z., Hall, W. T., McCredie, K. B., and Gallo, R. C., 1975, Growth and differentiation in culture of leukemic leukocytes from a patient with acute myelogenous leukemia and reidentification of a type C virus, *Proc. Nat. Acad. Sci. U.S.A.* **72**:4137.

Gallo, R. C., 1976, RNA tumor viruses and leukemia: Evaluation of present results supporting their presence in human leukemias, *in Modern Trends in Human Leukemia II* (R. Neth, R. C. Gallo, K. Mannweiler, and W. C. Moloney, eds.), pp. 431–450, J. F. Lehmanns Verlag, Munich.

Gallo, R. C., and Todaro, G. J., 1976, Oncogenic RNA viruses, *in Seminars in Oncology* (J. W. Yarbro, R. S. Bornstein, and M. J. Mastrangelo, eds.), pp. 81–95, Grune & Stratton, New York.

Gallo, R. C., Miller, N. R., Saxinger, W. C., and Gillespie, D., 1973, Primate RNA tumor virus-like DNA synthesized endogenously by RNA-dependent DNA polymerase in virus-like particles from fresh human acute leukemic blood cells, *Proc. Nat. Acad. Sci. U.S.A.* **70**:3219.

Gallo, R. C., Gallagher, R. E., Miller, N. R., Mondal, H., Saxinger, W. C., Mayer, R. J., Smith, R. G., and Gillespie, D. H., 1974, Relationships between components in primate RNA tumor viruses and in the cytoplasm of human leukemic cells: Implications to leukemogenesis, *Cold Spring Harbor Symp. Quant. Biol.* **34**:933.

Gallo, R. C., Saxinger, W. C., Gallagher, R. E., Gillespie, D. H., Reitz, M. S., Ruscetti, F., and Wong-Staal, F., 1977, Some ideas on the origin of leukemia in man and recent evidence for the presence of acquired and endogenous type-C viral related sequences, *in Origins of Human Cancer* (H. H. Hiatt, J. D. Watson, and J. A. Winston, eds.), Cold Spring Harbor Press, Cold Spring Harbor, New York (in press).

Gillespie, D., and Gallo, R. C., 1975, RNA processing and the origin and evolution of RNA tumor viruses, *Science* **188**:802.

Gillespie, D., and Gallo, R. C., 1976, New concepts on human myelogenous leukemia based on studies of the simian RNA tumor virus family, *in Proceedings of International Comparative Leukemia Lymphoma Meeting* (J. Clemmesen and D. S. Yohn, eds.), pp. 576–581, Karger, Basel.

Gillespie, D., Gillespie, S., Gallo, R. C., East, J., and Dmochowski, L., 1973, Genetic origin of RD114 and other RNA tumor viruses assayed by molecular hybridization, *Nature New Biol.* **244**:51.

Gillespie, D., Gallagher, R. E., Smith, R. G., Saxinger, W. C., and Gallo, R. C., 1975a, On the evidence for type-C RNA tumor virus information and virus-related reverse transcriptase in animals and in human leukemia cells, *in Fundamental Aspects of Neoplasia* (A. A. Gottlieb, O. J. Plescia, and D. H. L. Bishop, eds.), pp. 3–27, Springer-Verlag, Berlin and New York.

Gillespie, D., Saxinger, W. C., and Gallo, R. C., 1975b, Information transfer in cells infected by RNA tumor virus and extension to human neoplasia, *Prog. Nucleic Acid Res. Mol. Biol.* **15**:1.

Gillespie, D., Gillespie, S., and Wong-Staal, F., 1975c, RNA–DNA hybridization applied to cancer research: Special reference to RNA tumor viruses, *Methods Cancer Res.* **11**:205.

Haywood, W. S., and Hanafusa, H., 1975, Recombination between endogenous and exogenous RNA tumor virus genes as analyzed by nucleic acid hybridization, *J. Virol.* **122**:1367.

Hehlman, R., Kufe, D., and Spiegelman, S., 1972, RNA in human leukemic cells related to the RNA of a mouse leukemia virus, *Proc Nat. Acad. Sci. U.S.A.* **69**:435.

Huebner, R., and Todaro, G. J., 1969, Oncogenes of RNA tumor viruses as determinants of cancer, *Proc. Nat. Acad. Sci. U.S.A.* **64**:1087.

Kalter, S. S., Helmke, R. J., Panigel, M., Heberling, R. L., Felsburg, P. J., and Axelrod, L. R., 1973a, Observations of apparent C type particles in baboon *(Papio cynocephalus)* placentas, *Science* **179**:1332.

Kalter, S., Helmke, R., Heberling, R., Panigel, M., Fowler, A., Strickland, J., and

Hellman, A., 1973b, C type particles in normal human placentas, *J. Nat. Cancer Inst.* **50**:1081.

Kang, C. Y., and Temin, H., 1973, Lack of sequence homology among RNAs of avian leukosis-sarcoma viruses, reticuloendotheliosis viruses, and chicken endogenous RNA-directed DNA polymerase activity, *J. Virol.* **12**:1314.

Kawakami, T., Huff, S., Buckley, P., Dungworth, D., Snyder, S., and Gilden, R., 1972, C type virus associated with gibbon lymphosarcoma, *Nature New Biol.* **235**:170.

Kawakami, T., Buckley, P., McDowell, Y., and De Paoli, A., 1973, Antibodies to simian C type virus antigen in sera of gibbons *(Hylobates* sp.), *Nature New Biol.* **246**:105.

Kufe, K., Hehlmann, R., and Spiegelman, S., 1972, Human sarcomas contain RNA related to the RNA of a mouse leukemia virus, *Science* **175**:182.

Kurth, R., Teich, N. M., Weiss, R., and Oliver, R. T. D., 1977, Natural human antibodies reactive with primate type-C viral antigens, *Proc. Nat. Acad. Sci. U.S.A.* **74**:1237–1241.

Lai, M. M., Duesberg, P. H., Horst, J., and Vogt, P., 1973, Avian tumor virus RNA: A comparison of three sarcoma viruses and their transformation-defective derivatives by oligonucleotide fingerprinting and DNA–RNA hybridization, *Proc. Nat. Acad. Sci. U.S.A.* **70**:2266.

Lapin, B. A., 1973, The epidemiologic and genetic aspects of an outbreak of leukemia among Hamadryes baboons of the Sukhumi monkey colony, *Bibliotheca Haematologica,* No. 39 (R. Dutcher and L. Chieco-Bianchi, eds.), pp. 263–268, Karger, Basel.

Larsen, C. J., Marty, M., Hamelin, R., Peries, J., Boiron, M., and Tavitian, A., 1975, Search for nucleic acid sequences complementary to a murine oncornaviral genome in poly(A)-rich RNA of human leukemic cells, *Proc. Nat. Acad. Sci. U.S.A.* **72**:4900.

Levy, J., 1973, Xenotropic viruses: Murine leukemia virus associated with NIH Swiss, N2B, and other strains, *Science* **182**:1151.

Lieber, M. M., Benveniste, R. E., Livingston, D. M., and Todaro, G. J., 1973, Mammalian cells in culture frequently release type C viruses, *Science* **182**:56.

Lieber, M. M., Sherr, C. J., Todaro, G. J., Benveniste, R. E., Callahan, R., and Coon, H. G., 1975, Isolation from the Asian mouse *Mus caroli* of an endogenous type C virus related to infectious primate type C viruses, *Proc. Nat. Acad. Sci. U.S.A.* **72**:2315.

Lowy, D., Rowe, W., Teich, N., and Hartley, J., 1971, Murine leukemia virus high frequency activation *in vitro* by 5-iododeoxyuridine and 5-bromodeoxyuridine, *Science* **174**:155.

Mak, T. W., Manaster, J., Howatson, A. F., McCulloch, E. A., and Till, J. E., 1974, Particles with characteristics of leukoviruses in cultures of marrow cells from leukemic patients in remission and relapse, *Proc. Nat. Acad. Sci. U.S.A.* **71**:4336.

Mak, T. W., Kurtz, S., Manaster, J., and Housman, D., 1975, Viral-related information in oncornavirus-like particles isolated from cultures of marrow cells from leukemic patients in relapse and remission, *Proc. Nat. Acad. Sci. U.S.A.* **72**:623.

Mayer, R. J., Smith, R. G., and Gallo, R. C., 1974, Reverse transcriptase in normal rhesus monkey placenta, *Science* **185**:864.

Mellors, R. C., and Mellors, J. W., 1976, Antigen related to mammalian type-C RNA viral p30 proteins is located in renal glomeruli in human systemic lupus erythematosus, *Proc. Nat. Acad. Sci. U.S.A.* **73**:233.

Melnick, J. L., Altenburg, B., Arnstein, P., Mirkovic, R., and Tevethia, S., 1973, Transformation of baboon cells with feline sarcoma virus, *Intervirology* **1**:286.

Metzgar, R. S., Mohanakumar, T., and Bolognesi, D. P., 1976, Relationships between membrane antigens of human leukemic cells and oncogenic RNA virus structural components, *J. Exp. Med.* **143**:47.

Miller, N. R., Saxinger, W. C., Reitz, M. S., Gallagher, R. E., Wu, A. M., Gallo, R. C., and Gillespie, D., 1974, Systematics of RNA tumor viruses and virus-like particles of human origin, *Proc Nat. Acad. Sci. U.S.A.* **71**:3177.

Mondal, H., Gallagher, R. E., and Gallo, R. C., 1974, RNA-directed DNA polymerase from human leukemic blood cells and from primate type C virus-producing cells: High and low molecular weight forms with variant biochemical and immunological properties, *Proc. Nat. Acad. Sci. U.S.A.* **71**:1194.

Nayak, D., Murray, P., and Goldblast, D., 1974, Endogenous guinea pig virus: Equability of virus-specific DNA in normal, leukemic, and virus-producing cells, *Proc. Nat. Acad. Sci. U.S.A.* **71**:1164.

Neiman, P., 1972, Rous sarcoma virus nucleotide sequences in cellular DNA, *Science* **178**:750.

Neiman, P., 1973a, Measurement of endogenous leukosis virus nucleotide sequences in the DNA of normal avian embryos by RNA–DNA hybridization, *Virology* **53**:196.

Neiman, P., 1973b, Measurement of RD114 virus nucleotide sequences in feline cellular DNA, *Nature New Biol.* **244**:62.

Neiman, P., Wright, S., McMillin, S., and MacDonnell, D., 1974, Nucleotide sequence relationships of avian RNA tumor viruses, *J. Virol.* **13**:837.

Nooter, K., Aarssen, A. M., Bentvelzen, P., and d'Groot, F. G., 1975, Isolation of an infectious C type oncornavirus from human leukemic bone marrow cells, *Nature (London)* **256**:595.

Panem, S., Prochownik, E. V., Reale, R. R., and Kirsten, W. H., 1975, Isolation of C type virions from a normal human fibroblast strain, *Science* **189**:297.

Paran, M., Sachs, L., Barak, Y., and Resnitzky, P., 1970, *In vitro* induction of granulocyte differentiation in hematopoietic cells from leukemic and nonleukemic patients, *Proc. Nat. Acad. Sci. U.S.A.* **67**:1542.

Paran, M., Gallo, R. C., Richardson, L. S., and Wu, A. M., 1973, Adrenal corticosteroids enhance production of type C virus induced by 5-iodo-2'-deoxyuridine from cultured mouse fibroblasts, *Proc. Nat. Acad. Sci. U.S.A.* **70**:2391.

Prochownik, E. V., Panem, S., and Kirsten, W. H., 1977, Primate type C virus-related particles in normal human cells: Isolation of two infectious components from a strain of fetal lung fibroblasts, submitted for publication.

Rauscher, F. J. 1962, A virus-induced disease of mice characterized by erythrocytopoiesis and lymphoid leukemia, *J. Nat. Cancer Inst.* **29**:515.

Reitz, M. S., Smith, R. G., Roseberry, E. A., and Gallo, R. C., 1974, DNA-directed and RNA-primed DNA synthesis in microsomal and mitochondrial fractions of normal human lymphocytes, *Biochem. Biophys. Res. Commun.* **57**:934.

Reitz, M. S., Miller, N. R., Wong-Staal, F., Gallagher, R. E., Gallo, R. C., and Gillespie, D. H., 1976, Primate type C virus nucleic acid sequences (woolly monkey and baboon types) in tissues from a patient with acute myelogenous leukemia and in viruses isolated from cultured cells of the same patient, *Proc. Nat. Acad. Sci. U.S.A.* **73**:2113.

Rous, P., 1911, Transmission of a malignant new growth by means of a cell free filtrate, *JAMA* **56**:198.

Sarin, P. S., and Gallo, R. C., 1974, RNA directed DNA polymerase, *in International Review of Science*, Chap. 8, Vol. 6 (K. Burton, ed.), Butterworth, Oxford.

Sarngadharan, M. G., Sarin, P. S., Reitz, M. S., and Gallo, R. C., 1972, Reverse transcriptase activity of human leukemic cells: Purification of the enzyme, response to AMV 70S RNA, and characterization of the DNA product, *Nature New Biol.* **240**:67.

Sarngadharan, M. G., Allaudeen, H. S., and Gallo, R. C., 1976, Reverse transcriptase of RNA tumor viruses and animal cells, *in Methods of Cancer Research*, Vol. 12 (H. Busch, ed.), pp. 3–47, Academic Press, New York.

Schidlovsky, G., and Ahmed, M., 1973, C type particles in placentas and fetal tissues of rhesus monkeys, *J. Nat. Cancer Inst.* **51**:225.

Schlom, J., and Spiegelman, S., 1971, Simultaneous detection of reverse transcriptase and high molecular weight RNA unique to the oncogenic RNA viruses, *Science* **174**:840.

Scolnick, E. M., and Bumgarner, S. J., 1975, Isolation of infectious xentropic mouse type C virus by transfection of a heterologous cell with DNA from a transformed mouse cell, *J. Virol.* **15**:1293.

Scolnick, E. M., and Parks, W., 1974, Harvey sarcoma virus: A second murine type C sarcoma virus with rat genetic information, *J. Virol.* **13**:1211.

Scolnick, E. M., Rands, E., Williams, D., and Parks, W., 1973, Studies on the nucleic acid sequences of Kirsten sarcoma virus: A model for formation of a mammalian RNA-containing sarcoma virus, *J. Virol.* **12**:458.

Scolnick, M., Parks, W., Kawakami, T., Kohne, D., Okabe, H., Gilden, R., and Hatanaka, M., 1974, Primate and murine type C viral nucleic acid association kinetics: Analysis of model systems and natural tissues, *J. Virol.* **13**:363.

Seman, G., and Seman, C., 1968, Electron-microscopic search for virus particles in patients with leukemia and lymphoma, *Cancer* **22**:1033.

Sherr, C. J., and Todaro, G. J., 1974, Type C virus antigens in man. Antigens related to endogenous primate virus in human tumors, *Proc. Nat. Acad. Sci. U.S.A.* **71**:4703.

Sherr, C. J., and Todaro. G. J., 1975, Primate type C virus p30 antigen in cells from humans with acute leukemia, *Science* **187**:855.

Snyder, S., and Theilen, G., 1969, Transmissable feline fibrosarcoma, *Nature (London)* **221**:1074.

Snyder, H. W., Pincus, T., and Fleissner, E., 1976, Specificities of human immunoglobulins reactive with antigens in preparations of several mammalian type-C viruses, *Virology* **75**:60.

Spiegelman, S., 1976, Molecular evidence for the association of RNA tumor viruses with human mesenchymal malignancies, *in Modern Trends in Human Leukemia II* (R. Neth, R. C. Gallo, K. Mannweiler, and W. C. Moloney, eds.), pp. 391–429, J. F. Lehmanns Verlag, Munich.

Steele, L. K., Laube, H., and Chandra, P., 1977, Biochemical and serological characteristics of reverse transcriptase from human spleen in a case of childhood myelofibrotic syndrome, *Cancer Letters* (in press).

Stephenson, J. R., and Aaronson, S. A., 1976, Search for antigens and antibodies cross-reactive with type C viruses of the woolly monkey and gibbon ape in animal models and in humans, *Proc. Nat. Acad. Sci. U.S.A.* **73**:1725.

Strand, M., and August, J. T., 1974, Type C RNA virus gene expression in human tissue, *J. Virol.* **14**:1584.

Tavitian, A., Larsen, C. J., Hamelin, R., and Boiron, M., 1976, Murine and simian C-type viruses: Sequences detected in the RNA of human leukemic cells by the c-DNA probes, *in Modern Trends in Human Leukemia II* (R. Neth, R. C. Gallo, K. Mannweiler, and W. C. Moloney, eds.), pp. 451–455, J. F. Lehmanns Verlag, Munich.

Teich, N. M., Weiss, R. A., Salahuddin, S. Z., Gallagher, R. E., Gillespie, D. H., and Gallo, R. C., 1975, Infective transmission and characterization of a C type virus released by cultured human myeloid leukemia cells, *Nature (London)* **256**:551.

Temin, H., 1971, The protovirus hypothesis, *J. Nat. Cancer Inst.* **46**:3.

Theilen, G., Gould, D., Fowler, M., and Dungworth, D., 1971, C type virus in tumor tissue of a woolly monkey (lagothrix) with fibrosarcoma, *J. Nat. Cancer Inst.* **47**:881.

Tihon, C., and Green, M., 1973, Cyclic AMP-amplified replication of RNA tumor viruslike particles in Chinese hamster ovary cells, *Nature New Biol.* **244**:227.

Todaro, G. J., and Gallo, R. C., 1973, Immunological relationship of DNA polymerase from human acute leukemia cells and primate and mouse leukemia virus reverse transcriptase, *Nature (London)* **244**:206.

Todaro, G. J., Lieber, M. M., Benveniste, R. E., Sherr, C. J., Gibbs, C. J., and Gajdusek, D. C., 1975, Infectious primate type C viruses: Three isolates belonging to a new subgroup from the brains of normal gibbons, *Virology.* **67**:335.

Tooze, J., 1973, The molecular biology of tumor viruses, *Cold Spring Harbor Monograph.*

Varmus, H. E., Bishop, J. M., Nowinski, R. C., and Sarker, N. H., 1972, Mammary tumor virus specific nucleotide sequences in mouse DNA, *Nature New Biol.* **238**:189.

Vosika, G. J., Krivit, W., Gerrard, J. M., Coccia, P. F., Nesbit, M. E., Coalson, J. J., and Kennedy, B. J., 1975, Oncornaviruslike particles from cultured bone marrow cells preceding leukemia and malignant histiocytosis, *Proc. Nat. Acad. Sci. U.S.A.* **72**:2804.

Weiss, R. A., 1973, Transmission of cellular genetic elements by RNA tumor viruses, *in Possible Episomes in Eukaryotes* (L. Silvestri, ed.), p. 130, North-Holland Publ., Amsterdam.

Witkin, S. S., Ohno, T., and Spiegelman, S., 1975, Purification of RNA-instructed DNA polymerase from human leukemic spleens, *Proc. Nat. Acad. Sci. U.S.A.* **72**:4133.

Wolfe, L., Deinhardt, F., Theilen, G., Kawakami, T., and Bustad, L., 1971, Induction of tumors in marmoset monkeys by simian sarcoma virus type 1 (Lagothrix): A preliminary report, *J. Nat. Cancer Inst.* **48**:1905.

Wong-Staal, F., Gallo, R. C., and Gillespie, D., 1975, Genetic relationship of a primate RNA tumor virus genome to genes in normal mice, *Nature (London)* **256**:670.

Wong-Staal, F., Gillespie, D., and Gallo, R. C., 1976, Proviral sequences of baboon endogenous type C RNA virus in DNA of leukemic tissues from seven patients with myelogenous leukemia, *Nature (London)* **262**:190.

Wu, A., and Gallo, R. C., 1975, Reverse transcriptase, *in Critical Reviews in Biochemistry* (G. D. Fasman, ed.), pp. 289–347, Chem. Rubber Publ. Co., Cleveland, Ohio.

Wu, A. M., Ting, R. C., and Gallo, R. C., 1972, Cordecypin inhibits induction of murine leukovirus production by 5-iodo-2'-deoxyuridine, *Proc. Nat. Acad. Sci. U.S.A.* **69**:3820.

# 12

# Immunological Aspects of Leukemia

Ronald B. Herberman

## 12.1. Introduction

For many years, much attention has been focused on immunological studies in leukemia. This level of attention and effort has been disproportionately high, relative to the clinical frequency of leukemia compared to other types of neoplastic diseases. This may be accounted for by several important factors: (a) A considerable proportion of tumors arising spontaneously or induced in experimental animals, especially rodents, are leukemias or lymphomas. (b) The neoplastic leukemic cells are directly accessible in the peripheral blood or bone marrow, and there has been little or no need to use disaggregation or other procedures to obtain high yields of neoplastic cells. In many instances, it is possible to obtain very large numbers of leukemic cells virtually uncontaminated by normal cells. (c) Compared to carcinomas or sarcomas, it has been relatively easy to obtain the normal cellular counterparts of the various types of leukemic cells. This has provided an unusual opportunity to compare the normal processes of cell differentiation and the normal cell surface markers to the neoplastic processes and leukemia-associated markers.

Because of the extensive interest in experimental leukemias, and the availability of good models for various forms of clinical disease, it has been possible to perform detailed immunological studies of problems in model systems and then to relate the experimental findings to the clinical situa-

RONALD B. HERBERMAN • Laboratory of Immunodiagnosis, National Cancer Institute, Bethesda, Maryland 20014.

tion. In each of the areas of research to be discussed in this chapter, this ability to go back and forth between the experimental models and the clinical situation has helped considerably to accelerate the progress in immunological research in leukemia.

In this chapter, some selected aspects of the large number of immunological studies will be summarized and commented upon. We will first describe the findings of normal cell surface markers on leukemic cells. These investigations are providing important clues to the origin of some types of leukemia, and actually appear to be adding a new dimension to the difficult problem of classification of leukemias. They are also helping us to understand the factors influencing the expression of these cell surface markers. The cell surface antigens which are particularly, or even uniquely, associated with leukemias are discussed next, along with information about their possible relationship to viruses or to embryonic antigens.

A major emphasis in this chapter has been placed on the studies of immunity in leukemic individuals. First, there was a need to discuss the information relating to immunodepression due to the neoplastic process itself and to therapy, since at the clinical level, most patients studied have been given intensive chemotherapy or other forms of therapy. Despite the immunodepression which has been described in experimental and clinical leukemias, there is extensive evidence for humoral and cell-mediated immune responses to leukemia-associated antigens, and these studies are selectively summarized.

Finally, some additional comments and information on the practical clinical applications of all these studies are made. There has been increasing interest in the use of immunologic procedures to aid in the diagnosis of leukemia, in the detection of relapse, and to assess prognosis. Furthermore, there has been a long and extensive interest in the application of immunology to the therapy of leukemia. Many of the pioneering studies on the immunotherapy of experimental tumors and clinical tumors have been done in leukemia.

## 12.2. Normal Cell Surface Markers and Leukemia-Associated Antigens

Leukemia cells may contain a wide variety of membrane antigens and other cell surface markers. These include normal histocompatibility antigens, markers characteristic of the normal subpopulation of cells from which they are derived, leukemia-associated antigens, fetal antigens or other antigens characteristic of a particular state of differentiation, chemotherapeutic agent-induced antigens, and, in tumors induced by viruses or in species with expression of endogenous type C viruses, virus-associated antigens. The complexity of these cell surface markers and antigens is important from several standpoints: (a) In studies of leukemia-associated antigens and the immune response to these antigens, it is essential to distinguish these specific antigens from the other types of antigens. (b) The various cell surface markers may provide very useful clues as to the derivation of the tumors and, in fact, may provide important aids to the classification of leukemias. (c) Variations in expression of certain antigens and other markers may provide information regarding physiologic processes affecting cell surface membranes.

Most of the information regarding membrane antigens and other cell surface markers has been obtained in studies of experimental leukemias in mice and rats. However, in the past few years, similar approaches have been successfully applied to the study of human leukemias.

## 12.2.1. Experimental Animal Systems

### 12.2.1.1. Normal Cell Surface Markers

Lymphoid cells have been found to contain several different membrane antigens and receptors, and these have been very useful in characterizing subpopulations of cells. In the mouse, the alloantigen theta ($\theta$), or Thy 1, has been shown to be a very characteristic marker of thymus-derived lymphocytes (T cells) (Raff, 1969). Bone-marrow-derived lymphocytes (B cells) can be identified by the presence of easily detectable, membrane-bound immunoglobulin, primarily IgM. In addition, some cells contain receptors for the activated form of the complement component C3 (Bianco et al., 1970) or for the Fc portion of immunoglobulin G (IgG). The complement receptor has been found on B cells and on monocytes, macrophages, and granulocytes (Lay and Nussenzweig, 1968). The Fc receptor has been shown to be present on monocytes and macrophages (Lay and Nussenzweig, 1968), B cells (Dickler and Kunkel, 1972), and on some T cells (Yoshida and Andersson, 1972).

A large number of transplantable mouse leukemias and lymphomas have been examined for the presence of these markers (Shevach et al., 1972c,d). About half the tumors studied had detectable $\theta$ antigen and were therefore characterized as being derived from T cells. Most of the other tumors had no detectable markers, indicating that they might be derived from "null cells" or that they had lost their identifying markers during the process of transformation or during passage. Very few of the mouse leukemias or lymphomas initially studied were shown to contain surface immunoglobulin or receptors for complement or IgG (Shevach et al., 1972c,d).

The main category of tumors with B-cell surface markers are those induced by Abelson leukemia virus. This virus produces lymphoid leukemias and plasma cell tumors. An initial study indicated that the lymphoid tumors had surface κ light chains, detectable by immunofluorescence, but lacked Fc or complement receptors (Sklar *et al.,* 1975). Since all the tumors studied were grown *in vivo,* it remained possible that the detected immunoglobulins were passively bound antibodies. However, in a subsequent study (Premkumar *et al.,* 1975), several cell lines were shown to synthesize surface immunoglobulin. Haran-Ghera and Peled (1973) induced lymphocytic leukemias in thymectomized SJL/J mice by administration of the carcinogen, dimethylbenzanthracene. The tumors were shown by immunofluorescence to contain surface immunoglobulin and receptors for Fc and complement (Linker-Israeli and Haran-Ghera, 1975). Thus the Abelson virus-induced tumors and these chemically induced tumors in thymectomized SJL/J mice appear to be derived from B cells, and stand out as the main representatives of that type of leukemia in mice.

Most spontaneous leukemias in AKR mice arise in the thymus and bear θ antigen (Reif and Allen, 1964). These AKR leukemias have been found to be derived from different subpopulations of T cells, with varying concentrations of θ antigen and "homing" patterns (Barker and Waksal, 1974). Two AKR leukemias have recently been described which possess both θ antigen and surface IgM (Greenberg and Zatz, 1975). The derivation of such cells with double markers, characteristic of both T and B cells, is quite unclear. There may be a subpopulation of normal cells with such characteristics, or the neoplastic cells may acquire an additional marker, which is normally not expressed. As discussed later, similar types of findings have been made with some human cells.

Thymus leukemia (TL) antigens (Boyse and Old, 1969) are particularly interesting membrane antigens, since in some mouse strains they may be normal T-cell differentiation antigens and in other strains they may be leukemia-associated antigens. In normal mice, TL antigens are restricted to thymocytes and expression is controlled by a genetic locus (Tla) linked to the H-2D histocompatibility locus. The TL antigens are expressed on the thymocytes of some mouse strains (TL+) but not in others (TL−). In TL− strains, TL antigens may be found on some leukemia cells and in such cases they may be considered leukemia-associated antigens. It has not been clearly shown that expression of TL antigen on leukemia cells, particularly in TL− strains, is indicative of derivation of the leukemia from thymocytes, or whether some non-T-cell leukemias may also express TL.

Very few leukemias of other experimental animal species have been characterized as to their possible derivation from a particular subpopulation of lymphoid cells. The L$_2$C leukemia of the guinea pig (Shevach *et al.*, 1972a) and the Murphy Sturm leukemia of the rat (Djeu *et al.*, 1974) have been shown to have B-cell characteristics. Herpes virus saimiri-induced leukemias in owl monkeys have been shown to form rosettes with sheep erythrocytes and lack complement receptors; they therefore have been considered to be derived from T cells (Wallen *et al.*, 1973).

## 12.2.1.2. Leukemia-Associated Antigens

Antigens specifically associated with leukemias have been studied most extensively on murine leukemias induced by type C leukemia viruses. Studies of these tumors are complicated, since the murine leukemia viruses (MuLV) bud through the cell surface membrane. Therefore, virus envelope antigens (VEAs) and cell surface antigens not present in the virus may both be detected on the surface of leukemia cells. The interrelationships between these categories of antigens have been difficult to define, and some antigens which have been thought to be true cell surface antigens may be shown to be virus antigens. In this section, the antigens which have been characteristic of virus-induced tumors, but which have appeared to be distinct from virus antigens, are discussed.

Leukemias induced by Gross leukemia virus have been shown to contain the G (Gross) cell surface antigen (Slettenmark-Wahren and Klein, 1962; Old *et al.*, 1965), which can be detected by antibodies in cytotoxicity or membrane immunofluorescence assays. Subsequently, the G antigen has been found to be a complex of Gross cell surface antigens (GCSA), and a given tumor may express one or more of these (Herberman, 1972; Aoki *et al.*, 1972). Mouse G-typing antisera contain antibodies to GCSAa, which is found on Gross virus-induced tumors in mice and rats, and to GCSAc, which is present in AKR but not in C58 leukemic mice. Rat G-typing antisera contain antibodies to GCSAa and also to GCSAb, which is a broadly distributed antigen found on leukemia cells induced both by Gross virus and by other types of MuLV. In addition, the rat antisera react with at least three other cell surface antigens, G$_L$, and G$_T$ (Nowinski and Peters, 1973), and G$_{IX}$ (see the following section). Tumors induced by radiation leukemia virus (Lieberman and Kaplan, 1959) have antigens similar to those on Gross virus leukemias (Ferrer and Kaplan, 1968) but the precise relationship has not been defined.

The cells of leukemias induced by Friend, Moloney, Rauscher, and also Graffi viruses have been found to contain a serologically detectable antigen (FMR antigen) that is distinct from the GCSAs (Old *et al.*, 1964; Levy *et al.*, 1968). Although the FMR antigen was thought to be a single antigen, recent studies have indicated that it, like the G antigen, is a complex of several antigens. Friend virus-induced leukemias of mice and rats, in addition to antigens shared by leukemias induced by Moloney or Rauscher viruses, also contain a type-specific F (Friend) antigen (Kuzumaki *et al.*, 1973; Ting and Herberman, 1974).

A variety of other antigens have been associated with murine leukemias. Aoki *et al.* (1970b) described the E antigen associated with several spontaneous leukemias in C57BL/6 mice, and absent in virus-induced leukemias of the same strain. The ML (mammary leukemia) antigen was found in several leukemias of DBA/2 mice and also in mammary tumors induced by mouse mammary tumor virus (Stück *et al.*, 1964a). Leclerc *et al.* (1970) have described the L antigen, which was found in many tumors induced by Moloney, Rauscher, Gross, and Graffi viruses, and also in the chemically induced leukemia, EL-4. The relationship of these cell surface antigens to MuLV in the leukemia cells has not been defined. Recently, Sato *et al.* (1973) described the X.1 antigen, detected serologically and also by transplantation protection experiments, which appeared to be associated with expression of a type of MuLV.

All the antigens described thus far have been detected by tests with humoral antibodies. Although it has been generally assumed that cell-mediated immunity is also directed against the same antigens, this has recently been shown not to be the case, at least in some systems. Cell-mediated cytotoxicity in C57BL/6 mice against leukemia cells has been shown to be associated with a murine virus-associated antigen, MEV-SAl (Herberman *et al.*, 1974a) and in W/Fu rats, to a rat endogenous virus-associated antigen (Nunn *et al.*, 1976).

The actual location of some of these cell surface antigens and their relationship to the envelopes of budding type C viruses have been studied in detail by the technique of immunoelectron microscopy, in which the binding of antibodies can be visualized by a ferritin marker (Hammerling *et al.*, 1968). Antibodies to GCSA reacted only with the cell surface and not with the viral envelope (Aoki *et al.*, 1970a). Conversely, antibodies to viral envelope antigens reacted only with sites of evident viral maturation. H-2 and $\theta$ antigens were found in patches on the cell membrane and on restricted areas of the viral surface (Aoki, 1971).

Some of the leukemia-associated antigens are easily shed from the cell surface and are present as soluble antigens in the plasma of leukemic animals. This has been described for both G (Aoki *et al.*, 1968) FMR antigens (Stück *et al.*, 1964b) and $G_{IX}$ antigens (Obata *et al.*, 1975). When antigen-negative cells were incubated with plasma containing soluble antigen, sufficient antigen adsorbed to the cell surface to render the cells susceptible to lysis by specific antibody plus complement. The presence of detectable levels of circulating antigen in the plasma of leukemic individuals has important implications for the possible development of diagnostic procedures for leukemia.

In addition to leukemias in mice and rats, the cell surface antigens associated with avian and feline leukemia virus-induced tumors have been extensively studied, and their characteristics are briefly summarized herein. Some strains of avian sarcoma viruses have been able to transform mammalian cells, and therefore studies with antigens associated with these viruses have been performed in rodents as well as in chickens. *In vivo* transplantation experiments demonstrated a tumor-associated transplantation antigen common to tumors induced by avian leukemia and sarcoma viruses. Inoculation of avian myeloblastosis virus in mice, which is not tumorigenic, was able to induce resistance against syngeneic Rous sarcoma virus-induced tumor cells (Bauer *et al.*, 1969). In this system, the role of virion constituents can be fairly conclusively ruled out, since no infectious virus or internal virion components have been detected in the mammalian tumors (Bauer, 1974). By immunoelectron microscopy with chicken cells, a group-specific cell surface antigen, common to leukemia and sarcoma cells and distinct from VEAs, was demonstrated (Gelderblom *et al.*, 1972). The cell surface antigen was also shown to be common to chicken, mouse, and hamster tumor cells transformed by avian tumor viruses (Kurth and Bauer, 1972).

A series of studies have been performed on the cell surface antigens associated with feline leukemia or sarcoma viruses (reviewed recently by Essex, 1975). The FOCMA (feline oncornavirus membrane antigen), detected by immunofluorescence, has been the antigen best studied. It has been shown that the FOCMA antigen is different from those induced by murine, avian, or simian viruses.

### 12.2.1.3. Virus-Associated Antigens

A central problem in the studies of the leukemias induced by type C viruses has been the discrimination between antigens associated with the virions themselves and true leukemia-associated cell surface antigens. As discussed earlier, a particular concern has been directed toward the VEAs since these are obvious on the cell surface in the area of budding virus. In addition, however, some evidence has been presented that internal (core) virion antigens may also be detected on the surface of leukemia cells. Therefore it is important to summarize the known characteristics of the virion antigens. These have been reviewed in considerable detail elsewhere (Lilly and Steeves, 1974; Bolognesi, 1974). The VEA has been shown to be mainly associated with a high molecular weight glycoprotein, with approximate weight of 69,000–71,000 daltons (Strand and August, 1973) and has been termed gp69/71 or gp70 or gp71. This molecule has been shown to carry a variety of antigenic specificities. It appears to contain the virus neutralization antigen (Lilly and Steeves, 1974). An interspecies-specific determinant (interspec II) has been associated with gp69/71 (Strand and August, 1974). In addition, VEA carries common group-specific antigens (Aoki et al., 1974) and individual type-specific antigens (Aoki et al., 1974; Lilly and Steeves, 1974). Recent studies have helped to define the relationship of gp69/71 to VEAs and leukemic cell surface antigens. The most extensively studied specificity has been $G_{IX}$, originally described as a cell surface alloantigen associated with Gross leukemia virus (Stockert et al., 1971). The $G_{IX}$ antigen was demonstrated on the cell surface of all Gross leukemia virus-induced tumors of mice and rats studied, and also on the surface of normal thymocytes, but not on the peripheral T cells, of some strains of mice. The expression of $G_{IX}$ on thymocytes was shown to be determined by two genes, and was independent of the expression of easily detectable infectious viruses in the positive strains. Recently, the $G_{IX}$ antigen has been shown to be a constituent of gp69/71 (Obata et al., 1975; Tung et al., 1975b; Del Villano et al., 1975). The incorporation of the viral genetic information responsible for $G_{IX}$ into the host genome of some mouse strains accounts for the interesting paradox of a leukemia-associated antigen being present in some normal cells as a differentiation antigen. As an extension of these studies, Tung et al. (1975a) showed that gp69/71 can also be expressed on thymocytes of some $G_{IX}$-negative strains, and as one would expect, the gp69/71 from those strains lacked the $G_{IX}$ specificity. By immunoelectron microscopy, Kennel and Feldman (1976) showed that the gp69/71 on thymocytes was uniformly distributed over the cell surface and was independent of virus particle production.

The other major virion antigens are carried on proteins in the viral core. The p30 is the major structural protein of type C viruses. The MuLV p30 molecule is highly immunogenic in heterologous species, but there has been very little evidence that mice can respond immunologically to it. The heterologous antisera detect at least two antigenic determinants on p30. One is specific for a given species and has been called group-specific or gs-1 antigen; the other is an interspecies antigen (gs-3) which is present on all mammalian type C viruses (Gilden et al., 1971; Strand and August, 1974). The other core proteins are proteins of 15,000 (p15), 12,000 (p12), and 10,000 (p10) daltons molecular weight. In addition, the viruses contain reverse transcriptase, which is an antigenic protein of 70,000 molecular weight. Since all of these internal proteins cannot be detected on intact virions, it was not expected that they would be present on the surface of infected or transformed cells. However, several recent studies have detected internal virion antigens on the cell surface. Yoshiki et al. (1973), using a membrane immunofluorescence technique, detected a cell surface antigen common to tumors induced by, and cells infected by, murine and feline type C viruses. The antiserum used was prepared against disrupted feline leukemia virus, and p30 could absorb out the activity against the cell surface antigen. In further studies by this group (Yoshiki et al., 1974; Ikeda et al., 1974) and other groups (Grant et al., 1974; Epstein and Knight, 1975a), the presence of p30 on the cell surface of some virus-infected or -transformed cells was documented. In the study by Grant et al. (1974), the possibility was raised that the p30 was simply adsorbed onto the cell surface from disrupted virions, since isolated p30 could be shown to adhere to the surface of cells. Others, however, felt that the p30 molecule was an integral part of the cell membrane (Yoshiki et al., 1974; Epstein and Knight, 1975a). In any event, the p30 was bound sufficiently close to the cell membrane to allow cytotoxicity by anti-p30 antisera plus complement. Hunsmann et al. (1976) tested a series of antisera to virus structural proteins against virus-infected or -transformed cells, by a cytotoxicity assay. Strong reactions were obtained with anti-gp69/71 and anti-p12 antisera. The anti-p12 showed type-specific reactivity and the anti-69/71, type and group specificities. The antisera to p10, p15, and p30 were cytotoxic against only one cell line, and even there the reactions were weaker than those produced by anti-p12 and anti-gp69/71. An immunoelectron microscopic study confirmed these results (Schwarz et al., 1976). The gp69/71 antigen was detected on the virus envelope and also on nonbudding areas of the cell surface. P12 antigen was absent on the virus particles and abundant on nonbudding areas of the cell surface. Schwarz et al. (1976) concluded that p12, as well as gp69/71, was an integral cell surface constituent.

These recent findings of a variety of virus structural proteins on the cell surface raise some intriguing possibilities regarding the relationship between these antigens and the leukemia-associated cell surface antigens. As discussed earlier, immunoelectron microscopy studies showed the independence of GCSA and other cell surface antigens from VEA, and this presumably indicates that the surface antigenic specificities are not part of the gp69/71 molecule. Now, however, the whole range of virion antigens must be considered. Ferrer (1973) suggested that the GCSAb specificity was present on p30. Anti-FMR cytotoxic antibodies could not be inhibited appreciably by intact virions but disrupted virions inhibited well (Lilly and Steeves, 1974). Epstein and Knight (1975b) demonstrated the presence of p30 in the sera of mice bearing a Moloney virus-induced leukemia, and found that p30 could inhibit the cytotoxicity of an antiserum produced in rats against syngeneic Moloney virus-induced lymphoma. However, the specificity of this antiserum for cell surface antigens other than p30 was not defined. Similarly, Knight et al. (1975) detected p30 in the sera of lymphoma-bearing rats and presented evidence that p30 was the main antigen detected by syngeneic cytotoxic antisera to Gross or Moloney leukemia virus-induced tumors. However, again, the precise cell surface antigen specificities recognized by these antisera were not defined. The antisera reacted with both Gross and Moloney virus-induced tumors and therefore might have recognized GCSAb. If so, this would confirm the earlier suggestion of Ferrer (1973).

The question of the relationship between the cell surface antigens and virion antigens has also been approached by studies of cell lines following the loss of cell surface antigen or virus expression. By immuno-selection, Ferrer and Gibbs (1969) obtained rat cell lines which appeared to have lost their radiation leukemia virus-associated cell surface antigens. Concomitantly, the lines also ceased to express detectable levels of virus. Ioachim et al. (1974) obtained a similar pattern of results with two Gross virus-induced lymphomas. However, some studies have detected a divergence among the various markers. Freedman et al. (1975) developed cell lines which were nonproducers of Friend leukemia virus, lacked FMR antigen, but did express VEA and gp69/71. The study of Fenyö and Klein (1976) also showed that immunoselected Moloney virus-induced cell lines diverged in their expression of Moloney cell surface antigen (MCSA) and virion antigens, and their findings are more difficult to reconcile with some of those cited in the preceding paragraph. The selected lines appeared to have lost MCSA, but expression of p12, p15, p30, and gp69/71 appeared unchanged.

With the availability of the isolated virion antigens and of specific antisera to these, and with the intense recent interest in the relationship of these antigens to cell surface antigens, one would anticipate that the question, although still rather unsettled, will be resolved in the near future.

Before leaving this area, it should also be noted that the problem of cell surface antigens associated with MuLV is not confined to leukemias induced by leukemia viruses. A number of studies have demonstrated that spontaneous mouse and rat leukemias and other tumors, and leukemias induced by X-irradiation or chemical carcinogens may express endogenous type C viruses (e.g., Lieberman and Kaplan, 1959; Huebner and Todaro, 1969; Odaka, 1975) and virus-associated antigens (e.g., Pearson et al., 1972; Nowinski and Klein, 1975; Herberman, 1972; Colnaghi and Della Porta, 1973; Herberman et al., 1974a; Aoki et al., 1975; Nunn et al., 1976). In view of this, it will be important to consider carefully the possibility that any mouse or rat leukemia-associated antigen is actually due to type C virus expression.

### 12.2.1.4. Embryonic Antigens

Some cell surface antigens that are present on tumor cells and undetectable on normal adult cells, and hence can be considered tumor-associated antigens, may also be present on cells during the normal course of embryonic development. Embryonic antigens have been found in several murine leukemias induced by MuLV or of other origin (Hanna et al., 1971; Ting et al., 1972; Ishimoto and Ito, 1972; Ting and Herberman, 1974) and in avian oncornavirus-induced tumors (Kurth and Bauer, 1973). In most studies, embryonic antigens have been detected by antisera raised against fetal tissues. However, Ting and Herberman (1974) found that a syngeneic mouse antiserum against a Friend virus-induced leukemia reacted with embryonic antigens. It had been thought for a period of time that the tumor-associated cell surface antigens on virus-induced tumors might be embryonic antigens. However, in the studies with the Friend virus-induced leukemia (Ting and Herberman, 1974) and with other virus-induced tumors (Ting et al., 1972), the embryonic antigens were shown to be distinct from the type- or group-specific tumor-associated antigens. The embryonic antigens have been shown to be heterogeneous, but each appears to be broadly distributed on a variety of tumors, including those of different morphologic type and origin.

The possible role of embryonic antigens needs to be particularly considered with tumor antigens which are associated with type C virus expression, since MuLV gs antigen (i.e., p30) has been found in early mouse embryos (Huebner et al., 1970; Hilgers et al., 1974). Therefore, some embryonic antigens may actually be viral-associated antigens, although this has not yet been documented.

The L antigen, present on some murine leukemias, has been suggested to be an embryonic antigen (Fenyö et al., 1974). However, this was based only on the reactivity of NIH Swiss 3T3 and $S^+L^-$ cells with anti-L serum. Although these cell lines were derived from embryonic fibroblasts, they may carry a variety of other types of antigens, including endogenous type C virus-associated antigens (as noted in similar cells by Aoki et al., 1975).

### 12.2.1.5. Antigens Induced by Chemotherapeutic Agents

Increased immunogenicity of several mouse leukemias has been induced following in vivo treatment of the tumors with chemotherapeutic agents (Bonmassar et al., 1970; Houchens et al., 1976). When virus-induced leukemias were used, the virus-associated transplantation antigens were retained but the tumors also acquired additional antigenic specificities as a result of the drug treatment. Since chemotherapeutic agents are widely used for the therapy of leukemia, antigens induced by these agents need to be considered.

### 12.2.1.6. Relationship between Leukemia Antigens and Histocompatibility Antigens

A concept attracting much current attention is that cell surface antigens associated with virus infection or with tumors may actually be modified H-2 or other major histocompatibility complex antigens (reviewed by Doherty *et al.*, 1976). The cytotoxic reactivity of immune T cells has been shown, in some systems, to be restricted to syngeneic target cells or to cells sharing some H-2 antigens. Two recent studies with mouse virus-induced leukemias have supported this hypothesis (Gomard *et al.*, 1976; Blank *et al.*, 1976). However, Holden *et al.* (1977) have found that, under some conditions, immune T cells can react well with allogeneic leukemia cells and that the association of tumor antigens with histocompatibility antigens is not a universal phenomenon.

The evidence for a physical association between virus or tumor antigens with H-2 antigens has been mainly indirect. One direct method for analyzing this is to determine whether the antigens can be separated during the course of purification. Davies *et al.* (1967, 1974) found that TL antigen and an antigen associated with the EL-4 mouse leukemia could be physically separated from H-2 antigens. Martyré *et al.* (1973) and Law and Appella (1973) partially purified FMR antigen and could not separate this specificity from H-2 antigens. However, it is quite possible that further purification, or alternate methods of isolation, would separate the two specificities.

### 12.2.1.7. Variation in Expression of Leukemia-Associated Antigens

Studies with a variety of experimental leukemias have indicated that the quantitative expression of leukemia-associated antigens can vary considerably among cell lines and can even vary in the same line according to the phase in the cell cycle and in response to exposure to humoral antibodies. Klein *et al.* (1966) performed an extensive study on a number of mouse leukemias induced by Moloney leukemia virus, and showed a wide range in the expression of Moloney virus-associated cell surface antigen. Some tumors with low but detectable (by absorption experiments) quantities of antigen were shown to be resistant to immune rejection *in vivo* and to cytotoxic antibodies *in vitro*. Such studies indicate that the failure to detect antigens by direct tests does not necessarily mean that the antigens are absent, and that more sensitive techniques are usually needed to detect small quantities of cell surface antigens.

Cikes and Friberg (1971) studied the expression of Moloney virus-associated cell surface antigen (MCSA) and H-2 antigen during different phases of the cell cycle and found that the two types of antigens were temporally coexpressed, with maximal sensitivity to cytotoxicity in the Gl phase. Lerner *et al.* (1971) studied another Moloney virus-induced leukemia and obtained similar results. However, they felt the phenomenon was due to differences in sensitivity to lysis and not fluctuations in antigen levels. In response to this, Cikes and Klein (1972) showed by absorption experiments that MCSA and H-2 were expressed in higher amonts in Gl. The parallel fluctuation of the leukemia-associated antigen and H-2 might be taken as an indication of a physical association between them. However, Cikes *et al.* (1973) also showed that with prolonged passage of Moloney leukemias, MCSA increased whereas H-2 antigen expression decreased.

Initial studies attempting to immunize TL-negative strains of mice against their own TL+ leukemias were unsuccessful; leukemia cells recovered from these mice were found to have changed to TL− (Boyse *et al.*, 1963). However, return of the tumor to nonimmune mice led to a rapid reexpression of TL antigen. This reversible loss of TL antigen was termed antigenic modulation, and this could be induced *in vitro* by exposure at 37°C of cells to anti-TL antibodies (Old *et al.*, 1968). The loss of antigen from the cell surface was shown to require metabolic activity, and capping of the antigens was ordinarily seen (Stackpole *et al.*, 1974). However, modulation was shown to occur with monovalent antibody, without cap formation (Stackpole *et al.*, 1974).

Since the initial demonstration of antigenic modulation with TL antigen, this phenomenon has been shown to occur with a variety of normal and tumor-associated cell surface antigens. Aoki and Johnson (1973) were able to induce the modulation of GCSAa *in vivo* in both actively and passively immunized mice. Ortaldo *et al.* (1974) showed that fetal antigens on a mouse Rauscher virus-induced leukemia could be modulated, and that the loss of antigen was usually not complete but rather just a quantitative decrease.

## 12.2.2. Human Leukemia

### 12.2.2.1. Normal Cell Surface Markers

In the past few years, many studies of the cell surface markers on human leukemia cells have been performed. As in the experimental leukemias, markers associated with normal subpopulations of lymphoid cells have also been detected on leukemic cells, and these markers appear very useful for classifying the leukemias and for understanding some aspects of their biology.

Normal human T cells have been found to have receptors for sheep erythrocytes, and when these cell types are mixed together, they spontaneously form rosettes, which are frequently called E rosettes (Jondal *et al.*, 1972). Minowada *et al.* (1972) showed that the MOLT cell line, derived from a patient with acute lymphocytic leukemia (ALL), formed E rosettes. Since then, many investigators have shown that the lymphoblasts from some, but not all, patients with ALL form E rosettes (Borella and Sen, 1973; Belpomme *et al.*, 1974; Kersey *et al.*, 1974). Blast cells from some patients with ALL have also been shown to react with specific anti-T-cell antisera (Kersey *et al.*, 1974; Schlossman *et al.*, 1976). Among the ALL patients with T-cell markers, one had very high numbers of circulating blasts (Borella and Sen, 1973), but no other particular clinical features were noted (Belpomme *et al.*, 1974; Kersey *et al.*, 1974).

Although some ALLs have T-cell markers and appear to be derived from T lymphocytes, the blast cells from the majority of ALL patients lack these markers. The derivation of these tumors is not clear. Since these leukemias also usually lack complement receptors and surface immuno-globulins (Shevach *et al.*, 1972b; Wilson and Nossal, 1971; Smith *et al.*, 1973; Belpomme *et al.*, 1974), it has been suggested that they were also derived from T cells, but were not at the proper state of differentiation for expression of T-cell markers. However, recent studies with alloanti-sera (Fu *et al.*, 1975) and with a heterologous anti-p23,30 antiserum (Schlossman *et al.*, 1976), which react primarily with B cells, were reactive with ALL blast cells lacking T-cell markers.

The leukemia cells in Sézary's syndrome have been found to form E rosettes and react with anti-T-cell antisera (Broome *et al.*, 1973; Brouet *et al.*, 1973; Edelson *et al.*, 1974). However, T-cell markers have not been detected on the cells in some cases (Braylan *et al.*, 1975).

Chronic lymphocytic leukemia (CLL) cells have been shown usually to bear surface immunoglobulin (Aisenberg *et al.*, 1973), complement receptors (Shevach *et al.*, 1972b,c), and Fc receptors (Dickler *et al.*, 1973; Belpomme *et al.*, 1974), and to react with anti-B-cell sera (Greaves and Brown, 1973; Ishii *et al.*, 1975). Therefore most cases of CLL appear to be derived from B cells. It is thus of interest to note that many human lymphocytic leukemias have B-cell markers in contrast to the rarity of lymphocytic leukemias in mice with such markers. In some cases, how-ever, B-cell markers were not detected (e.g., Piessens *et al.*, 1973). A few such cases of CLL without B-cell markers have been shown to have T-cell markers (e.g., Insel *et al.*, 1975). In addition, cells from some patients with atypical forms of lymphocytic leukemia formed E rosettes and also had complement receptors (Shevach *et al.*, 1974; Lin and Hsu, 1976). Simi-larly, the MOLT cell line from a patient with ALL had both types of receptors (West and Herberman, 1974). It remains unclear whether an additional marker is produced abnormally by transformed lymphocytes or whether such cells with double markers are derived from a normal cell type with the same characteristics (Shevach *et al.*, 1974).

In contrast to all the attention given to normal cell surface markers on lymphocytic leukemias, there have been very few comparable studies of the myelogenous leukemias. This is easily explained by the lack of many immunologic markers for such cells. Schlossman *et al.* (1976) found that their anti-p23,30 serum, which reacted mainly with B cells, also reacted with most AML cells tested. However, the significance of this observation in regard to derivation of AML remains unclear.

### 12.2.2.2. Leukemia-Associated Antigens

Over the past several years, a number of investigators have attempted to produce specific antisera to human leukemia-associated antigens by immunization of heterologous species. Viza *et al.* (1970) prepared papain-solubilized materials from AML, CML, and CLL cells and used these to immunize rabbits. After absorptions of the antisera, they appeared to detect several leukemia-associated specificities by precipitation reactions and cytotoxicity. In further studies with one antiserum prepared against an AML cell extract, the detected antigen appeared to be present in fetal sera and in the sera of patients with all types of leukemia and Hodgkin's disease, but was not detected in normal sera (Harris *et al.*, 1971). Although the data in these brief reports appear quite promising, it is difficult to determine how extensive the specificity controls were. Yata *et al.* (1970) immunized rabbits with a homogenate of ALL cells, after being made "tolerant" to normal leukocytes by repeated inoculations during the neonatal period. The resulting antiserum gave one precipitin line in gel diffusion with acute and chronic lymphocytic and myelogenous leukemias and with lymphomas. It also reacted with normal thymocytes and some peripheral lymphocytes, and was therefore not leukemia specific. Mann *et al.* (1971, 1974) immunized rabbits with papain-solubilized cell membrane components from the lymphoid tissue culture line, Raji, derived from a patient with Burkitt's lymphoma. The resulting antiserum was cytotoxic for ALL and AML cells but not for normal leukocytes, remission leuko-cytes, or bone marrow cells. The antigen was not detected on embryonic kidney cell lines, but appeared after these lines were infected with MuLV or SV40. However, the antigen was not detected on mouse cell lines infected with the same viruses. Therefore the antigen appeared to be specific for an antigen common to human acute leukemia- and virus-infected human cells. However, in individual patients with leukemia, there was not a correlation between the proportion of morphologic blasts and of cells sensitive to the antibody. The antigen appeared to circulate in the sera of patients in relapse.

Bentwich *et al.* (1972) raised antisera against intact CLL cells. After absorptions, the antisera had cytotoxic reactivity with CLL cells and with some normal lymphocytes of newborns, but did not react with normal adult lymphocytes. However, it was not determined whether the antisera reacted with other types of leukemia cells.

Mohanakumar *et al.* (1974) used a somewhat different approach for immunization by inoculating leukemia cells into nonhuman primates. The pattern of specificity of the absorbed antisera was also different from those of the rabbit antisera prepared by other workers or themselves. Antisera produced against CLL cells detected an antigen common to ALL and CLL cells, and absent on myeloid leukemias. Antisera to myeloid leukemia cells gave the opposite pattern, reacting with AML and CML cells and not with lymphocytic leukemias. Metzgar *et al.* (1974) were able to solubilize the antigens detected by the primate antisera, by the use of trypsin or 3 M KCl extraction.

Greaves *et al.* (1975) prepared antisera in rabbits to ALL and attempted to block recognition of normal lymphocytes by precoating the cells with antitonsil antibodies. After absorption, the reactivity of the antisera was evaluated by membrane immunofluorescence. Positive results were obtained with lymphoblasts from some, but not all, patients with ALL; negative results were seen with CLL and CML cells, and with normal adult lymphocytes and fetal thymocytes. Of considerable interest was the fact that the ALL cells lacking this antigen were those with T-cell markers. Weak reactions were obtained with some AML cells and with cells from CML in blast crisis; however, this reactivity could be selectively removed by absorption with AML cells. Further studies with this absorbed antiserum revealed it to be quite specific for ALL cells lacking T-cell markers and for acute undifferentiated leukemias (Brown *et al.*, 1975a,b). As part of the detailed analysis of specificity, the antigen was shown to be undetectable on fetal cells, activated lymphocytes, enzyme-treated lymphocytes, normal bone marrow cells, and virus-infected cells. Of all the reagents developed thus far, this antiserum appears to be the most specific and applicable for diagnostic procedures. It is particularly impressive that such good specificity was seen with immunofluorescence, since this permits the examination of even weak reactions with individual cells.

All these antisera were prepared in heterologous species. Mann *et al.* (1975) raised cytotoxic antisera in ALL patients by immunization with Raji cells. The antisera reacted with the autologous leukemia cells, allogeneic ALL cells, but also with some AML cells; very infrequent reactions with normal cells were seen. The specificities of the antibodies were not further defined.

Klein *et al.* (1974) detected a nuclear antigen by anticomplement immunofluorescence in the nuclei of AML cells and designated it LANA (leukemia-associated nuclear antigen). The antibody to LANA was found in 73% of sera from AML patients, in an intermediate proportion of other types of leukemia and lymphoma, and in a small proportion of normal adults.

In summarizing these results, it is quite encouraging that apparently leukemia-specific antisera can be produced or found. Thus far there have been very few attempts at clinical applications of these reagents for initial diagnosis, or particularly for monitoring of patients during the course of therapy. However, one might anticipate that the results of such important studies will be available in the near future.

### 12.2.2.3. Possible Virus-Associated Antigens

The possible expression of type C virus-associated antigens, particularly those of MuLV, in human leukemia has been a subject of interest for many years. Fink *et al.* (1965) prepared heterologous antisera to Rauscher leukemia virus and to viruslike particles in human leukemic plasma, and used these in immunofluorescence studies of human bone marrow specimens. Positive reactions were obtained with bone marrows from erythroleukemia and also with marrow cells from a variety of other blood dyscrasias and malignancies. Bates *et al.* (1969) obtained similar results. Both in this study and in a study by Yohn *et al.* (1968), the reactivity of the antisera could be removed by absorption with normal bone marrow. It is therefore unlikely that these studies were detecting virus-associated antigens.

In a very recent detailed study, Metzgar *et al.* (1976a) reported that all leukemic cells from CML and some acute myelomonocytic leukemia (AMML) donors were lysed by rabbit antisera to purified Friend leukemia virus (FLV) gp69/71; cells from AML, ALL, and CLL patients, and normal and remission lymphocytes were unaffected. Although the authors strongly suggested that common antigens to FLV were being detected, the antiserum could not be inhibited by normal platelets and granulocytes. It therefore seems possible that the antiserum contained an antibody to normal marrow elements in addition to the viral specificity. Another antiserum to intact FLV also reacted with CLL cells, as well as CML and AMML cells, and this was thought to be related to p30 antigens and not to leukocyte or platelet antigens. Also of interest was the finding that FLV and FLV gp69/71 were able to absorb out all the cytotoxic reactivity of their nonhuman primate antisera to human myeloid leukemia antigens. In a further report Metzgar *et al.* (1976b) showed that a goat antiserum to feline leukemia virus reacted with cells from many patients with all morphological types of leukemia, and not with normal lymphocytes. Goat anti-simian sarcoma virus and anti-gibbon ape leukemia virus sera reacted with CLL and ALL cells. Gibbon ape leukemia virus was able to inhibit the cytotoxicity of primate anti-CLL antiserum against CLL target cells. The patterns of reactivity were quite complex, and were interpreted as indicating a multiplicity of leukemia-associated antigens. These results are intriguing, but their implications for the relationship between human leukemias and oncogenic viruses remain to be determined. These investigators are currently evaluating the clinical usefulness of these antiviral reagents for diagnosis and for classification of leukemias.

Another line of evidence that has been considered, suggestive of a virus association with human acute leukemia, is the frequent finding of humoral or cell-mediated reactivity of nonleukemic individuals against leukemic cells. As is discussed later in more detail, some relatives of leukemia patients and some unrelated normal donors have been found to have antibodies or cellular immunity (in cytotoxicity, migration inhibition, and lymphocyte proliferation assays) against leukemia-associated antigens. These data are consistent with, but certainly do not prove, the hypothesis that the reactivity is a result of horizontal transmission of an infectious agent, possibly a virus. It should be noted that these data could have other explanations, including sensitization to cross-reacting bacterial or other ubiquitous antigens.

## 12.3. Immunosuppression in Leukemia

### 12.3.1. Experimental Animal Systems

Depressed immunologic competence of animals bearing primary or transplantable leukemias has been noted by many investigators. Effects on humoral antibody responses and on the ability to mount a cell-mediated immune response have been described, and these have been attributed to a variety of mechanisms. A generally depressed ability to respond immunologically would be expected to have an important bearing on the development of effective immunity to leukemia-associated antigens and on effective resistance of the host to progressive tumor growth. Therefore, before discussing studies of immunity to leukemia antigens, it is important to review the immunological background in which such reactions might take place or be depressed. The following is not meant to be a comprehensive review on the subject of immune depression in cancer, which has been done quite recently by Stutman (1975).

The ability of leukemic animals to produce specific antibodies in response to antigens has been studied mainly in regard to the effects of type C leukemia viruses on humoral immunity. These virus-related effects are discussed later. The effects of the disease itself on antibody production have not been extensively studied. The main model employed has been the spontaneous leukemias arising in AKR mice. Since this form of leukemia is caused by an oncogenic leukemia virus, it is difficult to be certain that the observed deficits are due to the leukemia rather than to the presence of infectious virus. Despite this potential limitation, some early reports indicated no deficiency in preleukemic AKR mice, when viruses are already being expressed. Metcalf and Moulds (1967) noted only a slight delay and a somewhat lower peak in the response of preleukemic AKR mice to primary immunization with sheep erythrocytes. In AKR mice with leukemia present, the response to sheep erythrocytes was then severely depressed (Metcalf and Moulds, 1967; Ram et al., 1973). Frey-Wettstein and Hays (1970) also found that antibody responses in preleukemic AKR mice were normal, and furthermore that the immunoglobulin levels were normal. To analyze the depression that occurs with overt leukemia in AKR mice, Roman and Golub (1976) studied the *in vitro* response of AKR spleen cells to sheep erythrocytes and to a thymus-independent antigen. Both types of responses were markedly depressed. Cells from the leukemic mice were shown to suppress the antibody responses of normal syngeneic and semiallogeneic cells, but not of allogeneic cells. This suppression by leukemic cells required direct contact with the normal cells, and occurred when the leukemic cells were added at any time during the culture period. The suppression could be reversed by the addition of irradiated allogeneic cells. The precise mechanism for this type of suppression and whether the leukemic cells themselves rather than nonleukemic suppressor cells or other factors are responsible, remain to be determined. One factor which may be partially responsible for the depressed antibody responses, at least *in vivo*, is depressed antigen uptake by macrophages or reticuloendothelial cells (Ram et al., 1974).

Much more attention has been directed toward depression of cell-mediated immunity in leukemia. Preleukemic AKR mice were found to have depressed responses in macrophage migration inhibition tests with tuberculin (Frey-Wettstein and Hays, 1970). Zatz et al. (1973a) reported that lymphocyte proliferative responses to phytohemagglutinin (PHA) decreased in preleukemic AKR mice by 6 months of age. In studies of leukemic mice, they noted differences between two types of tumors, which they called type A and type B (Zatz et al., 1973b). With type A leukemia, which included thymic enlargement, there was normal responsiveness to PHA. In contrast, with type B, in which the thymus was atrophic, PHA reactivity was markedly depressed. They postulated that in this type of leukemia, there was destruction of the T-cell pool. Nagaya (1973) also noted some decrease in lymphoproliferative responses of preleukemic AKR mice to concanavalin A (Con A), but actually observed an increased response to PHA. The reason for this latter difference from the study of Zatz et al. (1973a) is not clear. Nagaya (1973) did find marked depression in reactions to both PHA and Con A in leukemic mice. Monkeys with herpes virus saimiri-induced leukemia or lymphoma have also been shown to have markedly depressed responses to PHA and Con A (Wallen et al., 1975).

Until recently, there were no adequate explanations for the

depressed cell-mediated reactivity of leukemic and other tumor-bearing individuals. One mechanism which can account for the depressed lymphoproliferative response to mitogens and tumor-associated antigens is the presence of suppressor cells in tumor-bearing hosts (reviewed by Kirchner et al., 1977). This phenomenon has been extensively studied in rats bearing the syngeneic Gross virus-induced leukemia (C58NT)D (Glaser et al., 1975). Rats with progressively growing tumors were found to have depressed lymphoproliferative responses to PHA and no detectable responses to tumor cells. After removal of suppressor cells on rayon adherence columns from the spleens of progressors, good reactivity to mitogens and to tumor cells was detected. The role of suppressor cells was documented by the addition of cells from progressor rats to the mixture of tumor cells with reactive cells from regressors, which resulted in strong inhibition of the response. These results clearly indicated that lymphocytes from rats bearing progressively growing leukemias do have the ability to recognize and to be stimulated in vitro by tumor cells or by mitogens, but that their proliferative response is abrogated or strongly inhibited by suppressor cells. In this system, the suppressor cells were shown to have the characteristics of macrophages (Glaser et al., 1975; Oehler et al., 1977) rather than the more commonly considered suppressor T cell. Such suppressor macrophages have been found within tumors themselves, as well as the lymphoid organs of tumor bearers (Holden et al., 1976).

Another factor to be considered for the depressed cellular immunity in leukemic hosts is immunosuppression by the tumor itself or by products of the tumor. Only low concentrations of the rat leukemia (C58NT)D caused proliferation of normal allogeneic or syngeneic immune lymphocytes, and this could be attributed to inhibitory properties of higher doses of the tumor cells (Bonnard and Herberman, 1975). The active factor has been shown to be a contaminating parvovirus in the tumor, the Kilham rat virus (KRV). This virus has been a consistent contaminant of (C58NT)D and other rat tumors. KRV, isolated from tumor cells, when added to in vitro cultures has markedly inhibited the proliferative response of normal lymphocytes to Con A, allogeneic lymphocytes, and to the tumor itself. It appears that KRV can grow preferentially in actively dividing cells, and that its effects on proliferative responses are largely related to cytopathic infection of the stimulated blast cells. A similar inhibitory phenomenon has been seen with some mouse leukemias (Bonnard et al., 1976). RBL-5, a Rauscher virus-induced leukemia, and a subline of EL-4, a chemically induced leukemia, were found to suppress proliferative responses to allogeneic lymphocytes strongly, and also to interfere with the generation of cytotoxic effector cells. This suppression was shown to be due to another parvovirus, minute virus of mice (MVM). MVM is a consistent contaminant of these and of some other mouse leukemias.

In considering factors which may interfere with the cell-mediated immune response of tumor-bearing individuals, serum-blocking factors are most frequently thought of (reviewed recently by Baldwin *et al.*, 1974). In a number of tumor systems, serum factors have been shown to interfere specifically or nonspecifically with immune reactions to tumor antigens. With leukemias, serum antibodies have been shown frequently to cause immunologic enhancement (Feldman, 1973). Recently, Ting and Herberman (1975) showed that a mixture of X-irradiated FBL-3 tumor cells (a Friend virus-induced leukemia) with anti-FBL-3 serum resulted in a block of *in vivo* immunogenicity, and this may be one of the mechanisms by which specific interference with serum occurs. Serum has also been reported to block cytotoxicity in the $^{51}$Cr release assay against (C58NT)D (Shellam and Knight, 1974). However, in our studies, we have had considerable difficulty in demonstrating specific serum blocking in this assay. Serum factors from tumor-bearing rats are another mechanism for inhibition of lymphoproliferative responses (Glaser *et al.*, 1975). In that study, however, the inhibition was not specific, since stimulation by PHA was also suppressed. One possible type of nonspecific inhibitory factor, which has been reported to be elevated in the sera of tumor-bearing individuals, is immunoregulatory $\alpha$-globulin. This protein has been found to inhibit lymphoproliferative responses of immune rats to tumor antigen (Glaser and Herberman, 1974) and the cytotoxic reactivity of mice immune to FBL-3 leukemia cells (Glaser *et al.*, 1976b).

Another major area of interest has been the immune suppression caused by murine leukemia viruses. This area has recently been reviewed (Ceglowski and Friedman, 1973; Friedman *et al.*, 1976). Many studies have indicated that the tumor viruses themselves can impair the immune response. The effects of these viruses on antibody response to sheep erythrocytes have been most extensively studied, but marked depression of humoral responses to a variety of other antigens has been seen. Cell-mediated immune responses to allografts and to microbial antigens have also been found to be depressed by murine leukemia viruses. These viruses can also impair macrophage function (Levy and Wheelock, 1975). However, despite the many studies in this area, very little is yet known about the effects of leukemia viruses on the immune response to the tumor virus antigens and to the cell surface antigens associated with the tumors.

## 12.3.2. Human Leukemia

In considering the competence of the immune system in patients with leukemia, one major difficulty is that most of the patients are treated with chemotherapeutic agents which are themselves immunosuppressive. It is therefore desirable to discuss first the effects of the disease itself on the immune responses and then to consider the superimposed effects of therapy. However, in some studies it is not possible to separate these variables.

### 12.3.2.1. Studies in Untreated Patients

Serum immunoglobulin levels in untreated patients with acute leukemia have been reported by several investigators to be in the normal range (e.g., Gooch and Fernbach, 1971). However, some studies found low IgG levels (Chandra, 1972) or IgA levels (McKelvey and Carbone, 1965). Antibody production has generally not been studied in acute leukemia prior to therapy. Chronic lymphocytic leukemia (CLL) is a disease of B cells (as discussed earlier) and is often accompanied by decreased serum immunoglobulins (Ultmann et al., 1959; Scamps et al., 1971). Antibody production in response to antigenic stimulation has also been found to be depressed in CLL patients (Larson and Tomlinson, 1953).

In regard to cell-mediated immunity, few studies on patients with acute leukemia have been performed prior to any therapy. Dupuy et al. (1971) studied 50 patients with untreated acute leukemia and found that 96% had positive delayed hypersensitivity skin reactions to at least one of a battery of recall antigens, but the number of positive skin tests and the size of the reactions were less than in controls. Santos et al. (1973) performed a similar study on 24 untreated patients, primarily adults with AML, and found that 10 were anergic, i.e., unreactive to any of the battery of recall antigens. In those patients not totally anergic, the number of antigens reacted to were less than in normal controls. Therefore, some deficit in cell-mediated immunity appears to exist in acute leukemia, but the extent of the deficit seems to vary over a wide range, and probably depends on the age of the patient and the type of leukemia.

In CLL, delayed hypersensitivity reactions to recall antigens and skin sensitization to dinitrochlorobenzene seem to be unimpaired in the majority of untreated cases (Block et al., 1969). In contrast, these and many other investigators (Nowell, 1960; Oppenheim et al., 1965; Rubin et al., 1969) have noted a markedly impaired in vitro lymphoproliferative response of CLL patients to PHA. Decreased proliferative responses in mixed lymphocyte cultures have also been noted (Smith et al., 1973). A further characteristic of the response to PHA of lymphocytes from CLL patients is a delayed peak, at 7 days instead of the usual 3 days (Oppenheim et al., 1965; Rubin et al., 1969; Bouroncle et al., 1969). A recent study by Wybran et al. (1973) showed that these abnormal responses could be accounted for by dilution of normally reactive T cells by the unreactive CLL cells.

The mechanisms causing decreased immunologic function in leukemia have not been extensively studied or defined. However, the recent studies of Waldmann *et al.* (1976) point to a possible role of suppressor cells in causing hypogammaglobulinemia in thymoma and multiple myeloma. In the thymoma patients, suppressor T cells could inhibit production of immunoglobulins by normal lymphocytes. However, in the myeloma patients, and similar to the findings in rodent leukemias (discussed earlier), the suppression was mediated by non-T cells with the properties of monocytes (Broder *et al.*, 1975). It will be of considerable interest to look for suppressor cells in patients with acute or chronic leukemia who have evidence of immune depression.

### 12.3.2.2. Effects of Therapy on Immune Responses in Leukemic Patients

Leventhal *et al.* (1974) recently reviewed the effects of chemotherapy on immune responses in acute leukemia, and in the present discussion, only some selected points will be made. Sen and Borella (1973) studied the proportions and absolute levels of T and B cells in children with acute leukemia, in remission after prolonged, continuous chemotherapy. In addition to depression of total lymphocyte counts, B cells were disproportionately low. After cessation of therapy, there was a rebound in B-cell levels, reaching a plateau at 2–3 months. T-cell levels rose more slowly, only reaching normal levels after 1 year.

The usual therapeutic regimens for acute leukemia have been found to cause more depression in B-cell function than in T-cell function. Depressed levels of immunoglobulins and poor primary and secondary antibody responses have been noted (Leventhal *et al.*, 1974; Schieffer *et al.*, 1976). During intensive induction chemotherapy for acute leukemia, depressed delayed hypersensitivity reactions (Hersh *et al.*, 1971) and lymphoproliferative responses (Hersh and Oppenheim, 1967) have been noted. Poor reactivity at this time was associated with poor prognosis (Hersh *et al.*, 1971). However, after patients have gone into remission and are maintained on cyclic chemotherapy, only minimal depression in cell-mediated immunity has been detected. Char *et al.* (1973) found very few patients to be anergic to recall antigen skin tests. At 10–20 days after completion of a course of therapy, rebound to higher than normal lymphoproliferative responses to antigens has been noted (Cheema and Hersh, 1971; Harris and Stewart, 1972). The occurrence of this rebound appeared to be associated with good prognosis. In CLL, induction of remission with whole-body irradiation (Kagan and Johnson, 1967) or with chemotherapy (Bouroncle *et al.*, 1969) resulted in a return to normal of lymphoproliferative responses.

## 12.4. Immune Responses to Experimental Leukemias

There has been a very large number of studies of the humoral and cell-mediated immune responses to leukemias in experimental animals. To summarize and interrelate these studies adequately would require a separate, detailed review, and such reviews have been published elsewhere (e.g., Herberman, 1974; Lamon, 1974; Ting and Herberman, 1976). This is not attempted here, but rather, we will briefly summarize some selected aspects of these studies, with particular emphasis on the *in vivo* significance of some of the *in vitro* reactions and on the potential applications to the understanding of the immune responses to human leukemia.

### 12.4.1. Humoral Immune Responses

Most of the antisera used in serologic studies of transplantable leukemias have been obtained from hyperimmune animals or at one or relatively few time points after inoculation of tumor cells. There have been very few detailed studies of the kinetics of antibody response to tumor-associated cell surface antigens, and of the relationship of antibody levels to tumor growth.

Herberman and Oren (1971) found that upon inoculation of the Gross virus-induced leukemia (C58NT)D into syngeneic W/Fu rats, there was a biphasic cytotoxic response, regardless of whether the tumor regressed or progressed. The first peak occurred 10–15 days after tumor cell inoculation and was due to 19S antibodies. The second peak occurred at 30–40 days and was due to 7S antibodies. In rats with regressing tumors, the level of antibodies declined to low concentrations after 50 days. In rats with progressively growing tumors, the first peak was the same as in regressor animals; however, the level of 7S antibody did not fall, but remained stable or continued to rise.

Similar results were obtained in studies of the Friend virus-induced leukemia FBL-3 in C57BL/6 mice (Herberman *et al.*, 1975f). The antibody response in regressors was biphasic; a first peak was seen at 10–14 days, no antibody was detected at 20–25 days, and then the antibody level rose progressively for at least 60 days. In progressors, antibodies were first detected at 7 days and the levels rose progressively until death.

In these studies of virus-induced tumors, the level of antibodies was correlated with the presence of actively growing tumor cells. It is important to note that no evidence was obtained in these leukemias for *in vivo* absorption of antibodies and resultant depression of the levels of circulating antibodies by the growing tumors, as has been seen in other types of tumor systems. In these systems, production of antibodies actually may be dependent on the continuing presence of tumor antigen in the host.

In addition to the induction of antibodies by immunization with tumor cells, it is becoming increasingly clear that natural or spontaneously appearing antibodies may be seen, with reactivity against a variety of tumor-associated or virus-associated antigens. One of the first studies of this type was by Aoki *et al.* (1966), who showed that older normal C57BL/6 mice developed antibodies to Gross cell surface antigen. Of considerable interest, these natural antibodies were only detected in strains of mice resistant to Gross leukemia. Recently, considerable evidence has been obtained for the widespread occurrence in mice of antibodies to endogenous type C viruses (Ihle *et al.*, 1973; Aaronson and Stephenson, 1973; Nowinski and Kaehler, 1974). These antibodies appear to be directed against the virus envelope antigens, gp69/71, gp43, and p15 (Lee and Ihle, 1975). It is not yet clear what the relationship of these antibodies is to the development of leukemia in various strains of mice.

Essex, Hardy, and their associates have performed an extensive series of studies on the natural appearance in cats of antibodies to FOCMA, a cell surface antigen associated with feline leukemia virus (FeLV), and on the relationship of these antibodies to the natural history of feline leukemia. Cats with naturally occurring leukemia have low or absent antibodies to FOCMA (Essex *et al.*, 1975a). Conversely, cats that are naturally exposed to FeLV and remain healthy develop persistently high titers of antibody to FOCMA (Essex *et al.*, 1975b). The inability of some cats exposed to leukemia to develop high titers of antibodies to FOCMA was shown to be a predictive indicator of the subsequent development of leukemia (Essex *et al.*, 1975c).

## 12.4.2. Cell-Mediated Immune Responses

The cell-mediated immune response to leukemia is quite complex, with evidence for involvement of T cells, non-T lymphocytes, and macrophages (Herberman, 1974). In terms of factors of importance to *in vivo* resistance against tumor growth, T cells appear to play the predominant role. Berenson *et al.* (1975) have shown in the FBL-3 mouse leukemia system that T cells were needed for effective adoptive transfer. Similarly, Glaser *et al.* (1976a) found that T cells, and not complement receptor-bearing cells or macrophages, were essential for adoptive transfer of resistance against the rat leukemia (C58NT)D.

One of the principal *in vitro* assays for the study of T-cell immunity to leukemia-associated antigens has been the $^{51}$Cr release cytotoxicity assay. One of the main points of apparent lack of correlation between *in vitro* reactivity in this assay and *in vivo* resistance against tumor growth was the much more transient detection of cytotoxicity after immunization. However, recent studies have provided a simple answer to this. In *in vivo* experiments to demonstrate resistance to tumor growth, the challenge with tumor cells actually represents the second exposure of the immune host to tumor-associated antigens. A key factor in resistance to challenge may be the ability of the host to mount a rapid secondary immune response, particularly in the region of challenge. In three different tumor systems, rapid development of T-cell-dependent cytotoxic reactivity after secondary tumor challenge has been demonstrated (Holden *et al.*, 1975; Ting *et al.*, 1976; Glaser and Herberman, 1976).

Another area of considerable interest and potential importance for *in vivo* resistance to tumor growth is the occurrence of natural cell-mediated cytotoxicity in mice and rats against a variety of leukemias (Herberman *et al.*, 1975e; Kiessling *et al.*, 1975a; Zarling *et al.*, 1975; Sendo *et al.*, 1975; Nunn *et al.*, 1976). Mice of most strains develop this reactivity, with a peak at 5–10 weeks of age, which declines to low levels thereafter. The natural cell-mediated cytotoxicity was found to have specificity, with reactivity against several antigens (Herberman *et al.*, 1975e). High cytotoxic reactivity was found in nude mice (Herberman *et al.*, 1975e), and initially the effector cells were found to have no detectable cell surface markers (Herberman *et al.*, 1975d; Kiessling *et al.*, 1975b; Nunn *et al.*, 1976). However, more recent studies have indicated that the effector cells may be pre-T cells, with a low density of $\theta$ antigen and Fc receptors (Herberman *et al.*, unpublished observations). There are several preliminary indications that the natural cell-mediated cytotoxicity may play a significant *in vivo* role. Kiessling *et al.* (1975c) found a correlation between levels of natural reactivity in different strains of mice and the relative resistance to growth of transplantable leukemia cells. We have recently found that some leukemia cells which are very sensitive to natural cell-mediated cytotoxicity grew less well in nude mice than in conventional mice of the same strain, and that tumor growth was also impeded in 5- to 8-week-old mice compared to 3-month-old mice. Several groups (Kumar *et al.*, 1976; Gallagher *et al.*, 1976; Bonmassar and Cudkowicz, 1976) have drawn attention to the possible relationship between the phenomenon of genetic resistance to bone marrow and natural *in vivo* resistance to leukemia. Studies are needed to compare directly the effector cells and other characteristics of bone marrow resistance.

## 12.5. Clinical Studies on Immune Response to Leukemia-Associated Antigens

### 12.5.1. Humoral Antibodies

In contrast to the number of studies of antibodies in rodents to syngeneic leukemias and of heterologous antibodies to human leukemia-associated antigens (discussed earlier), there have been very few detailed and well-documented reports of specific antibodies in the sera of leukemia patients to such antigens. Seligmann *et al.* (1954) found that 8 of 54 sera from patients with acute leukemia had precipitation reactions with lysates of leukocytes. However, the specificity of the apparent antibodies was not explored. Greenspan *et al.* (1963) did not find antibodies in the sera of leukemia patients, but obtained positive reactions with the sera of six people who worked with materials from leukemia patients. It was postulated that a virus was responsible for the antibody formation. To demonstrate specificty, some absorptions were performed, but they were not extensive. Doré *et al.* (1967) studied the sera of 29 patients with acute leukemia by a variety of tests for serum antibodies using the autologous blast cells as antigens: cytotoxicity, membrane immunofluorescence, complement fixation, and immune adherence. Eight positive results were obtained in at least one of the assays. However, there was no correlation among the various tests, and no evidence was offered for the specificity of any of the reactions. Similarly, the reactions observed by Maruyama *et al.* (1968) against leukemia cells and against cell lines derived from leukemia patients were not shown to be specific. Yoshida and Imai (1970) tested the sera of 30 patients with leukemia for antibodies to autologous leukemia cells by the immune adherence technique. They found many positive reactions, with titers higher in remission than in relapse. The nature of the antigens was uncertain, since the sera of some normal individuals also gave positive reactions to low titer. In addition, only 20% of the leukemic cells had detectable antigenic sites. Herberman and Fahey (1968) found cytotoxic antibodies in the sera of leukemia patients which reacted with tissue culture cell lines derived from leukemic and other individuals. In chronic lymphocytic and myelogenous leukemias, there was an inverse correlation between the incidence of positive reactions and titers and the leukocyte counts of the patients (Herberman and Nam, 1971). However, the majority of normal and other controls had positive reactions, and actually had higher antibody titers than those seen in acute and chronic leukemia. By absorption experiments, the antigen detected on the lymphoid cell lines was found not to be tumor specific, being detectable in low concentration on normal peripheral blood leukocytes (Herberman, 1969). Bias *et al.* (1972) found cytotoxic antibodies in the sera of three normal individuals which reacted with acute lymphocytic leukemia cells and not with a panel of normal leukocytes. Absorption of the sera with leukemic cells removed the cytotoxic activity, whereas absorption with the same volume of normal cells did not. Although these results indicate that a tumor-associated antigen may be involved, it is still quite possible that the detected antibodies were similar or identical to those previously described by Herberman and Fahey (1968). Many more normal leukocytes than blast cells were required to remove cytotoxic reactivity of those sera (Herberman, 1969). Mann *et al.* (1974) performed a similar type of study, testing sera of 39 acute leukemia patients for complement-dependent cytotoxicity against allogeneic leukemic cells. Only five sera, all from patients in remission, had significantly positive activity. One of these five sera was found to react also against normal lymphocytes, but the others reacted only with leukemic target cells. No absorption studies were done to define the specificity of the positive patients' sera. However, an interesting study was done in which all the sera were tested for their ability to inhibit the cytotoxicity of the more extensively characterized heterologous antiserum to acute leukemia-associated antigens. Only sera lacking cytotoxic activity and obtained during relapse had inhibitory activity. The authors concluded that the inhibition was due to circulating leukemia-associated antigen or antigen–antibody complexes, and that this might account for the lack of detectable antibody in the sera of most patients.

Mitchell *et al.* (1973) used a different approach for detection of antibodies. They tested the sera of 25 patients with acute leukemia for antibodies cytophilic for macrophages. All the sera had antibodies which attached to macrophages and rendered them reactive to autologous tumor cells and to allogeneic leukemic cells of the same histologic type. There was only one instance of cross-reactivity with a different type of leukemia. There was also no reactivity against remission leukocytes from one patient. Absorption studies with fairly large numbers of normal leukocytes resulted in no removal of activity, whereas leukemic cells were able to absorb. This study appears to present rather strong evidence for specific antibodies in the sera of most acute leukemia patients against leukemia-associated antigens. However, there have been no further reports on the characterization of this phenomenon, and the work has yet to be confirmed by other laboratories.

Gutterman *et al.* (1973b) reported that the blast cells of eight patients with acute myelogenous leukemia were coated with immunoglobulins, primarily IgG. The presence of immunoglobulin coating correlated with the ability of the patients' sera to block the stimulation of lymphocytes by autologous blast cells. The mechanisms for these events have not been elucidated. There was no evidence presented that the immunoglobulins coating the blast cells represented specific antibodies, nor that the inhibitory serum factors were immunologically specific. In contrast to the frequency of the phenomenon in the acute myelogenous leukemia patients, no blast cells from patients with acute lymphocytic leukemia were coated with immunoglobulin. Metzgar *et al.* (1975) performed a similar study, detecting various classes of immunoglobulins on the surface of leukemic cells from some patients with acute or chronic lymphocytic or myelogenous leukemia. In contrast, remission cells from such patients gave negative reactions. To determine the possible specificity of the adsorbed immunoglobulins, acid eluates were prepared from some cells. The eluted immunoglobulins were cytotoxic for leukemic cells, supporting the concept that they were specific antibodies. Although they reacted strongest with leukemic cells from patients with the same type of leukemia, there was some reactivity with leukemic cells of different morphologic types.

Hersey *et al.* (1973) reported the detection of antibodies in the sera of a high proportion of patients with acute myelogenous leukemia which could mediate the cytotoxicity of allogeneic myeloblasts by normal lymphoid cells (i.e., antibody-dependent cell-mediated cytotoxicity). Preliminary results suggested that these antibodies might show useful clinical correlations. However, further analysis of the sera indicated that they contained anti-HLA antibodies and failed to react with autologous leukemia cells (MacLennan, personal communication).

In reviewing all of this information regarding possible antibody responses of patients to human leukemia-associated antigens, one is left with a rather confusing picture. It seems clear that many sera from leukemic patients, and also some control sera, contain antibodies which can react with leukemic cells. However, a variety of specificities appear to be detected, including normal leukocyte antigens and histocompatibility antigens. It remains to be more clearly determined what proportion of the observed reactions are actually directed against leukemia-associated antigens and which of the various procedures are detecting the same specificities.

## 12.5.2. Cell-Mediated Immune Responses

Although studies of cell-mediated immune responses of leukemia patients to possible leukemia-associated antigens were begun only a few years ago, this area has developed rapidly and there is now a considerable body of evidence, obtained by a variety of procedures, for cellular immunity to leukemia-associated antigens. The approaches taken for these studies have included *in vivo* skin tests for delayed hypersensitivity and *in vitro* assays of lymphocyte proliferation, leukocyte migration inhibition, and lymphocyte-mediated cytotoxicity.

### 12.5.2.1. Skin Reactions to Leukemia Antigens

Skin tests with tumor cells or tumor extracts have been used as an *in vivo* measure of delayed hypersensitivity. In a preliminary study of patients with acute leukemia, Oren and Herberman (1971) found skin reactivity of some patients to autologous membrane extracts of leukemic cells. When less than 3 mg protein/ml were used in the tests, the reactions appeared to be specific for leukemia. Biopsies of many of the positive reactions showed typical histologic features of delayed hypersensitivity. Char *et al.* (1973) extended these studies to 53 patients with ALL and 25 patients with AML. The patients were tested with membrane extracts of autologous and allogeneic blast and remission cells. Positive results were elicited in many of the leukemia patients by blast cell extracts but not by extracts of remission or normal cells. In the tests with allogeneic extracts, considerable evidence for the leukemia-associated specificity of the reactions was obtained. There was only reactivity to blast cells of the same histological type. In both ALL and AML patients, a significantly higher incidence of reactions to autologous and allogeneic blast extracts was seen in patients in remission, when compared to those in bone marrow relapse. Serial responses of patients to autologous blast extracts were usually related to clinical status, being positive in remission and negative when a patient relapsed.

Several other groups have also studied skin reactions to leukemia materials. In contrast to these studies with membrane extracts, some investigators have employed intact cells. In small numbers of patients, Gutterman *et al.* (1973a) obtained uniformly negative reactions with viable autologous cells, and Santos *et al.* (1973) obtained negative results with mitomycin C-treated leukemic cells. In a larger study, Baker *et al.* (1974) obtained positive reactions in almost half the acute leukemic patients tested to autologous X-irradiated blast cells. However, there was no correlation of reactivity to clinical status. They obtained very few positive results with membrane extracts, with extracts similar to those used by Char *et al.* (1973). The reasons for the differences among these studies are not clear.

All these tests were performed with particulate membrane extracts or whole cells. Some initial attempts have been made to solubilize the leukemia antigens and use these for skin tests. Gutterman *et al.* (1973a) obtained some positive reactions to crude 3 M potassium chloride extracts. In collaborative studies with Dr. Ariel Hollinshead, we have tested separated fractions from sonicated membrane extracts (Herberman *et al.*, 1975c; Hollinshead and Herberman, 1975). In both ALL and AML, it was possible, by a sequence of column chromatographic procedures followed by gradient polyacrylamide gel electrophoresis, to partially purify the skin-reactive antigens. The blast antigens associated with ALL also appeared to be present in early human fetal thymus cells, indicating that the ALL-associated skin-reactive antigens may be embryonic antigens (Hollinshead and Herberman, 1975).

One major problem in the tests with the leukemic blast materials was that the antigens did not appear to be equally represented in all extracts.

For example, in the studies of Char *et al.* (1973), some allogeneic preparations gave positive reactions in more than half the appropriate leukemia patients, whereas others were poorly reactive or nonreactive. Partly as an attempt to obtain large amounts of standard antigenic test materials, extracts were prepared from human lymphoid tissue culture cell lines, derived from leukemia, other tumors, and normal leukocytes (Herberman *et al.*, 1974b). Extracts of some of these lines have given positive skin reactions in leukemia patients (Herberman *et al.*, 1974b,1975b; Herberman, 1977), but there have been some inexplicable differences in reactivity of ALL patients from different areas. The Raji cell line extracts, derived from a patient with Burkitt's lymphoma, gave positive reactions in 40% of American patients with ALL and in several patients with AML, whereas very few French or Canadian ALL patients have reacted to the same preparations. These differences may be related to the treatment protocols used by the various institutions. It should be noted that the antigens detected on the cultured cells had considerably broader specificity than the blast cell extracts, since patients with various types of leukemia and lymphoma, and with nasopharyngeal carcinoma, reacted to the same cell line extracts.

### 12.5.2.2. Lymphoproliferative Responses to Leukemia Antigens

*In vitro* studies of cell-mediated reactivity to leukemia antigens were first performed with the autologous mixed lymphocyte tumor interaction. Cryopreserved leukemic blast cells have been inactivated by X-irradiation or mitomycin C and mixed with lymphocytes from the patients, obtained after therapy. In several studies, stimulation of the lymphocytes to undergo increased DNA synthesis and incorporation of [³H]thymidine have been observed (Fridman and Kourilsky, 1969; Viza *et al.*, 1969; Powles *et al.*, 1971; Leventhal *et al.*, 1972; Gutterman *et al.*, 1973b; Anderson *et al.*, 1974).

The specificity of the antigens detected is not completely clear. Several workers have incubated remission bone marrow cells with autologous peripheral blood lymphocytes of leukemia patients. Most of these tests were negative, although some positive results have been obtained (Leventhal *et al.*, 1972; Gutterman *et al.*, 1974a). Gutterman *et al.* (1974a) suggested that the positive results were due to small numbers of leukemic blasts in the marrow, and raised the possibility of using this assay to detect minimal residual disease. These conclusions were based on the finding that 5 of 8 patients who gave positive results subsequently relapsed, whereas of 17 unreactive patients, 15 remained in complete remission.

Despite these interesting results, one still cannot conclude with certainty that the antigens recognized are leukemia specific. This is particularly true since it has been shown recently that T cells of normal individuals can be stimulated by autologous non-T peripheral blood mononuclear cells (Opelz et al., 1975). It will be of interest to determine whether some of the stimulation seen with leukemic cells is due to differentiation antigens on normal blast cells as well as on leukemic blasts. No studies have yet been reported on attempts to stimulate lymphocytes of normal or nonleukemic individuals by autologous bone marrow cells.

One dissenting note in stimulation studies in acute leukemia was offered by Schweitzer et al. (1973). They observed some stimulation by autologous blast cells, but did not feel that the assay could be reliably used to detect cell-mediated immunity.

### 12.5.2.3. Migration Inhibition Assays

In the past few years, assays of migration inhibition of macrophages or of leukocytes have become increasingly popular for detection of cell-mediated immunity to human tumor-associated antigens. However, there have been very few studies reported on the use of these assays in human leukemia. Hilberg et al. (1973) performed an indirect migration inhibition assay, measuring the production of migration inhibitory factor by use of guinea pig macrophages. One of two patients with ALL in remission and some of the patients' relatives reacted to homogenates of blast cells but not to homogenates of normal leukocytes. Anderson et al. (1974) also used an indirect assay to study reactivity of acute leukemia patients and family members to intact leukemic blasts. Four of six patients in remission and 5 of 12 HL-A identical siblings gave positive results. More extensive studies will certainly have to be done for the adequate evaluation of the specificity and significance of these results.

### 12.5.2.4. Cell-Mediated Cytotoxicity

Assays of cell-mediated cytotoxicity probably have been the most popular and widely used assays for studies of cell-mediated immunity to human tumor-associated antigens. However, most of these studies were performed with solid tumors, and little attention has been directed toward human leukemias. All of the studies in leukemia have utilized a short-term $^{51}Cr$ release cytotoxicity assay. The initial studies were performed in this laboratory (Rosenberg et al., 1972; Leventhal et al., 1972; Herberman et al., 1972). Testing of autologous reactivity of leukemia patients showed positive results in 8 of 20 ALL patients and in 6 of 19 AML patients. No reactions were seen against autologous remission target cells. The reactions against the blast target cells did not correlate with clinical state. There was at least as much reactivity during bone marrow relapse as there was when the patients were in remission. Anderson *et al.* (1974) observed that five of six patients in remission reacted against their autologous blast cells.

In order to study allogeneic cell-mediated cytotoxicity in leukemia using freshly harvested cells, and to have available comparable normal cells as controls for those from the leukemia patients, some experiments have been performed with identical twins, one member of each pair having leukemia (Rosenberg *et al.*, 1972). Leukemia-associated antigens were detected on the cells of 7 out of 10 leukemic patients. In these tests against allogeneic target cells, a broader specificity was detected than in the autologous studies, since reactions were seen against remission cells of the leukemic patients, as well as against blast cells. However, the pattern of reactivity against blast cells and remission cells of the same patients was different, and it was thought likely that the remission cells contained antigens different from those of the blast cells. The finding of leukemia-associated antigens on remission cells is reminiscent of the finding of some tumor-associated antigens on morphologically normal cells of mice infected with leukemia virus (as discussed earlier).

A considerable number of normal individuals, including unrelated normal adults, reacted against the target cells from leukemia patients, but they did not react against their own lymphocytes or against allogeneic normal lymphocytes (Rosenberg *et al.*, 1972; Herberman *et al.*, 1972; Anderson *et al.*, 1974). This finding is also analogous to the natural cell-mediated cytotoxicity in mice and rats against tumor-associated antigens (as discussed earlier).

### 12.5.2.5. Correlations among Assays of Cell-Mediated Immunity

Cellular immunity to antigens on autologous blast cells was measured in 20 patients by three assays: skin tests, $^{51}$Cr release cytotoxicity, and mixed lymphocyte tumor cell interaction (Leventhal *et al.*, 1972). As already noted, the results of skin tests correlated with the clinical state. The *in vitro* assays in this study did not correlate with the stage of disease, with as many tests positive in relapse as in remission. The two *in vitro* assays also did not correlate with each other. The reasons for the lack of correlations are not clear. It is possible that each assay is measuring different antigens. Studies with isolated, soluble antigens are now feasible and should help to decide this issue. The assays may also be measuring different phases of the immune response, and different subpopulations of lymphoid cells may be responsible for the various effects.

## 12.6. Practical Clinical Applications of Immunology to Leukemia

### 12.6.1. Diagnostic and Prognostic Tests

One of the important and potential practical applications of immunologic studies is the development of immunodiagnostic techniques for human leukemia. Immunologic assays might help in distinguishing among the various types of acute leukemia, and this would assist in the selection of proper agents for therapy. There is a particular need for sensitive methods to monitor patients with acute leukemia during the course of therapy and, while in remission, to detect small numbers of leukemic blast cells in the bone marrow and to distinguish these from normal stem cells clearly.

In the section on human leukemia antigens, several reagents were discussed which appear promising for these important applications. Detection of leukemia-associated antigens on individual cells in the bone marrow or detection of elevated levels of circulating leukemia-associated antigens might provide a rational basis for continued or altered therapy. For these practical applications, however, markers which are not leukemia specific but are quantitatively altered could also be employed. Mori *et al.* (1975a,b) developed antisera to ferritin in leukemic cells and in normal placentas, and used these to detect elevated circulating levels of ferritin in many patients with acute leukemia or with CML in blast crisis. However, studies have not yet been reported on the correlation of serum levels with clinical course. Lysozyme, detected either enzymatically or immunologically, appears to be a particularly distinctive marker for monocytic and monomyelocytic leukemias (Osserman and Lawlor, 1966). Lysozyme and another cationic antigenic protein (CLA) of leukocytes have been detected in the urine of some patients with CML (Tischendorf *et al.*, 1973).

In addition to antigenic markers which might be useful in immunodiagnosis, some aspects of the immune response of patients may have diagnostic or prognostic significance. Hersh *et al.* (1975) performed skin tests for delayed hypersensitivity in acute leukemia patients shortly after the onset of chemotherapy and found that anergy was correlated with a poorer chance of remission induction. However, in patients who achieve remission, general cell-mediated immune competence does not appear to be an important prognostic factor (Char *et al.*, 1973). Skin tests with extracts of autologous or allogeneic leukemic cells in those patients correlated fairly well with clinical status, with loss of reactivity at around the time of early bone marrow relapse (Char *et al.*, 1973). In addition, positive reactions to allogeneic leukemic extracts correlated with a longer duration of remission (Leventhal *et al.*, 1973). Gutterman *et al.* (1975) found good prognosis in AML patients to be correlated with a vigorous lymphoproliferative response to autologous leukemia cells, inhibition of that response by autologous serum, presence of IgG coating of leukemia cells, and positive reactions in a migration inhibition assay with autologous leukemia cells.

## 12.6.2. Immunotherapy

There has been much interest in the use of immunotherapy in acute leukemia. The types of approaches and the results of many trials have been reviewed in depth (Henderson and Leventhal, 1972; Hersh *et al.*, 1973). Most of the recent attention has centered around the use in acute leukemia of *Mycobacterium bovis*, BCG (Bacille–Calmette–Guérin), with or without the addition of allogeneic irradiated leukemic cells. The efficacy of this form of therapy remains controversial. Some trials with ALL (summarized most recently by Mathé *et al.*, 1976) and AML (Powles *et al.*, 1973; Gutterman *et al.*, 1974b) have indicated a significant improvement in remission duration and survival in patients receiving immunotherapy. However, other trials, including some careful, well-controlled ones, have given essentially negative results (Medical Research Council, 1971; Children's Cancer Study Group A, 1973; Freeman *et al.*, 1973; Poplack *et al.*, 1975).

It is not clear why there has been a wide divergence in results among the immunotherapy trials. One important factor may be that most of the trials have been empirical, without assessment of the antigenicity and immunogenicity of the BCG and cells used for immunization, and without immunological monitoring of the immune response to therapy. More extensive immunologic testing might help in the design of future immunotherapy trials in which allogeneic blast cells are used for immunization. Some leukemic blasts can be identified as poorly antigenic (Char *et al.*, 1973; MacLennan *et al.*, 1975) and such materials could be excluded from the trial.

In addition, one would anticipate that monitoring of patients during the course of therapy would be helpful in determining the immunogenicity of different forms and schedules of therapy. However, the major difficulty at present is to identify the test or tests which could provide the important information. Joseph *et al.* (1976) noted an increase in the levels of "null" cells in ALL patients receiving immunotherapy. Powles *et al.* (1971) observed that inoculation of patients with acute leukemia with autologous irradiated blast cells produced a transient increase in their *in vitro* lymphoproliferative response to the tumor cells, and proposed that such testing could assist in determining optimum dosage and schedules for immunotherapy trials. Serial skin tests were performed on patients with ALL undergoing immunotherapy with BCG and allogeneic ALL blast cells (Leventhal *et al.*, 1973). These tests did not provide clear evidence for immunization, even against the HL-A antigens of the donor cells. However, there was a correlation between skin reactivity against the extracts of donor cells and the duration of remission. In France, immunologic assays were used to study ALL patients receiving the immunotherapy of Dr. Georges Mathé (Oldham *et al.*, 1976). This study revealed the expected immunosuppression during the intensive continuous chemotherapy. However, no striking differences in immune reactivity were seen in patients receiving immunotherapy. The group of patients on long-term immunotherapy was not detectably hyperresponsive as measured by skin reactivity to microbial antigens, by primary sensitization *in vivo* to puryl chloride, or by response to PHA *in vitro*. These patients did have a significantly higher incidence of positive delayed hypersensitivity reactions to allogeneic leukemia extracts, compared to the other groups at the same institution. However, the length of time after remission and the interval after chemotherapy were different between the groups. When the long-term immunotherapy patients were compared with patients at another French institution, in long-term remission after chemotherapy alone, the incidence of positive skin tests was similar for both groups (Herberman *et al.*, 1975a,b). ALL patients who were given immunotherapy with Raji cells, a cultured cell line derived from Burkitt's lymphoma, were shown to develop cytotoxic antibodies and increased lymphoproliferative responses to the immunizing cells (Sacks *et al.*, 1975). However, the clinical aspects of the trial were unsuccessful, so that the significance of the induction of these immune reactions cannot be adequately assessed. In trials of immunotherapy of AML patients, inoculation of allogeneic AML blasts was shown to lead to production of alloantibodies (Klouda *et al.*, 1975) and to cell-mediated cytotoxicity against the donor cells (Taylor *et al.*, 1976). These results provide some evidence for immunogenicity of the materials and schedules used, but do not indicate specific increases in sensitization to leukemia-associated antigens.

The data summarized here are somewhat fragmentary and inconclusive. No test has stood out as an index of successful immunotherapy. However, the efforts at monitoring in the course of randomized, controlled trials, in which suitable control individuals are available, have not been sufficient. One might still anticipate that such immunologic studies would help to design more rational immunotherapy trials.

## References

Aaronson, S. A., and Stephenson, J. R., 1973, Independent segregation of loci for activation of biologically distinguishable RNA C-type virus in murine cells, *Proc. Nat. Acad. Sci. U.S.A.* **70**:2055–2058.

Aisenberg, A., Bloch, K., and Long, J., 1973, Cell-surface immunoglobulins in chronic lymphocytic leukemia and allied disorders, *Am. J. Med.* **55**:184–191.

Anderson, P. W., Klein, D. L., Bias, W. B., Mullins, G. M., Burke, P. J., and Santos, G. W., 1974, Cell-mediated immunological reactivity of patients and siblings to blast cells from adult acute leukemias, *Israel J. Med. Sci.* **10**:1033–1051.

Aoki, T., and Johnson, P. A., 1973, Suppression of G (Gross) leukemia cell surface antigens: A kind of antigenic modulation, *J. Nat. Cancer Inst.* **49**:183–189.

Aoki, T., Boyse, E. A., and Old, L. J., 1966, Occurrence of natural antibody to the G (Gross) leukemia antigen in mice. *Cancer Res.* **25**:1415–1419.

Aoki, T., Boyse, E. A., and Old, L. J., 1968, Wild-type Gross leukemia virus. I. Soluble antigen (GSA) in the plasma and tissues of infected mice, *J. Nat. Cancer Inst.* **41**:89–96.

Aoki, T., Boyse, E. A., Old, L. J., de Harven, E., Hammerling, U., and Wood, H. A., 1970a, G (Gross) and H-2 cell surface antigens: Location on Gross leukemia cells by electron microscopy with visually labeled antibody, *Proc. Nat. Acad. Sci. U.S.A.* **65**:569–576.

Aoki, T., Stück, B., Old, L. J., Hammerling, U., and de Harven, E., 1970b, E antigen: A cell-surface antigen of C57BL leukemia, *Cancer Res.* **30**:244–251.

Aoki, T., Herberman, R. B., Johnson, P. A., Liu, M., and Sturm, M. M., 1972, Wild-type Gross leukemia virus: Classification of soluble antigens (GSA), *J. Virol.* **10**:1208–1219.

Aoki, T., Huebner, R., Chang, K., Sturm, M., and Liu, M., 1974, Diversity of envelope antigens on murine type-C RNA viruses, *J. Nat. Cancer Inst.* **52**:1189–1197.

Aoki, T., Herberman, R. B., and Liu, M., 1975, Heterogeneity of surface antigens on endogenous type C virus-producing cell sublines derived from a clonal line of BALB/3T3 cells, *Intervirology* **5**:31–42.

Baker, M. A., Taub, R. N., Brown, S. M., and Ramachandar, K., 1974, Delayed cutaneous hypersensitivity in leukemic patients to autologous blast cells, *Br. J. Hematol.* **27**:627–633.

Baldwin, R. W., Embleton, M. J., Price, M. R., and Robins, A., 1974, Immunity in the tumor-bearing host and its modification by serum factors, *Cancer* **34**:1452–1460.

Barker, A., and Waksal, S., 1974, Thymus-derived lymphocyte differentiation and lymphocytic leukemias, *Cell. Immunol.* **12**:140–149.

Bates, H. A., Bankole, R. O., and Swaim, W. R., 1969, Immunofluorescence studies in human leukemia, *Blood* **34**:430–440.

Bauer, H., 1974, Virion and tumor cell antigens of C-type RNA tumor viruses, *Adv. Cancer Res.* **20**:275–315.

Bauer, H., Bubenik, J., Graf, T., and Allgaier, C., 1969, Induction of transplantation resistance to Rous sarcoma isograft by avian leukosis virus, *Virology* **39**:482–490.

Belpomme, D., Dantchev, D., Durusquec, E., Grandjon, D., Huchet, R., Pouillart, P., Schwarzenberg, L., Amiel, J. L., and Mathé, G., 1974, T and B lymphocyte markers on the neoplastic cell of 20 patients with acute and 10 patients with chronic lymphoid leukemia, *Biomedicine* **20**:109–118.

Bentwich, Z., Weiss, D., Sulitzeanu, D., 1972, Antigenic changes on the surface of lymphocytes from patients with chronic lymphocytic leukemia, *Cancer Res.* **32**:1375–1383.

Berenson, J. R., Einstein, A. B., Jr., and Fefer, A., 1975, Syngeneic adoptive immunotherapy and chemotherapy of Friend leukemia: Requirement for T cells, *J. Immunol.* **115**:234–238.

Bianco, C., Patrick, R., and Nussenzweig, V., 1970, A population of lymphocytes bearing a membrane receptor for antigen–antibody–complement complexes, *J. Exp. Med.* **132**:702–720.

Bias, W. B., Santos, G. W., Burke, P. J., Mullins, G. M., and Humphrey, R. L., 1972, Cytotoxic antibody on normal human serums reactive with tumor cells from acute lymphocytic leukemia, *Science* **178**:304–306.

Blank, K. J., Freedman, H. A., and Lilly, F., 1976, T-lymphocyte response to Friend virus-induced tumor cell lines in mice of strains congenic at H-2, *Nature (London)* **260**:250–252.

Block, J. B., Haynes, H. A., Thompson, W. L., and Neiman, P. E., 1969, Delayed hypersensitivity in chronic lymphocytic leukemia, *J. Nat. Cancer Inst.* **42**:973–980.

Bolognesi, D. P., 1974, Structural components of RNA tumor viruses, *in Advances in Virus Research*, Vol. 19 (M. Lauffer, F. B. Bang, K. Maramorosch, and K. M. Smith, eds.), pp. 315–359, Academic Press, New York.

Bonmassar, E., and Cudkowicz, G., 1976, Suppression of allogeneic lymphomas in spleens of irradiated mice: Importance of the D end of the complex, *J. Immunol.* **117**:697–700.

Bonmassar, E., Bonmassar, A., Vadlamudi, S., and Goldin, A., 1970, Immunological alteration of leukemic cells *in vivo* after treatment with an antitumor drug, *Proc. Nat. Acad. Sci. U.S.A.* **66**:1089–1095.

Bonnard, G. D., and Herberman, R. B., 1975, Suppression of lymphocyte proliferative response by murine lymphoma cells, *in Immune Recognition* (A. S. Rosenthal, ed.), pp. 817–828, Academic Press, New York.

Bonnard, G. D., Manders, E. K., Campbell, D. A., Jr., Herberman, R. B., and Collins, M. J., Jr., 1976, Immunosuppressive activity of a subline of the mouse EL-4 lymphoma. Evidence for minute virus of mice causing the inhibition, *J. Exp. Med.* **143**:187–205.

Borella, L., and Sen, T. A., 1973, T-cell surface markers on lymphoblasts from acute lymphocytic leukemia, *J. Immunol.* **3**:1257–1260.

Bouroncle, B. A., Clausen, K. P., and Aschenbrand, J. F., 1969, Studies of the delayed response of phytohemagglutinin (PHA) stimulated lymphocytes in 25 chronic lymphatic leukemia patients before and during therapy, *Blood* **34**:166–178.

Boyse, E. A., and Old, L. J., 1969, Some aspects of normal and abnormal cell surface genetics, *Annu. Rev. Genet.* **3**:269–301.

Boyse, E. A., Old, L. J., and Luell, S., 1963, Antigenic properties of experimental leukemias. II. Immunological studies *in vivo* with C57BL/6 radiation-induced leukemias, *J. Nat. Cancer Inst.* **31**:987.

Braylan, R., Variakojis, D., and Yachnin, S., 1975, The Sézary syndrome lymphoid cell: Abnormal surface properties and mitogen responsiveness, *J. Haematol.* **31**:553–564.

Broder, S., Humphrey, R., Durm, M., Blackman, M., Meade, B., Goldman, C., Strober, W., and Waldmann, T., 1975, Impaired synthesis of polyclonal (nonparaprotein) immunoglobulins by circulating lymphocytes from patients with multiple myeloma, *N. Engl. J. Med.* **293**:887–892.

Broome, J. D., Zucker-Franklin, D., Weiner, M. S., Bianco, C., and Nussenzweig, V., 1973, Leukemic cells with membrane properties of thymus-derived (T) lymphocytes in a case of Sézary's syndrome: Morphologic and immunologic studies, *Clin. Immunol. Immunopathol.* **1**:319–329.

Brouet, J. C., Flandrin, G., and Seligmann, M., 1973, Indications of the thymus-derived nature of the proliferative cells in six patients with Sézary's syndrome, *N. Engl. J. Med.* **289**:341–344.

Brown, G., Capellaro, D., and Greaves, M., 1975a, Leukemia-associated antigens in man, *J. Nat. Cancer Inst.* **55**:1281–1289.

Brown, G., Hogg, N., and Greaves, M., 1975b, Candidate leukemia-specific antigen in man, *Nature (London)* **258**:454–456.

Ceglowski, W. S., and Friedman, H., 1973, *Virus Tumorigenesis and Immunogenesis*, p. 414, Academic Press, New York.

Chandra, R. K., 1972, Serum immunoglobulin levels in children with acute lymphoblastic leukemia and their mothers and sibs, *Arch. Dis. Child.* **47**:618–621.

Char, D. H., Lepourhiet, A., Leventhal, B. G., and Herberman, R. B., 1973, Cutaneous delayed hypersensitivity responses to tumor associated and other antigens in acute leukemia, *Int. J. Cancer* **12**:409–419.

Cheema, A. R., and Hersh, E. M., 1971, Patient survival after chemotherapy and its relationship to *in vitro* lymphocyte blastogenesis, *Cancer* **28**:857–862.

Children's Cancer Study Group A, 1973, BCG in the treatment of acute lymphoblastic leukemia, *Proc. Am. Assoc. Cancer Res.* **14**:45.

Cikes, M., and Friberg, S., Jr., 1971, Expression of H-2 and Moloney leukemia virus-determined cell-surface antigens in synchronized cultures of a mouse cell line, *Proc. Nat. Acad. Sci. U.S.A.* **68**:566–569.

Cikes, M., and Klein, G., 1972, Quantitative studies of antigen expression in cultured murine lymphoma cells. I. Cell-surface antigens in "synchronous" cultures, *J. Nat. Cancer Inst.* **49**:1599–1606.

Cikes, M., Friberg, J. R., and Klein, G., 1973, Progressive loss of H-2 antigens with concomitant increase of cell-surface antigen(s) determined by Moloney leukemia virus in cultured Moloney leukemias, *J. Nat. Cancer Inst.* **50**:347–362.

Colnaghi, M. I., and Della Porta, G., 1973, Evidence for virus-related and unrelated antigens on murine lymphomas induced by chemical carcinogens, *J. Nat. Cancer Inst.* **50**:173–180.

Davies, D. A. L., Boyse, E. A., Old, L. J., and Stockert, E., 1967, Mouse isoantigens: Separation of soluble TL (thymus-leukemia) antigen from soluble H-2 histocompatibility antigen by column chromatography. *J. Exp. Med.* **125**:549–562.

Davies, D. A. L., Baugh, V. S. G., Buckham, S., and Manstone, A. J., 1974, Separation of the specific antigen of a mouse lymphoma from histocompatibility antigens, *Eur. J. Cancer* **10**:781–786.

Del Villano, B., Nave, B., Crocker, B., Lerner, R., and Dixon, F., 1975, The oncornavirus glycoprotein gp 69/71: A constituent of the surface of normal and malignant thymocytes, *J. Exp. Med.* **141**:172–187.

Dickler, H. B., and Kunkel, H. G., 1972, Interaction of aggregated γ-globulin with B lymphocytes, *J. Exp. Med.* **136**:191–201.

Dickler, H. B., Siegal, F. P., Bentwich, Z. H., and Kunkel, H. G., 1973, Lymphocyte binding of aggregated IgG and surface Ig staining in chronic lymphocyte leukemia, *Clin. Exp. Immunol.* **14**:97–106.

Djeu, J. Y., Glaser, M., Kirchner, H., Huang, K. Y., and Herberman, R. B., 1974, The effect of specific anti-rat thymocyte serum on cell-mediated tumor immunity and other lymphocyte functions, *Cell. Immunol.* **12**:164–169.

Doherty, P. C., Blanden, R. V., and Zinkernagel, R. M., 1976, Specificity of virus-immune effector T cells for H-2K or H-2D compatible interactions: Implications for H-antigen diversity, *Transplant. Rev.* **29**:89–124.

Doré, J. F., Motta, R., Markoley, L., Hrsak, I., Colas de la Nove, H., Seman, G., de Vassal, F., and Mathé, G., 1967, New antigens in leukemic cells, and antibody in the serum of leukemic patients, *Lancet* **2**:1396–1398.

Dupuy, J. M., Kourilsky, F. M., Fradelizzi, D., Feingold, N., Jacquillat, C., Bernard, J., and Dausset, J., 1971, Depression of immunologic reactivity of patients with acute leukemia, *Cancer* **27**:323–331.

Edelson, R. L., Kirkpatrick, C. H., Shevach, E. M., Schein, P. S., Smith, R. W., Green, I., and Lutzner, M. A., 1974, Preferential cutaneous infiltration by neoplastic thymus-derived lymphocytes: Morphologic and functional studies, *Ann. Intern. Med.* **80**:685–706.

Epstein, L. B., and Knight, R. A., 1975a, Studies on mouse Moloney virus-induced tumors: I. The detection of p30 as a cytotoxic target on murine Moloney leukaemic spleen cells, and on an *in vitro* Moloney sarcoma line by antibody-mediated cytotoxicity, *Br. J. Cancer* **31**:499–512.

Epstein, L. B., and Knight, R. A., 1975b, Studies on mouse Moloney virus-induced tumors: II. Detection of p30 in the serum of mice with Moloney leukaemia by *in vitro* blocking of complement-dependent antibody-mediated cytotoxicity, *Br. J. Cancer* **31**:513–523.

Essex, M., 1975, The immune response to oncornavirus infections, *in Viruses, Evolution and Cancer* (E. Kurstak and K. Maramorosch, eds.), pp. 513–548, Academic Press, New York.

Essex, M., Cotter, S. M., Hardy, W. D., Jr., Hess, P., Jarrett, W., Jarrett, O., Mackey, L., Laird, H., Perryman, L., Olsen, R. G., and Yohn, D. S., 1975a, *J. Nat. Cancer Inst.* **55**:463–467.

Essex, M., Jakowski, R. M., Hardy, W. D., Jr., Cotter, S. M., Hess, P., and Sliski, A., 1975b, Feline oncornavirus-associated cell membrane antigen. III. Antibody titers in cats from leukemia cluster households, *J. Nat. Cancer Inst.* **54**:637–641.

Essex, M., Sliski, A., Cotter, S. M., Jakowski, R. M., and Hardy, W. D., Jr., 1975c, Immunosurveillance of naturally occurring feline leukemia, *Science* **190**:790–792.

Feldman, J. D., 1973, Immunological enhancement: A study of blocking antibodies, *Adv. Immunol.* **15**:167–214.

Fenyö, E. M., and Klein, G., 1976, Independence of Moloney virus-induced cell-surface antigen and membrane-associated virion antigens in immunoselected lymphoma sublines, *Nature (London)* **260**:355–357.

Fenyö, E., Grundner, G., and Klein, E., 1974, Virus-associated surface antigens on L cells and Moloney lymphoma cells, *J. Nat. Cancer Inst.* **52**:743–750.

Ferrer, J. F., 1973, Cell-surface and virion-envelope antigens shared by radiation leukemia virus (Rad LV) and other murine C-type viruses, *Int. J. Cancer* **12**:378–386.

Ferrer, J., and Gibbs, F., 1969, Concomitant loss of specific cell-surface antigen and demonstrable type-C virus particles in lymphomas induced by radiation leukemia virus in rats, *J. Nat. Cancer Inst.* **43**:1317–1330.

Ferrer, J., and Kaplan, H., 1968, Antigenic characteristics of lymphomas induced by radiation leukemia virus in mice and rats, *Cancer Res.* **28**:2522–2528.

Fink, M. A., Malmgren, R. A., Karon, M., and Orr, H. C., 1965, Immunofluorescence studies in human leukemia, in *Methodological Approaches to the Study of Leukemias,* pp. 187–196, The Wistar Institute Press, Philadelphia.

Freedman, A. H., Lilly, F., and Steeves, R., 1975, Antigenic properties of cultured tumor cell lines derived from spleens of Friend virus-infected BALB/c and BALB/c-H-2^b mice, *J. Exp. Med.* **142**:1365–1375.

Freeman, C. B., Harris, R., Geary, C. G., Leyland, M. J., MacIver, J. E., and Delamore, I. W., 1973, Active immunotherapy used alone for maintenance of patients with acute myeloid leukaemia, *Br. Med. J.* **4**:571–573.

Frey-Wettstein, M., and Hays, E. F., 1970, Immune response in preleukemic mice, *Infect. Immun.* **2**:398–403.

Fridman, W. H., and Kourilsky, F. M., 1969, Stimulation of lymphocytes by autologous leukemic cells in acute leukemia, *Nature (London)* **224**:277–279.

Friedman, H., Specter, S., Kamo, I., and Kateley, J., 1976, Immunosuppressive factors from tumor cells, *Ann. N.Y. Acad. Sci.* **276**:417–430.

Fu, S. M., Winchester, R. J., and Kunkel, H. G., 1975, The occurrence of the HL-B alloantigens on the cells of unclassified acute lymphoblastic leukemias, *J. Exp. Med.* **142**:1334–1338.

Gallagher, M. T., Lotzova, E., and Trentin, J. J., 1976, Genetic resistance to marrow transplantation as a leukemia defense mechanism, *Biomedicine* **25**:1–3.

Gelderblom, H., Bauer, H., and Graf, T., 1972, Cell-surface antigens induced by avian RNA tumor viruses: Detection by immunoferritin technique, *Virology* **47**:416–425.

Gilden, R. V., Oroszlan, S., and Huebner, R. J., 1971, Coexistence of intraspecies and interspecies specific antigenic determinants on the major structural polypeptide of mammalian C-type viruses, *Nature New Biol.* **231**:107–108.

Glaser, M., and Herberman, R. B., 1974, The effect of immunoregulatory α-globulin (IRA) on *in vitro* proliferation of rat lymphocytes to syngeneic Gross virus-induced lymphoma, *J. Nat. Cancer Inst.* **53**:1767–1769.

Glaser, M., and Herberman, R. B., 1976, Secondary cell-mediated cytotoxic response to challenge of rats with syngeneic Gross virus-induced lymphoma, *J. Nat. Cancer Inst.* **56**:1211–1215.

Glaser, M., Kirchner, H., and Herberman, R. H., 1975, Inhibition of *in vitro* lymphoproliferative responses to tumor-associated antigens by suppressor cells from rats bearing progressively growing Gross leukemia virus-induced tumors, *Int. J. Cancer* **16**:384–393.

Glaser, M., Lavrin, D. H., and Herberman, R. B., 1976a, *In vivo* protection against syngeneic Gross virus-induced lymphoma in rats: Comparison with *in vitro* studies of cell-mediated immunity, *J. Immunol.* **116**:1507–1511.

Glaser, M., Ting, C. C., and Herberman, R. B., 1976b, *In vitro* inhibition of cell-mediated cytotoxicity against syngeneic Friend virus-induced leukemia by immunoregulatory alpha globulin, *J. Nat. Cancer Inst.* **55**:1477–1479.

Gomard, E., Duprez, V., Henin, Y., and Levy, J. P., 1976, An H2 region product is determinant in the immune cytolysis of syngeneic tumor cells by anti-MSV T lymphocytes, *Nature (London)* **260**:707–709.

Gooch, W. M., and Fernbach, D. J., 1971, Immunoglobulins during the course of acute leukemia in children, *Cancer* **28**:984–990.

Grant, J. P., Bigner, D. D., Fischinger, P. J., and Bolognesi, D. P., 1974, Expression of murine leukemia virus structural antigens on the surface of chemically induced murine sarcomas, *Proc. Nat. Acad. Sci. U.S.A.* **71**:5037–5041.

Greaves, M. F., and Brown, G., 1973, A human B-lymphocyte-specific antigen, *Nature New Biol.* **246**:116–118.

Greaves, M. F., Brown, G., Rapson, N. T., and Lister, J. A., 1975, Antisera to acute lymphoblastic leukemia cells, *Clin. Immunol. Immunopathol.* **4**:67–84.

Greenberg, R., and Zatz, M., 1975, Spontaneous AKR lymphoma with T- and B-cell characteristics, *Nature (London)* **257**:314–316.

Greenspan, I., Brown, E. R., and Schwartz, S. O., 1963, Immunologically specific antigens in leukemic tissues, *Blood* **21**:717–727.

Gutterman, J. U., Hersh, E. M., Freireich, E. J., Rossen, R. D., Butler, W. T., McCredie, K. B., Bodey, G. P., Sr., Rodriguez, V., and Mavligit, G. M., 1973a, Cell-mediated and humoral response to acute leukemia cells and soluble leukemia antigen—Relationship to immunocompetence and prognosis, *Nat. Cancer Inst. Monogr.* **37**:153–156.

Gutterman, J. U., Rossen, R. D., Butler, W. T., McCredie, K. B., Bodey, G. P., Freireich, E. J., and Hersh, E. M., 1973b, Immunoglobulin on tumor cells and tumor-induced lymphocyte blastogenesis in human acute leukemia, *N. Engl. J. Med.* **288**:169–173.

Gutterman, J. U., Mavligit, G., Burgess, M. A., McCredie, K. B., Hunter, C., Freireich, E. J., and Hersh, E. M., 1974a, Brief communication: Immunodiagnosis of acute leukemia: Detection of residual disease, *J. Nat. Cancer Inst.* **53**:389–392.

Gutterman, J. U., Rodriguez, V., Mavligit, G., Burgess, M. A., Hersh, E. M., McCredie, K. B., Reed, R., Smith, T., Bodey, G. P., Sr., and Freireich, E. J., 1974b, Chemo-immunotherapy of adult acute leukaemia. Prolongation of remission in myeloblastic leukaemia with B.C.G., *Lancet* **2**:1405–1409.

Gutterman, J. U., Mavligit, G., Rossen, R., Butler, W. T., McBride, C. M., McCredie, K. B., Freireich, E. J., and Hersch, E. M., 1975, Tumor immunity in human acute leukemia and solid tumors: A multifaceted study of cell-mediated and humoral response to autologous tumor cells and soluble tumor antigen and the correlation with prognosis, in *Immunological Aspects of Neoplasia* (Univ. Texas M.D. Anderson Hosp., 26th Annual Symposium on Fundamental Cancer Res.), pp. 343–365, Williams & Wilkins, Baltimore, Maryland.

Hammerling, U., Aoki, T., De Harven, E., Boyse, E. A., and Old, L. J., 1968, Use of hybrid antibody with an anti-G and anti-ferritin specificities in locating cell surface antigens by electron microscopy, *J. Exp. Med.* **128**:1461–1473.

Hanna, M. G., Tennant, R. W., and Coggin, J. H., Jr., 1971, Suppressive effect of immunization with mouse fetal antigens on growth of cells infected with Rauscher leukemia virus and on plasma cell tumor, *Proc. Nat. Acad. Sci. U.S.A.* **68**:1748–1752.

Haran-Ghera, N., and Peled, A., 1973, Thymus and bone marrow derived lymphatic leukemia in mice, *Nature (London)* **241**:396–398.

Harris, J. E., and Stewart, T. H. M., 1972, Recovery of mixed lymphocyte reactivity (MLR) following cancer chemotherapy in man, in *Proceedings of the Sixth Leucocyte Culture Conference* (M. R. Schwarz, ed.), pp. 555–559, Academic Press, New York.

Harris, R., Viza, D., Todd, R., Phillips, J., Sugar, R., Jennison, R. F., Marriott, G., and Gleeson, M. H., 1971, Detection of human leukaemia-associated antigens in leukaemic serum and normal embryos, *Nature (London)* **233**:556–557.

Henderson, E. S., and Leventhal, B., 1972, Immunotherapy of leukemia, in *Cancer Chemotherapy II, The 22nd Hahnemann Symposium* (I. Brodsky, S. B. Kahn, and J. H. Moger, eds.), pp. 327–345, Grune & Stratton, New York.

Herberman, R. B., 1969, Studies on the specificity of human cytotoxic antibody reactive with cultures of lymphoid cells, *J. Nat. Cancer Inst.* **42**:69–75.

Herberman, R. B., 1972, Serological analysis of cell surface antigens of tumors induced by murine leukemia virus, *J. Nat. Cancer Inst.* **48**:265–271.

Herberman, R. B., 1974, Cell-mediated immunity to tumor cells, in *Advances in Cancer Research*, Vol. 19 (G. Klein and S. Weinhouse, eds.), pp. 207–263, Academic Press, New York.

Herberman, R. B., 1977, Cell-mediated immunity to leukemia associated antigens in experimental models and in man, in *Modern Trends in Human Leukemia II* (R. Neth, R. C., Gallo, K. Mannweiler, and W. C. Moloney, eds.), pp. 195–206, J. F. Lehmanns Verlag, Munich.

Herberman, R. B., and Fahey, J. L., 1968, Cytotoxic antibody in Burkitt's tumor and normal human serum reactive with cultures of lymphoid cells, *Proc. Soc. Exp. Biol. Med.* **127**:938–940.

Herberman, R. B., and Nam, J. M., 1971, Cytotoxic antibody reactive with cultures of lymphoid cells: Occurrence in disease and normal human sera, *J. Nat. Cancer Inst.* **47**:489–494.

Herberman, R. B., and Oren, M. E., 1971, Immune response to Gross virus-induced lymphoma. I. Kinetics of cytotoxic antibody response, *J. Nat. Cancer Inst.* **46**:391–396.

Herberman, R. B., Rosenberg, E. B., Halterman, R. H., McCoy, J. L., and Leventhal, B. G., 1972, Cellular immune reactions to human leukemia, *Nat. Cancer Inst. Monogr.* **35**:259–266.

Herberman, R. B., Aoki, T., Nunn, M., Lavrin, D. H., Soares, N., Gazdar, A., Holden, H., and Chang, K. S. S., 1974a, Specificity of $^{51}$Cr-release cytotoxicity by lymphocytes immune to murine sarcoma virus, *J. Nat. Cancer Inst.* **53**:1103–1111.

Herberman, R. B., McCoy, J. L., and Levine, P. H., 1974b, Immunological reactions to tumor-associated antigens in Burkitt's lymphoma and other lymphomas, *Cancer Res.* **34**:1222–1227.

Herberman, R. B., Char, D. H., Oldham, R. K., and Leventhal, B. G., 1975a, The prognostic value of studies of specific cell-mediated immunity in acute leukemia, *in Advances in the Biosciences 14. Workshop on Prognostic Factors in Human Leukemia* (T. M. Fliedner and S. Perry, eds.), pp. 431–440, Friedr. Vieweg und Sohn, Braunschweig, West Germany.

Herberman, R. B., Char, D., Oldham, R., Levine, P., Leventhal, B. G., McCoy, J. L., Ho, H. C., and Chau, J. C. W., 1975b, Cell-mediated immunity in human adult leukemia, *in Comparative Leukemia Research, Leukemogenesis, 1973* (Y. Ito and R. M. Satcher, eds.), pp. 649–656, University of Tokyo Press, Tokyo; Karger, Basel.

Herberman, R. B., Lepourhiet, A., Hollinshead, A., Char, D., McCoy, J. L., and Leventhal, B. G., 1975c, Humoral and cell-mediated immunity in human acute leukemia, *in Immunological Aspects of Neoplasia*, pp. 423–438, Williams & Wilkins, Baltimore, Maryland.

Herberman, R. B., Nunn, M. E., Holden, H. T., and Lavrin, D. H., 1975d, Natural cytotoxic reactivity of mouse lymphoid cells against syngeneic and allogeneic tumors. II. Characterization of effector cells, *Int. J. Cancer* **16**:230–239.

Herberman, R. B., Nunn, M. E., and Lavrin, D. H., 1975e, Natural cytotoxic reactivity of mouse lymphoid cells against syngeneic and allogeneic tumors. I. Distribution of reactivity and specificity, *Int. J. Cancer* **16**:216–229.

Herberman, R. B., Ting, C. C., Holden, H. T., Glaser, M., and Lavrin, D., 1975f, Dynamics of immune responses to tumor associated antigens, *in Proceedings of the XIth International Cancer Congress* (P. Bucalossi, U. Veronesi, and N. Cassenelli, eds.), pp. 258–263, Excerpta Medica, Amsterdam.

Hersey, P., MacLennan, I. C. M., Campbell, A. C., Harris, R., and Freeman, C. B., 1973, Cytotoxicity against human leukemic cells. I. Demonstration of antibody-dependent lymphocyte killing of human allogeneic myoblasts, *Clin. Exp. Immunol.* **14**:159–166.

Hersh, E. M., and Oppenheim, J. J., 1967, Inhibition of *in vitro* lymphocyte transformation during chemotherapy in man, *Cancer Res.* **27**:98–109.

Hersh, E. M., Whitecar, J. P., Jr., McCredie, K. B., Bodey, G. P., Sr., and Freireich, E. J., 1971, Chemotherapy, immunocompetence, immunosuppression and prognosis in acute leukemia, *N. Engl. J. Med.* **285**:1211–1216.

Hersh, E. M., Gutterman, J. U., and Mavligit, G., 1973, *Immunotherapy of Cancer in Man. Scientific Basis and Current Status*, p. 141, Charles C. Thomas, Springfield, Illinois.

Hersh, E. M., Gutterman, J. U., Mavligit, G., McCredie, K. B., Bodey, G. P., Sr., and Freireich, E., 1975, Immunocompetence, immunological deficiency, and prognosis of established cancer, *in Immunological Aspects of Neoplasia* (Univ. Texas M.D. Anderson Hosp., 26th Annual Symposium on Fundamental Cancer Res.), pp. 293–303, Williams & Wilkins, Baltimore, Maryland.

Hilberg, R. W., Balcerzak, S. P., and LoBuglio, A. F., 1973, A migration inhibition-factor assay for tumor immunity in man, *Cell. Immunol.* **7**:152–158.

Hilgers, J., Decleve, A., Galesloot, J., and Kaplan, H., 1974, Murine leukemia virus group-specific antigenic expression in AKR mice, *Cancer Res.* **34**:2553–2561.

Holden, H. T., Kirchner, H., and Herberman, R. B., 1975, Secondary cell-mediated cytotoxic response to syngeneic mouse tumor challenge, *J. Immunol.* **115**:327–331.

Holden, H. T., Haskill, J. S., Kirchner, H., and Herberman, R. B., 1976, Two functionally distinct anti-tumor effector cells isolated from primary murine sarcoma virus-induced tumors, *J. Immunol.* **177**:440–446.

Holden, H. T., Landolfo, S., and Herberman, R. B., 1977, T-cell dependent reactivity against tumor-associated antigens on allogeneic target cells, *Transplant. Proc.* **9**:1149–1152.

Hollinshead, A. C., and Herberman, R. B., 1975, Identification and characterization: Cell-membrane antigens associated with the blast phase of human acute leukemia, in *Comparative Leukemia Research Leukemogenesis, 1973* (Y. Ito and R. M. Sutcher, eds.), pp. 339–348, University of Tokyo Press, Tokyo; Karger, Basel.

Houchens, D. P., Bommassar, E., Gaston, M. R., Kende, M., and Goldin, A., 1976, Drug-mediated immunogenic changes of virus-induced leukemia *in vivo*, *Cancer Res.* **36**:1347–1352.

Huebner, R. J., and Todaro, G. J., 1969, Oncogenesis of RNA tumor viruses as determinants of cancer, *Proc. Nat. Acad. Sci. U.S.A.* **64**:1087–1094.

Huebner, R., Kelloff, G., Sarma, P., Lane, W., Turner, H., Gilden, R. V., Oroszlan, S., Meier, H., Myers, D. D., and Peters, R. L., 1970, Group-specific antigen expression during embryogenesis of the genome of the C-type RNA tumor virus: Implications for ontogenesis, *Proc. Nat. Acad. Sci. U.S.A.* **67**:366–376.

Hunsmann, G., Claviez, M., Moennig, U., Schwarz, H., and Shafer, W., 1976, Properties of mouse leukemia viruses. X. Occurrence of viral structural antigens on the cell surface as revealed by a cytotoxicity test, *Virology* **69**:157–168.

Ihle, J. N., Yurconic, M., Jr., and Hanna, M. G., Jr., 1973, Autogenous immunity to endogenous RNA tumor virus: Radioimmune precipitation assay of mouse serum antibody levels, *J. Exp. Med.* **138**:194–208.

Ikeda, H., Pincus, T., Yoshiki, T., Strand, M., August, J. T., Boyse, E. A., and Mellors, R. C., 1974, Biological expression of antigenic determinants of murine leukemia virus proteins gp 69/71 and p30, *J. Virol.* **14**:1274–1280.

Insel, R., Melewicz, F. M., Iavia, M., and Blach, C. M., 1975, Morphology surface markers and *in vitro* responses of a human leukemic T cell, *Clin. Immunol. Immunopathol.* **4**:382–391.

Ioachim, H., Keller, S., Dorsett, B., and Pearse, A., 1974, Induction of partial immunologic tolerance in rats and progressive loss of cellular antigenicity in Gross virus lymphoma, *J. Exp. Med.* **139**:1382–1394.

Ishii, Y., Koshiba, H., Veno, H., Maeyama, I., Takami, T., Ishibashi, F., and Kikuchi, K., 1975, Characterization of human B-lymphocyte-specific antigens, *J. Immunol.* **114**:466–469.

Ishimoto, A., and Ito, Y., 1972, Presence of antibody against mouse fetal antigen in the sera of C57BL/6 mice immunized with Rauscher leukemia, *Cancer Res.* **32**:2333–2337.

Jondal, M., Holm, G., and Wigzell, H. J., 1972, Surface markers on human T and B lymphocytes. I. A large population of lymphocytes forming nonimmune rosettes with sheep red blood cells, *J. Exp. Med.* **136**:207–215.

Joseph, R. R., Belpomme, D., and Mathé, G., 1976, Short Communication: Increase in "null" cells in acute lymphocytic leukemia in remission on long-term immunotherapy, *Br. J. Cancer* **33**:567–570.

Kagan, R. A., and Johnson, R. E., 1967, Evaluation of therapy in chronic lymphocytic leukemia using *in vitro* lymphocyte transformation, *Radiology* **88**:352–359.

Kennel, S., and Feldman, J., 1976, Distribution of viral glycoprotein gp69/71 on cell surfaces of producer and nonproducer cells, *Cancer Res.* **36**:200–207.

Kersey, J., Nesbit, M., and Luckasen, J., 1974, Acute lymphoblastic leukemic and lymphoma cells with thymus-derived (T) markers, *Mayo Clinic Proc.* **49**:584–587.

Kiessling, R., Klein, E., and Wigzell, H., 1975a, "Natural" killer cells in the mouse. I. Cytotoxic cells with specificity for mouse Moloney leukemia cells. Specificity and distribution according to genotype, *Eur. J. Immunol.* **5**:112–117.

Kiessling, R., Klein, E., Pross, H., and Wigzell, H., 1975b, "Natural" killer cells in the mouse. II. Cytotoxic cells with specificity for mouse Moloney leukemia cells. Characteristics of the killer cell, *Eur. J. Immunol.* **5**:117–121.

Kiessling, R., Petranyi, G., Klein, G., and Wigzell, H., 1975c, Genetic variation of *in vitro* cytolytic activity and *in vivo* rejection potential of nonimmunized semisyngeneic mice against a mouse lymphoma line, *Int. J. Cancer* **15**:933–940.

Kirchner, H., Glaser, M., Holden, H. T., Fernbach, B. R., and Herberman, R. B., 1977, Suppressor cells in tumor-bearing mice and rats, *Biomedicine* **24**:371–373.

Klein, G., Klein, E., and Haughton, G., 1966, Variation of antigenic characteristics between different mouse lymphomas induced by the Moloney virus, *J. Nat. Cancer Inst.* **36**:607–621.

Klein, G., Steiner, M., Wiener, F., and Klein, E., 1974, Human leukemia-associated anti-nuclear reactivity, *Proc. Nat. Acad. Sci. U.S.A.* **71**:685–689.

Klouda, P. T., Lawler, S. D., Powles, R., Oliver, R. T. D., and Grant, C. K., 1975, HL-A antibody in patients with acute myelogenous leukemia treated by immunotherapy, *Transplantation* **19**:245–250.

Knight, R. A., Mitchison, N. A., and Shellam, G. R., 1975, Studies on a Gross-virus-induced lymphoma in the rat. II. The role of cell-membrane associated and serum p30 antigen in the antibody and cell-mediated response, *Int. J. Cancer* **15**:417–428.

Kumar, V., Trentin, J., and Cudkowicz, G., 1976, Discussion, *Ann. N.Y. Acad. Sci.* **276**:39–44.

Kurth, R., and Bauer, H., 1972, Common tumor-specific surface antigens on cells of different species transformed by avian RNA tumor viruses, *Virology* **49**:145–149.

Kurth, R., and Bauer, H., 1973, Avian oncornavirus-induced tumor antigens of embryonic and unknown origin, *Virology* **56**:496–504.

Kuzumaki, N., Takeichi, N., Sendo, F., Kodama, T., and Kobayashi, H., 1973,

Correlation between various cell-surface antigens induced by mouse leukemia virus in the rat: Serological analysis, *Int. J. Cancer* **11**:575–585.

Lamon, E. W., 1974, The immune response to virally determined tumor associated antigens, *Biochim. Biophys. Acta* **355**:149–176.

Larson, D. L., and Tomlinson, L. J., 1953, Quantitative antibody studies in man. III. Antibody response in leukemia and other malignant lymphomas, *J. Clin. Invest.* **32**:317–321.

Law, L. W., and Appella, E., 1973, Immunologic properties of solubilized tumour antigen from an RNA virus-transformed neoplasm, *Nature (London)* **243**:83–87.

Lay, W. H., and Nussenzweig, V., 1968, Receptors for complement on leukocytes, *J. Exp. Med.* **128**:991–1007.

Leclerc, J. C., Levy, J. P., Varet, B., Oppenheim, S., and Senik, A., 1970, Antigenic analysis of L strain cells: A new murine leukemia-associated antigen, "L," *Cancer Res.* **30**:2073–2079.

Lee, J., and Ihle, J., 1975, Autogenous immunity to endogenous RNA tumor virus: Reactivity of natural immune sera to antigenic determinants of several biologically distinct murine leukemia viruses, *J. Nat. Cancer Inst.* **55**:831–838.

Lerner, R. A., Oldstone, M. B., and Cooper, N. R., 1971, Cell-cycle dependent immune lysis of Moloney virus-transformed lymphocytes: Presence of viral antigen, accessibility to antibody, and complement activation, *Proc. Nat. Acad. Sci. U.S.A.* **68**:2584–2588.

Leventhal, B. G., Halterman, R. H., Rosenberg, R. B., and Herberman, R. B., 1972, Immune reactivity of leukemic patients to autologous blast cells, *Cancer Res.* **32**:1820–1825.

Leventhal, B. G., LePourhiet, A., Halterman, R. H., Henderson, E. S., and Herberman, R. B., 1973, Immunotherapy in previously treated acute lymphatic leukemia, *Nat. Cancer Inst. Monogr.* **39**:177–187.

Leventhal, B. G., Cohen, P., and Triem, S. C., 1974, Effect of chemotherapy on the immune response in acute leukemia, *Israel J. Med. Sci.* **10**:866–887.

Levy, J. P., Leclerc, J. C., Varet, B., and Oppenheim, E., 1968, Study of the antigenic specificity of Graffi leukemic cells, *J. Nat. Cancer Inst.* **41**:743–750.

Levy, M. H., and Wheelock, E. F., 1975, Impaired macrophage function in Friend virus leukemia: Restoration by statolon, *J. Immunol.* **114**:962–965.

Lieberman, M., and Kaplan, H. S., 1959, Leukemogenic activity of filtrates from radiation-induced lymphoid tumors of mice, *Science* **130**:387–388.

Lilly, F., and Steeves, R., 1974, Antigens of murine leukemia viruses, *Biochim. Biophys. Acta* **355**:105–118.

Lin, P. S., and Hsu, C. C. S., 1976, Human leukaemic T cells with complement receptors, *Clin. Exp. Immunol.* **23**:209–213.

Linker-Israeli, M., and Haran-Ghera, N., 1975, Cell-surface markers on murine lymphomas, *Immunochemistry* **12**:585–588.

MacLennan, I. C. M., Gale, D. G. L., and Wood J., 1975, Resistance of certain leukaemic myeloblasts to immunological attack, *Int. J. Cancer* **15**:995–999.

Mann, D. L., Halterman, R., Rogentine, G. N., and Leventhal, B. G., 1971, Detection of an acute leukemia-associated antigen, *Science* **174**:1136–1137.

Mann, D. L., Ulmer, C., Lepourhiet, A., Leventhal, B., and Halterman, R., 1974,

Studies on the immunologic reactivity of sera from acute leukemia patients, *Prog. Exp. Tumor Res.* **19**:102–109.

Mann, D. L., Leventhal, B., and Halterman, R., 1975, Brief communication: Human antisera detecting leukemia-associated antigens on autochthonous tumor cells, *J. Nat. Cancer Inst.* **54**:345–347.

Martyré, M. C., Halle-Pannenko, O., and Jolles, P., 1973, Characterization and partial purification of normal and tumor-associated transplantation antigens of Rauscher leukemia cells, *Eur. J. Cancer* **9**:757–761.

Maruyama, K., Dmochowski, L., Bowen, J. M., and Hales, R. L., 1968, Studies of human leukemia and lymphoma cells by membrane immunofluorescence and mixed hemadsorption tests, *Texas Rep. Biol. Med.* **26**:545–565.

Mathé, G., Delgado, M., Pouillart, P., Belpomme, D., Joseph, R., Schwarzenberg, L., Schneider, M., Cattan, A., Musset, M., Misset, J. L., and Jasmin, C., 1976, 1975 current results of the first 100 cytologically typed acute lymphoid leukemia submitted to BCG active immunotherapy, *Cancer Immun. Immunother.* **1**:77–86.

McKelvey, E., and Carbone, P. P., 1965, Serum immune globulin concentrations in acute leukemia during intensive chemotherapy. *Cancer* **18**:1292–1297.

Medical Research Council, 1971, Treatment of acute lymphoblastic leukemia. Comparison of immunotherapy (B.C.G.), intermittent methotrexate, and no therapy after a five-month intensive cytotoxic regimen (Concord trial), *Br. Med. J.* **4**:189–194.

Metcalf, D., and Moulds, R., 1967, Immune responses in preleukemic and leukemic mice. *Int. J. Cancer* **2**:53–58.

Metzgar, R. S., Mohanakumar, T., Green, R. W., Miller, D. S., and Bolognesi, D. P., 1974, Human leukemia antigens: Partial isolation and characterization, *J. Nat. Cancer Inst.* **52**:1445–1453.

Metzgar, R. S., Mohanakumar, T., and Miller, D. S., 1975, Membrane-bound immunoglobulins on human leukemic cells: Evidence for humoral immune responses of patients to leukemia-associated antigens, *J. Clin. Invest.* **56**:331–338.

Metzgar, R. S., Mohanakumar, T., and Bolognesi, D. P., 1976a, Relationships between membrane antigens of human leukemic cells and oncogenic RNA virus structural components, *J. Exp. Med.* **143**:47–63.

Metzgar, R. S., Mohanakumar, T., and Bolognesi, D. P., 1976b, Antigenic relationships between murine, feline and primate RNA tumor viruses and membrane antigens of human leukemic cells, *in Comparative Leukemia Research 1975*, Bibl. Haematol., No. 43 (J. Clemmesen and D. S. Yohn, eds.), pp. 549–554, Karger, Basel.

Minowada, J., Ohnuma, T., and Moore, G. E., 1972, Brief communication: Rosette-forming human lymphoid cell lines. I. Establishment and evidence for origin of thymus-derived lymphocytes, *J. Nat. Cancer Inst.* **49**:891–895.

Mitchell, M. S., Mokyr, M. M., Aspnes, G. T., and McIntosh, S., 1973, Cytophilic antibodies in man, *Ann. Intern. Med.* **79**:333–339.

Mohanakumar, T., Metzgar, R. S., and Miller, D. S., 1974, Human leukemia cell antigens: Serologic characterization with xenoantisera, *J. Nat. Cancer Inst.* **52**:1435–1444.

Mori, W., Asakawa, H., and Taguchi, T., 1975a, Antiplacental ferritin antiserum for cancer diagnosis, *Ann. N.Y. Acad. Sci.* **259**:446–449.

Mori, W., Asakawa, H., and Taguchi, T., 1975b, Antiserum against leukemia cell ferritin as a diagnostic tool for malignant neoplasms, *J. Nat. Cancer Inst.* **55**:513–518.

Nagaya, H., 1973, Thymus function in spontaneous lymphoid leukemia. II. *In vitro* response of "preleukemic" and leukemic thymus cells to mitogens, *J. Immunol.* **111**:1052–1061.

Nowell, P. C., 1960, Phytohemagglutinin, an initiator of mitosis in cultures of normal human leukocytes, *Cancer Res.* **20**:462–470.

Nowinski, R. C., and Kaehler, S. L., 1974, Antibody to leukemia virus. Widespread occurrence in inbred mice, *Science* **185**:869–871.

Nowinski, R. C., and Klein, P. A., 1975, Anomalous reactions of mouse alloantisera with cultured tumor cells. II. Cytotoxicity is caused by antibodies to leukemia viruses, *J. Immunol.* **115**:1261–1268.

Nowinski, R. D., and Peters, E., 1973, Cell surface antigens associated with murine leukemia virus: Definition of the $G_L$ and $G_T$ antigenic systems, *J. Virol.* **12**:1104–1117.

Nunn, M. E., Djeu, J. Y., Glaser, M., Lavrin, D. H., and Herberman, R. B., 1976, Natural cytotoxic reactivity of rat lymphocytes against syngeneic Gross virus-induced lymphoma, *J. Nat. Cancer Inst.* **56**:393–399.

Obata, Y., Ikeda, H., Stockert, E., and Boyse, E., 1975, Relation of $G_{IX}$ antigen of thymocytes to envelope glycoproteins of murine leukemia virus, *J. Exp. Med.* **141**:188–197.

Odaka, T., 1975, Strain-dependent expression of endogenous mouse-tropic leukemia viruses in chemically induced murine leukemias, *Int. J. Cancer* **16**:622–628.

Oehler, J. R., Campbell, D. A., Jr., and Herberman, R. B., 1977, *In vitro* inhibition of lymphoproliferative responses to tumor-associated antigens and of lymphoma cell proliferation by rat splenic macrophages, *Cell. Immunol.* **28**:355–370.

Old, L. J., Boyse, E. A., and Stockert, E., 1964, Typing of mouse leukemias by serological methods, *Nature (London)* **201**:777–779.

Old, L., Boyse, E. A., and Stockert, E., 1965, The G (Gross) leukemia antigen, *Cancer Res.* **25**:813–819.

Old, L. J., Stockert, E., Boyse, E. A., and Kim, J. H., 1968, Antigenic modulation. Loss of TL antigen from cells exposed to TL antibody. Study of the phenomenon *in vitro*, *J. Exp. Med.* **127**:523–540.

Oldham, R. K., Weiner, R. S., Mathé, G., Breard, J., Simmler, M. C., Carde, P., and Herberman, R. B., 1976, Cell-mediated immune responsiveness of patients with acute lymphocytic leukemia in remission, *Int. J. Cancer* **17**:326–377.

Opelz, G., Kiuchi, M., Takasugi, M., and Terasaki, P., 1975, Autologous stimulation of human lymphocyte subpopulations, *J. Exp. Med.* **142**:1327–1333.

Oppenheim, J. J., Whang, J., and Frei, E., III, 1965, Immunologic and cytogenetic studies of chronic lymphocytic leukemic cells, *Blood* **26**:121–132.

Oren, M. E., and Herberman, R. B., 1971, Delayed cutaneous hypersensitivity reactions to membrane extracts of human tumor cells, *Clin. Exp. Immunol.* **9**:45–56.

Ortaldo, J. R., Ting, C. C., and Herberman, R. B., 1974, Modulation of fetal antigen(s) in mouse leukemia cells, *Cancer Res.* **34**:1366–1371.

Osserman, E. F., and Lawlor, D. P., 1966, Serum and urinary lysozyme (muramidase) in monocytic and monomyelocytic leukemia, *J. Exp. Med.* **124**:921–952.

Pearson, G., Orr, T., Redmon, L., and Bergs, U., 1972, Membrane immunofluorescence studies on cells producing rat C-type virus particles, *Int. J. Cancer* **10**:14–19.

Piessens, U., Schur, P., Maloney, W., and Churchill, W. H., 1973, Lymphocyte surface immunoglobulins. Distribution and frequency in lymphoproliferative diseases, *N. Engl. J. Med.* **288**:176–180.

Poplack, D. G., Graw, R. G., Pomeroy, T. C., Henderson, E. S., and Leventhal, B. G., 1975, Chemotherapy (CT) vs. chemotherapy and immunotherapy (CT + IMT) in childhood acute lymphatic leukemia, *Proc. Am. Assoc. Cancer Res.* **16**:230.

Powles, R. L., Balchin, L. A., Hamilton Fairley, G., and Alexander, P., 1971, Recognition of leukemia cells as foreign before and after autoimmunization, *Br. Med. J.* **1**:486–489.

Powles, R. L., Crowther, D., Bateman, C. J. T., Beard, M. E. J., McElwain, T. J., Russell, J., Lister, T. A., Whitehouse, J. M. A., Wrigley, P. F. M., Pike, M., Alexander, P., and Hamilton Fairley, G., 1973, Immunotherapy for acute myelogenous leukemia, *Br. J. Cancer* **28**:365–376.

Premkumar, E., Potter, M., Singer, P. A., and Sklar, M. D., 1975, Synthesis, surface deposition and secretion of immunoglobulins by Abelson virus-transformed lymphosarcoma cell lines, *Cell* **6**:149–159.

Raff, M., 1969, Theta isoantigen as a marker of thymus-derived lymphocytes in mice, *Nature (London)* **224**:378–379.

Ram, M. D., Kohn, R. R., and Novak, D., 1973, Immune response to sheep red cells in AKR mouse leukemia, *Am. J. Pathol.* **72**:39–51.

Ram, M. D., Kohn, R. R., and Novak, D., 1974, Antigen distribution in AKR mouse leukemia, *J. Nat. Cancer Inst.* **52**:1505–1514.

Reif, A. E., and Allen, J. M., 1964, The AKR thymic antigen and its distribution in leukemias and nervous tissue, *J. Exp. Med.* **120**:413–433.

Roman, J. M., and Golub, E. S., 1976, Leukemia in AKR mice. I. Effects of Leukemic cells on antibody-forming potential of syngeneic and allogeneic normal cells, *J. Exp. Med.* **143**:482–495.

Rosenberg, E. B., Herberman, R. B., Levine, P. H., Halterman, R. H., McCoy, J. L., and Wunderlich, J. R., 1972, Lymphocyte cytotoxicity reactions to leukemia-associated antigens in identical twins, *Int. J. Cancer* **9**:648–658.

Rubin, A. D., Havemann, K., and Dameshek, W., 1969, Studies in chronic lymphocytic leukemia: Further studies of the proliferative abnormality of the blood lymphocyte, *Blood* **33**:313–320.

Sacks, K. L., Olwen, Y. C., Mann, D. L., Simon, R., Johnson, G. E., Poplack, D. G., and Leventhal, B. G., 1975, A clinical trial of chemotherapy and RAJI immunotherapy in advanced acute lymphatic leukemia, *Cancer Res.* **35**:3715–3720.

Santos, G. W., Mullins, G. M., Bias, W. B., Anderson, P. N., Graziano, K. D., Klein,

D. L., and Burke, P. J., 1973, Immunologic studies in acute leukemia, *Nat. Cancer Inst. Mongr.* **37**:69–75.

Sato, H., Boyse, E. A., Aoki, T., Iritani, C., and Old, L. J., 1973, Leukemia-associated transplantation antigens related to murine leukemia virus, *J. Exp. Med.* **138**:593–606.

Scamps, R. A., Streeter, A. M., and O'Neill, B. J., 1971, Immunoglobulin levels in chronic lymphocytic leukemia, *Med. J. Aust.* **1**:535–542.

Schieffer, C. A., Lichtenfeld, J. L., Wiernik, P. H., Mardiney, M. R., and Joseph, J. M., 1976, Antibody response in patients with acute nonlymphocytic leukemia, *Cancer* **37**:2177–2182.

Schlossman, S., Chess, L., Humphreys, R., and Strominger, J. L., 1976, Distribution of Ia-like molecules on the surface of normal and leukemic human cells, *Proc. Nat. Acad. Sci. U.S.A.* **73**:1288–1292.

Schwarz, H., Hunsmann, G., Moennig, U., and Shäfer, W., 1976, Properties of mouse leukemia viruses. XI. Immunoelectron microscopic studies on viral structural antigens on the cell surface, *Virology* **69**:169–178.

Schweitzer, M., Melief, C. J. M., and Eijsvoogel, V. P., 1973, Failure to demonstrate immunity to leukemia-associated antigens by lymphocyte transformation *in vitro, Int. J. Cancer* **11**:11–18.

Seligmann, M., Grabar, P., and Bernard, J., 1954, Mise en évidence dans le serum de sujets atteints de leucose aigüe d'anticorps precipitants anti-leucocytaires (Leucoprecipitaines), *C. R. Heb.* **239**:1559–1561.

Sen, L., and Borella, L., 1973, Expression of cell surface markers on T and B lymphocytes after long-term chemotherapy of acute leukemia, *Cell. Immunol.* **9**:84–95.

Sendo, F., Aoki, T., Boyse, E. A., and Buafo, C. K., 1975, Natural occurrence of lymphocytes showing cytotoxic activity to BALB/c radiation-induced leukemia RL♂ 1 cells, *J. Nat. Cancer Inst.* **55**:603–609.

Shellam, G. R., and Knight, R. A., 1974, Antigenic inhibition of cell-mediated cytotoxicity against tumour cells, *Nature (London)* **252**:330–332.

Shevach, E., Ellman, L., Davie, J. M., and Green, I., 1972a, L2C guinea pig lymphatic leukemia: A "B" cell leukemia, *Blood* **39**:1–12.

Shevach, E. M., Herberman, R. B., Frank, M. M., and Green, I., 1972b, Receptors for complement and immunoglobulin on human leukemic cells and human lymphoblastoid cell lines, *J. Clin. Invest.* **51**:1933–1938.

Shevach, E., Herberman, R., Lieberman, R., Frank, M. M., and Green, I., 1972c, Receptors for immunoglobulin and complement on mouse leukemias and lymphomas, *J. Immunol.* **108**:325–328.

Shevach, E. M., Stobo, J. D., and Green, I., 1972d, Immunoglobulin and Θ-bearing murine leukemias and lymphomas, *J. Immunol.* **108**:1146–1151.

Shevach, E., Edelson, R., Frank, M., Lutzner, M., and Green, I., 1974, A human leukemia cell with both B and T cell receptors, *Proc. Nat. Acad. Sci. U.S.A.* **71**:863–866.

Sklar, M. C., Shevach, E. M., Green, I., and Potter, M., 1975, Transplantation and preliminary characterization of lymphocyte surface markers of Abelson virus-induced lymphomas, *Nature (London)* **253**:550–552.

Slettenmark-Wahren, B., and Klein, E., 1962, Cytotoxic and neutralization tests with serum and lymph node cells of isologous mice with induced resistance against Gross lymphomas, *Cancer Res.* **22**:947–954.

Smith, J. L., Clein, G. P., Barker, C. R., and Collins, R. D., 1973, Characterization of malignant mediastinal lymphoid neoplasm (Sternberg sarcoma) as thymic in origin, *Lancet* **1**:74–76.

Smith, M., Browne, E., and Slungaard, A., 1973, The impaired responsiveness of chronic lymphatic leukemia lymphocytes to allogeneic lymphocytes, *Blood* **41**:505–509.

Stackpole, C., Jacobson, J., and Lardis, M., 1974, Antigenic modulation *in vitro* fate of thymus-leukemia (TL) antigen–antibody complexes following modulation of mouse leukemia cells and thymocytes, *J. Exp. Med.* **140**:939–953.

Stockert, E., Old, L., and Boyse, E., 1971, The $G_{IX}$ system. A cell surface associated with murine leukemia virus; implications regarding chromosomal integration of the viral genome, *J. Exp. Med.* **133**:1334–1355.

Strand, M., and August, J. T., 1973, Structural proteins of oncogenic ribonucleic acid viruses. Interspec II, a new interspecies antigen, *J. Biol. Chem.* **248**:5627–5633.

Strand, M., and August, J. T., 1974, Structural proteins of mammalian oncogenic RNA viruses: Multiple antigenic determinants of the major internal protein and envelope glycoprotein, *J. Virol.* **13**:171–180.

Stück, B., Boyse, E., Old, L., and Carswell, E., 1964a, A new antigen found in leukemias and mammary tumours of the mouse, *Nature (London)* **203**:1033–1034.

Stück, B., Old, L., and Boyse, E., 1964b, Occurrence of soluble antigen in the plasma of mice with virus-induced leukemia, *Proc. Nat. Acad. Sci. U.S.A.* **52**:950–958.

Stutman, O., 1975, Immunodepression and malignancy, *in Advances in Cancer Research,* Vol. 22 (G. Klein, S. Weinhouse, and A. Haddow, eds.), pp. 261–422, Academic Press, New York.

Taylor, G. M., Harris, R., and Freeman, C. B., 1976, Cell-mediated cytotoxicity as a result of immunotherapy in patients with acute myeloid leukemia, *Br. J. Cancer* **33**:137–143.

Ting, C. C., and Herberman, R. B., 1974, Serological analysis of the immune response to Friend virus-induced leukemia, *Cancer Res.* **34**:1676–1683.

Ting, C. C., and Herberman, R. B., 1975, Specific afferent interference by antiserum of *in vivo* immunity, *Nature (London)* **253**:801–802.

Ting, C. C., and Herberman, R. B., 1976, Humoral host defense mechanisms against tumors, *in International Review of Experimental Pathology,* Vol. 15 (G. W. Richter and M. A. Epstein, eds.), pp. 93–152. Academic Press, New York.

Ting, C. C., Lavrin, D. H., Shiu, G., and Herberman, R. B., 1972, Expression of fetal antigens in tumor cells, *Proc. Nat. Acad. Sci. U.S.A.* **69**:1664–1668.

Ting, C. C., Kirchner, H., Rodrigues, D., Park, J. Y., and Herberman, R. B., 1976, Cell-mediated immunity to Friend virus-induced leukemia. III. Characteristics of secondary cell-mediated cytotoxic response, *J. Immunol.* **116**:244–252.

Tischendorf, F. W., Ledderose, G., Wilmanns, W., and Tischendorf, M. M., 1973,

Cationic leukocyte antigen in urine of patients with chronic myelocytic leukemia, *Nature (London)* **245**:379–380.

Tung, J., Fleissner, E., Vitella, E., and Boyse, E., 1975a, Expression of murine leukemia virus envelope glycoprotein gp 69/71 on mouse thymocytes, *J. Exp. Med.* **142**:518–523.

Tung, J., Vitella, E., and Fleissner, E., 1975b, Biochemical evidence linking the $G_{IX}$ thymocyte surface antigen to the gp 69/71 envelope glycoprotein of murine leukemia virus, *J. Exp. Med.* **141**:198–205.

Ultmann, J. E., Fish, W., Osserman, E., and Gellhorn, A., 1959, The clinical implications of hypogammaglobulinemia in patients with chronic lymphatic leukemia and lymphocytic lymphosarcoma, *Ann. Intern. Med.* **51**:501–516.

Viza, D. C., Bernard-Degani, R., Bernard, C., and Harris, R., 1969, Leukemia antigens, *Lancet* **2**:493–494.

Viza, D., Davies, D. A. L., and Harris, R., 1970, Solubilization and partial purification of human leukaemic specific antigens, *Nature (London)* **227**:1249–1251.

Waldmann, T. A., Broder, S., Krakauer, R., MacDermott, R. P., Durm, M., Goldman, C., and Meade, B., 1976, The role of suppressor cells in the pathogenesis of common variable hypogammaglobulinemia and the immunodeficiency associated with myeloma, *Fed. Proc.* **35**:2067–2072.

Wallen, W. C., and Neubauer, R. H., Rabin, H., and Cicmanec, J., 1973, Nonimmune rosette formation by lymphoma and leukemia cells from herpesvirus saimiri-infected owl monkeys, *J. Nat. Cancer Inst.* **51**:967–975.

Wallen, W. C., Rabin, H., Neubauer, R. H., and Cicmanec, J. L., 1975, Depression in lymphocyte response to general mitogens by owl monkeys infected with herpesvirus saimiri, *J. Nat. Cancer Inst.* **54**:679–685.

West, W., and Herberman, R. B., 1974, A human lymphoid cell line with receptors for both sheep red blood cells and complement, *Cell. Immunol.* **14**:139–145.

Wilson, J. D., and Nossal, G. J. V., 1971, Identification of human T and B lymphocytes in normal peripheral blood and in chronic lymphocytic leukemia, *Lancet* **2**:788–791.

Wybran, J., Chantler, S., and Fudenberg, H. H., 1973, Isolation of normal T cells in chronic lymphatic leukemia, *Lancet* **1**:126–129.

Yata, J., Klein, G., Kobayashi, N., Furukawa, T., and Yanagisawa, M., 1970, Human thymus-lymphoid tissue antigen and its presence in leukaemia and lymphoma, *Clin. Exp. Immunol.* **7**:781–792.

Yohn, D. S., Horoszewicz, J. S., Ellison, R. R., Mittelman, A., and Chai, L. S., 1968, Immunofluorescent studies in human leukemia, *Cancer Res.* **28**:1692–1702.

Yoshida, T. O., and Imai, K., 1970, Autoantibody to human leukemic cell membrane as detected by immune adherence, *Rev. Eur. Etud. Clin. Biol.* **15**:61–65.

Yoshida, T. O., and Andersson, B., 1972, Evidence for a receptor recognizing antigen-complexed immunoglobulin on the surface of activated mouse thymus lymphocytes, *Scand. J. Immunol.* **1**:401–408.

Yoshiki, T., Mellors, R., and Hardy, W., 1973, Common cell-surface antigen associated with murine and feline C type RNA leukemia viruses, *Proc. Nat. Acad. Sci. U.S.A.* **70**:1878–1882.

Yoshiki, T., Mellors, R. C., Hady, W. D., Jr., and Fleissner, E., 1974, Common cell

surface antigen associated with mammalian C-type RNA viruses, *J. Exp. Med.*
   **139**:925–942.
Zarling, J. M., Nowinski, R. C., and Bach, F. H., 1975, Lysis of leukemia cells by
   spleen cells of normal mice. *Proc. Nat. Acad. Sci. U.S.A.* **72**:2780–2784.
Zatz, M. M., Goldstein, A. L., and White, A., 1973a, Lymphocyte populations of
   AKR/J mice. I. Effect of aging on migration patterns, response to PHA, and
   expression of theta antigen, *J. Immunol.* **111**:1514–1518.
Zatz, M. M., White, A., and Goldstein, A. L., 1973b, Lymphocyte populations of
   AKR/J mice. II. Effect of leukemogenesis on migration patterns, response to
   PHA, and expression of theta antigen, *J. Immunol.* **111**:1519–1525.

# Antihemophilic Factor

Oscar D. Ratnoff

## 13.1. Introduction

Antihemophilic factor (AHF, factor VIII) was first described as an agent in normal plasma that corrects the defective coagulation of patients with classic hemophilia (hemophilia A). It is a complex molecule that participates in the intrinsic pathway of thrombin formation and supports aggregation of platelets by the antibiotic, ristocetin, and retention of platelets by glass bead filters. The plasma of individuals with hemophilia contains normal amounts of protein immunologically related to AHF (AHF-like antigens), as detected by heterologous antiserum, and retains the platelet-related properties of AHF.

A deficiency of procoagulant AHF is also found in von Willebrand's disease, an autosomal dominant trait in which the bleeding time is prolonged and plasma is often deficient in AHF-like antigens and in the capacity to support ristocetin-induced platelet aggregation and retention of platelets by glass bead filters. Thus, the plasma of patients with von Willebrand's disease appears to be truly deficient in AHF whereas that of classic hemophilia contains an AHF-like protein that is deficient in procoagulant activity.

These observations suggest that AHF may be composed of at least two parts. One, functionally deficient in both classic hemophilia and von Willebrand's disease, is responsible for the coagulant properties of the AHF molecule, and is synthesized under the influence of a gene on the X

OSCAR D. RATNOFF • Department of Medicine, Case Western Reserve University School of Medicine, and University Hospitals of Cleveland, Cleveland, Ohio 44106. Career Investigator of the American Heart Association.

chromosome. The other, deficient only in von Willebrand's disease, contains AHF-like antigens, supports the platelet-related reactions of AHF, and is synthesized under the direction of an autosomal gene. The two subcomponents, probably parts of the same molecule, can be dissociated, facilitating study of the AHF molecule.

This chapter reviews our current knowledge concerning AHF and its disorders. Inevitably, clarity requires much repetition, so that the reader can understand one section independent of others. The literature concerning AHF has blossomed during the last 10 years, so that only a sample of the information available can be provided.

## 13.2. Assays for Antihemophilic Factor

*The procoagulant properties of AHF* (AHF$_{COAG}$, VIII$_{COAG}$, etc.) are assayed by measuring the capacity of plasma or its fractions to correct the coagulative defect of known hemophilic plasma. Modifications of the partial thromboplastin time[65,204] or thromboplastin generation test[289] are widely used to quantify the titer of procoagulant AHF. Such assays are standardized in comparison to pooled normal plasma,[313,408] or, less happily, to lyophilized preparations of normal plasma.[373] The normal range of procoagulant AHF in our own experience, measured by a modification of the partial thromboplastin time, is provided in Table I; 1 unit of procoagulant AHF is defined as the amount detected in 1 ml of a pool of 24 or 25 normal male plasmas.[408]

*The concentration of AHF-like antigens* (AHF$_{ANT}$, VIII$_{ANT}$, etc.) recognized by heterologous antiserum is usually measured by semiquantitative immunoelectrophoresis.[408] Other techniques that have been used include radioimmunoassay,[86,136,170,190] quantitative polyacrylamide gel electrophoresis of reduced subunits of AHF,[392] or estimation of the ability of AHF-like antigens to block the anticoagulant properties of heterologous antiserum to AHF.[36,408] Values for the concentration of AHF-like antigens in plasmas tested in our own laboratory are provided in Table I. Again, 1 unit of AHF-like antigens is defined as the amount detected in 1 ml of pooled normal plasma, but there is no *a priori* reason for assuming that the unitage of procoagulant AHF and AHF-like antigens can be equated.

*The property of AHF that supports ristocetin-induced platelet aggregation* (AHF$_{VWF}$, VIII$_{VWF}$, von Willebrand's factor, etc.) can be assayed qualitatively by adding the antibiotic to the subject's platelet-rich plasma and measuring the degree of platelet aggregation turbidimetrically.[165] A more quantitative assay can be performed by adding ristocetin to normal washed platelets in the presence of measured amounts of plasma or its

**Table I.** Normal Values for Some Properties of Antihemophilic Factor

| I. | Procoagulant activity[308] | | units/ml | |
|---|---|---|---|---|
| | Male | Range | 0.43–2.16 | 97 subjects |
| | | Geometric mean | 0.95 | |
| | | Geometric SD | +38%, −28% | |
| | Female | Range | 0.41–2.15 | 177 subjects |
| | | Geometric mean | 0.98 | |
| | | Geometric SD | +36%, −26% | |
| II. | Precipitating AHF-like antigens (in plasma)[308] | | units/ml | |
| | Male | Range | 0.33–2.15 | 66 subjects |
| | | Geometric mean | 0.97 | |
| | | Geometric SD | +31%, −24% | |
| | Female | Range | 0.44–2.07 | 147 subjects |
| | | Geometric mean | 0.90 | |
| | | Geometric SD | +40%, −28% | |
| III. | Ristocetin aggregation[394] | | units/100 ml | |
| | | Geometric mean | 92.4 | 20 subjects |
| | | Geometric SD | ±23% | |
| IV. | Platelet retention by glass bead filter | | % platelets retained by glass bead filters | |
| | Bowie's method[63] | Mean | 89.9 | 34 subjects |
| | | 95% of values | >65% | |
| | Salzman's method[335,367] | Mean | 46.7% | 100 subjects |
| | | 95% of values | >30% | |

AHF-rich fractions. [394] The platelets need not be viable; for example, paraformaldehyde-fixed platelets may be used.[5] Normal values for AHF$_{VWF}$, derived from data of Weiss, are provided in Table I.

*Platelet retention by glass bead filters* (platelet "adhesiveness") can be measured by comparing the platelet count of venous blood, with or without added anticoagulant, before and after it has trickled through a column of glass beads under standardized conditions.[63,150,335,367] This technique does not distinguish between adhesion of platelets to the glass beads and retention of platelet aggregates in the interstices of the filter. Although the literature often refers to the results of this test as a measure of platelet adhesiveness, this caveat should be kept in mind. Representative normal values are provided in Table I.

## 13.3. The Site of Synthesis of AHF

Early studies suggested that AHF is synthesized by the reticuloendothelial (RE) system[359] or by splenic[287] or lymphoid[404] tissue. But blockade of the RE system with methyl palmitate did not decrease the plasma titer of procoagulant AHF.[116] Moreover, a patient with the Swiss type of agammaglobulinemia, who had severe functional and morphologic abnormalities of the RE system and an almost total absence of lymphocytes and plasma cells in lymphoid tissues, bone marrow and blood, had a normal titer of procoagulant AHF.[231] Furthermore, splenectomy is not associated with a decreased titer of this clotting factor.[326]

On theoretic grounds, Owen *et al.*[274] proposed that AHF is synthesized by vascular endothelium. Studies of Hoyer[173] and Bloom[50] demonstrated that vascular endothelial cells contain AHF-like antigens recognized by indirect immunofluorescence. Jaffe[179] provided direct evidence that endothelial cells synthesize AHF-like antigens. The synthesized material, like plasma AHF, could be broken down by reducing agents to subunits with a molecular weight of 225,000.[181] The agent synthesized by endothelial cells supported platelet retention by glass bead filters and platelet aggregation by ristocetin.[180] In similar experiments by Bloom,[350] the AHF-like agent synthesized by endothelial cells migrated more anodally than normal plasma AHF upon electrophoresis.

The techniques currently available do not allow us to say whether the procoagulant portion of AHF is also synthesized by endothelial cells, and Bloom *et al.*[52] suggest that this is not the case. Intriguingly, procoagulant AHF appears to generate when the plasma of a patient with the CRM+ variant of classic hemophilia (Section 13.10.7) or perfusates of normal liver are perfused through rabbit spleens.[37] Compatible with this view, Tuddenham *et al.*[379] demonstrated that cultures of fetal spleen, and probably fetal liver, synthesized AHF-like antigens. These two studies do not rule out an endothelial origin for this protein.

An AHF-like agent with procoagulant activity has been extracted from porcine and canine kidney tissue by Barrow and Graham.[21,22] The relationship of this substance to plasma AHF is not understood; it has a molecular weight of about 25,000, much smaller than that attributed to the procoagulant subcomponent of AHF, and antiserum against hog kidney AHF-like material did not inactivate procoagulant AHF in human plasma. Nevertheless, a human circulating anticoagulant directed against AHF was neutralized by kidney preparations.

## 13.4. Purification of AHF

Since the first description of AHF, repeated attempts have been made to separate this agent from normal plasma in purified form. Procoagulant activity ascribed to the presence of AHF was detected in the precipitated euglobulin fraction of normal plasma,[278] in the fibrinogen-rich fractions of plasma insoluble in the presence of 8% ethanol,[49,78,211] 11% ether,[192] 33% ammonium sulfate,[45,387] phosphate and citrate buffers,[41] or neutral amino acids such as glycine[386] and in the insoluble residue of thawed, frozen plasma.[288] The AHF-like material in these precipitates has been further purified by extraction in various ways[49,192,263,354,358] or by chromatography on ion exchange resins,[89,249] reducing its content of fibrinogen and other impurities.

A major step in the purification of AHF came from the observation that AHF was excluded by gels retaining components of plasma with molecular weights less than 1,000,000–2,000,000.[156,184,189,316] Preparations purified as much as 16,000-fold could be separated from fractions of plasma insoluble in the presence of 3% ethanol and 10% polyethylene glycol and then filtered through 4% agarose.[184,407] Chromatography of AHF preparations upon diethylaminoethyl cellulose has also been exploited successfully.[345] A number of variations of these basic procedures have been described.[26,133,154,228,235,256]

## 13.5. Chemical and Physical Properties of AHF

The protein nature of AHF has been established by its inactivation by such proteases as plasmin,[95,387] trypsin,[198] and, under appropriate conditions, thrombin.[281,327] It migrates upon electrophoresis as an α-globulin,[19,214] although its mobility varies under different conditions. Its average concentration in plasma has been estimated to be 8–10 mg/liter.[86]

The sedimentation constant of AHF is disputed; estimates range from about 14S to 40S,[153,156,189,208] suggesting that aggregation may occur during refrigerated centrifugation; the molecular radius of AHF is said to be 390 Å.[155] The molecular weight of AHF is equally uncertain; most investigators believe it to be 1,000,000–2,000,000, but values as high as 8,000,000 and as low as 600,000 or less have been proposed.[154,189,208, 228,345,396]

AHF is a glycoprotein[155,208,228,345] and can be precipitated with con-canavalin A, which reacts with specific carbohydrate groups.[189] Its carbo-hydrate content has been estimated to be 5–10%,[54,228,345] and it loses its procoagulant activity when treated with glycolytic enzymes.[14] Although Hershgold et al.[154] have proposed that AHF contains as much as 11% lipid, our own preparations[316] and those of Legaz[208] contained no more that traces. The amino acid composition of AHF has been analyzed by Hershgold,[154] Marchesi,[228] Shapiro,[345] Legaz,[208] and their co-workers (Table II). The procoagulant properties of AHF have been linked to the presence of thiol groups at or near the active site.[13]

The procoagulant activity of AHF is erratically labile upon storage of

**Table II.** Composition of AHF[a]

| Amino acids | Hershgold[153] | Marchesi[228] | Shapiro[345] | Legaz[208] |
|---|---|---|---|---|
| Lysine | 0.508 | 0.437 | 0.492 | 0.399 |
| Histidine | 0.173 | ND | 0.272 | 0.225 |
| Arginine | 0.436 | 0.358 | 0.484 | 0.399 |
| Aspartic acid | 0.791 | 1.03 | 0.834 | 0.854 |
| Theonine | 0.508 | 0.461 | 0.511 | 0.601 |
| Serine | 0.630 | 0.700 | 0.666 | 0.708 |
| Glutamic acid | 1.032 | 0.946 | 1.149 | 0.899 |
| Proline | 0.521 | 0.644 | 0.600 | 0.612 |
| Glycine | 0.660 | 0.772 | 0.675 | 0.629 |
| Alanine | 0.543 | 0.506 | 0.497 | 0.438 |
| Half-cystine | 0.235 | Present | 0.619 | 0.657 |
| Valine | 0.596 | 0.639 | 0.778 | 0.758 |
| Methionine | 0.099 | 0.087 | 0.127 | 0.084 |
| Isoleucine | 0.317 | 0.345 | 0.319 | 0.337 |
| Leucine | 0.684 | 0.488 | 0.689 | 0.652 |
| Tyrosine | 0.230 | 0.193 | 0.178 | 0.202 |
| Phenylalanine | 0.265 | 0.253 | 0.253 | 0.270 |
| Tryptophan | ND | ND | ND | 0.247 |
| % protein | 76 | | | |
| % CHO (approx.) | 10 | 5 | 5 | 5.8 |
| % lipid (approx.) | 11–12 | <5 | — | 5 (?) |

[a]Values in nanomoles per gram of protein.
[b]ND = not determined.

bank blood[282] or plasma[360] at 4°C; plasma AHF is more stable at −30°C.[149] Procoagulant activity[213] and the capacity to support ristocetin-induced platelet aggregation[246] are quickly decreased when plasma is heated at 56°C, but AHF-like antigens detected by heterologous antiserum survive incubation at 60°C for 60 min.[407] Serum is devoid of procoagulant AHF,[128,277] presumably because this agent is inactivated by thrombin, but it contains normal concentrations of AHF-like antigens.[407]

Whether more than one species of AHF is present in the plasma of normal individuals is not certain. Meyer *et al.*[245a] detected only one subcomponent upon two-dimensional agarose gel electrophoresis, whereas Sultan and Siméon[369] and Zimmerman *et al.*[406] observed heterogeneity with this method and by ion exchange chromatography. A related unanswered question is whether differences exist among the AHF molecules of different normal individuals. Edson and Swinehart[96] reported antigenic heterogeneity among different normal individuals. We have tried to establish the heterogeneity of normal AHF by many techniques without success.[292]

## 13.5.1. Subcomponents of AHF

The substructure of AHF has been the subject of intense study. When purified preparations are reduced and subjected to sodium dodecyl sulfate (SDS) polyacrylamide gel electrophoresis, a major band with a molecular weight of 200,000–240,000 is regularly observed.[208,228,345] When the reduced subunits were subjected to ultracentrifugation, the molecular weight was estimated to be 105,000, as though the carbohydrate content of preparations of AHF may have interfered with measurements of molecular weight by SDS polyacrylamide gel electrophoresis.[208] Presumably, then, AHF consists of a number of subunits held together with disulfide bonds. Reduction of AHF inactivates its procoagulant activity, but under appropriate conditions the subunits retain their antigenicity and their ability to support ristocetin-induced platelet aggregation.[15]

More intriguingly, preparations of AHF may be dissociated in the presence of detergents[275] or high concentrations of various salts.[275,374,396,397] For example, after filtration of AHF through 4–8% agarose in the presence of 0.24–0.25 M calcium chloride, two subcomponents of AHF can be distinguished. One subcomponent, excluded from such gels, contains the bulk of the protein[275,397] and precipitating AHF-like antigens recognized by heterologous antiserum,[320] and supports ristocetin-induced platelet aggregation (AHF$_{VWF}$),[393] but has little or no procoagulant activity. The second subcomponent, retarded by the gel, has a molecular weight estimated by SDS polyacrylamide gel electrophoresis and agarose gel filtration to be 200,000–240,000,[319,322] and by sucrose gradient ultracentrifugation possibly 150,000.[322] This subcomponent does not possess AHF-like precipitating antigens, nor does it support ristocetin aggregation, but it contains most of the AHF procoagulant activity and this can be further enhanced by incubation with thrombin.[81,321] The AHF-like nature of the procoagulant activity of the low molecular weight subcomponent is supported by its neutralization of human antibodies against AHF and its consequent inactivation. A low molecular weight subcomponent with coagulant activity can also be separated from preparations of AHF by the addition of small amounts of thrombin[81,121,396] or by clotting recalcified cryoprecipitates rich in AHF.[121]

The question has been raised whether the high and low molecular weight subcomponents of AHF are part of a single molecule or are, in fact, two separate entities.[26,405] Dissociation of the subcomponents has been reported in experiments utilizing, for example, insolubilized human antibodies. The low molecular weight subcomponent is absorbed to the antibody, leaving a soluble residue containing the precipitating antigen. In another approach, McDonald et al.[233] separated procoagulant AHF from AHF-like antigens by adsorption of the former to solid phase ethylene maleic anhydride polyelectrolytes. These various experiments do not exclude the possibility that a loosely joined complex was dissociated by the experimental procedures, and in any event contrary results have been published.[55] Moreover, no dissociation of procoagulant AHF and AHF-like antigens was detected when plasma or its fractions were subjected to agarose gel immunoelectrophoresis.[48]

Immunologic studies with antiserums specific for the high and low molecular weight subcomponents appear to demonstrate that they are part of a single molecule.[319] Indeed, some investigators hold that in nature the subcomponents are held together by covalent bonds and that the apparent ease with which they are separated on agarose columns is the artifactual result of proteolysis by plasma enzymes.[209,236,372] But the two subcomponents appear to reassociate when calcium ions are removed by dialysis[80] and we have been able to dissociate AHF into its subcomponents despite the presence of a mixture of protease inhibitors.[293] Firkin and Howard[110] reported an interesting variant of this experiment. Insolubilized antiserum to preparations of precipitating AHF-like antigen devoid of procoagulant AHF activity was incubated with normal plasma. This procedure depleted the plasma of proportional amounts of AHF-like antigens, procoagulant AHF, and the property of AHF supporting aggregation of platelets by ristocetin (AHF$_{VWD}$), as if all were properties of the same molecule. Firkin and Howard then washed the insolubilized antigen–antibody complex that formed with 0.25 M calcium chloride, presumably depleting it of procoagulant AHF. When the complex was then mixed with normal plasma, the latter was disproportionately depleted of procoagulant AHF, as if a procoagulant fraction had dissociated from plasma AHF and then combined with the AHF-like antigens of the insoluble antigen–antibody complex.

These observations support the view that the high and low molecular weight subcomponents of AHF are held together by noncovalent bonds, analogous to the structure of the first component of complement (C1). Since classic hemophilia is inherited as an X-chromosome-linked disorder, and von Willebrand's disease as an autosomal dominant trait, a reasonable inference is that the synthesis of the low molecular weight subcomponent is directed by an X chromosomal gene, and that of the high molecular weight subcomponent by an autosomal gene, as proposed by Graham.[127]

Experiments of van Mourik et al.[255] appear to demonstrate that AHF can also be dissociated into several subunits by dialysis against low ionic strength buffers. Since the subunits were recognized by their precipitation with rabbit antiserum, they were presumably derived from molecules containing the high molecular weight subcomponent that can be separated by gel filtration in the presence of 0.25 M calcium chloride.

## 13.6. The Antigenicity of AHF Preparations

In 1957, Shanberge and Gore[344] described the preparation of antiserum in rabbits that inhibited the procoagulant properties of AHF. A satisfactory precipitating antiserum to AHF was subsequently elicited in rabbits by Zimmerman et al.[408] and others. Such antiserums also inhibit the properties of AHF that support ristocetin-induced platelet aggregation (AHF$_{vWD}$)[248] and the retention of platelets by glass bead filters.[232,248] Antiserums to normal AHF vary widely in their capacity to inhibit procoagulant AHF, in contrast to the relative ease of producing precipitating antibodies.[55,349] On the other hand, antibodies have been produced in the rabbit,[245] duck,[172] and goat[129] that were neutralized by the plasmas of patients with the variant of hemophilia designated CRM+ (see Section 13.10.7), and not that of CRM− individuals, as if directed against a specific site on the procoagulant part of AHF.

Relatively specific antiserums have been prepared against the high and low molecular weight subcomponents of AHF separated by gel filtration in the presence of 0.25 M calcium chloride.[319] The antiserum against the low molecular weight subcomponent inhibited procoagulant AHF but did not form precipitates with whole AHF, whereas the reverse was true of antiserum prepared against the high molecular weight subcomponent. Nonetheless, cross-antigenicity between the subcomponents could be demonstrated by antiserum absorption experiments.

## 13.7. Functions of AHF

### 13.7.1. Procoagulant Activity

How AHF participates in the generation of thrombin is only vaguely understood (Fig. 1). The clotting time of hemophilic blood is usually prolonged[402] and the partial thromboplastin time of plasma, nearly always. These defects reflect impaired conversion of prothrombin to thrombin.[2,66] The one-stage prothrombin time is normal in hemophilia, indicating that the extrinsic pathway of clotting is not impaired.[305] These observations localize the action of AHF to an early step of the intrinsic pathway of thrombin formation, preceding the participation of Stuart Factor (factor X).

In the test tube, the first recognized events in the intrinsic pathway are the activation of Hageman factor (factor XII) by certain negatively charged agents and, consequent upon this, the proteolytic activation of plasma thromboplastin antecedent (PTA, factor XI). In plasma, this reaction requires participation of a plasma prekallikrein (Fletcher factor) and high molecular weight kininogen (Fitzgerald factor). Since hereditary

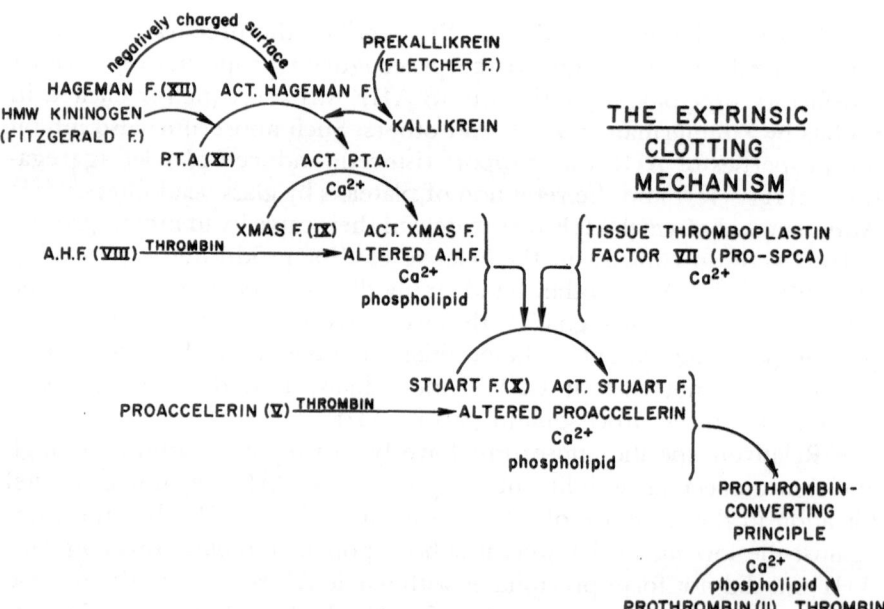

**Fig. 1.** The intrinsic and extrinsic pathways of thrombin formation. (PTA = plasma thromboplastin antecedent; Xmas F = Christmas factor; AHF = antihemophilic factor). (Reprinted with permission from Stanbury.[362a])

deficiencies of Hageman factor, prekallikrein, or high molecular weight kininogen are not associated with a bleeding tendency, perhaps other ways of activating PTA exist in nature. Activated PTA, in turn, changes Christmas factor (factor IX) from an inert to a clot-promoting state, but only if calcium ions are present. Again the mildness of hereditary PTA deficiency suggests that other mechanisms may exist to activate Christmas factor *in vivo*.

AHF participates with activated Christmas factor to convert Stuart factor to its active form, via a proteolytic reaction. The enzymatic site responsible for this limited proteolysis of Stuart factor is almost certainly on the Christmas factor molecule.[90] No firm evidence has arisen to suggest an enzymatic role for AHF. Activated Stuart factor, in concert with proaccelerin (factor V), phospholipid, and calcium ions, changes prothrombin to thrombin, the enzyme responsible for converting fibrinogen to fibrin.[339]

The nature of the interaction of activated Christmas factor and AHF is unknown, but it requires the presence of calcium ions and phospholipid micelles, to which both factors are adsorbed.[25,39,152,163] Perhaps AHF forms a bridge that enables Christmas factor to combine optimally with Stuart factor via calcium links, in parallel to the way proaccelerin potentiates the release of thrombin from prothrombin by activated Stuart factor.

The action of AHF is greatly potentiated if it has first been altered by thrombin.[304,307] Although some investigators believe that this step is a *sine qua non* for the activation of Stuart factor,[306] it is more likely that activation can proceed slowly in the absence of AHF or AHF can function, albeit poorly, without being altered by thrombin, since platelet-deficient plasma will clot. Just how thrombin alters AHF is not known, although its effect has been localized to the low molecular weight subcomponent of the molecule.[81] The molecular change brought about by thrombin is uncertain. It does not induce a clearly recognizable change in the AHF or its reduced subcomponents, although it presumably brings about some form of limited proteolysis[208,345]; I have already noted that some investigators have detected low molecular weight procoagulant AHF fragments after treatment of plasma or its AHF-containing subcomponents with thrombin (Section 13.5.1). Continued action of thrombin inactivates AHF.[282,327]

In sum, then, AHF appears to be a necessary cofactor for the enzymatic activation of Stuart factor by activated Christmas factor.

## 13.7.2. Ristocetin-Induced Platelet Aggregation

Ristocetin is an antibiotic elaborated by *Nocardia lurida* that was introduced primarily for the treatment of gram-positive infections.[329] Its use was accompanied by an unacceptably high incidence of severe thrombocytopenia[115] related to its capacity to aggregate platelets.[114] In the process, both ADP and ATP are slowly released from the platelets.[191,398]

In 1971, Howard and Firkin[165] reported that, in contrast to its action upon normal or hemophilic platelet-rich plasma, ristocetin induced little or no aggregation of platelets in the platelet-rich plasma of patients with von Willebrand's disease. Subsequently, Weiss et al.[398] demonstrated that the defect in von Willebrand's disease plasma could be corrected by addition of purified AHF[398] or the high molecular weight subcomponent of AHF separated by gel filtration in the presence of 0.24 M calcium chloride[393]; the procoagulant low molecular weight subcomponent did not support ristocetin-induced platelet aggregation. Confirming the role of AHF, Meyer et al.[247] observed that antiserum to this clotting factor blocked ristocetin aggregation of normal platelet-rich plasma. Weiss[394] has devised a quantitative assay for the agent supporting ristocetin aggregation (AHF$_{VWF}$).

Green et al.[137] reported binding between ristocetin and AHF. The effect of ristocetin apparently depends on the presence of specific receptor sites on platelets, probably membrane glycoproteins that also bind thrombin.[183,271] The mechanisms involved in aggregation are poorly understood.[389] The receptor sites are functionally absent in the platelets of individuals with the Bernard–Soulier syndrome, a hereditary disorder in which platelets are unusually large and functionally defective, and appear to be deficient in a membrane glycoprotein[72]; such platelets do not aggregate upon addition of ristocetin even though AHF is present.[166,398] Other qualitative abnormalities of platelets have been inconsistently associated with impaired platelet aggregation.[398]

Ristocetin, in concentrations higher than those that bring about aggregation of platelets, precipitates fibrinogen in plasma and in the canaliculi of platelets.[65] Although this suggests the possibility that alteration of the fibrinogen-like material in platelets by ristocetin is a necessary step in the aggregation of these cells, it must be borne in mind that paraformaldehyde-fixed platelets undergo aggregation,[5] and the platelets of a patient with congenital afibrinogenemia aggregated normally.[165]

Failure of ristocetin-induced platelet aggregation is an important diagnostic feature of von Willebrand's disease, but the test may give normal results in mildly affected cases or in patients whose titers of AHF have increased during stress (see Section 13.11.1).

Although ristocetin-induced platelet aggregation is a function of the high molecular weight subcomponent of AHF, the site on the molecule responsible for this phenomenon is different from that which reacts with precipitating antiserum against AHF, as clearly demonstrated, for example, by its heat lability,[246] and its sensitivity to human circulating anticoagulants against AHF.[376] Variants of von Willebrand's disease have been described in which ristocetin-induced aggregation is impaired despite the presence of normal concentrations of AHF-like precipitating antigens (Section 13.11.4).

### 13.7.3. Platelet Retention by Glass Bead Columns and Platelet Adhesion to Subendothelial Structures

The platelets in heparinized blood adhere to glass surfaces,[251,403] a process requiring the presence of fibrinogen.[140] The phenomenon of retention of platelets by columns of glass beads is more complex. When blood is filtered through such columns, the number of platelets in the effluent is less than that in the original sample.[150] Platelet retention is observed only if the red blood cells have not been separated from the platelets and plasma.[150] At first, the erythrocytes were thought to furnish adenosine diphosphate (ADP), required for platelet retention.[112,151] More recent evidence implicates the platelets themselves as a source of ADP.[238,254] Thus, the role of the red cells is unclear. Additionally, AHF is needed for retention of platelets, at first suggested because the phenomenon was impaired in von Willebrand's disease,[335,409] and demonstrated by the repair of this defect by purified AHF.[59] Additionally, impaired retention can be induced by treating normal plasma with heterologous antiserum to AHF.[59] Nonetheless, platelet retention is normal in hemophilia, as though the phenomenon were unrelated to the procoagulant site on the AHF molecule.[335]

A likely course of events has been suggested by McPherson and Zucker.[237] Salzman[335] and Mason and Conway[230] believed that retention reflected both adhesion of platelets to glass and aggregation of platelets to each other. McPherson and Zucker proposed that during filtration of blood through columns of glass beads, some platelets stick to the glass and release ADP. Other platelets then adhere to these platelets, a process requiring AHF.

Platelets in normal blood stick to exposed rabbit subendothelial structures.[27] Again, studies in von Willebrand's disease indicate that AHF is a requisite for this phenomenon.[378] Presumably, these observations are related to the prolonged bleeding time of patients with this disease (see Section 13.11.1).

## 13.8. The AHF-like Properties of Platelets

Mann[222] and Seibert et al.[342] demonstrated that normal human platelets possessed AHF-like procoagulant activity and that this property was absent from hemophilic platelets. The defect could be corrected by exposing hemophilic plasma to normal platelet-deficient plasma, as if the AHF were adsorbed to the platelet surface.

The function of platelet-bound membranes is not known. Megakaryocytes[50] and both normal and hemophilic platelet membranes were shown to contain equivalent amounts of AHF-like precipitating antigens, whereas these were usually, but not always, deficient in von Willebrand's disease[79,138,167,261,349] and from a single patient with thrombasthenia.[167] Further, Jaffe and Nachman[182] described a protein in normal platelets that binds AHF-like antigens. AHF-like antigens and $AHF_{VWF}$ (the property supporting ristocetin-induced platelet aggregation) have also been detected in subcellular granule fractions of platelets.[261] The platelets of individuals with Bernard–Soulier syndrome (Section 13.7.2), which fail to aggregate upon addition of ristocetin, contain AHF-like antigens.[167]

Normal platelets are aggregated by addition of thrombin to platelet-rich plasma. Ardlie and Reardon[11] proposed that this action of thrombin is dependent on the presence of AHF. The platelets of individuals with von Willebrand's disease aggregate upon addition of thrombin, making this suggestion unlikely.

## 13.9. Variations in AHF in Physiologic and Nonhereditary Pathologic States

The wide variation in the titer of procoagulant AHF and AHF-like antigens in normal individuals has already been noted (Table 1). Among normal siblings, the variation in procoagulant AHF is said to be less than that among unrelated individuals, and a child's titer is determined by that of his parents.[286] Individuals with blood group A have a higher titer of procoagulant AHF than those of blood group O.[299]

Under basal conditions, the titer of procoagulant AHF is relatively constant from year to year.[308] AHF titers probably rise with age, although this is not entirely clear.[82,106,286,299] The mechanisms controlling the plasma titer of procoagulant AHF are complex. Experimental electrical stimulation of the dog brain increased or decreased AHF depending on the site stimulated, as though the titer were partially under neural control[141]; similar conclusions have been derived from human studies.[226] Both procoagulant AHF and AHF-like precipitating antigens increase in normal pregnancy,[31,186,368] during stress,[31] or after exercise[324] or the administration of sympathomimetic agents,[175] the latter two a $\beta$-adrenergic effect.[77,113,177] The rise in titer in procoagulant AHF after exercise or epinephrine is not diminished by splenectomy,[297,326] a disputed point.[351] The titer of procoagulant AHF is probably the same in normal men and women.[299] It increases in women taking oral contraceptive agents[103] which may account for our contemporary observation that the mean titer is slightly higher in normal women than in normal men. The titer of procoagulant AHF is also increased after administration of prednisone.[178]

Sarji *et al.*[337] have reported a striking sex difference in the amount of the agent in normal plasma that supports aggregation of platelets by ristocetin ($AHF_{VWD}$), fasting males having twice the concentration as females. Further, in males the concentration appeared to increase with age. A correlation was also detected between the level of $AHF_{VWD}$ and the fasting blood glucose, although postprandial hyperglycemia paradoxically reduced the titer.

The titer of procoagulant AHF increases after surgical procedures,[7] and X-irradiation,[356] in febrile,[98] hyperthyroid,[99,157,352] or hypergammaglobulinemic[285,395] states (perhaps explaining the high titer of AHF in Bantu[244] and Australian aborigines[285]), and in individuals with atherosclerosis.[83] Similar increases have been noted both in procoagulant titers and in the concentration of AHF-like antigens in renal failure,[97,104] severe preeclampsia,[169] diabetes,[100,147] malignancy,[7,148,330] and hepatic disease.[132,239] The rise in the concentration of AHF-like antigens may be disproportionately high. Sultan and Siméon[369] reported that the elevated AHF-like antigens in acute viral hepatitis migrated abnormally upon two-dimensional immunoelectrophoresis.

In individuals believed to be undergoing disseminated intravascular coagulation, procoagulant AHF titers may decrease whereas the concentration of AHF-like antigens remains unaltered.[30] Perhaps this reflects inactivation of procoagulant activity by thrombin; human serum, which is deficient in procoagulant AHF, has normal concentrations of AHF-like antigens.[408] Perhaps, too, under these conditions AHF is inactivated by plasmin liberated during intravascular coagulation, since this enzyme inactivates procoagulant AHF.[95,387] A decrease in the titer of procoagulant AHF may also be observed in macroglobulinemia, myelosclerosis, aplastic anemia,[264] and hypothyroidism[102,352]; the mechanisms responsible are not known.

Circulating anticoagulants against AHF in nonhemophilic patients and acquired von Willebrand's disease are discussed in Sections 13.10.6 and 13.12.

## 13.10. Classic Hemophilia

Classic hemophilia is an X-chromosome-linked hemorrhagic disorder limited to males but transmitted by female carriers, themselves usually asymptomatic. Extrapolating from our own experience[314] and that of others,[186] it occurs about once in 10,000 male births.

### 13.10.1. The Nature of the Defect in Hemophilic Plasma

Although Liston,[219] in 1839, had hinted that blood clotting might be impaired in patients with hemophilia-like disease, it was not until 1893 that Wright[402] demonstrated that the clotting time of whole blood was prolonged. Some time later, Addis,[2] who may really have examined Christmas disease blood, added the additional information that the conversion of prothrombin to thrombin was impaired. Only with the studies of Frank and Hartmann,[111] Bendien and van Creveld,[28] Govaerts and Gratia,[123] and Patek and Stetson[277] was the defect sharply localized to the patients' plasma. Frank and Hartmann attributed impaired clotting to an inhibitory property of plasma, and Govaerts and Gratia to abnormal stability of platelets resulting from a defect in plasma. Patek and Stetson,[277] however, could not confirm that the clotting abnormality was related to a platelet defect. They found that normal plasma contained an agent that corrected the abnormal clotting without intervention of platelets. They were uncertain whether what is now known as AHF was deficient in the plasma of affected patients or was present in an aberrant or unavailable, nonfunctional form. Thereafter, the prevalent view ascribed hemophilia to a deficiency of AHF, although this concept had its critics.[377]

In 1957, Shanberge and Gore[344] provided immunologic evidence that hemophilic plasma contained a species of AHF recognized by heterologous antiserum to this agent. Despite some supporting evidence,[38,154,284,380] this important observation was not accepted until the early 1970s, when confirmatory observations were reported by several investigators.[36,364,408] An agent resembling AHF has been identified by immunologic[36,364,408] or physical[346,392] means in the plasma of all hemophiliacs tested. Indeed, it appears to be present, on the average, at somewhat higher concentrations than in normal plasma.[314]

To my knowledge, no certain method is yet available to distinguish the AHF-like protein present in hemophilic plasma from that in normal plasma except by its deficient procoagulant activity. Like normal AHF, the AHF-like protein of hemophiliacs appears to be a glycoprotein.[279] Bennett et al.[29] and Bouma et al.[58] prepared antiserum in rabbits against the fraction of hemophilic plasma analogous to that containing normal AHF. Such antiserums were immunologically identical to those produced by injection of normal AHF, and inactivated the procoagulant properties of normal AHF. In contrast, Kernoff and Rizza[193,195] evoked antiserum that induced precipitating antibodies but had little or no inhibitory effect upon procoagulant AHF. The reason for the difference between these observations is not clear, although the antigenic material used by Kernoff and Rizza was relatively crude.

The AHF-like material in hemophilic plasma, like that of normal individuals, can be dissociated by reduction to subunits with a molecular weight of 200,000–240,000[29,316]; the isoelectric point of these subunits is similar to that of normal AHF.[316] In three hemophilic plasmas, Poon *et al.*[291] demonstrated the presence of both high and low molecular weight subcomponents in the AHF-like material separated by agarose gel chromatography in the presence of 0.25 M calcium chloride. Conceivably, in other cases, the low molecular weight portion of the molecule that normally bears procoagulant activity is deleted in whole or in part, and perhaps this was the case in the studies of Kernoff and Rizza just quoted.

### 13.10.2. The Hereditary Nature of Classic Hemophilia and Detection of the Carrier State

Hemophilia is a striking example of an X-chromosome-linked disorder; one remarkable exception has been reported.[124] The Babylonian Talmud, compiled in the sixth century A.D., quotes a Rabbi Judah who exempted from circumcision the male offspring of a woman whose sons had bled to death after circumcision.[331] In 1803, John Otto[273] of Philadelphia described a family in which a bleeding diathesis was limited to males but transmitted by females. Much later, Legg[210] added the essential observation that the daughters of hemophiliacs carried the disease to their offspring.

An explanation for the peculiar sex-linked inheritance of hemophilia was provided by Morgan[252] in studies of fruit flies. Sex, he pointed out, was determined by the inheritance of a special pair of chromosomes, designated X and Y. An individual inheriting an X chromosome from each parent is female, whereas one who inherits an X chromosome from its mother and a Y from its father is male. The defect in classic hemophilia is attributable to an abnormality of a gene on the X chromosome. In a heterozygous female, bleeding is usually absent because of the presence of the normal X chromosome, whereas in a hemizygous male the disorder is experienced because the only X chromosome is abnormal. Rarely, the union of a heterozygous female and a hemizygous male has resulted in the birth of a daughter homozygous for the abnormal X chromosome, and she has exhibited all the features of classic hemophilia.[243,253]

The titer of functional AHF is approximately the same in the plasma of normal men and women, even though there are two X chromosomes in the somatic cells of females and only one in males. The Lyon hypothesis[40,220,270] provides a rational explanation of this unexpected finding. At an early stage of embryonal development, one of the pair of X chromosomes in each female somatic cell becomes inactive; its shriveled remains are visible as the Barr body. Once inactivation has taken place, the same X chromosome remains functional through succeeding divisions of the embryonal cells. In this way, the female is a mosaic, some of whose cells contain functional X chromosomes derived from her mother, and the others from her father. Since the inactivation of the X chromosome is a random event, the proportion of functional X chromosomes of maternal and paternal origin varies from female to female. An excellent discussion of this subject in relation to hemophilia has been provided by Barrow and Graham.[23]

Based on these considerations, it is not surprising that, on the average, the titer of procoagulant AHF in the plasma of female carriers of classic hemophilia is about half that of normal women. The variation in titer, both among carriers and normal women, however, is such that only about half the carriers can be identified at the 95% level of certainty by measuring procoagulant AHF alone,[314] although more optimistic reports have been published.[266] In a few instances, the titer of procoagulant AHF in individuals thought to be heterozygous is so low that symptoms similar to those of hemophilia occur.[234]

The carrier state may be identified with much greater precision by simultaneous measurement of procoagulant AHF and AHF-like antigens detected by heterologous antiserums. The abnormal X chromosome of carriers, like those of patients with hemophilia, directs the synthesis of AHF-like antigens, and thus the concentration of such antigens is not reduced in carriers. Comparison of the relative titer of procoagulant AHF and the concentration of AHF-like antigens permits identification of the vast majority of obligate carriers.[33,36,44,407] The technique of logarithmic discriminant analysis is most effective in separating carriers from normal women[57,314] and in our experience with 67 obligate carriers, we were able to identify 63, or 94%, at a level of certainty that would have misidentified 5% of normal women as carriers.[314] Most investigators have had comparable experiences (e.g., Eyster[107] and Panicucci[276]), whereas others have had less impressive results (e.g., Holmberg[161]).

The utility of this approach for the detection of carriers is supported by studies of daughters of carriers. Such daughters, if they themselves have no sons, are at 50% risk of being carriers themselves. We have identified 34 of 75 such women as carriers; correcting for the 6% error in detecting the carrier state in obligate carriers, 36 or 48% of our subjects appeared to be carriers.

In about one-third of families (70 of 205 families in our own experience), a single male is affected and there are no other known relatives with hemophilia.[241] Such sporadic cases are more likely to be severe than those associated with a positive family history.[365] Were hemophilia due to a lethal gene, that is, one in which affected individuals do not have offspring, one might expect that in two-thirds of cases the mothers of individuals with isolated cases of hemophilia would be carriers, and in one-third, the disorder would have arisen as the result of mutation in the ovum from which the patient developed. But experience tells us that this is not the case in hemophilia, for affected individuals often have children. In fact, 31 of 39 (79%) mothers of patients with isolated cases have been identified as carriers because the titer of procoagulant AHF was significantly lower than the concentration of AHF-like antigens; the corrected value would be 85%.[314] Thus, only a small fraction of hemophilia appears to be the result of a fresh mutation. Similar data have been published by others. [47,147,276] A recent estimate of the mutation rate is $1.2 \times 10^{-5}$.[20] Our own data suggest approximately the same rate.[315]

In one interesting family, the grandmother and several other female relatives of the patient's mother appear to be normal, whereas the the mother has the characteristics of a carrier.[33] In this family, mutation may have occurred in the sperm or ovum from which the patient's mother had developed.

In providing eugenic advice to female relatives of hemophiliacs, one may have confidence in reporting positive results in tests for the carrier state. The converse is not true, and women in whom tests are negative should be warned that these do not exclude the carrier state.

### 13.10.3. Clinical Picture

In the severest form of hemophilia, in which no measurable AHF is found in procoagulant assays, the newborn infant bleeds profusely from circumcision, but only rarely from the umbilical stump[17]; AHF does not cross the placenta. [145,309] Rarely, massive hemorrhage, hemoperitoneum, intracranial bleeding[17] or bleeding into the scalp of the newborn child[201] may occur. As the baby starts to crawl, he is soon covered with ecchymoses and hematomas.[300] The eruption of teeth brings about protracted bleeding from biting wounds of the tongue and frenum. As the infant learns to walk—and fall—he experiences hemarthrosis, and the recurrence of this complication, most often localized in decreasing frequency, to the knees, elbows, ankles, wrists, hips, and shoulders,[359] leads to destruction of joint surfaces, atrophy of supporting muscles, crippling arthritis, and ankylosis.[300] Why impaired coagulation may result in hemarthrosis, though this complication does not occur in thrombocytopenia, is an unsolved puzzle. Periarticular hematomas or subperiosteal or intraosseous hemorrhage may bring pressure upon adjacent bone with the development of huge pseudocysts of bone, particularly the femur; the cysts are often the sites of fracture or infection.[363] Bleeding into tendons may result in flexion deformities of the elbow and tallipes equinus of the ankle. Subcutaneous hematomas reducing hematocrit by a third or more may arise spontaneously. Indeed, no part of the body is immune, and the hemophiliac may sustain hematuria, usually of renal origin,[298] hemothorax,[71] orbital or ocular hemorrhage,[53] epistaxis, retroperitoneal bleeding, or peripheral nerve damage.[70] Gastrointestinal bleeding, sometimes unexplained but often a concomitant of peptic ulcer[75] is not unusual. Intracranial[341] or intraspinal[359] hemorrhage or obstruction of the pharynx[359] or airway[207] by bleeding is often the cause of death. Gingival bleeding results in poor oral hygiene, and dental extractions are followed by protracted hemorrhage. Disastrous hemorrhage may ensue after any surgical procedure and most injuries, although death from exsanguination is rare.

Fortunately, not all hemophiliacs are so direly affected.[202,212,359] In perhaps one-half the cases, the titer of functional AHF ranges from about 1% of the average normal to as high as 48%, and the severity of symptoms is proportionately less. In patients with titers of about 5% or more, spontaneous bleeding is unusual, and the patient is handicapped only by bleeding after dental extractions, surgery, or injury. Moreover, the symptoms of severe hemophiliacs may ameliorate as the patients survive into adult life, either because the growing muscle mass is protective, the patients learn to avoid injury, or for more subtle reasons, and patients may survive into late adult life.[197] Not unexpectedly, hemophiliacs and their families are subject to great psychological stresses,[310,359] and patients often report that bleeding episodes are related to emotional crises. Some evidence has accumulated that a successful, mature adjustment to their precarious situation is accompanied by a decreased frequency of handicapping bleeding.[3]

### 13.10.4. Laboratory Diagnosis

The diagnosis of severe classic hemophilia is readily established. The clotting time of whole blood and the partial thromboplastin time of plasma[204] are greatly prolonged, and the bleeding time, that is, the duration of bleeding from a deliberately incised wound, is normal. The clotting defect is localized to the steps of the intrinsic pathway preceding the participation of Stuart factor, for the prothrombin time is normal.[305] Specific assays for clotting factors participating in the early intrinsic pathway are used to establish that the patient's plasma is deficient in procoagulant AHF, and to quantify the degree of the deficiency.

In milder cases, the clotting time and even the partial thromboplastin time may be normal; the diagnosis is suggested by the deficiency of procoagulant AHF.[241,242,400] Rarely, demonstration that the concentration of AHF-like antigens is disproportionately higher than that of procoagulant AHF, and that the properties of AHF that support ristocetin-induced platelet aggregation and retention of platelets by glass bead filters are normal is necessary for diagnosis. Indeed, in the mildest cases, careful attention to the family history and examination of other family members may be needed to provide reassurance that the diagnosis is classic hemophilia and not von Willebrand's disease.

### 13.10.5. Therapy

The principal means of treatment for episodes of bleeding in patients with classic hemophilia is based on the observations of Feissly[109] and Patek and Stetson[277] that the defect in coagulation can be corrected by transfusion of normal blood or plasma. Indeed, transfusion was successfully used as early as 1840.[203] An earlier vogue for the transfusion of fresh frozen stored plasma has been superceded by the intravenous infusion of concentrates of plasma rich in AHF. In general, two types of preparation are in common use in this country: frozen, stored cryoprecipitated AHF and lyophilized AHF.

AHF is poorly soluble at 0°C.[67,290] Pool et al.[288] froze plasma separated from freshly drawn blood and then allowed it to thaw overnight at 4°C. The insoluble "cryoprecipitate" was then separated by centrifugation and the supernatant plasma was returned to the blood cells for use in nonhemophilic patients. Such cryoprecipitates, containing perhaps 40–75% of the plasma's AHF, are widely used in therapy. Cryoprecipitates have the disadvantage that they must be kept frozen, and cannot readily be transported. A number of lyophilized preparations of AHF have now become available. In general, the AHF of plasma is separated either by addition of neutral amino acids or by cryoprecipitation, and the precipitates are then lyophilized. Since these preparations are separated from large pools of plasma, they carry with them a higher risk of inducing hepatitis than frozen cryoprecipitates, and we have seen a number of instances of this disorder. Nonetheless, lyophilized preparations are popular because they can be administered at locations other than the specialized center, and allow the patient much more mobility. They have made possible home transfusion by the patient or his family, encouraging early transfusion, decreased absenteeism, and decreased dependence on the hospital.[135]

After an initial period during which procoagulant activity may disappear more rapidly,[1,351] probably because it is distributed through extravascular spaces, the half-disappearance time of infused AHF is approximately 10–14 hr[44,64,381]; AHF-like antigens usually[32] disappear more slowly, but exceptions have been described.[215] Thus, maintenance of effective hemostasis requires repeated infusions during the episode of bleeding. A typical regimen for soft tissue bleeding or hematuria consists of an initial infusion of one bag of cryoprecipitate (perhaps 70 units of procoagulant AHF on the average) for every 4 kg of body weight, followed by one bag for every 8 kg every 12 hr until signs of bleeding have abated. The usual hemarthrosis may be treated by a single outpatient infusion of 1½ bags of cryoprecipitate for each 4 kg of body weight, accompanied, in the absence of contraindications, by orally administered prednisone, 80 mg/day for 3 days and 40 mg for 2 days in adults, and proportionately less in children.[199]

The availability of concentrated AHF preparations has made possible many types of surgical procedures, including those designed to restore damaged joint function. In preparation for surgery, one bag of cryoprecipitate for every 2 kg of body weight is infused just before incision, followed by one bag for every 4 kg, 6 and 12 hr after the initial infusion, and then one bag for each 8 kg every 12 hr until wound healing seems well established. A similar regimen is used in individuals who have sustained intracranial bleeding.

Dental extractions should be performed only under the joint supervision of an oral surgeon and a hematologist. In severe hemophilia, we give the patient a single transfusion of one bag of cryoprecipitate for every 4 kg of body weight, followed by oral administration of 4 g of ε-aminocaproic acid (Amicar) every 4 hr for 10 days[388]; proportionately smaller doses of ε-aminocaproic acid are used in children, approximately 1 g/3 kg of body weight a day. In milder cases, we usually omit the infusion of cryoprecipitate.[390]

In addition to the administration of concentrates of AHF, other measures may be useful to control bleeding. Gentle pressure to accessible wounds, possibly combined with the local application of powdered bovine thrombin (Topical Thrombin, Parke, Davis Co.), may provide hemostasis. The affected part should be immobilized and cooled with ice packs. Bleeding from the tongue may be ameliorated by having the patient suck on a Popsicle, providing local cooling.[302]

Perhaps the most important part of the care of patients with hemophilia is nurturing of normal emotional and intellectual development.[3,310] The mother of a hemophiliac is obsessed by guilt, and his father has an often ill-concealed hostility toward his wife, who brought about their son's affliction. As a result, the parents tend to be overprotective, and they should be warned to allow their son as much freedom as is compatible with safety. Further, schooling may be sporadic, and the bleeder may reach adult life unprepared to earn a living. The family should be reminded that, properly encouraged, hemophiliacs have become physicians, lawyers, teachers, and merchants, overcoming their handicap. During adolescence, the bleeder often throws aside his family's protective shield and indulges in risk-taking behavior; my patients have raced sports cars, dropped from parachutes, ridden motorcycles, and participated in demolition derbys in their zeal to display their normality. Careful rearing, with a minimum of restraint, may help to curb these activities.

Aspirin, because it interferes with the hemostatic functions of platelets, must be avoided by patients with any bleeding disorder. They and their families should learn to examine the labels of commercially available analgesic preparations, most of which contain aspirin. Acetaminophen is a useful substitute.

### 13.10.6. Circulating Anticoagulants against AHF in Hemophilia and Nonhemophilic States

A much-to-be feared complication of classic hemophilia is the development of resistance to the beneficial effects of transfusion. This complication, perhaps originally observed by Weil[391] but not understood until the studies of Lawrence,[206] is the result of the appearance of IgG antibodies to AHF, so-called circulating anticoagulants, in the patients' plasmas. These antibodies arise in patients who have previously been transfused, as if the AHF in the infused material were antigenically distinct from that of normal AHF; two exceptional cases in infants who have never been transfused have been reported.[144] The antibodies are usually of the $IgG_4$ subclass[8,328] and neither fix complement nor form precipitates with AHF. In disagreement with earlier data,[347,348] the antibodies appear to be polyclonal in nature.[295]

These anti-AHF antibodies seem to be directed against the procoagulant properties of AHF in the low molecular weight subcomponent that is separated by agarose gel filtration in the presence of high concentrations of salt.[291] They do not inhibit the property of AHF that induces retention of platelets by glass filters[232] and the plasma contains normal or increased amounts of AHF-like antigens detected by rabbit antiserums.[58,160,314,408] This phenomenon is compatible with the observations of Zimmerman[405] that insoluble human antibodies to AHF will dissociate procoagulant AHF from AHF-like antigens detected by heterologous antiserums. Further, Hougie et al.[164] observed that human anti-AHF antibodies did not inhibit the property of plasma supporting ristocetin-induced platelet aggregation. This is not always the case, however, for Thomson et al.[376] have described circulating anticoagulants that appeared to inhibit ristocetin-induced platelet aggregation, one more example of the dissociation between AHF-like antigen and the agent responsible for the ristocetin phenomenon.

Circulating anticoagulants have been detected in about 7–12% of all hemophiliacs,[68,174,188] but in as many as 20% of those with severe hemophilia.[366] Although there is evidence that they are more likely to appear in those individuals repeatedly transfused with AHF, I have seen one infant in whom a circulating anticoagulant against AHF was detected after his first cource of cryoprecipitate therapy. Why some hemophiliacs develop circulating anticoagulants whereas others remain unaffected is unknown. In several families under my care, more than one hemophiliac has developed circulating anticoagulants, a relationship Allain et al.[6] suggests is not due to chance.

In one interesting hemophiliac, abnormalities of platelet function, including a prolonged bleeding time and impaired clot retraction, platelet aggregation by ADP, thrombin, and collagen, and impaired retention of platelets by glass bead columns, coincided with the appearance of a circulating anticoagulant.[74] I am unfamiliar with other similar cases.

Rarely, circulating anticoagulants similar in nature to those observed in classic hemophilia have been detected in the plasma of nonhemophilic patients, both male and female. Such antibodies occasionally appear postpartum, or in association with systemic lupus erythematosus, various chronic cutaneous disorders, or the dysproteinemias.[119,229] In other patients, the circulating anticoagulants seem to develop in relationship to therapy with penicillin,[229] and we have seen one and perhaps two patients in whom a causal relationship to treatment with diphenylhydantoin was suggested.[294] In still other patients, usually middle-aged or elderly, no apparent cause for the development of circulating anticoagulants has been detected.[229] The plasma of patients with acquired circulating anticoagulants is usually devoid of procoagulant AHF, although occasionally a low titer can be detected when the circulating anticoagulant is weak. The patients have symptoms suggestive of severe classic hemophilia, and may die as a result of bleeding.

The treatment of patients with circulating anticoagulants directed against AHF is difficult. Unless the titer of the anticoagulant is very low, the administration of preparations containing human AHF, even in massive doses, is usually futile, and an anamnestic rise in the titer of the circulating anticoagulant usually, but not always, ensues. AHF of animal origin has been used, particularly in Great Britain,[43] but thrombocytopenia may complicate therapy, and antibodies against the heterologous protein soon appear, vitiating further therapy.[325] Porcine AHF is much less susceptible to human circulating anticoagulants than that of bovine origin,[35] and would be the preferred agent were it not for the induction of thrombocytopenia.

Numerous attempts have been made to inhibit the formation of human antibodies against AHF by such agents as corticosteroids, azathiaprine, or cyclophosphamide.[134,212,328] The results reported are unimpressive. More recently, some success in controlling episodes of bleeding has come from the use of preparations of the vitamin-K-dependent clotting factors that contain activated Stuart factor.[202] Presumably, these preparations provide hemostasis by initiating clotting at a point in the intrinsic pathway distal to the participation of AHF. The use of these preparations is, however, potentially dangerous,[311] and should be reserved for life-threatening situations.

Fortunately, in some cases the titer of the circulating anticoagulant gradually diminishes, and when the antibody disappears it may not recur even though hemophiliacs are retreated. In one woman in whom an anticoagulant had appeared postpartum and then disappeared, the anticoagulant did not recur after a subsequent pregnancy[229]; this patient later had evidence of lupus erythematosus.

### 13.10.7. The Heterogeneous Nature of Classic Hemophilia

As might be anticipated, the relatively clear picture of classic hemophilia that I have presented has been fogged by the discovery of a number of variant forms of this disorder. The earliest type of heterogeneity that was recognized was the variation in severity of the clinical picture, a variation paralleled by the titer of procoagulant AHF found in plasma.[126,242] In general, all affected individuals within a family have similar titers of procoagulant AHF,[302] but among families with mild disease some exceptions have been found.[317]

Another form of heterogeneity has been described under the name "Heckathorn's disease." In contrast to most hemophiliacs,[302] the affected individuals in Mr. Heckathorn's family had variable titers of procoagulant AHF from time to time, not in proportion to the severity of symptoms.[317] The disorder was inherited in an X-chromosome-linked manner and, as in the usual case of classic hemophilia, AHF-like antigens and the capacity to support ristocetin-induced platelet aggregation (AHF$_{VWD}$) were normal.

In one notable family, classic hemophilia appeared to be inherited as an autosomal dominant trait.[124] The explanation of this unusual inheritance is not known.

The most intriguing form of heterogeneity is that first described by Hoyer and Breckenridge.[171] In a minority of hemophiliacs, plasma contains antigens that inhibit human antibodies against AHF; that is, they have material in their plasma that cross-reacts with the circulating anticoagulant (CRM+). These antigens are heat labile, like procoagulant AHF,[172] and by inference are localized to the low molecular weight subcomponent of AHF separated by agarose gel filtration in the presence of high concentrations of salt. Such antigens cannot be detected in the vast majority of hemophiliacs, who are therefore CRM−. Presumably, therefore, the antigenic sites reacting with the circulating anticoagulant differ from the site on the low molecular weight subcomponent usually impaired in the disease. Although other investigators have made similar observations,[91,108,160,245] Biggs[42] believes that some antigenic material related to AHF can be demonstrated by appropriate techniques in the plasma of CRM− patients. Despite reports to the contrary, the members of any one family are either all CRM+ or CRM−; that is, the presence of cross-reacting material is an inherited characteristic.

## 13.11. Von Willebrand's Disease

In 1926, von Willebrand[385] described an unusual clotting disorder, affecting both males and females, in a family who lived on the Åland Islands in the Baltic sea. The disorder, which varied in intensity from individual to individual, was inherited as an autosomal dominant trait. The bleeding time was long in affected individuals, whereas the clotting time of whole blood was normal; von Willebrand attributed the disorder to an abnormality in platelet function. What was probably the same syndrome had been observed earlier by Minot.[250] In 1953, three groups of investigators reported that they had studied patients with similar symptoms in whom the bleeding time was prolonged and the titer of procoagulant AHF was abnormally low.[4,205,303] Restudy of the Åland Island patients demonstrated that they, too, had a decreased titer of procoagulant AHF.[187]

Patients with von Willebrand's disease may bleed upon injury or after surgical procedures or dental extractions.[162] In most patients, the bleeding tendency is otherwise mild. I have never observed hemarthrosis, although this has been described.[142] Epistaxis and cutaneous bruising may occur in moderately severely affected individuals. Menorrhagia is commonplace, as is bleeding at, or more often several days after, childbirth, despite a rise in the titer of procoagulant AHF, often to normal levels, in most[368] but not all[401] pregnant patients. Gastrointestinal bleeding may be a troublesome and sometimes lethal problem, although a lesion is seldom demonstrated. In studies of relatives of patients with von Willebrand's disease, one may find individuals who can be identified as affected by laboratory tests, but who may have no clinical bleeding. As a result, in some instances the disorder appears to be inherited as an autosomal recessive trait.[24,355,384]

### 13.11.1. The Nature of von Willebrand's Disease

In contrast to classic hemophilia the concentration of precipitating AHF-like antigens is decreased as much or even more relative to the decreased titer of procoagulant AHF.[217,364,380,408] The bleeding tendency of patients with von Willebrand's disease is often milder than in hemophiliacs in whom the titer of procoagulant AHF is comparable, suggesting that the deficiency of procoagulant AHF is not the sole cause of bleeding. Two striking defects in platelet function have been detected. When normal or hemophilic blood is filtered through columns of glass beads, a high proportion of platelets is retained by the filter (Section 13.7.3). In contrast, retention of platelets by glass bead filters is usually decreased in von Willebrand's disease, in rough parallel to the degree of deficiency of AHF and the prolongation of the bleeding time.[260,335,409] Bouma,[59] Weiss,[399] and Bowie[62] demonstrated that this defect could be corrected by addition of purified AHF or the analogous fraction of hemophilic blood to the blood of patients with von Willebrand's disease. Thus, the abnormality in platelet retention is related to the deficiency of AHF and does not reflect an anomaly of the platelets. In agreement with this, platelet retention is normal in patients with circulating anticoagulants against AHF.[56]

A second defect of platelet function, first described by Howard and Firkin,[165] is impaired aggregation of platelets by ristocetin, an abnormality corrected by addition of purified AHF[398] or its high molecular weight subcomponent.[393] In contrast, aggregation of platelets by ADP, collagen, thrombin, and epinephrine, and release of PF3, the procoagulant activity of platelets, are normal.[389] Although the defect in ristocetin-induced aggregation appears to be related to the deficiency of AHF-like antigens in plasma, there may be poor correlation between the concentration of these proteins and the ability of the plasma of patients with von Willebrand's disease to sustain ristocetin-induced platelet aggregation, as though the antigenic sites on the molecule and the portion of the molecule needed for ristocetin-induced platelet aggregation differed.[216,371]

Still another abnormality in von Willebrand's disease was first studied by Nilsson.[265] When patients with hemophilia are transfused with normal plasma or concentrates containing AHF, the titer of procoagulant AHF rises to the anticipated level and then rapidly decreases with a half-disappearance time of 10–12 hr (Section 13.10.5). In von Willebrand's disease, on the other hand, after the transfusion of material containing AHF, the titer of procoagulant AHF often rises above the anticipated level, reaching a peak in 6–8 hr, and then declines at a much slower rate than in hemophiliacs[265]; exceptions have been observed.[24] The concentration of AHF-like antigens, however, usually decreases rapidly, with a half-disappearance time of about 12 hr[34,105]; these results parallel studies of the transience of the correction of defective platelet function.[62] Exceptionally, the concentration of AHF-like antigens has decreased more slowly[276,381] or risen again coincident with the rise in titer of procoagulant AHF.[196] Perhaps in these cases the concentration of antigenic materials was influenced by the effects of stress on this agent (Section 13.9). Both in our own studies and those of others,[196,259] the procoagulant AHF activity that evolved after transfusion in von Willebrand's disease had the high molecular weight of normal AHF.[34] Bloom, however, reported that clotting activity was associated with a low molecular weight entity,[51] and Muntz and Ekert[105,259] have reported that it lacks the property of supporting ristocetin-induced platelet aggregation (AHF$_{VWD}$).

How AHF brings about the unexpected rise in procoagulant AHF titer is an enigma. The effector of this response is present in hemophilic plasma[84,265] and in normal serum[46]; one explanation is that the stimulus may reside in the noncoagulant portion of the AHF molecule. Whether increased synthesis of AHF occurs, or whether this protein in transferred from extravascular spaces or catabolized abnormally slowly is not known.

The pathogenesis of the prolonged bleeding time in patients with von Willebrand's disease is not clear. The immediate temptation is to ascribe the long bleeding time to the deficiency of AHF in plasma. But there is poor correlation among the bleeding time, the titer of procoagulant AHF, the concentration of AHF-like antigens, and the capacity of plasma to aggregate ristocetin-induced platelet aggregation.[18,216] After the transfusion of material containing AHF, at most only a transient correction of the bleeding time is observed, not parallel with the rise in AHF-like antigens or the agent supporting ristocetin-induced platelet aggregation (AHF$_{VWD}$) or platelet retention by glass bead filters.[46,62,84,371] Moreover, under some conditions of stress, including pregnancy,[88,312,368] or after exercise[46,101] or administration of epinephrine,[323] 1-deamino-8-D-vasopressin[225] or triiodothyronine,[157] the plasma titer of procoagulant AHF may rise to normal levels. Nonetheless, the bleeding time may remain abnormally long even though the concentration of AHF-like antigens and platelet retention by glass bead columns may also become normal; in one case, the AHF-like antigens migrated abnormally upon immunoelectrophoresis.[336] Ristocetin-induced platelet aggregation may also be normal under stress[318]; an exception has been reported.[332]

Since AHF-like antigens are present in normal vascular endothelium,[50,173] it is tempting to ascribe a local function for AHF in hemostasis, a role that is impaired in von Willebrand's disease. In agreement with this view, Holmberg et al.[158] found that the vascular endothelial cells of some, but not all, patients with von Willebrand's disease were deficient in AHF-like antigens. This defect was not corrected by transfusion of cryoprecipitates rich in AHF, perhaps explaining the ineffectiveness of such therapy in shortening the bleeding time in this disorder.[223] In addition, Potter et al.[296] could not find immunologically recognizable AHF-like antigens in the dermal blood vessels of two patients with the disease.

Observations of this nature have led Caen and Sultan[73] to suggest that the basic abnormality in von Willebrand's disease is impaired synthesis by endothelial cells of "von Willebrand's factor," that is, the agent associated with the high molecular weight subcomponent of AHF that supports ristocetin-induced platelet aggregation. Tschopp et al.[378] found that platelets in the whole blood of patients with von Willebrand's disease did not adhere normally to rabbit vascular subendothelial tissue, in agreement with studies in patients in which platelets appeared to adhere poorly to a stab wound[54] and, presumably as a consequence, contained more platelets than normally.

Considerable speculation has generated concerning the fact that heterozygotes for von Willebrand's disease may have very low titers of procoagulant AHF and equally low concentrations of AHF-like antigens. One attractive hypothesis is that the impaired synthesis of the high molecular weight subcomponent of AHF, containing AHF-like antigens, is due to repression by a mutant gene.[382]

### 13.11.2. Diagnosis

The diagnosis of von Willebrand's disease is based on the family history, the prolonged bleeding time, the low titer of procoagulant AHF, the parallel decrease in the concentration of AHF-like antigens, and the impaired aggregation of platelets by ristocetin. Sometimes diagnosis is difficult because of the great variability in the pattern of clinical and laboratory findings among different affected individuals within a single family, or from time to time in the same individual.[85] Tests for decreased retention of platelets by glass bead columns are not generally available and are at best erratic, while the response to transfusion, however helpful diagnostically, should not be measured unless the procedure is needed therapeutically because of the risk of hepatitis. Thus, in any given case, not all of these features may be present; a large number of variants of von Willebrand's disease have been described (Section 13.11.4).

### 13.11.3. Therapy

The treatment of episodes of bleeding in patients with von Willebrand's disease is less than satisfactory. Transfusion of plasma or AHF-rich fractions of plasma has only a transient and often trivial effect upon the prolonged bleeding time, not paralleling either the AHF procoagulant titer or the concentration of AHF-like antigens; cryoprecipitated AHF appears to be more effective than lyophilized AHF preparations.[139, 283,361] Nonetheless, such therapy, provided in a manner similar to that used for treatment of bleeding in hemophilia, may provide hemostasis during surgical procedures in some, but unfortunately not all, patients. Nor does such therapy appear to alter the course of gastrointestinal bleeding, which usually abates only slowly; transfusions of whole blood or packed red blood cells may be needed to prevent hypovolemic shock. In my own limited experience[308] and that of Noller,[267] transfusions are usually not needed during the immediate postpartum period but may be required during subsequent vaginal bleeding in the succeeding days. Fortunately, in most patients with von Willebrand's disease, the bleeding tendency is so mild that transfusion of AHF-containing concentrates may either be unnecessary or required only on the day of surgery, as in one of our patients subjected to mastectomy. Dental extractions do not usually require transfusion; we prescribe 24 g of ε-aminocaproic acid per day for 10 days, in divided doses, in adults, and proportionately less in children. Whether this maneuver is responsible for the benign outcome of this procedure is not certain.

Glueck and Flessa[118] have suggested that the bleeding tendency of women with von Willebrand's disease may ameliorate upon administration of oral contraceptive agents, and others[16,221] report a similar experience, although the mechanisms responsible are disputed.

As in the case of classic hemophilia, the patients should avoid all aspirin-containing products which appear to aggravate the bleeding tendency and to prolong the bleeding time.[301]

### 13.11.4. Variants of von Willebrand's Disease

In its usual form, von Willebrand's disease is inherited as an autosomal dominant trait. In a few reported families, the disorder appears to be the homozygous condition for an autosomal recessive disorder.[370,384] This may be only a semantic distinction, however, for the heterozygotes in such families can be identified in the laboratory, and it is well recognized that the clinical picture presented among affected different members of a given family may be extremely variable. Thus it is not surprising that homozygotes may have serious symptoms whereas their heterozygote relatives may be asymptomatic.

Another form of heterozygosity can be detected in some cases of von Willebrand's disease by examining the pattern of laboratory abnormalities. Thus, patients have been observed in whom the bleeding time is prolonged, the titer of procoagulant AHF is decreased, and adhesion of platelets to glass is impaired, yet the concentration of precipitating AHF-like antigens in plasma is normal.[56,159] In some of these individuals, plasma may not support ristocetin-induced platelet aggregation normally, as though the AHF-like protein were functionally defective.[194,246,280,371] Further, procoagulant AHF and the concentration of AHF-like antigens may be normal, but the plasma does not support ristocetin-induced platelet aggregation; the AHF-like protein in these patients appears to be deficient in carbohydrates.[60,131,279,375] In other individuals, ristocetin-induced platelet aggregation may be normal although procoagulant AHF titers are diminished.[168,200] Sometimes the electrophoretic mobility of the AHF-like protein is abnormal[194,280,371] or the protein may behave aberrantly on gel filtration.[130]

Circulating anticoagulants have been described in patients thought to have von Willebrand's disease. For example, a boy had characteristics of classic hemophilia complicated by the presence of antibodies against procoagulant AHF. But this boy's mother and a sister had long bleeding times, as though the true diagnosis was a variant form of von Willebrand's disease.[218] Rarely, other patients with von Willebrand's disease have had inhibitors of ristocetin-induced platelet aggregation in plasma.[224,338]

Some caution must be exercised in interpreting the significance of these variants, for affected relatives may have laboratory findings typical of von Willebrand's disease.[216] A similar heterogeneity in genetically related swine with von Willebrand-like disease has been observed.[61] These variants do tell us, however, that one cannot equate the AHF-like antigens detected by heterologous antiserum with the site on the AHF molecule that supports ristocetin-induced platelet aggregation (Section 13.5.1).

Cramer et al.[87] recently reported that 9 of 39 patients thought to have von Willebrand's disease had slightly reduced plasma levels of Hageman factor (factor XII). This has not been true in a small group of patients under our care.[333]

## 13.12. Acquired von Willebrand's Disease

Occasionally, a disorder clinically indistinguishable from von Willebrand's disease may become manifest in an individual previously without symptoms of a bleeding tendency and without a family history of this disorder. In such patients the bleeding time has been prolonged, the titer of procoagulant AHF and, when these have been measured, the concentration of precipitating AHF-like antigens have been reduced, and the platelet-supporting functions of plasma attributed to AHF impaired. This strange anomaly has been observed in association with systemic lupus erythematosus,[353] with monoclonal gammopathy,[176,227] or with diffused elevation of the immunoglobulins.[176] In one case, the disorder appeared transiently after ingestion of a pesticide containing lindane, pyrethrium, acetone, and kerosene.[383] In one individual with idiopathic monoclonal gammopathy, a circulating inhibitor was detected that blocked the platelet-aggregating effect of ristocetin and, more weakly, inactivated procoagulant AHF.[146] Similar inhibitors were described in a patient who had lymphosarcoma[143] and another under treatment with chlorpropamide for diabetes mellitus.[362] Anticoagulant activity has not been described in other cases.

## 13.13. Combined Deficiency of Antihemophilic Factor and Proaccelerin

Since the original description by Oeri et al.,[269] coexistent deficiencies of AHF and proaccelerin (factor V) have been described in at least 25 individuals in 18 families. This unusual disorder occurs with about equal frequency in each sex. Analysis of genetic data suggests that this combined defect is inherited as an autosomal recessive trait.[357] Parental consanguinity was present in at least 8 of the 18 families, suggesting the rarity of the abnormal genes. Of many proposed explanations for the existence of this disorder, two seem most attractive. Perhaps a single gene controls synthesis of a precursor common to both AHF and proaccelerin. Alternatively, a single gene may regulate the blood level of these two clotting factors. Neither hypothesis, however, is supported by data.

Whatever the genetic defect in combined deficiencies of AHF and proaccelerin, it seems unrelated to von Willebrand's disease. In several patients, plasma contained normal amounts of antigen related to AHF, the condition observed in classic hemophilia.[117,120,408] The results of transfusion of normal or hemophilic plasma have been inconclusive. In some patients, there was no delayed rise in the titer of procoagulant AHF,[185,343] whereas in others, a rise similar to that seen in von Willebrand's disease was detected.[240,334]

## 13.14. Combined Deficiency of Antihemophilic Factor and Plasma Thromboplastin Antecedent

Several patients have been described in whom mild[12] or severe[340] deficiencies of procoagulant AHF and plasma thromboplastin antecedent (PTA, factor XI) have coexisted. All the reported cases have been in males. In one family the concentration of AHF-like antigens was significantly higher than the titer of procoagulant AHF, the situation typical of classic hemophilia,[12] whereas in another the deficiency of AHF was attributed to von Willebrand's disease.[122] In all likelihood, the combination of AHF and PTA deficiencies is coincidental and does not represent a reflect genetic defect.

## 13.15. Animal Models of Hemophilia and von Willebrand's Disease

Diseases resembling classic hemophilia clinically, in the laboratory, and in their mode of inheritance have been studied in dogs,[69,93,125] horses,[10,268] and cats.[272] The disorder varies in severity among different colonies of affected animals, but is uniform in related animals. As in human hemophilia, the concentration of AHF-like antigens detected by heterologous antiserum is normal despite the deficiency in procoagulant AHF.[94]

Disorders comparable to human von Willebrand's disease have also been described in swine[76,257,258] and dogs.[92] Again, as in human von Willebrand's disease, these diseases are inherited as autosomal dominant traits, although heterozygote swine are usually only detected in the laboratory. The concentration of AHF-like antigens is decreased in parallel to procoagulant AHF,[94] the bleeding time may be prolonged, impaired ristocetin-induced aggregation of *human* platelets and impaired platelet retention by glass bead columns may be detected, and a delayed rise in the titer of procoagulant AHF follows the transfusion of normal plasma or serum.[62,258]

The existence of these unusual animals has allowed genetic and physiologic investigation not appropriate in human subjects, much of which is reviewed in a recent volume.[9]

ACKNOWLEDGMENTS

Otherwise unpublished studies were supported by Grant No. HL 01661 from the National Heart, Lung, and Blood Institute, the National Institutes of Health, United States Public Health Service, and in part by grants from the American Heart Association.

## References

1. Abildgaard, C. F., Cornet, J. A., Fort, E., and Schulman, J., 1964, The *in vivo* longevity of antihaemophilic factor (factor VIII), *Br. J. Haematol.* **10**:225.
2. Addis, T., 1911, The pathogenesis of hereditary haemophilia, *J. Pathol. Bacteriol.* **15**:427.
3. Agle, D. P., 1964, Psychiatric studies of patients with hemophilia and related states, *Arch. Intern. Med.* **114**:76.
4. Alexander, B., and Goldstein, R., 1953, Dual hemostatic defect in pseudo-hemophilia, *J. Clin. Invest.* **32**:551 (Abstract).

5. Allain, J. P., Cooper, H. A., Wagner, R. H., and Brinkhous, K. M., 1975, Platelets fixed with paraformaldehyde: A new reagent for assay of von Willebrand factor and platelet aggregating factor, *J. Lab. Clin. Med.* **85**:318

6. Allain, J. P., Muller, J. Y., and Frommel, D., 1976, Genetic factors governing immune response to factor VIII in hemophilia A, Abstracts, XI Congr. World Federation of Hemophilia, p. 41.

7. Amundsen, M. A., Spittell, J. A., Jr., Thompson, J. H., Jr., and Owen, C. A., Jr., 1963, Hypercoagulability associated with malignant disease and with the postoperative state. Evidence for elevated levels of antihemophilic globulin, *Ann. Intern. Med.* **58**:608.

8. Anderson, B. R., and Terry, W. D., 1968, Gamma G4-globulin antibody causing inhibition of clotting factor VIII, *Nature (London),* **217**:174.

9. Animal Models of Thrombosis and Hemorrhagic Diseases, 1976, U.S. Dept. of Health, Education, and Welfare, DHEW Publication No. (NIH) 76-982.

10. Archer, R. K., and Allen, B. V., 1972, True haemophilia in horses, *Vet. Rec.* **91**:655.

11. Ardlie, N. G., and Reardon, M. F., 1974, Nature of hemophilia and von Willebrand's disease, *Circulation* **50** (Suppl. 3):281.

12. Attock, B., Wilson, E., and Dormandy, K., 1975, Low ratios of factor VIII clotting activity to factor VIII related antigen in a family with combined deficiencies of factors VIII and IX, *Br. J. Haematol.* **30**:132 (Abstract).

13. Austen, D. E. G., 1970, Thiol groups in the blood clotting action of factor VIII, *Br. J. Haematol.* **19**:477.

14. Austen, D. E. G., and Bidwell, E., 1972, Carbohydrate structure in factor VIII, *Thromb. Diath. Haemorth.* **28**:464.

15. Austen, D. E. G., Carey, M., and Howard, M. A., 1975, Dissociation of factor VIII-related antigen into subunits, *Nature (London)* **253**:55.

16. Bachner, V., Etzel, F., Schander, K., and Egli, H., 1975, Diagnostic criteria and long-term therapy of bleeding disorders in von Willebrand's disease, *Thromb. Res.* **6**:119.

17. Baehner, R. L., and Strauss, H. S., 1966, Hemophilia in the first year of life, *N. Engl. J. Med.* **275**:524.

18. Barbui, T., Battista, R., and Dini, E., 1974, Relationship between ristocetin-induced platelet aggregation and factor VIII (activity and antigen) in von Willebrand's disease, *Blut* **29**:260.

19. Barkhan, P., Lai, M., and Stevenson, M., 1963, Antihaemophilic factor (factor VIII): An α-2 globulin, *Br. J. Haematol.* **9**:499.

20. Barrai, I., Cann, H. M., Cavalli-Sforza, L. L., and deNicola, P., 1968, The effect of parental age on rates of mutation for hemophilia and evidence for differing mutation rates for hemophilia A and B, *Am. J. Hum. Gent.* **20**:175.

21. Barrow, E. M., and Graham, J. B., 1968, Kidney antihemophilic factor: Partial purification and some properties, *Biochemistry* **7**:3917.

22. Barrow, E. M., and Graham, J. B., 1971, Antihemophilic factor isolated from kidneys of normal and hemophilic dogs, *Am. J. Physiol.* **220**:1020.

23. Barrow, E. M., and Graham, J. B., 1974, Blood coagulation factor VIII (antihemophilic factor): With comments on von Willebrand's disease and Christmas disease, *Physiol. Rev.* **54**:23.

24. Barrow, E. M., Heindel, C. C., Roberts, H. R., and Graham, J. B., 1965,

Heterozygosity and homozygosity in von Willebrand's disease, *Proc. Soc. Exp. Biol. Med.* **118**:684.

25. Barton, P. G., 1967, Sequence theories of blood coagulation reevaluated with reference to lipid-protein interactions, *Nature (London)* **215**:1508.

26. Baugh, R., Brown, J., Sargeant, R., and Hougie, C., 1974, Separation of human factor VIII activity from the von Willebrand's antigen and ristocetin platelet aggregating activity, *Biochim. Biophys. Acta* **371**:360.

27. Baumgartner, H. R., Stemerman, M. B., and Spaet, T. H., 1971, Adhesion of platelets to subendothelial surface: Distinct from adhesion to collagen, *Experientia* **27**:283.

28. Bendien, W. M., and van Creveld, S., 1935, Investigation on haemophilia, *Acta Brev. Neerl.* **5**:135.

29. Bennett, B., Forman, W. B., and Ratnoff, O. D., 1973, Studies on the nature of antihemophilic factor (factor VIII): Further evidence relating the AHF-like antigens in normal and hemophilic plasmas, *J. Clin. Invest.* **52**:2191.

30. Bennett, B., Oxnard, S. C., Douglas, A. S., and Ratnoff, O. D., 1974, Studies in antihemophilic factor (AHF, factor VIII) during labor in normal women, in patients with premature separation of the placenta, and in a patient with von Willebrand's disease, *J. Lab. Clin. Med.* **84**:851.

31. Bennett, B., and Ratnoff, O. D., 1972, Changes in antihemophilic factor (AHF, factor VIII) procoagulant activity and AHF-like antigen in normal pregnancy, and following exercise and pneumoencephalography, *J. Lab. Clin. Med.* **80**:256.

32. Bennett, B., and Ratnoff, O. D., 1972, Studies on the response of patients with classic hemophilia to transfusion with concentrates of antihemophilic factor. A difference in the half-life of antihemophilic factor as measured by procoagulant and immunologic techniques, *J. Clin. Invest.* **51**:2593.

33. Bennett, B., and Ratnoff, O. D., 1973, Detection of the carrier state for classic hemophilia, *N. Engl. J. Med.* **288**:342.

34. Bennett, B., Ratnoff, O. D., and Levin, J., 1972, Immunologic studies in von Willebrand's disease. Evidence that the antihemophilic factor (AHF) produced after transfusions lacks an antigen associated with normal AHF and the inactive material produced by patients with hemophilia, *J. Clin. Invest.* **51**:2597.

35. Bennett, B., and Ratnoff, W. D., 1973, Immunologic relationships of antihemophilic factor of different species detected by specific human and rabbit antibodies, *Proc. Soc. Exp. Biol. Med.* **143**:701.

36. Bennett, E., and Huehns, E. R., 1970, Immunological differentiation of three types of haemophilia and identification of some female carriers, *Lancet* **2**:956.

37. Benson, R. E., and Dodds, W. J., 1975, Partial characterization of the factor VIII-stimulating material of rabbit liver perfusates: Relationship to rabbit plasma factor VIII, *Br. J. Haematol.* **31**:437.

38. Berglund, G., 1962, Studies of the inhibitory activity of specific antisera to some clotting factors in human plasma, *Br. J. Haematol.* **8**:204.

39. Bergsagel, D. E., and Hougie, C., 1956, Intermediate stages in the formation of blood thromboplastin, *Br. J. Haematol.* **2**:113.

40. Beutler, E., 1962, Biochemical abnormalities associated with hemolytic states,

*in Mechanisms of Anemia* (I. M. Weinstein and E. Beutler, eds.), p. 195, McGraw-Hill, New York.

41. Bidwell, E., 1955, The purification of bovine antihaemophilic globulin, *Br. J. Haematol.* **1**:35.

42. Biggs, R., 1974, The absorption of human factor VIII neutralizing antibody by factor VIII, *Br. J. Haematol.* **26**:259.

43. Biggs, R., 1976, *Human Blood Coagulation, Haemostasis and Thrombosis,* 2nd ed., Blackwell, Oxford.

44. Biggs, R., and Denson, K. W. E., 1963, The fate of prothrombin and factors VII, IX and X transfused to patients deficient in these factors, *Br. J. Haematol.* **9**:532.

45. Biggs, R., Douglas, A. S., and Macfarlane, R. G., 1953, The formation of thromboplastin in human blood, *J. Physiol.* **119**:89.

46. Biggs, R., and Matthews, J. M., 1963, The treatment of haemorrhage in von Willerbrand's disease and the blood level of factor VIII (AHG), *Br. J. Haematol.* **9**:203.

47. Biggs, R., and Rizza, C. R., 1976, The sporadic case of haemophilia A, *Lancet* **2**:431.

48. Bird, P., and Rizza, C. R., 1975, A method for detecting factor-VIII clotting activity associated with factor VIII-related antigen in agarose gels, *Br. J. Haematol.* **31**:5.

49. Blombäck, B., and Blombäck, M., 1956, Purification of human and bovine fibrinogen, *Ark. Kemi* **10**:415.

50. Bloom, A. L., Giddings, J. C., and Wilks, C. J., 1973, Factor VIII on the vascular intima: Possible importance in haemostasis and thrombosis, *Nature New Biol.* **241**:217.

51. Bloom, A. L., Peake, I. R., and Giddings, J. C., 1973, The presence and reactions of high and lower-molecular-weight procoagulant factor VIII in the plasma of patients with von Willebrand's disease after treatment: significance for a structural hypothesis for factor VIII, *Thromb. Res.* **3**:389.

52. Bloom, A. L., Shearn, S. A. M., Peake, I. R., and Giddings, J. C., 1976, The synthesis and differential localization of antigens related to factor VIII in vascular endothelium, Abstract, 16th International Congress on Hematology, p. 325.

53. Bonnet, M., Prost, J., and Favre-Gilly, J., 1964, Complications ophtalomogiques de l'hémophilie, *Hémostase* **4**:297.

54. Borchgrevink, C. F., 1961, Platelet adhesion *in vivo* in patients with bleeding disorders, *Acta Med. Scand.* **170**:231.

55. Bouma, B. N., de Graaf, S., Hordijk-Hos, J. M., van Mourik, J. A., and Sixma, J. J., 1975, Investigations on the relationship of factor VIII related antigen, factor VIII procoagulant activity and von Willebrand factor activity using insolubilized rabbit antiserum, *Thromb. Res* **7**:695.

56. Bouma, B. N., Sixma, J. J., de Graaf, S., Wiegerinck, Y., van Mourik, J. A., and Mochtar, I. A., 1973, Factor-VIII antigen and platelet retention in a glass bead column, *Br. J. Haematol.* **25**:645.

57. Bouma, B. N., van der Klaauw, M. M., Veltkamp, J. J., Starkenburg, A. E., van Tilburg, N. H., and Hermans, J., 1975, Evaluation of the detection ratio of hemophilia carriers, *Thromb. Res.* **7**:339.

58. Bouma, B. N., van Mourik, J. A., Wiegerinck, Y., Sixma, J. J., and Mochtar, I.A., 1973, Immunologic characterization of anti-haemophilic factor A related antigen in haemophilia A, *Scand. J. Haematol.* **11**:184.

59. Bouma, B. N., Wiegerinck, Y., Sixma, J. J., van Mourik, J. A., and Mochtar, I. A., 1972, Immunological characterisation of purified antihaemophilic factor A (factor VIII) which corrects abnormal platelet retention in von Willebrand's disease, *Nature New Biol.* **236**:104.

60. Bowie, E. J. W., Fass, D. N., Olson, J. D., and Owen, C. A., Jr., 1976, The spectrum of von Willebrand's disease revisited, *Mayo Clinic Proc.* **51**:37.

61. Bowie, E. J. W., Fass, D. N., and Owen, C. A., Jr., 1976, Variants of von Willebrand's disease in pigs, Abstract, 16th International Congress on Hematology, p. 331.

62. Bowie, E. J. W., and Owen, C. A., Jr., 1972, Platelet abnormalities in von Willebrand's disease, *Ann. N.Y. Acad. Sci.* **201**:400.

63. Bowie, E. J. W., Owen, C. A., Jr., Thompson, J. H., Jr., and Didisheim, P., 1969, Platelet adhesiveness in von Willebrand's disease, *Am. J. Clin. Pathol.* **52**:69.

64. Bowie, E. J. W., Thompson, J. H., Jr., and Owen, C. A., Jr., 1964, The stability of antihemophilic globulin and labile factor in human blood, *Mayo Clinic Proc.* **39**:144.

65. Breckenridge, R. T., and Ratnoff, O. D., 1962, Studies on the nature of the circulating anticoagulant directed against antihemophilic factor: With notes on an assay for antihemophilic factor, *Blood* **20**:137.

66. Brinkhous, K. M., 1939, A study of the clotting defect in hemophilia: The delayed formation of thrombin, *Am. J. Med. Sci.* **198**:509.

67. Brinkhous, K. M., 1954, Plasma antihemophilic factor. Biological and clinical aspects, *Sang* **25**:738.

68. Brinkhous, K. M., Roberts, H. R., and Weiss, A. E., 1972, Prevalence of inhibitors in hemophilia A and B, *Thromb. Diath. Haemorrh.* (Suppl.) **51**:315.

69. Brock, W. E., Buckner, R. G., Hampton, J. W., Bird, R. M., and Wulz, C. E., 1963, Canine hemophilia, *Arch. Pathol.* **76**:464.

70. Brower, T. B., and Wilde, A. H., 1966, Femoral neuropathy in hemophilia, *J. Bone Joint Surg. (Am.)* **48A**:487.

71. Burke, J. F., and Salzman, E. W., 1959, Spontaneous hemothorax in a hemophiliac, *JAMA* **169**:1623.

72. Caen, J. P., Nurden, A. T., Jeanneau, C., Michel, H., Tobelm, G., Levy-Toledano, S., Sultan, Y., Valensi, F., and Bernard, J., 1976, Bernard–Soulier syndrome: A new platelet glycoprotein abnormality. Its relationship with platelet adhesion to subendothelium and with the factor VIII von Willebrand protein, *J. Lab. Clin. Med.* **87**:586.

73. Caen, J. P., and Sultan, Y., 1975, Von Willebrand disease as an endothelial-cell abnormality, *Lancet* **2**:1129.

74. Call, K. E., Mull, M. M., and Hathaway, W. E., 1969, Platelet function in classic (AHF-deficiency) hemophilia: Report of a case with defective platelet function, *Blood* **33**:26.

75. Carron, D. B., Boon, T. H., and Walker, F. C., 1965, Peptic ulcer in the haemophiliac and its relation to gastrointestinal bleeding, *Lancet* **2**:1036.

76. Chan, J. Y. S., Owen, C. A., Jr., Bowie, E. J. W., Didisheim, P., Thompson, J.

H., Jr., Muhrer, M. E., and Zollman, P. E., 1968, Von Willebrand's disease "stimulating factor" in porcine plasma, *Am. J. Physiol.* **214**:129.

77. Cohen, R. J., Epstein, S. E., Cohen, L. S., and Dennis, L. H., 1968, Alterations of fibrinolysis and blood coagulation induced by exercise, and the role of beta-adrenergie-receptor stimulation, *Lancet* **2**:1264.

78. Cohn, E. J., Strong, L. E., Hughes, W. L., Jr., Mulford, D. J., Ashworth, J. N., Melin, M., and Taylor, F. H. L., 1946, Preparation and properties of serum and plasma proteins. IV. A system for the separation into fractions of the protein and lipoprotein components of biological tissues and fluids, *J. Am. Chem. Soc.* **68**:459.

79. Coller, B. S., Hirschman, R. J., and Gralnick, H. R., 1975, Studies on the factor VIII/von Willebrand factor antigen on human platelets, *Thromb. Res.* **6**:469.

80. Cooper, H. A., Griggs, T. R., and Wagner, R. H., 1973, Factor VIII recombination after dissociation by $CaCl_2$, *Proc. Nat. Acad. Sci. U.S.A.* **70**:2326.

81. Cooper, H. A., Reisner, F. F., Hall, M., and Wagner, R. H., 1975, Effect of thrombin treatment on preparations of factor VIII and the $Ca^{2+}$-dissociated small active fragment, *J. Clin. Invest.* **56**:751.

82. Cooperberg, A. A., and Teitelbaum, J., 1960, The concentration of antihaemophilic globulin (AHG) related to age, *Br. J. Haematol.* **6**:281.

83. Cooperberg, A. A., and Teitelbaum, J. I., 1961, The concentration of antihemophilic globulin (AHG) in patients with coronary artery disease, *Ann. Intern. Med.* **54**:899.

84. Cornu, P., Larrieu, M. J., Caen, J., and Bernard, J., 1960, Données nouvelles concernant la maladie de Willebrand (angiohémophilie), *Rev. Fr. Etud. Clin. Biol.* **6**:614.

85. Cornu, P., Larrieu, M. J., Caen, J., and Bernard, J., 1961, Maladie de Willebrand. Étude clinique, génétique et biologiques (a propos de 22 observations), *Nouv. Rev. Fr. Hematol.* **1**:231

86. Counts, R. B., 1975, Solid-phase immunoradiometric assay of factor-VIII protein, *Br. J. Haematol.* **31**:429.

87. Cramer, A. D., Melaragno, A. J., Phifer, S. J., and Hougie, C., 1976, Von Willebrand disease San Diego; a new variant, *Lancet* **2**12.

88. van Creveld, S., Kloosterman, G. L., Mochtar, I. A., and Koppe, J. G., 1962, Interchange between blood of mother and fetus in vascular hemophilia, *Biol. Neonat.* **4**:379.

89. van Creveld, S., Pascha, C. N., and Veder, H. A., 1961, The separation of AHF from fibrinogen.III, *Thromb. Diath. Haemorrh.* **7**:282.

90. Davie, E. W., and Fujikawa, K., 1975, Basic mechanisms in blood coagulation, *Annu. Rev. Biochem.* **14**:799.

91. Denson, K. W. E., Biggs, R., Haddon, M. E., Borrett, R., and Cobb, K., 1969, Two types of haemophilia (A+ and A−): A study of 48 cases, *Br. J. Haematol.* **17**:163.

92. Dodds, W. J., 1970, Canine von Willebrand's disease, *J. Lab. Clin. Med.* **76**:713.

93. Dodds, W. J., 1974, Hereditary and acquired hemorrhagic disorders in

animals, *in Progress in Hemostasis and Thrombosis Vol. 2* (T. H. Spaet, ed.), p. 215, Grune & Stratton, New York.

94. Dodds, W. J., 1975, Further studies of canine von Willebrand's disease, *Blood* **45**:221.

95. Donaldson, V. H., 1960, Effect of plasmin *in vitro* on clotting factors in plasma, *J. Lab. Clin. Med.* **56**:644.

96. Edson, J. R., and Swinehart, C. D., 1975, Antigenic differences in normal human factor VIII, Abstract, American Society of Hematology, 18th Annual Meeting, p. 162.

97. Egeberg, O., 1962, Blood coagulation in renal failure, *Scand. J. Clin. Lab. Invest.* **14**:163.

98. Egeberg, O., 1962, The effect of unspecific fever induction on the blood clotting system, *Scand. J. Clin. Lab. Invest.* **14**:471.

99. Egeberg, O., 1963, Influence of thyroid function in the blood clotting system, *Scand. J. Clin. Lab. Invest.* **15**:1.

100. Egeberg, O., 1963, The blood coagulability in diabetic patients, *Scand. J. Clin. Lab. Invest.* **15**:533.

101. Egeberg, O., 1963, The effect of muscular exercise on hemostasis in von Willebrand's disease, *Scand. J. Clin. Lab. Invest.* **15**:273.

102. Egeberg, O., 1964, Thyroid function and hemostasis, *Scand. J. Clin. Lab. Invest.* **16**:511.

103. Egeberg, O., and Owren, P. A., 1963, Oral contraceptives and blood coagulability, *Br. Med. J.* **1**:220.

104. Ekberg, M., and Nilsson, I. M., 1975, Factor VIII and glomerulonephritis, *Lancet* **1**:1111.

105. Ekert, H., and Firkin, B. G., 1975, Recent advances in haemophilia and von Willebrand's disease, *Vox Sang.* **28**:409

106. Elston, R. C., Graham, J. B., Miller, C. H., Reisner, H. M., and Bouma, B. N., 1976, Probabilistic classification of hemophilia A carriers by discriminant analysis, *Thromb. Res.* **8**:683.

107. Eyster, M. E., Jones, M. B., Moore, T., and Delli-Bovi, L., 1976, Carrier detection in classic hemophilia by combined measurement of immunologic (VIII AGN) and procoagulant (VIII AHF) activities, *Am. J. Clin. Pathol.* **65**:975.

108. Feinstein, D., Chong, M. N. Y., Kasper, C. K., and Rapaport, S. I., 1969, Hemophilia A: Polymorphism detectable by a factor VIII antibody, *Science* **163**:1071.

109. Feissly, R., 1923, Études sur l'hémophilie, *Bull. Mém. Soc. Med. Hop. Paris* **47**:1778.

110. Firkin, B. G., and Howard, M. A., 1976, On von Willebrand's disease (vWd), *Br. J. Haematol.* **32**:151.

111. Frank, E., and Hartmann, E., 1927, Über das Wesen und die therapeutische Korrektur der hämophilen Gerinnungstörung, *Klin. Wochenschr.* **6**:435.

112. Gaarder, A. M., Jonsen, J., Laland, S., Hellem, A. J., and Owren, P. A., 1961, Adenosine diphosphate in red cells as a factor in the adhesiveness of human blood platelets, *Nature (London)* **192**:531.

113. Gader, A. M. A., Clarkson, A. R., and Cash, J. D., 1973, The plasminogen

activator and coagulation factor VIII responses to adrenaline, noradrenaline, isoprenaline and salbutamol in man, *Thromb. Res.* **2**:9.

114. Gangarosa, E. J., Johnson, T. R., and Ramos, H. S., 1960, Ristocetin-induced thrombocytopenia: Site and mechanism of action, *Arch. Intern. Med.* **105**:83.

115. Gangarosa, E. J., Landerman, N. S., Rosch, P. J., and Herndon, E. G., Jr., 1958, Hematologic complications arising during ristocetin therapy. Relation between dose and toxicity, *N. Engl. J. Med.* **259**:156.

116. Gaynor, E., and Spaet, T. H., 1966, Failure of methylpalmitate induced reticuloendothelial blockade to affect plasma levels of factor VIII, *Blood* **28**:595.

117. Girolami, A., and Bareggi, G., 1974, Normal factor VIII antigen level in combined congenital deficiency of factor V and factor VIII, *Acta Haematol.* **51**:362.

118. Glueck, H. I., and Flessa, H. C., 1972, Control of hemorrhage in von Willebrand's disease and a hemophilic carrier with norethylnodrelmestranol, *Thromb. Res.* **1**:253.

119. Glueck, H., and Hong, R., 1965, A circulating anticoagulant in $\gamma_{1A}$-multiple myeloma: Its modification by penicillin, *J. Clin. Invest.* **44**:1866.

120. Gonzalez, M. F., Fox, K. R., Cimo, P. L., Natelson, E., and Moake, J. L., 1975, Platelet function in heterozygous combined deficiency of factors V and VIII, Abstract, American Society of Hematology, 18th Annual Meeting, p. 163.

121. Gordon, N. R., and Shulman, N. R., 1975, The effect of clotting on structure and function of human factor VIII, *Ann. N.Y. Acad. Sci.* **240**:79.

122. Gordon, S., Hewett, B., Raik, E., and Graham, S. J., 1976, Combined factor XI and factor VIII deficiency in one family, Abstract, 16th International Congress on Hematology, p. 236.

123. Govaerts, P., and Gratia, A., 1931, Contribution á l'étude de l'hémophilie, *Rev. Belge Sci. Med.* **3**:689.

124. Graham, J. B., Barrow, E. S., Roberts, H. R., Webster, W. P., Blatt, P. M., Buchanan, P., Cederbaum, A. I., Allain, J. P., Barrett, D. A., and Gralnick, H. R., 1975, Dominant inheritance of hemophilia A in three generation of women, *Blood* **46**:175.

125. Graham, J. B., Buckwalter, J. A., Hartley, L. J., and Brinkhous, K. M., 1949, Canine hemophilia. Observations on the course, the clotting anomaly, and the effect of blood transfusions, *J. Exp. Med.* **90**:97.

126. Graham, J. B., McLendon, W. W., and Brinkhous, K. M., 1953, Mild hemophilia: An allelic form of the disease, *Am. J. Med. Sci.* **225**:46.

127. Graham, J. B., McLester, W. D., Pons, K., Roberts, H. R., and Barrow, E. M., 1964, Genetics of vascular hemophilia and biosynthesis of the plasma anti-hemophilic factor, *in The Hemophilias* (K. M. Brinkhous, ed.), p. 263, University of North Carolina Press, Chapel Hill.

128. Graham, J. B., Penick, G. O., and Brinkhous, K. M., 1951, Utilization of antihemophilic factor during clotting of canine blood and plasma, *Am. J. Physiol.* **164**:710.

129. Gralnick, H. R., Abrell, E., and Bagley, J., 1971, Immunological studies of factor VIII (antihaemophilic globulin) in haemophilia A, *Nature New Biol.* **230**:16.

130. Gralnick, H. R., Coller, B. S., and Sultan, Y., 1975, Studies on the human factor VIII/von Willebrand factor protein. III. Qualitative defects in von Willebrand's disease, *J. Clin. Invest.* **56**:814.

131. Gralnick, H. R., Coller, B. S., and Sultan, Y., 1976, Carbohydrate deficiency of the factor VIII/von Willebrand factor protein in von Willebrand's disease variants, *Science* **192**:56.

132. Green, A. J., and Ratnoff, O. D., 1974, Elevated antihemophilic factor (AHF, factor VIII) procoagulant activity and AHF-like antigen in alcoholic cirrhosis of the liver, *J. Lab. Clin. Med.* **83**:189.

133. Green, D., 1971, A simple method for the purification of factor VIII (antihemophilic factor) employing snake venom, *J. Lab. Clin. Med.* **77**:153.

134. Green, D., 1971, Suppression of an antibody to factor VIII by a combination of factor VIII and cyclophosphamide, *Blood* **37**:381.

135. Green, D., 1973, *Hemophilia. A Manual of Outpatient Management*, Thomas, Springfield, Illinois.

136. Green, D., 1975, A double-antibody radioimmunoassay for the ristocetin aggregation factor, *Clin. Res.* **23**:274A (Abstract).

137. Green, D., Burns W., and Floyd, M., 1975, On the interaction between ristocetin and the ristocetin aggregation factor ($VIII_{RAF}$), Abstract, American Society of Hematology, p. 163.

138. Green, D., and Potter, E., 1974, Evidence for the presence of the von Willebrand factor on platelets, Abstract, American Society of Hematology, p. 88.

139. Green, D., and Potter, E. V., 1976, Failure of AHF concentrates to control bleeding in von Willebrand's disease, *Am. J. Med.* **60**:357.

140. Gugler, E., and Lüscher, E. F., 1965, Platelet function in congenital afibrino-genemia, *Thromb. Diath. Haemorrh.* **14**:361.

141. Gunn, C. G., and Hampton, J. W., 1967, CNS influence on plasma levels of factor VIII activity, *Am. J. Physiol.* **212**:124.

142. Hagedorn, B., 1971, von Willebrand's disease, *JAMA* **216**:991.

143. Handin, R. I., and Moloney, W. C., 1974, Antibody-induced von Willebrand's disease, Abstract, American Society of Hematology, p. 73.

144. Harmon, M. C., Zipursky, A., and Lahey, M. C., 1957, A study of hemophilia, *Am. J. Dis. Child.* **93**:375.

145. Hartmann, J. R., and Diamond, L. K., 1955, Natural history of 73 patients with hemophilia and related hemorrhagic diseases, *Am. J. Dis. Child.* **90**:594 (Abstract).

146. Hasiba, U., Lewis, J. H., and Spero, J. A., 1975, Circulating inhibitor to von Willebrand's factor, *Clin. Res* **23**:582A.

147. Hathaway, H. S., Lubs, M. L., Kimberling, W. J., and Hathaway, W. E., 1976, Carrier detection in classical hemophilia, *Pediatrics* **57**:251.

148. Hathaway, W. E., Hays, T., Downing, T., Borden, C., and Clarke, S., 1974, Hypercoagulability in childhood malignancies. Relationship of immunologic and biologic assays for factor VIII, *Circul. Res.* **22**:224A.

149. Hawkey, C. M., Anstall, H. B., and Grove-Rasmussen, M., 1962, A study of comparative antihemophilic factor levels in fresh frozen plasma *in vitro* and *in vivo*, *Transfusion* **2**:94.

150. Hellem, A. J., 1960, The adhesiveness of human platelets *in vitro, Scand. J. Clin. Lab. Invest.* **12**(Suppl. 51):1.

151. Hellem, A. J., Ödegaard, A. E., and Skålhegg, B. A., 1963, Investigation of adenosine diphosphate (ADP) induced platelet adhesiveness *in vitro*. Part I. The ADP-platelet reaction in various experimental conditions, *Thromb. Diath. Haemorrh.* **10**:61.

152. Hemker, H. C., Kahn, M. J. P., and Devilee, P. P., 1970, The adsorption of coagulation factors onto phospholipids. Its role in the reaction mechanism of blood coagulation, *Thromb. Diath. Haemorrh.* **24**:214.

153. Hershgold, E. J., 1974, Properties of factor VIII (antihemophilic factor), *in Progress in Hemostasis and Thrombosis*, Vol. 2 (T. H. Spaet, ed.), p. 99, Grune & Stratton, New York.

154. Hershgold, E. J., Davison, A. M., and Janszen, M. E., 1971, Isolation and some chemical properties of human factor VIII (antihemophilic factor), *J. Lab. Clin. Med.* **77**:185.

155. Hershgold, E. J., Silverman, L., Davison, A., and Janszen, M., 1967, Native and purified factor VIII: Molecular and electron microscopical properties and a comparison with hemophilic plasma, *Fed. Proc.* **26**:488 (Abstract).

156. Hershgold, E. J., and Sprawls, S., 1966, Molecular properties of purified human, bovine and porcine antihemophilic globulin (AHG), *Fed. Proc.* **25**:317 (Abstract).

157. Hoak, J. C., Wilson, W. R., Warner, E. D., Theilen, E. O., Fry, G. L., and Benoit, F. L., 1969, Effects of triiodothyronine-induced hypermetabolism on factor VIII and fibrinogen in man, *J. Clin. Invest.* **48**:768.

158. Holmberg, L., Mannucci, P. M., Turesson, I., Rugerri, Z. M., and Nilsson, I. M., 1974, Factor VIII antigen in the vessel walls in von Willebrand's disease and haemophilia A, *Scand. J. Haematol.* **13**:33.

159. Holmberg, L., and Nilsson, I. M., 1972, Genetic variants of von Willebrand's disease, *Br. Med. J.* **3**:317.

160. Holmberg, L., and Nilsson, I. M., 1973, Immunologic studies in haemophilia A, *Scand. J. Haematol.* **10**:12.

161. Holmberg, L., Nilsson, I., and Stolten, C., 1975, Fifteen-year follow-up of potential carriers of hemophilia A and their progeny, *in Haemophilia* (O. N. Ulutin and I. R. Peake, eds.), p. 47, American Elsevier, New York.

162. Horowitz, H. I., and O'Leary, D., 1965, von Willebrand's disease. A critical evaluation of diagnostic criteria, *N.Y. State J. Med.* **65**:2236.

163. Hougie, C., Denson, K. W. E., and Biggs, R., 1967, A study of the reaction product of factor VIII and factor IX by gel filtration, *Thromb. Diath. Haemorrh.* **18**:211.

164. Hougie, C., Sargeant, R. B., Brown, J. E., and Baugh, R. F., 1974, Evidence that factor VIII and the ristocetin aggregating factor (factor VIII$_{Rist}$) are separate molecular entities, *Proc. Soc. Exp. Biol. Med.* **147**:58.

165. Howard, M. A., and Firkin, B. G., 1971, Ristocetin—A new tool in the investigation of platelet aggregation, *Thromb. Diath. Haemorrh.* **26**:362.

166. Howard, M. A., Hutton, R. A., and Hardisty, R. M., 1973, Hereditary giant platelet syndrome. A disorder of a new aspect of platelet function, *Br. Med. J.* **2**:586.

167. Howard, M. A., Montgomery, D. C., and Hardisty, R. M., 1974, Factor-VIII-related antigen in platelets, *Thromb. Res.* **4**:617.

168. Howard, M. A., Sawers, R. J., and Firkin, B. G., 1973, Ristocetin: A means of differentiating von Willebrand's disease into two groups, *Blood* **41**:687.

169. Howie, P. W., Purdie, P. W., Begg, C. B., and Prentice, C. R. M., 1976, Use of coagulation tests to predict the clinical progress of preeclampsia, *Lancet* **2**:323.

170. Hoyer, L. W., 1972, Immunologic studies of antihemophilic factor (AHF, factor VIII). IV. Radioimmunoassay of AHF antigen, *J. Lab. Clin. Med.* **80**:822.

171. Hoyer, L. W., and Breckenridge, R. T., 1968, Immunologic studies of antihemophilic factor (AHF or factor VIII): Cross-reacting material in a genetic variant of hemophilia A, *Blood* **32**:962.

172. Hoyer, L. W., and Breckenridge, R. T., 1970, Immunologic studies of antihemophilic factor (AHF, factor VIII). II. Properties of cross-reacting material, *Blood* **35**:809.

173. Hoyer, L. W., de los Santos, R. P., and Hoyer, J. R., 1973, Antihemophilic factor. Localization in endothelial cells by immunofluorescent microscopy, *J Clin. Invest.* **52**:2737.

174. Ikkala, I., and Simonen, O., 1971, Factor VIII inhibitors and the use of blood products in paients with haemophilia A, *Scand. J. Haematol.* **8**:16.

175. Ingram, G. I. C., 1961, Increase in antihaemophilic globulin activity following infusion of adrenaline, *J. Physiol.* **156**:217.

176. Ingram, G. I. C., Kingston, P. J., Leslie, J., and Bowie, E. J. W., 1971, Four cases of acquired von Willebrand's syndrome, *Br. J. Haematol.* **21**:189.

177. Ingram, G. I. C., and Vaughan Jones, R., 1966, The rise in clotting factor VIII induced in man by adrenaline: Effect of $\alpha$ and $\beta$ blockers, *J. Physiol.* **187**:447.

178. Isacson, S., 1970, Effect of prednisolone on the coagulation and fibrinolytic systems, *Scand. J. Haematol.* **7**:212.

179. Jaffe, E. A., Hoyer, L. W., and Nachman, R. L., 1973, Synthesis of antihemophilic factor antigen by cultured human endothelial cells, *J. Clin. Invest.* **52**:2757.

180. Jaffe, E. A., Hoyer, L. W., and Nachman, R. L., 1974, Synthesis of von Willebrand factor by cultured human endothelial cells, *Proc. Nat. Acad. Sci. U.S.A.* **71**:1906.

181. Jaffe, E. A., and Nachman, R. L., 1975, Subunit structure of factor VIII antigen synthesized by cultured human endothelial cells, *J. Clin. Invest.* **56**:698.

182. Jaffe, E. A., and Nachman, R. L., 1976, Factor VIII binding protein in human platelets, *Clin. Res.* **23**:276A.

183. Jenkins, C. S. P., Phillips, D. R., Clemetson, K. J., Meyer, D., Larrieu, M.-J., and Lüscher, E. F., 1976, Platelet membrane glyoproteins implicated in ristocetin-induced aggregation. Studies of the proteins on platelets from patients with Bernard–Soulier syndrome and von Willebrand's disease, *J. Clin. Invest.* **57**:112.

184. Johnson, A. J., Newman, J., Howell, M. B, and Puszkin, S., 1967, Purification

of antihemophilic factor (AHF) for clinical and experimental use, *Thromb. Diath. Haemorrh.* Suppl. **26**:377.

185. Jones, J. H., Rizza, C. R., Hardisty, R. M., Dormandy, K. M., and Macpherson, I. C., 1962, Combined deficiency of factor V and factor VIII (antihaemophilic globulin). A report of 3 cases, *Br. J. Haematol.* **8**:120.

186. Jorpes, E., and Ramgren, O., 1962, The haemophilia situation in Sweden, *Acta Med. Scand.* **171** (Suppl. 379):23.

187. Jürgens, R., Lehmann, W., Wegelius, O., Eriksson, A. W., and Hiepler, E., 1957, Mitteilung über den Mangel an Antihämophilem Globulin (Faktor VIII) bei der Åländischen Thrombopathie (v. Willebrand-Jürgens), *Thromb. Diath. Haemorrh.* **1**:257.

188. Kasper, C. K., 1973, Incidence and cause of inhibitors amoung patients with classic hemophilia, *Thromb. Diath. Haemorrh.* **30**:263.

189. Kass, L., Ratnoff O. D., and Leon, M. A., 1969, Studies on the purification of antihemophilic factor (factor VIII). I. Precipitation of antihemophilic factor by concanavalin A, *J. Clin. Invest.* **48**:351.

190. Kasten, B. L., Vaitukaitis, J. L., and Gralnick, H. R., 1973, A new factor VIII radioimmunoassay, *Clin. Res.* **21**:558 (Abstract).

191. Kattlove, H. E., and Gomez, M. H., 1975, Studies on the mechanism of ristocetin-induced platelet aggregation, *Blood* **45**:91.

192. Kekwick, R. A., and Walton, P. L., 1965, Studies on the purification and stability of human antihaemophilic factor (factor VIII), *Br. J. Haematol.* **11**:537.

193. Kernoff, P. B. A., 1973, Affinity of factor VIII clotting activity for antigen detected immunologically, *Nature New Biol.* **244**:148.

194. Kernoff, P. B. A., Gruson, R., and Rizza, C. R., 1974, A variant of factor VIII related antigen, *Br. J. Haematol.* **26**:435.

195. Kernoff, P. B. A., and Rizza, C. R., 1973, The specificity of antibodies to factor VIII produced in the rabbit after immunization with human cryoprecipitate, *Thromb. Diath. Haemorrh.* **29**:652.

196. Kernoff, P. B. A., Rizza, C. R., and Kaelin, A. C., 1974, Transfusion and gel filtration studies in von Willebrand's disease, *Br. J. Haematol.* **28**:357.

197. Kerr, C. B., 1962, The elderly haemophiliac, *Australas. Ann. Med.* **11**:158.

198. Kirby, E. P., Martin, N., and Marder, V. J., 1973, Enzymatic degradaton of the antihemophilic factor (factor VIII), *Clin. Res.* **21**:559 (Abstract).

199. Kisker, C. T., and Burke, C., 1970, Double-blind studies on the use of steroids in the treatment of acute hemarthrosis in patients with hemophilia, *N. Engl. J. Med.* **282**:639.

200. Koutts, J., Stott, L., Sawers, R. J., and Firkin, B. G., 1974, Variant patterns in von Willebrand's disease, *Thromb. Res.* **5**:557.

201. Kozinn, P. J., Ritz, N. D., and Horowitz, A. W., 1965, Scalp hemorrhage as an emergency in the newborn, *JAMA* **194**:179.

202. Kurczynski, E. M., and Penner, J. A., 1974, Activated prothrombin concentrate for patients with factor VIII inhibitors, *N. Engl. J. Med.* **291**:164.

203. Lane, S., 1840, Haemorrhagic diathesis. Successful transfusion of blood, *Lancet* **1**:185.

204. Langdell, R. D., Wagner, R. H., and Brinkhous, K. M., 1953, Effect of

antihemophilic factor on one-state clotting tests, a presumptive test for hemophilia and a simple one-state antihemophilic factor assay procedure, *J. Lab. Clin. Med.* **41**:637.

205. Larrieu, M.-J., and Soulier, J. P., 1953, Déficit en facteur antihémophilique A chez une fille associeé à un trouble de saignement, *Rév. Hematol.* **8**:361.

206. Lawrence, J. S., and Johnson, J. B., 1942, The presence of a circulating anticoagulant in a male member of a hemophiliac family, *Trans. Am. Clin. Climatol. Assoc.* **57**:223.

207. Leatherdale, R. A. L., 1960, Respiratory obstruction in haemophilic patients, *Br. Med. J.* **1**:1316.

208. Legaz, M. E., Schmer, G., Counts, R. B., and Davie, E. W., 1973, Isolation and characterization of human factor VIII (antihemophilic factor), *J. Biol. Chem.* **248**:3946.

209. Legaz, M. E., Weinstein, M. J., Heldebrant, C. M., and Davie, E. W., 1975, Isolation, subunit structure, and proteolytic modification of bovine factor VIII, *Ann. N.Y. Acad. Sci.* **240**:43.

210. Legg, J. W., 1881, Report on haemophilia with a note on the hereditary descent of colour-blindness, *St. Bartholomew's Hosp. Rep.* **42**:303.

211. Lewis, J. H., Davidson, C. S., Minot, G. R., Soulier, J. P., Tagnon, H. J., and Taylor, F. H. L., 1946, Chemical, clinical and immunological studies on the products of human plasma fractionation: XXXII. The coagulation defect in hemophilia. An *in vitro* and *in vivo* comparison of normal and hemophilic whole blood, plasma and derived plasma protein fractions, *J. Clin. Invest.* **25**:870.

212. Lewis, J. H., Ferguson, J. H., and Arends, T., 1956, Hemorrhagic disease with circulating inhibitors of blood clotting: Anti-AHF and Anti-PTC in eight cases, *Blood* **11**:846.

213. Lewis, J. H., Soulier, J. P., and Taylor, F. H. L., 1946, Chemical, clinical and immunological studies on the products of human plasma fractionation. XXXIII. The coagulation defect in hemophilia: The effect *in vitro* and *in vivo* on the coagulation time in hemophilia of a prothrombin and fibrinogen-free normal plasma and its derived plasma fractions, *J. Clin. Invest.* **25**:876.

214. Lewis, J. H., Walters, D., Didisheim, P., and Merchant, W. R., 1959, Application of continuous flow electrophoresis to the study of the blood coagulation proteins and the fibrinolytic enzyme system. I. Normal human materials, *J. Clin. Inves.* **37**:1323.

215. Lian, E. C.-Y., 1976, The response to transfusion with factor VIII concentrate in patients with classic hemophilia, Abstract, XI Congress of the World Federation on Hemophilia, p. 54.

216. Lian, E. C.-Y., and Deykin, D., 1976, Diagnosis of von Willebrand's disease. A comparative study of diagnostic tests on nine families with von Willebrand's disease and its differential diagnosis from hemophilia and thrombocytopathy, *Am. J. Med.* **60**:344.

217. Lian, E. C.-Y., and Deykin, D., 1976, *In vivo* dissociation of factor VIII (AHF) activity and factor VIII-related antigen in von Willebrand's disease, *Am. J. Hematol.* **1**:71.

218. Lian, E. C.-Y., Diaz-Ewald, M., Deykin, D., and Harkness, D. R., 1975,

Circulating anticoagulant in a variant of von Willebrand's disease, *Clin. Res.* **23**:487A.

219. Liston, M. R., 1839, Haemorrhagic idiosyncrasy, *Lancet* **2**:137.

220. Lyon, M. F., 1968, Chromosomal and subchromosomal inactivation, *Annu. Rev. Genet.* **2**:31.

221. Mammen, E. F., 1975, von Willebrand's disease-history, diagnosis and management, *Sem. Thromb. Hemost.* **2**:61.

222. Mann, F. D., 1956, Reactivity of hemophilic plasma to platelet thromboplastin, *J. Lab. Clin. Med.* **48**:51.

223. Mannucci, P. M., Holmberg, L., Ruggeri, Z. M., and Nilsson, I. M., 1975, Mechanism of the prolonged bleeding time in von Willebrand's disease (vWd), *Thromb. Diath. Haemorrh.* **34**:607.

224. Mannucci, P. M., Meyer, D., Ciavarella, N., Ruggeri, Z. M., and Lavergne, J. M., 1976, Precipitating antibodies in von Willebrand's disease: Study of three cases, *Br. J. Haematol.* **33**:611.

225. Mannucci, P. M., Pareti, F. I., and Ruggeri, Z. M., 1974, Enhanced factor VIII activity in von Willebrand's disease, *N. Engl. J. Med.* **290**:1259.

226. Mannucci, P. M., Ruggeri, Z. M., and Gagnatelli, G., 1971, Nervous regulation of factor-VIII levels in man, *Br. J. Haematol.* **20**:195.

227. Mant, M. J., Hirsh, J., Gauldie, J., Bienenstock, J., Pineo, G. F., and Luke, K. H., 1973, Von Willebrand's syndrome presenting as an acquired bleeding disorder in association with a monoclonal gammopathy, *Blood* **42**:429.

228. Marchesi, S. L., Shulman, N. R., and Gralnick, H. R., 1972, Studies on the purification and characterization of human factor VIII, *J. Clin. Invest.* **51**:2151.

229. Margolius, A., Jr., Jackson, D. P., and Ratnoff, O. D., 1961, Circulating anticoagulants: A study of 40 cases and a review of the literature, *Medicine* **40**:145.

230. Mason, R. G., and Conway, W. F., 1971, Platelet retention in particle-filled columns: Effect of particle type, plasma proteins, and platelet reactivity, *Am. J. Clin. Pathol.* **55**:49.

231. Maurer, H. M., Valdes, O., Shumway, C. N., and Massie, F. S., 1969, Plasma activity of antihemophilic globulin (AHF) and other coagulation factors in Swiss type of agammaglobulinemia, *Blood* **34**:701.

232. Mazurier, C., Parquet-Gernez, A., and Goudemand, M., 1973, Action des anticorps anti-facteur VIII sur la rétention des plaquettes aux billes de verre, *Path-Biol.* **21** (Suppl. 72):75.

233. McDonald, V. E., Johnson, A. J., and Fields, J., 1976, Rapid, quantitative separation of factor VIII-AHF from factor VIII-vWF in human ACD plasma with solid-phase polyelectrolytes, Abstract, XIth Congress of the World Federation on Hemophilia, p. 22.

234. McGovern, J. J., and Steinberg, A. G., 1958, Antihemophilic factor deficiency in the female, *J. Lab. Clin. Med.* **51**:386.

235. McKee, P. A., 1970, Purification and electrophoretic analysis of human antihemophilic factor (factor VIII), *Fed. Proc.* **29**:647.

236. McKee, P. A., Andersen, J. C., and Switzer, M. C., 1975, Molecular structural studies of human factor VIII, *Ann. N.Y. Acad. Sci.* **240**:8.

237. McPherson, J., and Zucker, M. B., 1976, Platelet retention in glass bead columns: Adhesion to class and subsequent platelet–platelet interactions, *Blood* **47**:55.
238. McPherson, V. J., Zucker, M. B., Friedberg, N. M., and Rifkin, P. L., 1974, Platelet retention in glass bead columns: Further evidence for the importance of ADP, *Blood* **44**:411.
239. Meili, E. O., and Straub, P. W., 1970, Elevation of factor VIII in acute fatal liver necrosis, *Thromb. Diath. Haemorrh.* **24**:161.
240. Ménaché, D., 1968, A new case of combined deficiency of factor V and factor VIII, Abstract, XII Congress of the International Society of Hematology, p. 178.
241. Merskey, C., 1950, The laboratory diagnosis of haemophilia, *J. Clin. Pathol.* **3**:301.
242. Merskey, C., 1951, Haemophilia associated with normal coagulation time, *Br. Med. J.* **1**:906.
243. Merskey, C., 1951, The occurrence of haemophilia in the human female, *Q. J. Med.* **20**:299.
244. Merskey, C., Gordon, H., and Lackner, D., 1958, Diet, blood chemistry, blood coagulation and fibrinolysis in relation to coronary heart disease: An interracial study, *S. Afr. Med. J.* **32**:855.
245. Meyer, D., Dray, L., and Larrieu, M. J., 1970, Hémophilie. Les variants des Facteurs VIII et IX, *Nouv. Rev. Fr. Hematol.* **10**:619.
245a. Meyer, D., Dreyfus, M. D., and Larrieu, M. J., 1973, Willebrand factor: Immunologic and biologic study, *Pathol. Biol.* **21**(Suppl.):66.
246. Meyer, D., Jenkins, C. S. P., Dreyfus, M. D., Fressinaud, E., and Larrieu, M.-J., 1974, Willebrand factor and ristocetin. II. Relationship between Willebrand factor, Willebrand antigen and factor-VIII activity, *Br. J. Haematol.* **28**:579.
247. Meyer, D., Jenkins, C. S. P., Dreyfus, M., and Larrieu, M.-J., 1973, Experimental model for von Willebrand's disease, *Nature (London)* **243**:293.
248. Meyer, D., and Larrieu, M.-J., 1973, Le facteur Willebrand. Biologie et immunologie, *Nouv. Rev. Frç.* **13**:264.
249. Michael, S. E., and Tunnah, G. W., 1963, The purification of factor VIII (antihaemophilic globulin), *Br. J. Haematol.* **9**:236.
250. Minot, G. R., 1928, A familial hemorrhagic condition with prolongation of the bleeding time, *Am. J. Med. Sci.* **175**:301.
251. Moolten, S. E., and Vroman, L., 1949, The adhesiveness of blood platelets in thromboembolism and hemorrhagic disorders. I. Measurement of platelet adhesiveness by the glass-wool filter, *Am. J. Clin. Pathol.* **19**:701.
252. Morgan, T. H., 1929, *The Theory of the Gene*, Hafner, New York (1964 reprint).
253. Morita, H., Kagami, M., Ebata, Y., and Yoshimura, H., 1971, The occurrence of homozygous hemophilia in the female, *Acta Haematol.* **45**:112.
254. Morris, C. D. W., 1968, Observations on the effect of glass beads on platelet aggregation and its relation to platelet stickiness, *Thromb. Diath. Haemorrh.* **20**:345.
255. van Mourik, J. A., Bouma, B. N., LaBruyère, W. T., de Graaf, S., and

Mochtar, I. A., 1974, Factor VIII: A series of homologous oligomers and a complex of two proteins, *Thromb. Res.* **4**:155.

256. van Mourik, J. A., and Mochtar, I. A., 1970, Purification of human antihemophilic factor (factor VIII) by gel chromatography, *Biochim. Biophys. Acta* **221**:677.

257. Muhrer, M. E., Hogan, A. G., and Bogart, R., 1942, A defect in the coagulation mechanism of swine blood, *Am. J. Physiol.* **136**:355.

258. Muhrer, M. E., Lechler, E., Cornell, C. N., and Kirkland, J. L., 1965, Antihemophilic factor levels in bleeder swine following infusions of plasma and serum, *Am. J. Physiol.* **208**:508.

259. Muntz, R. H., Ekert, H., and Helliger, H., 1974, Properties of postinfusion factor VIII in von Willebrand's disease, *Thromb. Res.* **5**:111.

260. Murphy, E. A., and Salzman, E. W., 1972, Platelet adhesiveness in von Willebrand's disease: A cooperative study, *Thromb. Diath. Haemorrh.*, Suppl. **51**:341.

261. Nachman, R. L., and Jaffe, E. A., 1975, Subcellular-platelet factor VIII antigen and von Willebrand factor, *Clin. Res.* **23**:405A.

262. Newman, J., Johnson, A. J., and Harris, R. B., 1976, Estimation of molecular weights of factor VIII AHF and vWF in fresh plasma by ultrafiltration, Abstract, 16th International Congress on Hematology, p. 330.

263. Niemetz, J., Weiland, C., and Soulier, J. P., 1961, Préparation d'une fraction plasmatique humaine riche en facteur VIII (antihémophilique A) et pauvre en fibrinogène, *Nouv. Rev. Fr. Hematol.* **1**:880.

264. Niléhn, J.-E., 1962, On symptomatic antihaemophilic globulin (AHF) deficiency, *Acta Med. Scand.* **171**:491.

265. Nilsson, I. N., Blombäck, M., and Blombäck, B., 1960, The use of human antihaemophilic globulin (faction I-0) in haemophilia A and in von Willebrand's disease, *Acta Haematol.* **24**:116.

266. Nilsson, I. N., Blombäck, M., Thilén, A., and v. Francken, I., 1959, Carriers of hemophilia A. A laboratory study, *Acta Med. Scand.* **165**:357.

267. Noller, K. L., Bowie, E. J. W., Kempers, R. D., and Owen, C. A., Jr., 1973, von Willebrand's disease in pregnancy, *Obstet. Gynecol.* **41**:865.

268. Nossel, H. L., Archer, R. K., and Macfarlane, R. G., 1962, Equine haemophilia: Report of a case and its response to multiple infusions of heterospecific AHG, *Br. J. Haematol.* **8**:335.

269. Oeri, J., Matter, M., Isenschmid, H., Hauser, F., and Koller, F., 1954, Angeborener Mangel an Factor V (parahaemophilie) verbunden mit echter Haemophilie A bei zwei Brudern, *Mod. Probl. Paediatr.* **1**:575, *Ann. Paediatr,* Suppl. 58.

270. Ohno, S., 1969, Evolution of sex chromosomes in mammals, *Annu. Rev. Genet.* **3**:495.

271. Okumura, T., and Jamieson, G. A., 1976, Platelet glycocalicin: A single receptor for platelet aggregation induced by thrombin or ristocetin, *Thromb. Res.* **8**:701.

272. Osbaldiston, G. W., 1974, Hemophilia in the cat, *Bull. Am. Soc. Vet. Clin. Pathol.* **3**:64.

273. Otto, J. C., 1803, An account of an hemorrhagic disposition existing in certain families, *Med. Repository* **6**:1.

274. Owen, C. A., Jr., Bowie, E. J. W., Didisheim, P., and Thompson, J. H., Jr., 1966, Speculations on von Willebrand's disease, *Hemostase* **6**:1.

275. Owen, W. G., and Wagner, R. H., 1972, Antihemophilic factor: Separation of an active fragment following dissociation by salts or detergents, *Thromb. Diath. Haemorrh.* **27**:502.

276. Panicucci, F., Baicchi, U., Sagripanti, A., Pinori, E., and Bruno, V., 1975, Detection of carriers of haemophilia, *in Haemophilia* (O. N. Ulutin and I. R. Peake, eds.), p. 52, American Elsevier, New York.

277. Patek, A. J., Jr., and Stetson, R. J., 1936, Hemophilia. I. The abnormal coagulation of the blood and its relation to the blood platelets, *J. Clin. Invest.* **15**:531.

278. Patek, A. J., Jr., and Taylor, F. H. L., 1937, Hemophilia. II. Some properties of a substance obtained from normal human plasma effective in accelerating the clotting of hemophilic blood, *J. Clin. Invest.* **16**:113.

279. Peake, I. R., and Bloom, A. L., 1976, Normal and abnormal factor VIII-related protein: Differential precipitation by concanavalin A, Abstract, 16th International Congress on Hematology, p. 324.

280. Peake, I. R., Giddings, J. C., and Bloom, A. L., 1974, An abnormality of factor VIII-related protein (FVIIIRP)-possible variants of von Willebrand's disease, *Br. J. Haematol.* **28**:143 (Abstract).

281. Penick, G. D., 1957, Some factors that influence utilization of antihemophilic activity during clotting, *Proc. Soc. Exp. Biol. Med* **96**:277.

282. Penick, G. D., and Brinkhous, K. M., 1956, Relative stability of plasma antihemophilic factor (AHF) under different conditions of storage, *Am. J. Med. Sci.* **232**:434.

283. Perkins, H. A., 1967, Correction of the hemostatic defects in von Willebrand's disease, *Blood* **30**:375.

284. Piper, W., and Schreier, M. H., 1964, Über den immunologischen Nachweis von Faktor VIII-Protein im Bluterplasma und seine Bedeutung für das Verständnis der Häemophilie A, *Thromb. Diath. Haemorrh.* **11**:423.

285. Pitney, W. R., and Elliott, M. H., 1960, Plasma antihaemophilic-factor concentrations in the Australian aborigine and in conditions associated with hypergammaglobulinaemia, *Nature (London)* **185**:397.

286. Pitney, W. R., Kirk, R. L., Arnold, B. J., and Stenhouse, N. S., 1962, Plasma anti-haemophilic factor (factor VIII) concentrations in normal families, *Br. J. Haematol.* **8**:421.

287. Pool, J. H., 1966, Antihemophilic globulin (AHF, factor VIII) activity in spleen, *Fed. Proc.* **25**:317 (Abstract).

288. Pool, J. G., Hershgold, E. J., and Pappenhagen, A. R., 1964, High-potency antihaemophilic factor concentrate prepared from cryoglobulin precipitate, *Nature (London)* **203**:312.

289. Pool, J. G., and Robinson, J., 1959, Assay of plasma antihaemophilic globulin (AHG), *Br. J. Haematol.* **5**:17.

290. Pool, J. G., and Robinson, J., 1959, Observations on plasma banking and transfusion procedures for haemophilic patients using a quantitative assay for antihaemophilic globulin (AHG), *Br. J. Haematol.* **5**:24.

291. Poon, M.-C., Unpublished observations.

292. Poon, M-C., and Ratnoff, O. D., Unpublished observations.

293. Poon, M.-C., and Ratnoff, O. D., 1976, Evidence that functional subunits of antihemophilic factor (factor VIII) are linked by non- covalent bonds, *Blood* **48**:87.

294. Poon, M.-C., Saito, H., Ratnoff, O. D., Forman, W. B., and Wisnieski, J., 1977, Techniques for demonstration of the specificity of circulating anticoagulants against antihemophilic factor (factor VIII), with studies of two cases possibly related to diphenylhydantoin therapy, *Blood* **49**(3):477–482.

295. Poon, M.-C., Wine, A. C., Ratnoff, O. D., and Bernier, G. M., 1975, Heterogeneity of human circulating anticoagulants against antihemophilic factor (factor VIII), *Blood* **46**:409.

296. Potter, E. V., Chediak, J., and Green, D., 1976, Absence of ristocetin aggregation factor from the skin of a patient with von Willebrand's disease, *Lancet* **1**:514.

297. Prentice, C. R. M., Hassanein, A. A., McNicol, G. P., and Douglas, A. S., 1969, Studies on the haemostatic mechanism following exercise, *Br. J. Haematol.* **17**:611.

298. Prentice, C. R. M., Lindsay, R. M., Barr, R. D., Forbes, C. D., Kennedy, A. C., McNicol, G. P., and Douglas, A. S., 1971, Renal complications in haemophilia and Christmas disease, *Q. J. Med. n.s.* **40**:47.

299. Preston, A. E., and Barr, A., 1964, The plasma concentration of factor VIII in the normal population, II. The effects of age, sex and blood group, *Br. J. Haematol.* **10**:238.

300. Quick, A. J., 1953, Hemophilia, *Am. J. Med.* **14**:349.

301. Quick, A. J., 1967, The Minot–von Willebrand syndrome, *Am. J. Med. Sci.* **253**:520.

302. Quick, A. J., and Hussey, C. V., 1952, Hemophilia: Clinical and laboratory observations relative to diagnosis and inheritance, *Am. J. Med. Sci.* **223**:401.

303. Quick, A. J., and Hussey, C. V., 1953, Hemophilic condition in the female, *J. Lab. Clin. Med.* **42**:929.

304. Quick, A. J., Hussey, C. V., and Epstein, E., 1953, Activation of thromboplastinogen by thrombin, *Am. J. Physiol.* **174**:123.

305. Quick, A. J., Stanley-Brown, M., and Bancroft, F. W., 1935, A study of the coagulation defect in hemophilia and in jaundice, *Am. J. Med. Sci.* **190**:501.

306. Rapaport, S. I., Hjort, P. F., and Patch, M. J., 1965, Further evidence that thrombin-activation of factor VIII is an essential step in intrinsic clotting, *Scand. J. Clin. Lab. Invest.* **17** (Suppl. 84):88.

307. Rapaport, S. I., Schiffman, S., Patch, M. J., and Ames, S. B., 1963, The importance of activation of antihemophilic globulin and proaccelerin by traces of thrombin in the generation of intrinsic prothrombinase activity, *Blood* **21**:221.

308. Ratnoff O. D., Unpublished observations.

309. Ratnoff, O. D., 1958, Hereditary defects in clotting mechanisms, *Adv. Intern. Med.* **9**:107.

310. Ratnoff, O. D., 1960, *Bleeding Syndromes*, Charles C. Thomas, Springfield, Illinois.

311. Ratnoff, O. D., 1974, Prothrombin complex preparations: A cautionary note, *Ann. Intern. Med.* **81**:852.

312. Ratnoff, O. D., and Bennett, B., 1973, Clues to the pathogenesis of bleeding in von Willebrand's disease, *N. Engl. J. Med.* **289**:1182.

313. Ratnoff, O. D., Botti, R. E., Breckenridge, R. T., and Littell, A. S., 1964, Some problems in the measurement of antihemophilic activity, *in The Hemophilias* (K. M. Brinkhous, ed.), p. 3, University of North Carolina Press, Chapel Hill.

314. Ratnoff, O. D., and Jones, P. K., 1977, The laboratory diagnosis of the carrier state for classic hemophilia, *Ann. Int. Med.* (in press).

315. Ratnoff, O. D., Jones, P. K., and Steinberg, A. G., Unpublished observations.

316. Ratnoff, O. D., Kass, L., and Lang, P. D., 1969, Studies on the purification of antihemophilic factor (factor VIII). II. Separation of partially purified antihemophilic factor by gel filtration of plasma, *J. Clin. Invest.* **48**:957.

317. Ratnoff, O. D., and Lewis, J. H., 1975, Heckathorn's disease: Variable functional deficiency of antihemophilic factor (factor VIII), *Blood* **46**:161.

318. Ratnoff, O. D., and Saito, H., 1974, Bleeding in von Willebrand's disease, *N. Engl. J. Med.* **290**:1089 (Letter).

319. Ratnoff, O. D., Slover, C. C., and Poon, M.-C., 1976, Immunologic evidence that the properties of human antihemophilic factor (factor VIII) are attributes of a single molecular species, *Blood* **47**:657.

320. Rick, M. E., and Hoyer, L. W., 1973, Immunologic studies of antihemophilic factor (AHF, factor VIII). V. Immunologic properties of AHF subunits produced by salt dissociation, *Blood* **42**:737.

321. Rick, M. E., and Hoyer, L. W., 1974, Activation of low molecular weight fragment of antihaemophilic factor (factor VIII by thrombin, *Nature (London)* **252**:404.

322. Rick, M. E., and Hoyer, L. W., 1975, Molecular weight of human factor VIII procoagulant activity, *Thromb. Res.* **7**:909.

323. Rickles, F. R., Hoyer, L. W., Rick, M. E., and Ahr. D. J., 1976, The effect of epinephrine infusion in patients with von Willebrand's disease, *J. Clin. Invest.* **57**:1618.

324. Rizza, C. R., 1961, The effect of exercise on the level of antihemophilic globulin in human blood, *J. Physiol.* **156**:128.

325. Rizza, C. R., 1972, The management of patients with coagulation factor deficiencies, *in Human Blood Coagulation, Haemostasis and Thrombosis,* 2nd ed. (R. Biggs, ed.), p. 365, Blackwell, Oxford.

326. Rizza, C. R., and Eipe, J., 1971, Exercise, factor VIII and the spleen, *Br. J. Haematol.* **20**:629.

327. Rizza, C. R., and Walker, W., 1957, Inactivation of antihaemophilic globulin by thrombin, *Nature (London)* **180**:143.

328. Robboy, S. J., Lewis, E. J., Schur, P. H., and Colman, R. W., 1970, Circulating anticoagulants to factor VIII, Immunochemical studies and clinical response to factor VIII concentrates, *Am. J. Med.* **49**:742.

329. Romansky, M. J., Limson, B. M., and Hawkins, J. E., 1956–1957, Ristocetin. New antibiotic, laboratory and clinical studies: Preliminary report, *Antibiot. Ann.* 706.

330. Rosental, R. L., and Sloan, E., 1967, Elevated factor VIII (AHG) activity in acute leukemia. *Fed. Proc.* **26**:487 (Abstract).

331. Rosner, F., 1969, Hemophilia in the Talmud and Rabbinic writings, *Ann. Intern. Med.* **70**:833.

332. Royen, E. A. van, Flier, O. T. N., and ten Cate, J. W., 1974, Von Willebrand-factor activity in pregnancy, *Lancet* **2**:657 (Letter).

333. Saito, H., Ratnoff, O. D., and Pensky, J., 1976, Radioimmunoassay of human Hageman factor (factor XII), *J. Lab. Clin. Med.* **88**:506.

334. Saito, H., Shioya, M., Koie, K. Kamiya, T., and Katsumi, O., 1969, Congenital combined deficiency of factor V and factor VIII: A case report and the effect of transfusion of normal plasma and hemophilic blood, *Thromb. Diath. Haemorrh.* **22**:316.

335. Salzman, E. W., 1963, Measurement of platelet adhesiveness: A simple *in vitro* technique demonstrating an abnormality in von Willebrand's disease, *J. Lab. Clin. Med.* **62**:724.

336. Samama, M., Lecrubier, C., Conard, J., and Cazenave, B., 1976, Abnormal factor-VIII-related antigen, von Willebrand's disease, and pregnancy, *Lancet* **1**:151.

337. Sarji, K. E., Graves, J. M., and Colwell, J. A., 1975, Von Willebrand factor activity in normal subjects: Sex difference and variability, *Thromb. Res.* **7**:885.

338. Sarji, K. E., Stratton, R. D., Wagner, R. H., and Brinkhous, K. M., 1974, Nature of von Willebrand factor: A new assay and a specific inhibitor, *Proc. Nat. Acad. Sci. U.S.A.* **71**:2937.

339. Schiffman, S., Rapaport, S. I., and Chong, M. M. Y., 1966, The mandatory role of lipid in the interaction of factors VIII and IX, *Proc. Soc. Exp. Biol. Med.* **123**:736.

340. Schulz, K., Nowotny, P., Schmutzler, R., and Duckert, F., 1964, Kombinierter AHG- und PTA-Mangel, *Thromb. Diath. Haemorrh.* **10**:282.

341. Seeler, R. A., and Imana, R. B., 1973, Intracranial hemorrhage in patients with hemophilia, *J. Neurosurg.* **39**:181.

342. Seibert, R. H., Margolius, A., Jr., and Ratnoff, O. D., 1958, Observations on hemophilia, parahemophilia and coexistent hemophilia and parahemophilia, *J. Lab. Clin. Med.* **52**:449.

343. Seligsohn, U., and Ramot, B., 1969, Combined factor-V and factor-VIII deficiency: Report of 4 cases, *Br. J. Haematol.* **16**:475.

344. Shanberge, J. N., and Gore, I., 1957, Studies on the immunologic and physiologic activities of antihemophilic factor (AHF), *J. Lab. Clin. Med.* **50**:954 (Abstract).

345. Shapiro, G. A., Anderson, J. C., Pizzo, S. V., and McKee, P. A., 1973, The subunit structure of normal and hemophilic factor VIII, *J. Clin. Invest.* **52**:2198.

346. Shapiro, G. A., and McKee, P. A., 1970, Demonstration of a non-functional antihemophilic factor (factor VII) in classic hemophilia, *Clin. Res.* **18**:615 (Abstract).

347. Shapiro, S. S., and Carroll, K. S., 1968, Acquired factor VIII antibodies: Further immunologic and electrophoretic studies, *Science* **160**:786.

348. Shapiro, S. S., and Hultin, M., 1975, Acquired inhibitors to the blood coagulation factors, *Sem. Thromb. Haemos.* **1**:336.

349. Shearn, S. A. M., Giddings, J. C., Peake, I. R., and Bloom, A. L., 1974, A comparison of five different rabbit antisera to factor VIII and the demon-

stration of a factor VIII related antigen in normal and von Willebrand's disease platelets, *Thromb. Res.* **5**:585.

350. Shearn, S. A. M., Tuddenham, E. G. D., Peake, I. R., Giddings, J. C., and Bloom, A. L., 1976, Factor VIII related protein synthesized by endothelial cells, *Br. J. Haematol.* **33**:147 (Abstract).

351. Shulman, N. R., Cowan, D. H., Libre, E. P., Watkins, S. P., Jr., and Marder, V. J., 1967, The physiologic basis for therapy of classic hemophilia (factor VIII deficiency) and related disorders, *Ann. Intern. Med.* **67**:856.

352. Simone, J. V., Abildgaard, C. F., and Schulman, I., 1965, Blood coagulation in thyroid dysfunction, *N. Engl. J. Med.* **273**:1057.

353. Simone, J. V., Cornet, J. A., and Abildgaard, C. F., 1968, Acquired von Willebrand's syndrome in systemic lupus erythematosus, *Blood* **31**:806.

354. Simonetti, C., Casillas, G., and Pavlovsky, A., 1961, Purification du facteur VIII antihémophilique (FAH), *Hémostase* **1**:57.

355. Singer, K., and Ramot, B., 1956, Pseudohemophilia type B, *Arch. Intern. Med.* **97**:715.

356. Sise, H. S., Gautheir, J., Becker, R., and Bolger, J., 1961, Blood coagulation factors in total body irradiation, *Blood* **18**:702.

357. Smit Sibinga, C. T., Gökemeyer, V. D. M., ten Kate, L. P., and Bos-van Zwol, F., 1972, Combined deficiency of factor V and factor VIII. Report of a family and genetic analysis, *Br. J. Haematol.* **23**:467.

358. Soulier, J. P., 1959, Un nouvel adsorbant des facteurs de coagulation: la bentonite, *Rev. Hematol.* **14**:26.

359. Spaet, T. H., 1955, Recent progress in the study of hemophilia, *Stanford Med. Bull.* **13**:24.

360. Spaet, T. H., and Garner, E. S., 1955, Studies on the storage lability of human antihemophilic factor, *J. Lab. Clin. Med.* **46**:111.

361. Spurling, C. L., and Sacks, M. S., 1959, Inherited hemorrhagic disorder with antihemophilic globulin deficiency and prolonged bleeding time (vascualr hemophilia), *N. Engl. J. Med.* **261**:311.

362. Stableforth, P., Tamagnini, G. L., and Dormandy, K. M., 1976, Acquired von Willebrand syndrome with inhibitors both to factor VIII clotting activity and ristocetin-induced platelet aggregation, *Br. J. Haematol.* **33**:565.

362a. Stanbury, J. B., Wyngaarden, J. B., and Frederickson, D. S., 1977, *The Metabolic Basis of Inherited Disease*, 4th ed., McGraw-Hill, New York, in press.

363. Steel, M. M., Duthie, R. B., and O'Connor, B. T., 1969, Haemophilic cysts: Report of five cases, *J. Bone Joint Surg.* **51B**:614.

364. Stites, D. P., Hershgold, E. J., Perlman, J. D., and Fudenberg, H. H., 1971, Factor VIII detection by hemagglutination inhibition. Hemophilia A and von Willebrand's disease, *Science* **171**:196.

365. Strauss, H. S., 1967, The perpetuation of hemophilia by mutation, *Pediatrics* **39**:186.

366. Strauss, H. S., 1969, Acquired circulating anticoagulants in hemophilia A, *N. Engl. J. Med.* **281**:866.

367. Strauss, H. S., and Bloom, G. E., 1965, von Willebrand's disease. Use of a platelet-adhesiveness test in diagnosis and family investigation, *N. Engl. J. Med.* **273**:171.

368. Strauss, H. S., and Diamond, L. K., 1963, Elevation of factor VIII (antihe-

mophilic factor) during pregnancy in normal persons and in a patient with von Willebrand's disease, *N. Engl. J. Med.* **269**:1251.

369. Sultan, Y., and Siméon, J., 1974, L'électro-immunodiffusion double dimensionnelle. Moyen d'étude de la protéin plasmatique liée à l'activité coagulante du facteur VIII et à l'activité Willebrand, *Nouv. Rev. Fr. Hematol.* **14**:786.

370. Sultan, Y., Simeon, J., and Caen, J. P., 1975, Detection of heterozygotes in both parents of homozygous patients with von Willebrand's disease, *J. Clin. Pathol.* **28**:309.

371. Sultan, Y. Simeon, J., and Caen, J. P., 1976, Electrophoretic heterogeneity of normal factor VIII/von Willebrand protein, and abnormal electrophoretic mobility in patients with von Willebrand's disease, *J. Lab. Clin. Med.* **87**:185.

372. Switzer, M. E., and McKee, P. A., 1976, Studies on human antihemophilic factor. Evidence for a covalently linked subunit structure, *J. Clin. Invest.* **57**:925.

373. Thelin, G. M., 1968, Preparation and standardization of a stable AHF plasma, *Thromb. Diath. Haemorrh.* **19**:423.

374. Thelin, G. M., and Wagner, R. H., 1961, Sedimentation of plasma antihemophilic factor, *Arch. Biochem.* **95**:70.

375. Thomson, C., Forbes, C. D., and Prentice, C. R. M., 1974, Evidence for a qualitative defect in factor VIII-related antigen in von Willebrand's disease, *Lancet* **1**:594.

376. Thomson, C., Forbes, C. D., and Prentice, C. R. M., 1973, Relationship of factor VIII to ristocetin-induced platelet aggregation: Effect of heterologous and acquired factor VIII antibodies, *Thromb. Res.* **3**:363.

377. Tocantins, L. M., 1943, Demonstration of antithromboplastic activity in normal and hemophilic plasma, *Am. J. Physiol.* **139**:265.

378. Tschopp, T. B., Weiss, H. J., and Baumgartner, H. R., 1974, Decreased adhesion of platelets to subendothelium in von Willebrand's disease, *J. Lab. Clin. Med.* **83**:296.

379. Tuddenham, E. G. D., Shearn, S. A. M., Peake, I. R., Giddings, J. C., and Bloom, A. L., 1974, Factor-VIII-related antigen in the human foetus and its synthesis in tissue culture, *Br. J. Haematol.* **28**:143.

380. Uszyński, L., 1966, The immunological properties of factor VIII. I. Studies on the inhibitory activity of specific antisera to human antihemophilic globulin, *Thromb. Diath. Haemorrh.* **16**:559.

381. Uszyński, L., 1975, Biological half-life of factor VIII antigen and of antihemophilic globulin activity in hemophilia A and in von Willebrand's disease, *Acta Haematol. Pol.* **5**:189, quoted in *Blood* **46**:153.

382. Veltkamp, J. J., 1973, Factor VIII, *Lancet* **2**:803 (Letter).

383. Veltkamp, J. J., Stevens, P., Plass, M. V. D., and Loeliger, E. A., 1970, Production site of bleeding factor (acquired morbus von Willebrand), *Thromb. Diath. Haemorrh.* **23**:412.

384. Veltkamp, J. J., and van Tilburg, N. H., 1973, Detection of heterozygotes for recessive von Willebrand's disease by the assay of antihemophilic factor-like-antigen, *N. Engl. J. Med.* **289**:882.

385. von Willebrand, E. A., 1931, Über hereditare pseudohämophilie, *Acta Med. Scand.* **76**:521.

386. Wagner, R. H., McLester, W. D., Smith, M., and Brinkhous, K. M., 1964, Purification of antihemophilic factor (factor VIII) by amino acid precipitation, *Thromb. Diath. Haemorrh.* **11**:64.

387. Wagner, R. H., Pate, D., and Brinkhous, K. M., 1954, Further purification of antihemophilic factor (AHF) from dog plasma, *Fed. Proc.* **13**:445 (Abstract).

388. Walsh, P. N., Rizza, C. R., Matthews, J. M., Eipe, J., Kernoff, P. B. A., Coles, M. D., Bloom, A. L., Kaufman, B. N., Beck, P., Hanan, C. M., and Biggs, R., 1971, ε-Aminocaproic acid therapy for dental extractions in haemophilia and Christmas disease: A double blind controlled trial, *Br. J. Haematol.* **20**:463.

389. Walsh, R. T., 1975, The platelet in von Willebrand's disease: Interactions with ristocetin and factor VIII, *Sem. Thromb. Haemos.* **2**:105.

390. Webster, W. P., Roberts, H. R., and Penick, G. D., 1968, Dental care of patients with hereditary disorders of blood coagulation, in *Treatment of Hemorrhagic Disorders* (O. D. Ratnoff, ed.), p. 93, Harper & Row, New York.

391. Weil, P. E., 1906, Etude du sang chez les hémophiles, *Bull. Mem. Soc. Med. Hop. Paris* **23**:1001.

392. Weinstein, M. J., Deykin, D., and Davie, E. W., 1976, Quantitative determination of factor-VIII protein by two-stage gel electrophoresis, *Br. J. Haematol.* **33**:343.

393. Weiss, H. J., and Hoyer, L. W., 1973, von Willebrand's factor: Dissociation from antihemophilic factor procoagulant activity, *Science* **182**:1149.

394. Weiss, H. J., Hoyer, L. W., Rickles, F. R., Varma, A., and Rogers, J., 1973, Quantitative assay of a plasma factor, deficient in von Willebrand's disease, that is necessary for platelet aggregation—Relationship to factor VIII procoagulant activity and antigen content, *J. Clin. Invest.* **52**:2708.

395. Weiss, H. J., and Kochwa, S., 1968, Antihaemophilic globulin (AHG) in multiple myeloma and macroglobulinaemia, *Br. J. Haematol.* **14**:205.

396. Weiss, H. J., and Kochwa, S., 1970, Molecular forms of antihaemophilic globulin in plasma cryoprecipitate and after thrombin activation, *Br. J. Haematol.* **18**:89.

397. Weiss, H. J., Phillips, L. L., and Rosner, W., 1972, Separation of subunits of antihemophilic factor (AHF) by agarose gel chromatography, *Thromb. Diath. Haemorrh.* **27**:212.

398. Weiss, H. J., Rogers, J., and Brand, H., 1973, Defective ristocetin-induced platelet aggregation in von Willebrand's disease and its correction by factor VIII, *J. Clin. Invest.* **52**:2697.

399. Weiss, H. J., Rogers, J., and Brand, H., 1973, Properties of the platelet retention (von Willebrand) factor and its similarity to the antihemophilic factor (AHF), *Blood* **41**:809.

400. Wilkinson, J. F., Nour-Eldin, F., Israëls, M. C. G., and Barrett, K. E. B., 1961, Haemophilia syndromes. A survey of 267 patients, *Lancet* **2**:947.

401. Winckelman, G., Groh, R. Schneider, J., and Huber, P., 1967, Pregnancy and childbirth in von Willebrand's disease, *Germ. Med. Monthly* **120**:208.

402. Wright, A. E., 1893, On the method of determining the condition of blood coagulability for clinical and experimental purposes, and on the effect of the

administration of calcium salts in haemophilia and actual or threatened haemorrhage, *Br. Med. J.* **2**:223.

403. Wright, H. P., 1941, The adhesiveness of blood platelets in normal subjects with varying concentrations of anti-coagulants, *J. Pathol. Bacteriol.* **53**:255.

404. Zacharski, L. R., Bowie, E. J. W., Titus, J. L., and Owen, C. A., Jr., 1968, Synthesis of antihemophilic factor (factor VIII) by leukocytes: Preliminary report, *Mayo Clinic Proc.* **43**:617.

405. Zimmerman, T. S., and Edgington, T. S., 1973, Factor VIII coagulant activity and factor VIII-like antigen: Independent molecular entities, *J. Exp. Med.* **138**:1015.

406. Zimmerman, T. S., Edgington, T. S., Foroozan, P., and Roberts, J., 1975, The von Willebrand's disease antigen: Heterogeneity in plasma, *Clin. Res.* **23**:408A.

407. Zimmerman, T. S., Ratnoff, O. D., and Littell, A. S., 1971, Detection of carriers of classic hemophilia using an immunologic assay for antihemophilic factor (factor VIII), *J. Clin. Invest.* **50**:255.

408. Zimmerman, T. S., Ratnoff, O. D., and Powell, A. E., 1971, Immunologic differentiation of classic hemophilia (factor VIII deficiency) and von Willebrand's disease, with observations on combined deficiencies of antihemophilic factor and proaccelerin (factor V) and on an acquired circulating anticoagulant against antihemophilic factor, *J. Clin. Invest.* **50**:244.

409. Zucker, M. B., 1963, *In vitro* abnormality of the blood in von Willebrand's disease correctable by normal plasma, *Nature (London)* **197**:601.

# 14

# Research on the Biochemical Basis of Platelet Function

## Thomas C. Detwiler and Israel F. Charo

## 14.1. Introduction

Within the past few years there has been a great increase in platelet research by scientists with diverse interests. This is in part because of the relevance of platelet research to major health problems, but also because platelets have proved to be excellent subjects for research into many fundamental cell processes (e.g., contractility, secretion, prostaglandin synthesis, cell adhesion, and cytoplasmic regulatory mechanisms). In this chapter, we briefly summarize the current concepts of platelet function and evaluate the status of research into the biochemical basis of key platelet processes. Our emphasis is on topics that we believe represent the most active areas of platelet research at the molecular level. Reference citations are not complete, but have been selected to validate major points and to refer the reader to more detailed discussions. We regret that space does not permit us to acknowledge many of the key papers that have played such vital parts in developing our understanding of platelets.

THOMAS C. DETWILER and ISRAEL F. CHARO • Department of Biochemistry, State University of New York Downstate Medical Center, Brooklyn, New York 11203.

## 14.2. Current Concepts of Platelet Function

There are certain ideas that form a necessary base for any discussion of platelet function. We have briefly summarized these concepts without the critical evaluation that they deserve; they are developed in more detail in recent reviews (Marcus, 1969; Mustard and Packham, 1970; Smith and Macfarlane, 1974; Weiss, 1976). Because of the complexity of intact cells, even these basic conclusions should be accepted with reservations.

### 14.2.1. The Physiological Role of Platelets

Platelets are the agents of primary hemostasis. At the site of a vessel injury, platelets adhere to the damaged surface (adhesion) and to each other (aggregation), and then the aggregate contracts, forming a "hemostatic plug." This process largely precedes coagulation, although the activated platelets greatly accelerate coagulation and thrombin may be required for the final stage, contraction of the aggregate. Bleeding time (time to stop bleeding from severed capillaries) is the *in vivo* test of this role. The other side of the coin of the primary hemostatic mechanism is thrombosis, occlusion of a vessel by aggregated platelets, usually initiated at the site of some lesion. A related physiological role of platelets is the formation of a protective covering in areas of the vasculature where endothelial cells have been removed, allowing migration of new endothelial cells under the platelets until the lesion is healed.

There is currently much interest in the possibility that platelets are involved in vascular disease not only in the acute, thrombotic stage but also in the initial stages of atherosclerosis. Platelet factors that enhance growth of cultured smooth muscle and fibroblast cells have been reported (Ross *et al.*, 1974; Rutherford and Ross, 1976) and it is suggested that when platelets attach to regions freed of endothelial cells, they release a growth factor that causes smooth muscle cells to proliferate, thickening the vascular wall, an early step in atherosclerosis.

### 14.2.2. Platelet Morphology

A discussion of molecular biology should not be separated from considerations of morphology. This brief description of platelet morphology is taken primarily from a detailed description by White (1971).

Human platelets are anucleate, discoid cells about 2 $\mu$m in diameter. The major ultrastructural features essential to this discussion are shown schematically in Fig. 1 and are described in the legend. The essence of platelet function is the response to stimuli. Morphologically, the response includes a shape change from disk to sphere with long pseudopods and a

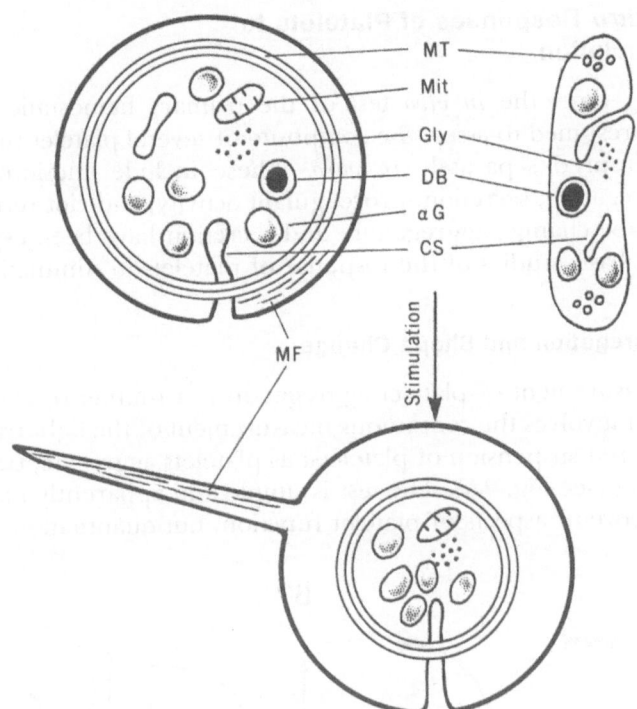

**Fig. 1.** Schematic representation of some ultrastructural features of platelets. The upper diagrams show two different sections of the typical discoid resting platelet. Although not obvious in thin sections, the many vacuoles observed in platelets are believed to be continuous with the outside by open canals, the canalicular system (CS), which makes platelets spongelike, with a much larger surface area than expected for their size. Platelets contain three major types of granules: (a) α granules (αG), which are lysosomelike and are characterized by a dense region, the nucleoid; (b) dense bodies (DB), which are characterized by electron opacity prior to staining and are believed to be the secretory granules; and (c) mitochondria (Mit). Microtubules (MT) form a prominent circumferential ring and microfilaments (MF) have been reported in the region between the membrane and microtubules. Glycogen particles (Gly) are another striking feature. The *lower diagram* represents a platelet several seconds after stimulation (e.g., by thrombin). The platelet is more spherical, but with many pseudopods. The pseudopods do not appear this long in thin sections, but scanning electron microscope studies suggest that they are actually much longer and thinner than depicted in this diagram. The pseudopods contain many microfilaments.

concomitant shrinkage of the ring of microtubules, with granules retained within the ring. This takes place within a few seconds of stimulation and is followed quickly by disappearance of dense bodies, the apparent secretory granules. The stimulated platelets aggregate, and within several minutes the aggregate becomes degranulated and contracts, forming a tight mass without clear delineation between platelets.

### 14.2.3. *In Vitro* Responses of Platelets to Stimulation

Bleeding time, the *in vivo* test of the primary hemostatic role of platelets, is presumed to assess the composite of several platelet functions that are measured separately *in vitro*. These include ahesion, shape change, aggregation, secretion, procoagulant activity, and clot retraction. Of these, shape change, aggregation, and secretion have been especially important in basic studies of the response of platelets to stimulation.

### 14.2.3.1. Aggregation and Shape Change

The measurement of platelet aggregation is a routine research and clinical test. It involves the continuous measurement of the light transmittance of a stirred suspension of platelets; as platelets aggregate, transmittance increases (see Fig. 2A). The test is simple and apparently measures the most important aspects of platelet function, but quantitation is diffi-

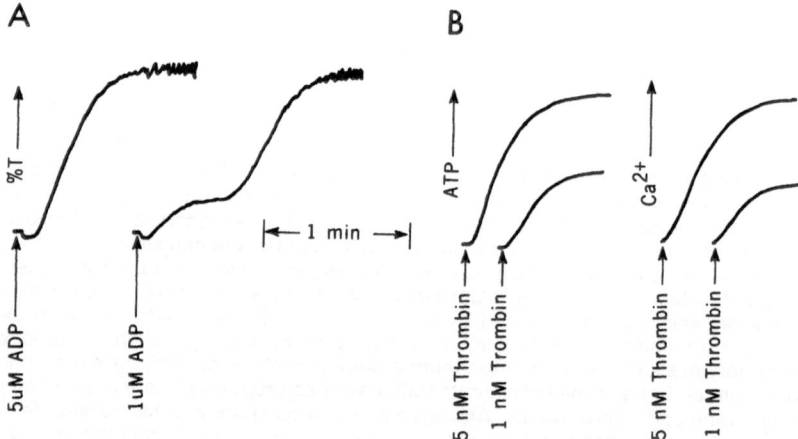

**Fig. 2.** Examples of the measurement of platelet aggregation and secretion. (A) These are typical traces of ADP-induced aggregation of platelets in platelet-rich plasma. Transmittance is measured using red light. Approximately 5 $\mu$mol ADP will cause complete aggregation, whereas 1–2 $\mu$mol ADP causes partial aggregation followed by a second wave of complete aggregation, which is due to secreted ADP. The usual parameters reported are the time to the beginning of aggregation and the extent of aggregation. The rate of aggregation is sometimes calculated as the slope of the curve, but this is clearly not a valid parameter since it will depend on extent as well as rate; time for half-maximal aggregation is more appropriate. (B) These are typical recordings of thrombin-induced secretion of ATP and $Ca^{2+}$ by washed platelets. Released ATP is measured by its luminescent reaction with luciferin and luciferase (Detwiler and Feinman, 1973b). Released $Ca^{2+}$ is measured with the metalochromic dye, murexide, in a dual wavelength spectrophotometer (Detwiler and Feinman, 1973a). These curves are evaluated with the parameters of (a) yield; (b) time to the inflection, which is a measure of the rate of stimulation; and (c) the first-order rate constant for the exponential part of the curve.

cult and interpretation is frequently ambiguous because transmittance cannot be directly related to a particular parameter of a particle suspension.

Crucial to our current concept of platelet function is the "second wave" of aggregation observed with low levels of ADP. This apparently is a reflection of the fact that the low concentration of ADP causes some platelets to aggregate and to secrete more ADP, which in turn causes more aggregation. Thus, the second wave of aggregation is a measure of secretion and the crucial role of ADP in platelet function is demonstrated. In fact, it was suspected that ADP was the primary aggregating agent, the direct cause of aggregation regardless of the stimulus, but this has been generally disproved (Mills and Macfarlane, 1975). Recent studies of the temporal relationship of aggregation and secretion (Charo, Feinman, and Detwiler, manuscript in preparation) have led us to question whether secreted substances *cause* second-wave aggregation. They suggest instead that secretion and second-wave aggregation are parallel events, so that the traditional explanation of biphasic aggregation must be reevaluated.

The slight decrease in transmittance that precedes aggregation is due to the change in shape from disk to spiny sphere and is one of the earliest responses to stimulation. By measuring right-angle scattered light, this measurement is much more easily and specifically measured (Michal and Born, 1971).

### 14.2.3.2. Secretion

In response to stimuli, platelets secrete their dense body contents, including ATP, ADP, 5-hydroxytryptamine (serotonin), and $Ca^{2+}$. This process has frequently been referred to as the "release reaction," but we prefer the term secretion, which is more consistent with the terminology of modern cell biology. Secretion has usually been measured by the release of preloaded [5-$^{14}$C]hydroxytryptamine or of adenine nucleotides, frequently as 260 nm absorbing material. At intervals after addition of the stimulus, secretion is stopped by addition of EDTA and cooling, the platelets are removed by centrifugation, and the released material is measured in the supernatant. Since this is not fully suitable for the reliable measurement of the time course of secretion, the continuous measurement of released ATP or $Ca^{2+}$ has been used more recently (Fig. 2B). The major advantage of these measurements over those of aggregation is that they produce a quantitative recording of a discrete platelet function, less dependent on external factors than is aggregation.

The responses shown in Fig. 2 (shape change, aggregation, and secretion) are substantially the same regardless of the stimulus, but there are important differences. For example, thrombin can cause secretion in the absence of appreciable aggregation, whereas ADP cannot. An important unanswered question, therefore, is whether all stimuli induce the same sequence of platelet responses.

### 14.2.4. Platelet Stimuli

Platelets are stimulated by diverse substances. The physiologically important ones include thrombin, a proteolytic enzyme; collagen, a structural protein; and ADP, a nucleotide. Stimuli of unknown physiological significance or of clearly nonphysiological origin include such diverse substances as antigen–antibody complexes, latex particles, polylysine, 5-hydroxtryptamine, and epinephrine. The mechanism for these is unknown.

### 14.2.5. Inhibitors of Platelet Function

The use of specific inhibitors has played an important role in the development of our understanding of platelet function. Two types of drugs are especially important to this discussion. Platelet responses to stimulation are inhibited by agents that elevate cAMP: These include dibutyryl cAMP, $PGE_1$ (which activates adenyl cyclase), and theophylline (which inhibits phosphodiesterase). Aspirin and indomethacin inhibit prostaglandin synthesis and have been crucial to establishing the importance of this pathway in platelet function. Aggregation is also inhibited by chelation of extracellular $Ca^{2+}$.

## 14.3. Membranes

A cell's plasma membrane may be considered to serve two broad functions. First, it packages the cell within a barrier with controlled permeability and transport; and second, it contains the surface elements with which a cell communicates with and responds to external agents and stimuli. There is little reason to suspect that the first function is appreciably different in platelets than in other cells, but the platelet has apparently unique interactions with many agents, or specific stimuli, so that its surface properties, including specific receptors, may be quite different from those of other cells.

### 14.3.1. Fluid Mosaic Model of Membranes

Although our understanding of biological membranes is in a state of rapid evolution, it is now generally accepted (but not proved) that membranes consist of discrete protein "particles" floating in a lipid "sea," the fluid mosaic model of Singer and Nicolson (1972). (For a lucid and authoritative review of cell membranes, see Weissmann and Claiborne, 1975.) Membrane proteins are classified as peripheral (easily dissociable from the membrane) and integral (dissociable only by disruption of the membrane, as with detergents). Most of the integral proteins are embedded in either the inside or the outside surface, whereas a few large proteins penetrate the entire membrane and are exposed on both sides. Those proteins exposed to the outside of a cell are glycoproteins with a high content of carbohydrate (50–80% carbohydrate in contrast to 2–10% carbohydrate of most glycoproteins), giving cell surfaces a carbohydrate coating. The proteins on the inner surface do not have large amounts of carbohydrate.

An important feature of this model is that the membrane proteins are not interconnected, but exist as separate particles that "float" freely in the lipid with the possibility of unlimited lateral mobility. Lateral migration of membrane particles is believed to be of fundamental importance (e.g., as in lymphocyte capping) and there is now considerable work on peripheral proteins associated with the inner membrane surface that may restrict lateral motion or add rigidity to membranes.

## 14.3.2. Platelet Membranes

Much less is known about the composition of platelet membranes than, for example, of red blood cell membranes. This is due in large part to the difficulty of obtaining sufficient quantities of uncontaminated preparations of platelet plasma membranes, in contrast to the relative ease of obtaining and manipulating large amounts of red cell membranes. The development of a method for the isolation of platelet plasma membranes free of granule membranes (Barber and Jamieson, 1970) was therefore a major contribution to work in this field.

### 14.3.2.1. Membrane Proteins

In recent years, the major work on platelet membranes has involved attempts to define the protein complement and to identify the proteins that are exposed to the outside, since these presumably include the receptors for various platelet stimuli and the points of adhesion and aggregation. Sodium dodecyl sulfate (SDS) acrylamide gel electrophoresis of isolated platelet membranes (Barber and Jamieson, 1971c; Nachman and Ferris, 1972; Phillips, 1972) has been used to resolve the total protein into 14–20 major bands of protein with molecular weights of from 10,000 to nearly 300,000. Three of these protein bands stain heavily for carbohydrate (Nachman and Ferris, 1972; Phillips, 1972), indicating glycoproteins with a high percentage of carbohydrate, as with surface proteins in other cells. The identification of proteins on the outside surface of the platelet membrane has been based on accessibility to lactoperoxidase-catalyzed radioiodination. Phillips (1972) observed at least seven bands of iodinated proteins when intact platelets were subjected to lactoperoxidase-catalyzed iodination; three of these bands correspond to the major glycoprotein bands, referred to as glycoproteins I, II, and III with molecular weights of 150,000, 118,000, and 92,000 daltons. [The exact molecular weights of these proteins have varied in other reports and band II has been further resolved into two bands, IIa and IIb (Tanner and Boxer, 1974; Phillips *et al.*, 1975), but the basic observations still seem valid.] Nachman *et al.* (1973) independently obtained qualitatively similar results and, in a different type of experiment, Pepper and Jamieson (1969) observed that trypsin treatment of platelet membranes released several different glyco-peptides. The carbohydrate compositions of these glycopeptides were different, with large amounts of *N*-acetylglucosamine and variable amounts of sialic acid (Pepper and Jamieson, 1969). This suggests a considerably more complex surface than on red blood cells, presumably a reflection of the more elaborate surface phenomena of platelets. Thus, the exterior surface of the platelet membrane contains large amounts of different glycoproteins that can be resolved into four bands by SDS acrylamide gel electrophoresis.

The membrane presumably contains hundreds of different proteins, many of which may be in concentrations too low to be detected on gels of total membrane protein or which may not be readily resolved into separate protein bands. Improved methods of protein resolution will certainly demonstrate many more surface proteins. Characterization of these proteins will be a difficult but essential step toward understanding platelet function. The proteins on the inside surface of the platelet membrane are as important as those on the outside, but nothing is known about their composition.

### 14.3.2.2. Studies with Lectins

Lectins are proteins that bind to specific carbohydrates, and have been used to examine membrane structure in a variety of cells (Lis and Sharon, 1973). Several groups have studied the effects of specific lectins on platelets, but no clear pattern has emerged. Erythroagglutinating phytohemagglutinin (E-PHA) induced secretion in washed platelets (Tollefsen *et al.*, 1974b), and lectins with specificities for galactose (*R. communis*) or *N*-acetylglucosamine (wheat germ agglutinin) induced both aggregation and secretion (Greenberg and Jamieson, 1974). Concanavalin A (glucose and mannose specific) has been reported to induce secretion but not aggregation (Greenberg and Jamieson, 1974). In contrast, Nachman *et al.* (1973) reported that concanavalin A caused aggregation, whereas trypsinized concanavalin A did not (Kaplan and Nachman, 1975). This is an interesting result because the trypsinized concanavalin A is probably monovalent (Burger and Noonan, 1970), suggesting that multiple sites of attachment may be necessary for aggregation.

## 14.4. Physiological Stimuli

The response of platelets to specific stimuli is basic to their function, and considerable effort has been directed to an understanding of mechanisms of the interactions of the stimuli with platelets. Although there is uncertainty about the extent to which responses to different stimuli are the same, the diversity of stimulating agents suggests that the initial events must be different. The status of research of the more extensively studied and presumably more physiologically significant stimuli is now discussed.

### 14.4.1. Thrombin

Thrombin, the most potent platelet stimulus, is the final proteolytic enzyme activated in the blood coagulation "cascade." It is one of a class of enzymes referred to as "serine proteases," enzymes characterized by an active serine that functions as a nucleophilic catalyst in the hydrolysis of peptides (for review, see Magnusson, 1971). It shares a high degree of structural homology with other serine proteases such as trypsin, chymotrypsin, plasmin, and factor Xa. Its catalytic specificity, similar to that of trypsin, is for arginyl and lysyl peptides and esters, but it has a high degree of specificity for protein substrates, hydrolyzing at an appreciable rate only 4 of the 100 or so trypsin-sensitive bonds in fibrinogen, one of its major physiological substrates.

#### 14.4.1.1. Thrombin Substrates on Platelets

Most studies of the mechanism of thrombin stimulation of platelets have involved attempts to identify the putative platelet surface protein whose hydrolysis by thrombin leads to platelet stimulation. Fibrinogen, the major plasma substrate of thrombin and a normal platelet constituent, is generally discounted because fibrinogen clotting activity does not parallel platelet stimulating activity (Davey and Luscher, 1967; Brown *et al.*, 1972).

There have been numerous attempts to identify other thrombin substrates in, or on, platelets. Typically, these studies have utilized the high resolving power of polyacrylamide gel electrophoretic separation of proteins to detect changes in protein composition accompanying thrombin treatment. This can be a powerful technique, but it has certain inherent problems. Since thrombin is a protease, it can be expected to have at least some proteolytic activity toward many proteins unrelated to physiological substrates, and only thrombin proven to be of the highest purity can be assumed to be free of contaminating proteases. Thus, only changes resulting from very brief treatment of intact platelets with low concentrations of highly purified thrombin are even suggestive of the physiological action of thrombin. (Maximum physiological effect is observed within a few seconds with 1 NIH unit/ml; e.g., see Detwiler and Feinman, 1973a; Phillips, 1974). On the other hand, the physiological substrate may be such a minor component of the total protein, or even of the membrane protein, that it might not be observed with conventional separation and detection procedures.

With these considerations in mind, several recent studies are noteworthy. Baenziger *et al.* (1971, 1972) observed that treatment of intact platelets with thrombin led to the disappearance of a 190,000-dalton protein from a membrane fraction. The change was observed only with thrombin treatment of intact platelets (not of isolated membranes), it required only 1 unit/ml of thrombin and changes were detected within 15 sec. It thus had characteristics consistent with a physiological thrombin substrate. However, it proved to be *released* from platelets, apparently intact, without evidence of proteolytic cleavage, so that its role as a thrombin substrate is in doubt. In a different approach, Phillips and Agin (1974) and Steiner (1973) studied the effect of thrombin on platelet proteins that had been radioactively labeled by lactoperoxidase-catalyzed iodination, permitting very sensitive detection of proteins presumably derived from the platelet surface (available to lactoperoxidase). Phillips and Agin (1974) found that although thrombin treatment of membranes isolated from labeled platelets caused a decrease in three glycoproteins and a 220,000-dalton polypeptide, thrombin treatment of intact platelets caused a decrease in only a single glycoprotein of 118,000 daltons. The change was very small and could be clearly shown only with a double isotope procedure. No appearance of a smaller peptide was observed.

### 14.4.1.2. Evidence for a Nonproteolytic Mechanism

Since neither of these approaches showed a concomitant increase in smaller proteins, thrombin substrates were not proven and thrombin-catalyzed proteolysis of a platelet membrane protein remains an unproven, though still reasonable, hypothesis. This is significant because recent studies indicate that the interaction of thrombin with platelets has some characteristics inconsistent with an enzyme-catalyzed reaction. This was initially emphasized by Detwiler and Feinman (1973a), who studied the kinetics of the thrombin-induced secretion of $Ca^{2+}$. They observed that the *extent* of stimulation as well as the *rate* of stimulation was dependent on thrombin concentration, indicating that thrombin did not "turn over" as, by definition, does a catalyst. Indeed, Tollefsen *et al.* (1974a) showed that thrombin binds tightly (but reversibly) to the platelet surface. Martin *et al.* (1975), therefore, reevaluated the enzymatic role of thrombin in platelet stimulation. They concluded that the enzyme specificity, the pH dependence, and the effect of a competitive inhibitor were consistent with a catalytic role of thrombin. However, pH and the competitive inhibitor had the same effects on the *extent* of stimulation as on the *rate* of stimulation, inconsistent with a catalytic mechanism. Thus, the mechansim appears to involve the catalytic site of thrombin, but not as a true catalyst, since there is apparently no thrombin turnover.

The reversible binding of thrombin to platelets reported by Tollefsen *et al.* (1974a) could be reconciled with the apparent lack of thrombin turnover only if the binding were exceptionally tight and with an extremely slow dissociation. But Martin *et al.* (1976) reported that binding reached equilibrium within at least 30 sec, possibly much faster, and that with concentrations of thrombin that caused only partial stimulation of platelets, 90% of the added thrombin was free in solution and potentially reactive toward platelets. An explanation of why this free thrombin does not react further with partially stimulated platelets is essential to an understanding of the mechanism of the reaction of thrombin with platelets.* A hypothetical model (Martin *et al.*, 1975; Detwiler *et al.*, 1975) is shown in equation (1), where T is thrombin, R is a platelet receptor, and $R^0$ is a modified

$$T + R \rightleftharpoons TR \rightleftharpoons TR^0 \tag{1}$$

receptor. This is written in the conventional form for an enzyme–substrate reaction; the essential feature is the *reversible* reaction of thrombin and receptor, with the extent of stimulation dependent on the equilibrium concentration of $TR^0$. Thus the reaction has aspects of both an enzyme-catalyzed reaction and an agonist–receptor equilibrium, and is consistent

---

*Tollefsen and Majerus (1976) suggest that their observed slow dissociation explains the lack of thrombin turnover. Although we question whether their experiments have adequately established slow dissociation, especially since Martin *et al.* (1976) observed more rapid dissociation using a more direct procedure, it should be noted that the rate of dissociation is irrelevant to the question of why the extent of stimulation depends on thrombin concentration *as long as the binding is sufficiently weak to leave most of the thrombin unbound,* as all binding studies have indicated.

with the following observations: (a) The extent of stimulation depends on thrombin concentration (Detwiler and Feinman, 1973a); (b) thrombin binding is an equilibrium with most thrombin free and active even with less than maximal stimulation (Tollefsen et al., 1974a; Martin et al., 1976); and (c) the reaction involves the active site of thrombin and is perturbed as a catalytic reaction (Davey and Luscher, 1967; Martin et al., 1975). The reversible hydrolysis of soybean trypsin inhibitor by trypsin (Laskowski, 1971) is a reasonable analogy of one possible mechanism and illustrates that there need not be appreciable hydrolysis of a substrate.

### 14.4.1.3. Binding of Thrombin to Platelets

Direct measurement of the binding of thrombin to platelets has given valuable insight into the thrombin–platelet reaction, but these studies are difficult to interpret (see Martin et al., 1976, for a discussion of some of the problems of interpretation). To some extent, results are dictated by the choice of methods, explaining some apparently contradictory results. For example, the rapid equilibrium reported by Martin et al. (1976) could never be observed using methods that involve dilution before isolation of the thrombin–platelet complex (Tollefsen et al., 1974a; Tollefsen and Majerus, 1976) or washing of the isolated thrombin–platelet complex (Tollefsen et al., 1974a; Tollefsen and Majerus, 1976; Mohammed et al., 1976) since these procedures eliminate any rapidly dissociable thrombin. The use of long incubations by these workers (15–30 min) also increases the possibility of thrombin being taken into the platelet, the simplest explanation for the obvious paradox reported by Mohammed et al. (1976) of (a) unlimited binding sites, (b) irreversible binding, and (c) only a small fraction of total thrombin bound. That is, their data are inconsistent with a thermodynamic equilibrium, and the dependence of amount bound on thrombin concentration must be due to a concentration-dependent slow *rate* of irreversible binding.

The major problem in interpretation of binding data is to distinguish specific binding (i.e., to a physiological "receptor") from nonspecific binding. The fact that irreversibly inhibited thrombin binds the same as active thrombin and competes with active thrombin for binding, but neither stimulates nor competes with active thrombin for stimulation (Tollefsen et al., 1974a), suggests that the major part of observed binding may not be to specific receptors. On the other hand, it has been reported that thrombin binding is specific for platelets (Tollefsen et al., 1974a), that prothrombin does not bind (Tollefsen et al., 1975), and that anion composition affects binding the same way it affects stimulation (Shuman and Majerus, 1975).

These observations suggest that measured binding is related to the physiological action of thrombin. Martin *et al.* (1976) observed that stimulation of platelets was closely correlated to binding of thrombin to a population of high affinity sites described by Tollefsen *et al.* (1974a). There are only about 500 of these high affinity sites per platelet, but 10,000–50,000 total thrombin binding sites. Thus, in most studies, binding to specific receptors might be completely masked by nonspecific binding.

### 14.4.1.4. Summary

Although thrombin is a proteolytic enzyme, its stimulation of platelets has not been attributed to proteolysis, and kinetic studies indicate that some aspects of the reaction are inconsistent with a catalytic mechanism. The reaction is consistent with the occupation theory of agonist–receptor reactions, and a mechanism combining aspects of an enzyme active site reaction and an agonist–receptor equilibrium has been proposed. Binding studies indicate equilibrium binding, with most thrombin free even at concentrations too low to give maximal stimulation, consistent with the equilibrium mechanism.

## 14.4.2. Collagen

Collagen may be the most important physiological platelet stimulus, since the primary hemostatic event is believed to be adhesion of platelets to collagen that has been exposed by vessel damage. Despite very extensive research on the collagen–platelet interaction, the mechanism is not known, and even fundamental questions remain unanswered. For example, studies designed to define the structural requirements for stimulation of platelets have led to such diverse conclusions as (a) the quaternary structure, or supramolecular organization, is essential (Jaffe and Deykin, 1974; Brass and Bensusan, 1974; Muggli and Baumgartner, 1973), or (b) a single peptide (from CNBr cleavage of collagen) without tertiary structure is active (Katzman *et al.*, 1973; Chiang *et al.*, 1975). There are two inherent problems that make the design of experiments and the interpretation of published results especially difficult. First, collagen is not a simple, homogeneous substance. Its chemical composition varies with the source; its physical state depends on how it has been treated and is usually not well defined. (Some of the important structural features of collagen are described in Fig. 3.) Second, there is no ideal parameter of the collagen–platelet interaction.

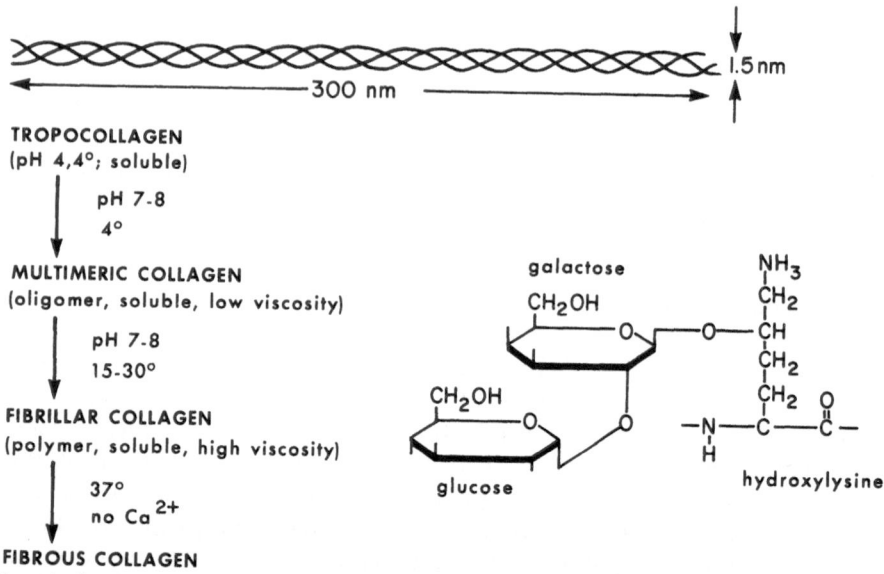

**Fig. 3.** Important structural features of collagen. The basic structural unit of collagen is tropocollagen, an approximately 290,000-dalton protein composed of three polypeptide chains. Each of the three chains of tropocollagen is a helix and they are wound around each other to form a three-stranded rod about 300 nm long and 1.5 nm in diameter. Collagen has a distinctive amino acid composition; about one-third of the residues are glycine, and there is a high content of proline and of the unusual amino acids hydroxyproline and hydroxylysine. Depending on the source, there is a variable content of carbohydrate in glycosidic linkage to hydroxylysine. The carbohydrate is either glucosyl galactose or just galactose without the terminal glucosyl unit.

Tropocollagen spontaneously associates in a specific end-to-end and side-by-side configuration to form a highly ordered fiber. Collagen is stabilized by covalent bonds between the three chains of tropocollagen and between tropocollagen units. The degree of cross-linking depends on physiological function and increases with age. The *in vitro* polymerization of soluble tropocollagen proceeds through more or less distinct stages. (The intermediate stages are not precisely defined and there is no general agreement on terminology as yet. For a detailed discussion of the polymerization scheme shown, see the recent review by Jaffe, 1977.) The course of these transitions can be substantially modified by controlling temperature and cation composition and by the use of specific inhibitors.

## 14.4.2.1. Measurement of the Collagen–Platelet Interaction

A survey of the collagen–platelet literature reveals that conclusions frequently depend on how the reaction is measured. The interaction of collagen with platelets has most often been measured by the aggregation of platelets or the secretion of 5-hydroxytryptamine or adenine nucleotides, but it is not clear whether these are separate and independent phenomena. Perhaps secretion is a consequence of aggregation, or aggregation a consequence of secretion. To avoid this type of uncertainty, many researchers have directly measured the adhesion of collagen to platelets. However, adhesion is not the same as stimulation of aggregation or secretion; it may not even be the first step, since it could involve a distinct type of binding. This is not the same problem as that of nonspecific binding of thrombin, since adhesion of platelets to collagen may be as physiologically significant as induction of aggregation; *stimulation* of platelets by collagen may simply be a by-product of the physiologically relevant process, *adhesion*.

### 14.4.2.2. Structural Requirements for Reaction of Collagen with Platelets

What are the essential physicochemical features of collagen necessary for the collagen–platelet interaction? Because of the complexity of collagen structure, this simple question still has no answer; there is some disagreement about basic observations and considerable controversy about their interpretation.

Wilner *et al.* (1968) demonstrated that heat denaturation, proteolytic degradation, or chemical modification of free amino groups abolished the ability of soluble collagen to aggregate platelets, suggesting that native structure was necessary and that $\epsilon$-amino groups of lysine had a special role. In contrast, esterification of carboxyl groups had no effect. Chesney *et al.* (1972) demonstrated that galactose oxidase-treated collagen failed to cause platelet aggregation, suggesting an essential role for accessible galactose residues. Although these data suggest that a native protein conformation is necessary to permit reaction of free amino groups and galactose with the platelet surface, an attractive alternative interpretation has been suggested by several groups who have emphasized the role of collagen *quaternary* structure (Jaffe and Deykin, 1974; Muggli and Baumgartner, 1973; Brass and Bensusan, 1974; Simons *et al.*, 1975). Since collagen spontaneously polymerizes, the effect of modifying the rate or extent of polymerization on collagen-induced aggregation or secretion was measured. To summarize briefly some rather detailed and elegant experiments, intermediate collagen polymers ("fibrillar collagen") caused aggregation or secretion without appreciable delay, whereas lower polymers ("multimeric collagen") caused aggregation or secretion only after a delay of several minutes. The delay observed with multimeric collagen could be correlated with the time required for formation of "fibrillar collagen." Significantly, treatment with galactose oxidase (Muggli and Baumgartner, 1973; Harper *et al.*, 1975) or modification of $\epsilon$-amino groups of lysine (R. Jaffe and D. Deykin, personal communication) not only impaired the ability of collagen to aggregate platelets, it also inhibited

polymerization. Thus, requirements for certain chemical groups on collagen are confirmed but with an interpretation based on requirements for
polymerization, not for direct reaction with platelets.

The major contradictions to this interpretation are the reports that an
isolated glycopeptide fragment of collagen can cause platelets to aggregate (Katzman *et al.*, 1973; Kang *et al.*, 1974) or secrete (Chiang *et al.*,
1975). This peptide represents only about 4% of a single chain of tropocollagen and has no tertiary (and thus no quaternary) structure. Although
this contradiction cannot yet be resolved, it should be remembered that
many unrelated agents cause platelets to aggregate, presumably by different mechanisms, so that such discrepancies might be expected.

### 14.4.2.3. Possible Role of Membrane Glycosyl Transferase

For the past 5 years, work on the collagen–platelet interaction has
been greatly influenced by the proposal of Jamieson *et al.* (1971) that
adhesion of collagen and platelets is through surface enzymes, colla-
gen:glycosyl transferases. Two platelet enzymes have been characterized,
collagen:*gluco*syl transferase (Barber and Jamieson, 1971a; Bosmann,
1971) and collagen:*galacto*syl transferase (Barber and Jamieson, 1971b;
Bosmann, 1971). These membrane-bound enzymes catalyze the reaction

$$UDPG + Collagen \rightarrow UDP + Collagen\text{-}G$$

where "G" is a glycosyl unit. The galactose is added to collagen hydroxyly-
sines freed of carbohydrate and the glucose to collagen galactose (see Fig.
3).

The hypothesis that collagen–platelet adhesion is mediated by colla-
gen:glucosyl transferase has been evaluated most extensively by Jamieson
and co-workers (for brief reviews see Jamieson, 1974a,b). The proposal is
simply that collagen adhesion to platelets is due to binding of the enzyme
to its acceptor, in essence formation of an enzyme–substrate complex of
the platelet glucosyl transferase and one of its substrates, collagen. In
support of this mechanism, there are close parallels between inhibition of
collagen adhesion and inhibition of transferase activity (though note that
such a correlation is not essential, since the proposed mechanism for
adhesion does not actually involve catalysis).

### 14.4.2.4. Summary

Collagen is a very complex and variable protein with an elaborate
supramolecular structure. One of the major problems of the collagen–
platelet reaction is identification of the structural features of collagen
essential for the reaction. The recent proposals of a requirement for a

specific supramolecular structure offer a new interpretation of requirements for certain chemical groups, but they do not yet explain what there
is about collagen that reacts with platelets. The hypothetical collagen–
glucosyl transferase complex as the mechanism for binding continues to
be an intriguing proposal.

### 14.4.3. ADP

Adenosine diphosphate (ADP) is one of the simplest and most extensively studied of the platelet stimuli. It is a primary aggregating agent and
is believed to play a major role in the important secondary aggregation
induced by other stimuli. This central role and the relatively simple
structure of ADP have generated much speculation about the mechanism
of ADP-induced platelet aggregation, and several models, mostly speculative, have been proposed, but none has found general acceptance (for a
discussion of the various proposals see Mustard and Packham, 1970).
Guccione et al. (1971; Mustard et al., 1975) proposed that ADP stimulates
aggregation by interaction with a membrane-bound nucleoside diphos-
phokinase, which phosphorylates added ADP by reaction with a platelet-
associated triphosphate as the high-energy source:

$$*\text{ADP} + \text{Platelet-ATP} \xrightarrow{\text{nucleotide diphosphokinase}} *\text{ATP} + \text{Platelet-ADP}$$

It is hypothesized that breakdown of the platelet-associated ATP somehow induces the state of "aggregability" or "stickiness," and full aggregation then follows. Born and Feinberg (1975) also measured the conversion
of [$^{14}$C]ADP to [$^{14}$C]ATP by platelets, and proposed a similar theory of
aggregation.

Nachman and Ferris have attempted to characterize the ADP receptor (Nachman and Ferris, 1974; Nachman, 1975). Reversible binding to
isolated membranes and to a preparation solubilized by freeze-thawing
was observed, and known inhibitors of ADP-induced aggregation (such as
ATP, AMP, and 2-chloroadenosine) blocked [$^{14}$C]ADP binding. Using
these cell-free preparations Nachman found that [$^{14}$C]ADP was not
metabolized to [$^{14}$C]ATP, as reported by Guccione et al. (1971) with intact
cells. However, the binding was extremely slow, requiring 60 min for
equilibration at 37°C. Since ADP stimulation requires only a few seconds,
it is uncertain whether this binding represents the ADP receptor for
platelet stimulation.

### 14.4.4. Conclusion

The most remarkable aspect of platelet stimuli is their diversity. Not
only are the three stimuli discussed herein different, but many other

nonphysiologic substances not obviously related to these are active. Much of the current work involves the characterization of and search for presumed receptors. Although this seems reasonable, no receptor has been identified and it is difficult to see how the many nonphysiologic stimuli could have specific receptors, so there is still some uncertainty whether the concept of "receptors" is valid. Determination of the mechanism for any of these stimuli will be a major step toward a full understanding of platelet function. It is interesting that each of the hypothetical mechanisms discussed involves some aspect of an enzyme–substrate complex.

## 14.5. Intracellular Regulatory Mechanisms

The responses of platelets to various stimuli are presumably initiated by reactions on the platelet surface followed by a series of intracellular events that couple the initial signal to the final responses. In this section we discuss the possible involvement in platelets of several intracellular regulatory mechanisms known to function in other cells.

### 14.5.1. Calcium

$Ca^{2+}$ is an important regulatory agent in many cells (for review, see Rasmussen *et al.,* 1972) and its role has been especially well characterized in the regulation of skeletal muscle contraction (Ebashi, 1976) and in secretion (Rubin, 1974). There is an absolute $Ca^{2+}$ requirement for platelet aggregation, but this involves *extra*cellular $Ca^{2+}$, whereas here we are concerned with the possibility of an intracellular regulatory role for $Ca^{2+}$. This has been studied primarily in terms of a single platelet response, secretion, a process that is triggered by $Ca^{2+}$ in most cells (Rubin, 1974), either by an influx of extracellular $Ca^{2+}$ or by a translocation of intracellular $Ca^{2+}$.

Direct investigation of the regulatory role of $Ca^{2+}$ in platelet secretion is complicated by two facts. First, extracellular $Ca^{2+}$ may be required for *stimulation* by several agents (collagen?), severely restricting experimental flexibility. Thus most information is on thrombin, a stimulus that does *not* require extracellular $Ca^{2+}$. Second, platelet secretion includes secretion of an exceedingly large amount of $Ca^{2+}$ (Murer, 1969; Detwiler and Feinman, 1973a), tending to mask the more subtle fluxes that could serve a regulatory role.

The role of $Ca^{2+}$ in platelet secretion has been most effectively studied with the divalent cation ionophore A23187, which transports divalent cations across membranes (Pressman, 1973). A23187 induces platelet secretion in the absence of extracellular $Ca^{2+}$ (Feinman and Detwiler, 1974; White et al., 1974; Massini and Luscher, 1974). Iono-phore- and thrombin-induced secretion have the same rate constants and yield (Feinman and Detwiler, 1974) and the same temperature dependence (Friedman and Detwiler, 1975). Drugs that affect late steps in thrombin-induced secretion have the same effect on A23187-induced secretion, whereas drugs that affect early steps of thrombin-induced secretion have no effect on secretion induced by A23187 (Friedman and Detwiler, 1975). Thus, A23187 apparently bypasses the initial thrombin reactions and directly triggers secretion. Since the reaction proceeds as well in the presence of EDTA* as of $Ca^{2+}$, the mechanism is presumed to involve a flux of a divalent cation from an intracellular reservoir. Direct evidence that $Ca^{2+}$ is the active cation was obtained by inhibiting secretion with an antagonist of intracellular $Ca^{2+}$ and demonstrating that the inhibited platelets were dependent on extracellular $Ca^{2+}$ (not $Mg^{2+}$) for iono-phore-induced secretion (Charo et al., 1976).

The source of this intracellular $Ca^{2+}$ flux is not known. Platelets have been reported to contain membrane-associated $Ca^{2+}$ pumps (Statland et al., 1969; Robblee et al., 1973a). White (1972) has suggested that a "dense tubular system" might be analogous to sarcoplasmic reticulum, and a thrombin-sensitive $Ca^{2+}$ pool in $\alpha$ granules has been reported (Sato et al., 1975), but there is no evidence that any of these is related to stimulus–response coupling.

## 14.5.2. Cyclic Nucleotides

### 14.5.2.1. cAMP

Adenosine 3′,5′-cyclic monophosphate (cAMP) is formed by the enzyme-catalyzed breakdown and cyclization of ATP and is degraded by a specific phosphodiesterase to 5′-AMP (AMP):

$$ATP \xrightarrow[\text{(PGE}_1\text{ activates)}]{\text{adenyl cyclase}} cAMP \xrightarrow[\text{(theophylline inhibits)}]{\text{phosphodiesterase}} AMP$$

Sutherland and Rall (1960), in now classic experiments, showed that cAMP acts as an intracellular messenger (the "second messenger") in cells responsive to circulating hormones (the "first messenger") that react with membrane-bound receptors. Since these original reports, cAMP has been

---

*There continue to be numerous reports that at low levels of stimulus there is a requirement for extracellular $Ca^{2+}$ for platelet secretion, but this almost certainly reflects a requirement for aggregation, which in effect amplifies the low stimulus. This question has been discussed in more detail by Feinman and Detwiler (1975). There is also a thrombin-induced influx of extracellular $^{45}Ca^{2+}$, but this has been shown to be after secretion (Robblee et al., 1973b).

found to be virtually ubiquitous, and the diverse effects of many hormones seem to be mediated by their activation of adenyl cyclase.

Marcus and Zucker (1965) first reported that cAMP was an inhibitor of platelet aggregation, an observation that has been substantiated by many groups. (Friedman and Detwiler, 1975, have pointed out that cAMP does not actually inhibit platelet responses, but inhibits transmission of membrane-initiated signals.) Intracellular cAMP can be raised* by agents that either activate adenyl cyclase, such as $PGE_1$, or those that inhibit phosphodiesterase, such as caffeine, theophylline, or papaverine. In general, either leads to inhibition of platelet aggregation and secretion, but the effect of cAMP on platelet function has proved to be quite complex. The overall question is whether the level of cAMP is correlated with platelet function and whether it changes in direct response to stimulating agents. When platelets are incubated with $PGE_1$, there is a dose-dependent increase in intracellular cAMP, which reaches a maximum within about 30 sec and then declines to a plateau at approximately 50% of the peak value, or two to four times the basal level. Incubation with $PGE_1$ *plus* a phosphodiesterase inhibitor (caffeine) causes a two- to tenfold greater increase in cAMP, which plateaus *at* its peak value (Haslam, 1973; McDonald and Stuart, 1973). Although the degree of elevation of cAMP may be roughly correlated with inhibition of platelet aggregation, the time of maximum inhibition lags behind the time of maximum accumulation of cAMP (Ball *et al.*, 1970). Thus inhibition of aggregation does not appear to be directly due to cAMP; it has been suggested that these results are consistent with cAMP activation of a protein kinase, with phosphorylation of some protein the immediate mechanism of inhibition.

If elevation of cAMP inhibits aggregation, is it possible that a decrease in cAMP *causes* aggregation? When certain platelet activators, such as ADP or epinephrine, are added to platelets that have been incubated with $PGE_1$ plus caffeine, a prompt fall in cAMP is, in fact, observed (Haslam and Taylor, 1971). This apparently represents an inhibition of adenyl cyclase, rather than activation of phosphodiesterase (Haslam, 1973), and studies using intact platelets (Brodie *et al.*, 1972) have reported that thrombin inhibits the $PGE_1$ activation of adenyl cyclase.

---

*There are several methods available for measuring cyclic AMP, but all reduce to two basic approaches, each with its own shortcomings: (a) Measurement of total cyclic AMP in platelet-rich plasma. This method ensures detection of the total cAMP change in PRP, but Haslam (1975) claimed that 75% of the cAMP in PRP is in the plasma, and so changes *within* the platelet may well go undetected. (b) Radioactive labeling of cAMP through incorporation of [$^{14}$C]adenine or [$^{14}$C]adenosine into platelet ATP. This method is quite sensitive, and allows one to work in PRP and see only *platelet* cAMP synthesis. However, there is always the danger that not all ATP pools will be equally labeled, and if one does not know the specific activity of the precursor pool, changes in [$^{14}$C]cAMP are difficult to interpret. Each of these techniques is widely seen in the platelet literature, and the reader is advised to note how each is being used in evaluating any result.

The more important question is whether aggregating agents affect *basal* levels of cAMP. Salzman and Neri (1969) reported that ADP and epinephrine induced a decrease in total cAMP in platelet-rich plasma, and they proposed that this is the trigger for aggregation. However, several other groups (McDonald and Stuart, 1973; Haslam and Taylor, 1971), using a variety of assay techniques, have been unable to detect this change in basal cAMP upon platelet stimulation.

There are two generally accepted major conclusions from the extensive work on platelet cAMP: (a) Elevation of cAMP is causally associated with inhibition of aggregation by an unknown, indirect mechanism. (b) Many aggregating agents clearly lower *elevated* cAMP, but probably do not lower basal levels. Thus, although cAMP may help regulate the poise of the stimulus–response mechanism, it apparently does not act as a direct coupling agent, or "trigger."

### 14.5.2.2. cGMP

In many tissues levels of guanosine 3',5'-cyclic monophosphate (cGMP) vary in the opposite direction to levels of cAMP (Hadden *et al.*, 1972), and thus an increase in cGMP has been proposed as a possible platelet "second messenger." An increase in intracellular cGMP has been noted in response to several stimuli (Haslam and McClenaghan, 1974; White *et al.* 1973; Chiang *et al.*, 1975), but it has not been possible to show that the elevation of cGMP *causes* platelet responses. Haslam (1975) has recently shown that acetylcholine-induced secretion in dog platelets is *not* accompanied by an elevation in cyclic GMP. Thus, changes in platelet cyclic GMP are not a general requirement for secretion; what role, if any, they do play in stimulation remains to be seen.

### 14.5.3. Prostaglandins, Endoperoxides, and Thromboxanes

Over the past several years there has been rapid and dramatic expansion in our understanding of the role of prostaglandins in platelet function. Historically, this developed from observations of the effect of aspirin on platelet aggregation. Aspirin had long been associated with gastrointestinal bleeding in patients with normal prothrombin times, but the mechanism was unclear. In 1967, Weiss and Aledort demonstrated that ingested aspirin caused both increased bleeding time and inhibition of "connective tissue"-induced platelet aggregation and secretion in normal volunteers. Smith and Willis (1970, 1971) subsequently demonstrated

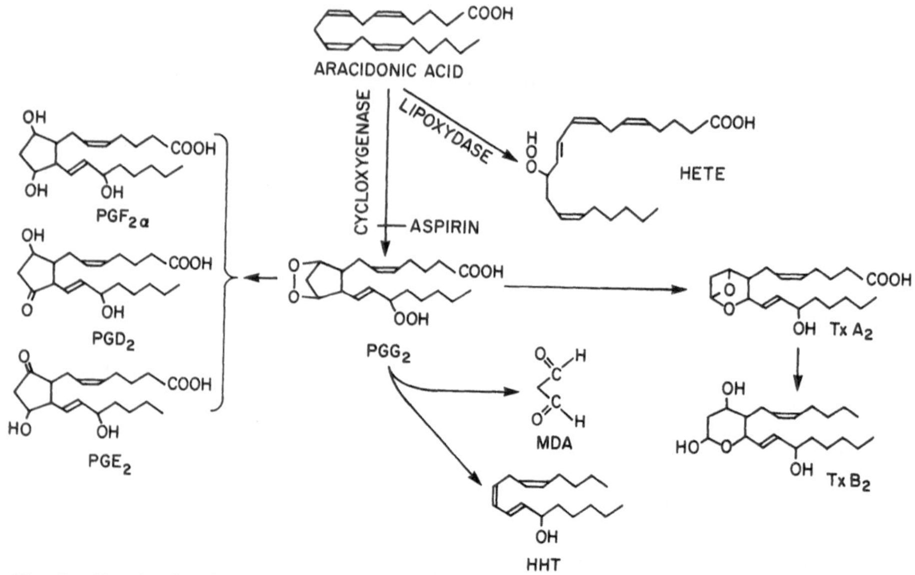

**Fig. 4.** Synthesis of prostaglandins, endoperoxides, and thromboxanes by platelets. In this scheme the prostaglandins $PGF_{2\alpha}$, $PGE_2$, and $PGD_2$ are shown on the left; the endoperoxide $PGG_2$ is in the center; and the thromboxanes $A_2$ and $B_2$ ($TxA_2$, $TxB_2$) are on the right. Arachidonic acid is the major precursor for prostaglandin synthesis in platelets, where it is mostly esterified to phospholipids (Marcus et al., 1969). The first step in prostaglandin synthesis is activation of a phospholipase that catalyzes the rate-determining step, hydrolysis of the arachidonate ester to free arachidonic acid. Free arachidonic acid can be oxygenated either by a lipoxydase to HETE, a compound of unknown function, or by cycloxygenase to prostaglandin $G_2$ ($PGG_2$), an endoperoxide that sits at a key branch point in prostaglandin biosynthesis. $PGG_2$ is itself a potent platelet aggregator. Endoperoxides have several possible fates; they may be secreted intact by the platelet (and presumably cause further aggregation), or they may be transformed to either stable prostaglandins or nonprostaglandin end products. The prostaglandins $F_{2\alpha}$, $E_2$, and $D_2$ are produced in small quantities by platelets; $E_2$ and $F_2\alpha$ are relatively inactive, but $D_2$ has recently been shown (Mills and MacFarlane, 1974) to be a more powerful activator of adenyl cyclase than $PGE_1$ and may be produced in greater quantity by other tissues. HHT is a nonprostaglandin of unknown function that is produced in parallel with malondialdehyde (MDA), a small molecule that is easily assayed and reflects total endoperoxide production (Smith et al., 1976b). Hamberg et al. (1975) isolated and identified thromboxane $A_2$; it is unstable ($t\frac{1}{2} = 30$ sec), is a potent platelet aggregator, and may be identical to substances previously known as "rabbit aorta contracting substance" (Piper and Vane, 1969). The degradation product of thromboxane $A_2$ is thromboxane $B_2$ (formerly called PHD), which has no established physiological role.

Our current understanding of these intermediates in platelets is based on the recent reports of Nugteren and Hazelhof (1973) and Hamberg, Samuelsson, and their colleagues (Hamberg and Samuelsson, 1973, 1974; Hamberg et al., 1974a,b, 1975). They identified endoperoxide intermediates in the synthesis of prostaglandins by fractions of sheep vesicular gland homogenates and by human platelets. Two of the endoperoxides, which they named prostaglandin $G_2$ ($PGG_2$) and prostaglandin $H_2$ ($PGGH_2$), were isolated and found to be potent platelet aggregating agents. These endoperoxides were synthesized and released by thrombin-stimulated platelets. Significantly, aspirin did not inhibit aggregation induced by $PGG_2$ and $PGH_2$, suggesting that the effect of aspirin may be to inhibit formation of $PGG_2$ and $PGH_2$ within the platelet. They quantitated the synthesis of prostaglandins from [$^{14}$C]arachidonic acid in platelets and found, surprisingly, that little label was recovered in the prostaglandins, but nearly all the radioactivity was found at the level of the endoperoxides, which were further metabolized to three nonprostaglandin products, HHT, HETE, and thromboxane $B_2$.

that thrombin stimulated prostaglandin synthesis in platelets, and that aspirin inhibited this process.

There now seems little doubt that prostaglandins, or intermediates in their biosynthesis, play a significant role in platelet function. Recent work has shown that although many prostaglandins themselves are biologically inert, unstable oxygenated intermediates in their synthesis are potent aggregating agents. It has been possible to identify these intermediates in intact platelets, and to demonstrate their production in response to typical platelet stimuli (e.g., thrombin and collagen).

The biosynthesis of prostaglandins and their intermediates is shown schematically in Fig. 4.

### 14.5.3.1. Evidence for the Importance of Prostaglandin Biosynthesis in Platelets

Platelets synthesize and secrete $PGE_2$ and $PGF_2\alpha$ when stimulated by thrombin (Smith and Willis, 1970), and Smith et al. (1973) observed that these prostaglandins were synthesized as aggregation was induced by collagen (single wave) and as the second wave of aggregation was beginning in epinephrine-induced secretion. Although this suggested a physiological role, these prostaglandins were relatively inactive toward platelets (Kloeze, 1967; Sekhar, 1970).

A clearer understanding of prostaglandin function came as a result of the suggestion by Willis and Kuhn (1973) that an *intermediate* in prostaglandin synthesis from arachidonic acid was the long sought factor whose activity was inhibited by aspirin. They showed that incubation of arachidonate with sheep vesicular gland concentrates (which synthesize prostaglandins) generated a "labile aggregation-stimulating substance" (LASS) that was a potent aggregator of platelets, and whose appearance preceded that of $PGE_2$. Furthermore, LASS-induced aggregation was *not* inhibited by aspirin or indomethacin, whereas arachidonic acid induced aggregation by an aspirin-inhibited process (Silver et al., 1973). Willis et al. (1974) isolated LASS and demonstrated its conversion to $PGE_2$ and $PGF_2\alpha$, indicating that LASS is an intermediate in the synthesis of prostaglandins from arachidonic acid. Hamberg and co-workers (1974a,b, 1975; Hamberg and Samuelsson, 1973), in an elegant series of experiments, isolated and identified an endoperoxide intermediate ($PGG_2$) in prostaglandin biosynthesis (see Fig. 4) and showed it to be a potent aggregator of human platelets. This endoperoxide is similar to the LASS compound described by Willis et al. (1974), and has recently been found to be a precursor for yet another biologically active compound, thromboxane $A_2$. Thromboxane $A_2$ is unstable ($t\frac{1}{2} = 30$ sec), will aggregate platelets in PRP, and is formed in platelets in response to stimuli. Thus, thromboxanes as well as the endoperoxides appear to be physiologically significant in platelets.

### 14.5.3.2. What Is the Role of Prostaglandin Biosynthesis in Platelets?

Although prostaglandin biosynthesis is clearly a significant part of platelet function, its exact role is not known. Significantly, thrombin can induce perfectly normal secretion and aggregation in aspirin- or indomethacin-treated platelets, which do *not* synthesize prostaglandins! What then *are* prostaglandins (or endoperoxides or thromboxanes) necessary for? Alternatively, one may ask what impairments are found in aspirin-treated platelets. Almost all known platelet responses to stimuli proceed unimpaired following aspirin or indomethacin treatment, with the exception of the second wave of aggregation induced by ADP and epinephrine. It seems likely that these two stimuli do *not* cause secretion directly, but rather induce primary aggregation, which in turn induces secretion. It is this aggregation-induced secretion that requires prostaglandin biosynthesis (Smith and Macfarlane, 1974). It should be emphasized that shape change and primary aggregation proceed normally in aspirin-treated platelets. An interesting observation is that whereas thrombin and collagen cause platelets to produce considerable amounts of prostaglandins and endoperoxides, ADP and epinephrine cause almost none. In fact, one must use 40 $\mu$M ADP to see any measurable prostaglandin synthesis, whereas only 1–2 $\mu$M ADP induces characteristic biphasic aggregation.

Several groups have attempted to analyze the role of endoperoxides in the regulation of platelets. Smith *et al.* (1975, 1976a) used arachidonic acid, fibrinogen, and ADP to induce aggregation of washed platelets,* and found that a combination of any two was both necessary and sufficient to produce full aggregation. Indomethacin blocked the effects of arachidonic acid, implying that a prostaglandin precursor was the active compound. This synergism among ADP, prostaglandin intermediates, and fibrinogen in inducing aggregation is perplexing and may have important physiological significance. Salzman (1976) showed that incubation of arachidonic acid with lysed platelets led to formation of an endoperoxide-like compound that decreased the intracellular cAMP level in intact platelets, and proposed that endoperoxides and $PGE_2$ induce secretion via this decrease in cAMP. Recently, however, Malmsten *et al.* (1976) found that cAMP inhibits the prostaglandin synthetase enzyme (cycloxygenase), thereby decreasing the formation of endoperoxides in collagen-stimu-

---

*Platelets are "washed" by resuspending them in buffer solution several times to remove plasma proteins. These washed platelets *cannot* ordinarily be aggregated by ADP unless fibrinogen is added (Harbury *et al.*, 1972).

lated platelets. They propose that a prostaglandin intermediate, and not cAMP, is the trigger for secretion. Obviously much further investigation will be necessary to sort out this highly complex area. The synthesis of stable analogs of the endoperoxides by Corey *et al.* (1975) may therefore be quite valuable.

In summary, the endoperoxides and thromboxanes are clearly potent platelet aggregators, and their discovery is certainly one of the most exciting advances in platelet research in recent years. However, our understanding of their role in platelet function is still rudimentary. For instance, such fundamental questions as whether endoperoxides and thromboxanes elicit their effects intracellularly and only in the platelet where they are synthesized remain unanswered. Elucidation of the role of prostaglandin biosynthesis in the response of platelets to various stimuli is now at the forefront of platelet research, and answers obtained here will have profound effects on our general understanding of cell biology.

### 14.5.4. Protein Kinases

Phosphorylation of specific proteins by protein kinases, especially by cAMP-dependent protein kinases, is an important regulator mechanism in many cells, and several recent studies have explored the possibility that it has an important role in the regulation of platelet function.

A cAMP-dependent kinase activation of phosphorylase has been demonstrated in intact platelets and in platelet extracts (Gear and Schneider, 1975; Chaiken *et al.*, 1975), and a cAMP-dependent protein kinase has been partially purified from platelets (Booyse *et al.*, 1976). The physiological significance of these kinases, if any, is not clear.

Lyons *et al.* (1975) loaded platelets with $^{32}PO_4$ (which labels the $\gamma$-phosphate of ATP) and found that radioactivity was quickly incorporated into many proteins separated by SDS acrylamide gel electrophoresis. Stimulation of the platelets by thrombin led to a significant increase in the labeling of two bands corresponding to proteins of 20,000 and 40,000 daltons. The concentration of thrombin required for maximal phosphorylation, the time course of phosphorylation, and the inhibition of thrombin-stimulated phosphorylation by $PGE_1$ and dibutyryl cAMP suggest that this phosphorylation is related to the physiological response of platelets to thrombin, but do not show that it is a cause of the response.

Phosphorylation of myosin light chains by a platelet protein kinase, which may play an important role in regulating contractility, has been demonstrated by Adelstein *et al.* (1973); this is discussed further in Section 14.6.2.

### 14.5.5. Conclusion

There are several types of regulation that may be presumed to be involved in platelet function. First is the self-regulation of a steady state condition. An example of this would be the feedback, allosteric regulation of the rate of glycolysis to balance ATP production against ATP utilization. At the other extreme is some type of "switch" or "trigger" that can change the platelet from a resting to an activated state. Between these two, there are apparently mechanisms for adjusting the "poise" or "balance" of the system, modifying its sensitivity to external stimuli. There has apparently been inadequate recognition of these different levels of regulation in platelet studies. For example, it is clear that with cAMP research many workers have been concerned with its role as a "triggering" agent, even though there is essentially no evidence for such a role, but convincing evidence that it regulates the sensitivity of platelets to stimulation.

Awareness of the different types of regulation is especially important when the many types of interaction between regulatory agents are considered (see, e.g., Rasmussen *et al.*, 1972). These regulatory interrelationships are especially well established for $Ca^{2+}$, cAMP, and protein kinase; the evidence is less for prostaglandins, probably because our knowledge of endoperoxides and thromboxanes is so new. To cite a single example of a possible interrelationship, an interaction between $Ca^{2+}$ and cAMP has been propsed for platelets (Day and Holmsen, 1971; also see discussion in Ciba Foundation Symposium 35, 1975) based on known interactions in other tissues. If platelets are activated by release of $Ca^{2+}$ from an intracellular vesicle (the "trigger"), and cAMP activates a pump that transfers $Ca^{2+}$ from the cytosol to the vesicle, cAMP would effectively modulate sensitivity to a stimulus. A decrease in cAMP would make platelets more sensitive and, in some circumstances, might seem to act as the "trigger."

There is as yet no definitive evidence for the exact role of any of the regulatory agents in platelets. Perhaps the best evidence is for a role for an intracellular $Ca^{2+}$ flux as the "trigger" for stimulation of platelets, but this is based in large part on analogies with other tissues and there is nothing known of the actual mechanism.

### 14.6. Contractility

Since Bettex-Galland and Luscher first demonstrated in 1959 that platelets contain an actomyosinlike complex, there have developed totally new concepts of the role of contractile processes in nonmuscle cells. (For a review of nonmuscle contractile proteins, see Pollard and Weihing, 1974.) It is now generally recognized that actin and myosin (or myosinlike proteins) are present in most, if not all, cells. Although there are important differences between the actomyosin complexes isolated from muscle and those isolated from platelets (or other nonmuscle cells), more significant are the remarkable similarities. Thus, much of the work on nonmuscle contractile proteins has involved comparisons with muscle contractile proteins.

Contractile proteins are usually extracted as actomyosin, a complex of many specialized proteins, the principal ones being actin and myosin; contractile force is generated through the interaction of *filaments* of actin and myosin. The fundamental characteristics of actin and myosin are shown in Fig. 5.

## 14.6.1. Platelet Actomyosin

Platelet actomyosin can be extracted and partially purified by methods essentially identical to those used for muscle actomyosin, indicating substantially similar physical properties. However, there are significant differences. The low MgATP activity and the dependence of this activity on ionic strenght, pH, cation composition, etc., are distinct from similar properties of skeletal muscle actomyosin but similar to those of actomyosin from smooth muscle and other nonmuscle sources (Bettex-Galland and Luscher, 1961; Abramowitz *et al.*, 1971, 1972a; Adelstein and Conti, 1972; Malik *et al.*, 1974a). The physiological significance of these differences is not clear, but it may be noted that low MgATPase of muscle actomyosins has been correlated with a slow rate of contraction (Barany, 1967). Comparisons have been extended to individual proteins of the actomyosin complex.

### 14.6.1.1. Platelet Myosin

Any thorough study of platelet contractile proteins requires purification of the component proteins, a task that proved more difficult than with the corresponding muscle proteins. Adelstein *et al.* (1971) were the first to demonstrate clearly the preparation of pure platelet myosin.* They found that the structure of platelet myosin is similar to that of muscle myosin: It has heavy chains of about 200,000 daltons; it binds to actin to form a complex that is dissociated by MgATP; and it aggregates at low ionic strength into thick filaments similar to those of muscle myosin, but smaller (Niederman and Pollard, 1975). Like smooth muscle myosin it

---

*Cohen *et al.* (1969) and Booyse *et al.* (1971b) also reported the purification of platelet myosin, but they did not assess purity by SDS acrylamide gel electrophoresis, the current standard criterion; in retrospect, their methods would be expected to result in appreciable actin contamination.

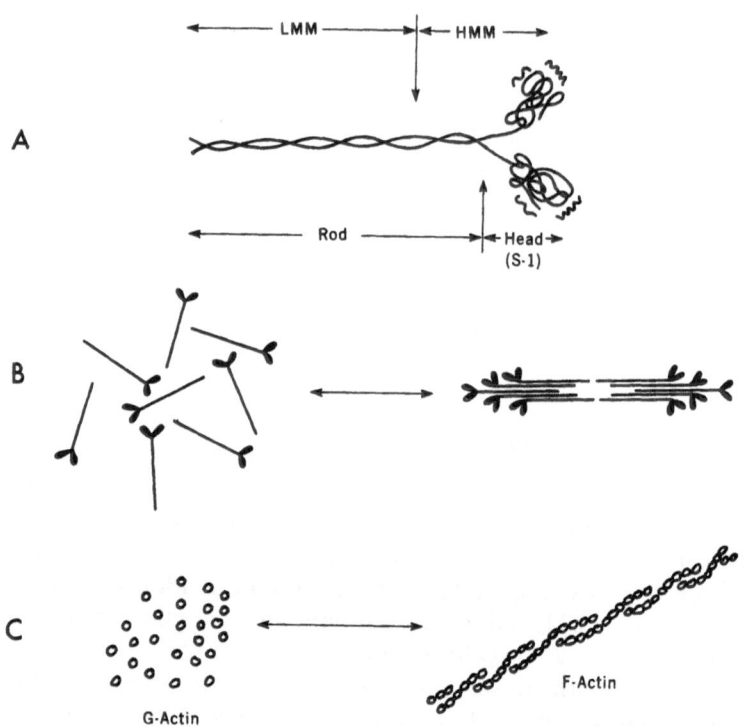

**Fig. 5.** Properties of purified actin and myosin. (A) Myosin is both a structural protein and an enzyme; the myosin-catalyzed hydrolysis of ATP yields the energy for contraction. It is a multisubunit protein composed of two heavy chains of about 200,000 daltons and four light chains. The light chains vary with the source of the myosin; skeletal muscle myosin has one chain of 16,000, two of 18,000, and one of about 25,000 daltons, whereas platelet myosin has two of 16,000 and two of 19,000 daltons. The heavy chains consist of a globular head and an $\alpha$-helical "rod." The $\alpha$ helices of the two heavy chains are coiled around each other to form the major structural aspect of the molecule, while the globular region binds the light chains and contains both the catalytic site and the actin binding site. There is a region in the heavy chain that is especially sensitive to proteolysis. Limited proteolysis can produce either "light meromyosins" (LMM) plus "heavy meromyosin" (HMM), which retains most properties of myosin except for those that depend on self-association at low ionic strength, or "rod" plus "head" (also referred to as subfragment-1), the smallest fragment with ATPase and actin binding capacity. (B) Myosin is soluble at high ionic strength, but at low ionic strength it aggregates in a specific way to form "thick" filaments, with the globular regions protruding and free to bind actin. In muscle, myosin exists in filamentous form, but this may not be true in nonmuscle cells. It is not clear what factors control filament formation *in vivo*. The defining features of myosin are (a) reversible binding to actin, (b) actin-activated ATPase activity, and (c) self-association to form filaments. (C) The actin monomer (G-actin) is a globular protein of about 45,000 daltons. The essential features of actin are its ability to polymerize into filaments (F-actin) and to bind to myosin, activating the myosin Mg-ATPase activity. Actin filaments are double helices, two strands of globular monomers coiled about each other. The filaments are about 6 nm in diameter and are identified electron microscopically by their ability to bind heavy meromyosin or myosin head to form "decorated" filaments with a distinctive repeating "arrowhead" structure. Other polymeric forms of actin are observed *in vitro* and may also exist *in vivo*. In muscle, but not in platelets and many other nonmuscle cells, actin exists almost entirely as F-actin. It is not known what controls filament formation *in vivo*.

has two light chains of 16,000 and two of 19,000 daltons (Pollard *et al.*, 1974). Adelstein *et al.* (1971) also reported that platelets contain appreciable amounts of two myosin fragments, myosin "rod" and myosin "head" (see Fig. 5). This was confirmed by Abramowitz *et al.* (1974), but only with platelets that had been stored for several days. It remains to be determined whether these fragments have a physiological role or represent an artifact of the isolation procedures.

### 14.6.1.2. Platelet Actin

Although it was until recently generally believed that actin is a highly conserved molecule, with no apparent difference between actins isolated from a wide variety of tissues and species (Bray, 1972), there are now several reports suggesting different types of platelet actin (Abramowitz *et al.*, 1972b, 1975; Spudich, 1972; Probst and Luscher, 1972; Gallagher *et al.*, 1976; Muszbeck *et al.* 1976). This has been investigated in detail only in our laboratory, where Abramowitz *et al.* (1972b) initially observed two forms of actin when they sought to explain why myosin that was separated from actomyosin complexes by conventional means always had a large, persistent actin contamination (e.g., see Adelstein *et al.*, 1971). Analysis of the actomyosin complex by sucrose gradient centrifugation revealed that about half the apparent actin was depolymerized by CaATP under conditions in which muscle actin would be polymerized. This protein was shown to be actin by its amino acid composition and its formation of 6-nm filaments that could be characteristically "decorated" by muscle heavy meromyosin. Thus two forms of actin have been identified: the first form (actin I) does not readily depolymerize *in vitro*, whereas the second form (actin II) is reversibly depolymerized by addition of CaATP. Comparison of the properties of these two forms with published procedures for the isolation of platelet actin suggests that other workers have selectively purified actin II (Gallagher *et al.*, 1976). There are several possible explanations for these two forms of actin. They may represent (a) the effects of trace substances that modify the polymerization properties of actin; (b) posttranslational covalent modification, or (c) distinct gene products. Significantly, different genes for human actin have recently been demonstrated (Elzinga *et al.*, 1976), indicating that all human cells, including megakaryocytes, have the genetic information for more than one type of actin.

### 14.6.1.3. Interaction of Actin and Myosin

The specific interaction of actin filaments and myosin filaments is presumably obligatory for contraction. Platelet myosin and actin interact to form complexes that are electron microscopically similar to the complexes of muscle myosin and actin (Adelstein et al., 1971), and hybrid complexes of platelet and muscle proteins have been demonstrated. A functional reflection of this interaction is the actin activation of myosin MgATPase activity. With skeletal muscle proteins, activation of 50-fold is typical, but with platelet proteins, activations of only four- to tenfold are reported (Adelstein et al., 1971; Probst and Luscher, 1972; Puszkin et al., 1975; Adelstein and Conti, 1975). In general, this low activation is also observed with other nonmuscle actomyosins. The experiments of Booyse et al. (1973), who studied activation of muscle or platelet myosin by muscle or platelet actin, suggest that the poor activation is due to properties of both actin and myosin. However, the significance of the low activation cannot be evaluated until platelet actin and myosin are better character-ized and the activation is studied in detail with a wide range of actin concentrations and under a variety of conditions. It is possible that with good preparations, conditions will be found for a much greater actin activation. Pollard (1975) has suggested a requirement for a "cofactor" protein.

### 14.6.1.4. Regulation of Platelet Actomyosin

There has been considerable effort to determine whether platelet actomyosin is regulated by $Ca^{2+}$ through an actin-linked troponin–tro-pomyosin system analogous to that in skeletal muscle. A protein similar to muscle tropomyosin has been isolated from platelets (Cohen and Cohen, 1972), and activation of actomyosin MgATPase activity by low concentra-tions of $Ca^{2+}$ has been reported (Adelstein and Conti, 1972; Cohen and Cohen, 1972; Hanson et al., 1973; Cohen et al., 1973). However, the $Ca^{2+}$ sensitivity is slight compared to the nearly complete $Ca^{2+}$ dependence in muscle actomyosin, and troponin has not been definitely identified in platelets. There is no a priori reason to suspect troponin in platelets, since of all the suggested functions for platelet contractile proteins, none obviously requires the elegant control (e.g., the ability to respond with millisecond twitches) of skeletal muscle. It also seems significant that actomyosin from smooth muscle, apparently a better model for platelet actomyosin than is skeletal muscle actomyosin, is not regulated by an actin-linked, troponin–tropomyosin type of mechanism (Bremel, 1974; Sobieszek and Small, 1976). There have also been suggestions of other possible mechanisms for the regulation of platelet actomyosin. For exam-ple, Adelstein et al. (1973) have demonstrated that platelets contain a protein kinase that phosphorylates the 20,000-dalton myosin light chains. Phosphorylation causes about a fivefold increase in MgATPase activity, but since it is not known whether the control myosin is partially phosphor-ylated, the potential regulation by phosphorylation may be much greater.

The physiological significance of this phosphorylation remains to be established. Platelet actomyosin has also been shown to have kinetic characteristics of allosteric ensymes (Malik *et al.*, 1974b), with $Ca^{2+}$ acting as an allosteric effector (Malik *et al.*, 1974c). No physiological role of allosteric regulation has yet been suggested, and the major current significance of this work seems to be what it can tell about the mechanism of myosin-catalyzed hydrolysis of ATP. It also seems likely that at least part of the regulation of platelet contractility is at the level of assembly of contractile filaments (see Section 14.6.2), so that direct regulation of actomyosin ATPase could be a minor regulatory mechanism.

## 14.6.2. Function of Platelet Contractile Proteins

Suggestions have been made for roles of platelet contractile proteins in such platelet phenomena as aggregation, secretion, pseuodopod formation, clot retraction, and maintenance of the disk shape, but there is no clear evidence for a direct involvement of contractile proteins in any of these processes. It is certainly significant that platelets contain large amounts of actin and myosin. Bettex-Galland and Luscher (1961) estimated that 15% of platelet protein was extracted as actomyosin, but from SDS gel electrophoresis of total platelet protein, the amount may be twice that high (Roger C. Lucas, personal communication). The relative amounts of actin and myosin have been estimated as a molar ratio of 10:10:1 (actin I–actin II–myosin) (Abramowitz *et al.*, 1975). For comparison, the molar ratio of skeletal muscle actomyosin is about 4:1 (actin–myosin).

Definition of the state and intracellular location of this large amount of actin and myosin is an essential step toward understanding their function. The striking conclusion from ultrastructural studies of contractile proteins in platelets is that resting platelets have very few structural features that can be attributed to actin or myosin, with the possible exception of 7.5-nm submembranous filaments (Zucker-Franklin, 1970; White, 1971) that may be actin filaments. However, when platelets are stimulated, microfilaments are observed parallel with the long axis of pseudopods (Zucker-Franklin, 1969), and in glycerinated (Zucker-Franklin and Grusky, 1972) or osmotically shocked (Behnke *et al.*, 1971) platelets, many actin filaments (decorated with heavy meromyosin) and myosin filaments were observed. This suggests that platelet stimulation involves formation of contractile filaments from nonfilamentous actin and myosin. Analogous situations have been observed in other cells (for a review see Tilney, 1975).

It has been reported that a portion of platelet actomyosin can be isolated with platelet membranes and that antibodies to platelet actomyosin react with the surface of intact platelets (Nachman *et al.*, 1967; Booyse *et al.*, 1971a). These experiments are difficult to interpret because (a) it would not be surprising if cytosolic actin or myosin adhered to membranes during preparation, especially because it might be expected that the inner surface of the membrane contains either actin or actin binding proteins, and (b) since the antibodies were made against acto-myosin, which is difficult to purify, nonspecific reactions cannot be excluded. (It is preferable to prepare antibodies to myosin, since acto-myosin is a complex of proteins and purity is difficult to achieve and to prove.) More recent studies with antibodies to purified myosin have failed to detect surface antigens on intact platelets (Pollard, 1975). The theories and interpretations based on the assumption of actomyosin on the platelet surface have, unfortunately, greatly exceeded the evidence for a surface location.

The presence of two forms of actin and the many different possible contractile functions of platelets suggest that no single mechanism will be found. For example, it has been suggested (Abramowitz *et al.*, 1975) that one form of actin might serve a primarily structural, or cytoskeleton, role and the other a contractile role. Additional proteins are almost certainly involved in the assembly, orientation, attachment, and regulation of contractile filaments. The recent discovery of a high molecular weight actin binding protein (distinct from myosin) (Lucas *et al.*, 1976) is of great potential significance.

### 14.6.3. Microtubules

Microtubules are a conspicuous aspect of platelet ultrastructure, forming a circumferential ring (Fig. 1). They are believed to function primarily as a cytoskeleton, but some type of participation in contractile processes cannot be excluded, since the microtubular ring appears to contract when platelets are stimulated. Tubulin, the subunit of microtubules, has recently been isolated from platelets (Castle and Crawford, 1975) by methods essentially the same as those used with other tissues. It bound colchicine and comigrated with brain tubulin on SDS gel electrophoresis. The isolation from platelets of a protein that bound a small amount of colchicine and activated myosin MgATPase was also reported (Puszkin *et al.*, 1971). This is an intriguing observation, but unfortunately the possible presence of actin was tested only by polymerizing actin under standard conditions, and it is now known that platelet actin has unusual polymerization properties. Castle and Crawford (1975) found that a very large contamination by actin was a special problem in the purification of platelet tubulin.

### 14.6.4. Summary

Platelets contain an exceptionally large amount of actomyosin. The myosin is similar to that from other nonmuscle cells, and the actin is observed in two different forms. Neither the cellular location nor the mechanism of regulation of platelet actomyosin has been clearly established. Although platelets have many functions that might involve contractility, there is no definitive evidence for the involvement of actomyosin in any platelet process.

## References

Abramowitz, J., Detwiler, T., Dow, J., and Stracher, A., 1971, Isolation and properties of a myosin-like protein from platelets, *Biophys. J.* **11**:108 (Abstract).

Abramowitz, J., Malik, M. N., Stracher, A., and Detwiler, T. C., 1972a, Studies on the contractile proteins from blood platelets, *Cold Spring Harbor Symp. Quant. Biol.* **37**:595.

Abramowitz, J., Stracher, A., and Detwiler, T. C., 1972b, The differential effect of Ca-ATP and Mg-ATP on platelet actomyosin, *Biochem. Biophys. Res. Commun.* **49**:958.

Abramowitz, J., Stracher, A., and Detwiler, T. C., 1974, Proteolysis of myosin during platelet storage, *J. Clin. Invest.* **53**:1493.

Abramowitz, J. W., Stracher, A., and Detwiler, T. C., 1975, A second form of platelet actin: Platelet microfilaments depolymerized by ATP and divalent cations, *Arch. Biochem. Biophys.* **167**:230.

Adelstein, R. S., and Conti, M. A., 1972, The characterization of contractile proteins from platelets and fibroblasts, *Cold Spring Harbor Symp. Quant. Biol.* **37**:599.

Adelstein, R. S., and Conti, M. A., 1975, Phosphorylation of platelet myosin increases actin-activated myosin ATPase activity, *Nature (London)* **256**:597.

Adelstein, R. S., Pollard, T. D., and Kuehl, W. M., 1971, Isolation and characterization of myosin and two myosin fragments from human blood platelets, *Proc. Nat. Acad. Sci. U.S.A.* **68**:2703.

Adelstein, R. S., Conti, M. A., and Anderson, W., Jr., 1973, Phosphorylation of human platelet myosin, *Proc. Nat. Acad. Sci. U.S.A.* **70**:3115.

Baenziger, N. L., Brodie, G. N., and Majerus, P. W., 1971, A thrombin-sensitive protein of human platelet membranes, *Proc. Nat. Acad. Sci. U.S.A.* **68**:240.

Baenziger, N. L., Brodie, G. N., and Majerus, P. W., 1972, Isolation and properties of a thrombin-sensitive protein of human platelets, *J. Biol. Chem.* **247**:2723.

Ball, G., Brereton, G. G., Fulwood, M., Ireland, D. M., and Yates, P., 1970, Effect of prostaglandin $E_1$ alone and in combination with theophylline or aspirin on collagen-induced platelet aggregation and on platelet nucleotides including 3':5'-cyclic monophosphate, *Biochem. J.* **120**:709.

Barany, M., 1967, ATPase of myosin correlated with speed of muscle shortening, *J. Gen. Physiol.* **50**:197.

Barber, A. J., and Jamieson, G. A., 1970, Isolation and characterization of plasma membranes from human blood platelets, *J. Biol. Chem.* **245**:6357.

Barber, A. J., and Jamieson, G. A., 1971a, Platelet collagen adhesion: Characterization of collagen glucosyltransferase of plasma membranes of human blood platelets, *Biochim. Biophys. Acta* **252**:533.

Barber, A. J., and Jamieson, G. A., 1971b, Characterization of membrane bound collagen galactosyltransferase of human blood platelets, *Biochim. Biophys. Acta* **252**:546.

Barber, A. J., and Jamieson, G. A., 1971c, Isolation of glycopeptides from low- and high-density platelet plasma membranes, *Biochemistry* **10**:4711.

Behnke, O., Kristensen, B. I., and Nielsen, L. E., 1971, Electron microscopical observations on actinoid and myosinoid filaments in blood platelets, *J. Ultrastruct. Res.* **37**:351.

Bettex-Galland, M., and Luscher, E. F., 1959, Extraction of an actomyosin-like protein from human thrombocytes, *Nature (London)* **184**:276.

Bettex-Galland, M., and Luscher, E. F., 1961, Thrombosthenin—A contractile protein from thrombocytes. Its extraction from human blood platelets and some of its properties, *Biochim. Biophys. Acta* **49**:536.

Booyse, F. M., Sternberger, L. A., Zschocke, D., and Rafelson, M. E., 1971a, Ultrastructural localization of contractile protein (thrombosthenin) in human platelets using an unlabeled peroxidase staining technique, *J. Histochem. Cytochem.* **19**:540.

Booyse, F. M., Hoveke, T. P., Zschocke, D., and Rafelson, M. E., Jr., 1971b, Human platelet myosin, *J. Biol. Chem.* **246**:4291.

Booyse, F. M., Hoveke, T. P., and Rafelson, M. E., 1973, Human platelet actin, *J. Biol. Chem.* **248**:4083.

Booyse, F. M., Marr, J., Yang, D.-C., Guiliani, D., and Rafelson, M. E., Jr., 1976, Adenosine cyclic 3',5'-monophosphate-dependent protein kinase from human platelets, *Biochim. Biophys. Acta* **422**:60.

Born, G. V. R., and Feinberg, H., 1975, Binding of adenosine diphosphate to intact human platelets, *J. Physiol.* **251**:803.

Bosmann, H. B., 1971, Platelet adhesiveness and aggregation: The collagen:glycosyl, polypeptide:*N*-acetylgalactosaminyl and glycoprotein:galactosyl transferases of human platelets, *Biochem. Biophys. Res. Commun.* **43**:1118.

Brass, L. F., and Bensusan, H. B., 1974, The role of collagen quaternary structure in the platelet:collagen interaction, *J. Clin. Invest.* **54**:1480.

Bray, D., 1972, Cytoplasmic actin: A comparative study, *Cold Spring Harbor Symp. Quant. Biol.* **37**:567.

Bremel, R., 1974, Myosin-linked calcium in vertebrate smooth muscle, *Nature (London)* **252**:405.

Brodie, G. N., Baenziger, N. L., Chase, L. R., and Majerus, P. W., 1972, The effects of thrombin on adenyl cyclase activity and a membrane protein from human platelets, *J. Clin. Invest.* **51**:81.

Brown, C. H., III, Bell, W. R., Schreiner, D. P., and Jackson, D. P., 1972, Effects of arvin on blood platelets. *In vitro* and *in vivo* studies, *J. Lab. Clin Med.* **79**:758.

Burger, M. M., and Noonan, K. D., 1970, Restoration of normal growth by covering of agglutinin sites on tumor cell surface, *Nature (London)* **228**:512.

Castle, A. G., and Crawford, N., 1975, Isolation of tubulin from pig platelets, *FEBS Lett.* **51**:195.

Chaiken, R., Pagano, D., and Detwiler, T. C., 1975, Regulation of platelet phosphorylase, *Biochim. Biophys. Acta* **403**:315.

Charo, I. F., Feinman, R. D., and Detwiler, T. C., 1976, Inhibition of platelet secretion by an antagonist of intracellular $Ca^{2+}$, *Biochem. Biophys. Res. Commun.* **72**:1462.

Chesney, C., McI., Harper, E., and Colman, R. W., 1972, Critical role of carbohydrate side chains of collagen in platelet aggregation, *J. Clin. Invest.* **51**:2693.

Chiang, T. M., Beachey, E. H., and Kang, A. H., 1975, Interaction of a chick skin collagen fragment ($\alpha$1-CB5) with human platelets, *J. Biol. Chem.* **250**:6916.

Ciba Foundation Symposium 35, 1975, *Biochemistry and Pharmacology of Platelets*, pp. 98–99, Elsevier, Amsterdam.

Cohen, I., and Cohen, C., 1972, A tropomyosin-like protein from human platelets, *J. Mol. Biol.* **68**:383.

Cohen, I., Bohak, Z., DeVries, A., and Katchalski, E., 1969, Thrombosthenin M. Purification and interaction with thrombin, *Eur. J. Biochem.* **10**:388.

Cohen, I., Kaminski, E., and DeVries, A., 1973, Actin-linked regulation of the human platelet contractile system, *FEBS Lett.* **34**:315.

Corey, E., Nicolaou, K., Machida, Y., Malmsten, C., and Samuelsson, B., 1975, Synthesis and biological properties of a 9,11-azo-prostanoid: Highly active biochemical mimic of prostaglandin endoperoxides, *Proc. Nat. Acad. Sci. U.S.A.* **72**:3355.

Davey, M. G., and Luscher, E. F., 1967, Actions of thrombin and other coagulant and proteolytic enzymes on blood platelets, *Nature (London)* **216**:857.

Day, H. J., and Holmsen, H., 1971, Concepts of the platelet release reaction, *Ser. Haematol.* **4**:3.

Detwiler, T. C., and Feinman, R. D., 1973a, Kinetics of the thrombin-induced release of Ca(II) by platelets, *Biochemistry* **12**:282.

Detwiler, T. C., and Feinman, R. D., 1973b, Kinetics of the thrombin-induced release of adenosine triphosphate by platelets. Comparison with release of calcium, *Biochemistry,* **12**:2462.

Detwiler, T. C., Martin, B. M., and Feinman, R. D., 1975, Stimulus–response coupling in the thrombin-platelet interaction, *in Biochemistry and Pharmacology of Platelets, Ciba Foundation Symposium 35 (New Series)*, pp. 77–91, Elsevier, Amsterdam.

Ebashi, S., 1976, Excitation–contraction coupling, *Annu. Rev. Physiol.* **39**:293.

Elzinga, M., Maron, B. J., and Adelstein, R. S., 1976, Human heart and platelet actins are products of different genes, *Science* **191**:94.

Feinman, R. D., and Detwiler, T. C., 1974, Platelet secretion induced by divalent cation ionophores, *Nature (London)* **249**:172.

Feinman, R. D., and Detwiler, T. C., 1975, Absence of a requirement for extracellular calcium for secretion from platelets, *Thromb. Res.* **7**:677.

Friedman, F., and Detwiler, T. C., 1975, Stimulus-secretion coupling in platelets. Effects of drugs on secretion of adenosine 5'-triphosphate, *Biochemistry* **14**:1315.

Gallagher, M., Detwiler, T. C., and Stracher, A., 1976, Two forms of platelet actin that differ from skeletal muscle actin, in *Cell Motility, Cold Spring Harbor Conferences on Cell Proliferation,* (R. Goldman, T. Pollard and J. Rosenbaum, eds.) Vol. 3, p. 475.

Gear, A. R. L., and Schneider, W., 1975, Control of platelet glycogenolysis: Activation of phosphorylase kinase by calcium, *Biochim. Biophys. Acta* **392**:111.

Greenberg, J. H., and Jamieson, G. A., 1974, The effects of various lectins on platelet aggregation and release, *Biochim. Biophys. Acta* **345**:231.

Guccione, M. A., Packham, M. A., Kinlough-Rathbone, R. L., and Mustard, J. F., 1971, Reactions of $^{14}$C-ADP and $^{14}$C-ATP with washed platelets from rabbits, *Blood* **37**:542.

Hadden, J. W., Hadden, E. M., Haddox, M. K., and Goldgerg, N. D., 1972, Guanosine 3':5'-cyclic monophosphate: A possible intracellular mediator of mitogenic influences in lymphocytes, *Proc. Nat. Acad. Sci. U.S.A.* **69**:3024.

Hamberg, M., and Samuelsson, B., 1973, Detection and isolation of an endoperoxide intermediate in prostaglandin biosynthesis, *Proc. Nat. Acad. Sci. U.S.A.* **70**:899.

Hamberg, M., and Samuelsson, B., 1974, Prostaglandin endoperoxides. Novel transformations of arachidonic acid in human platelets, *Proc. Nat. Acad. Sci. U.S.A.* **71**:3400.

Hamberg, M., Svensson, J., Wakabayashi, T., and Samuelsson, B., 1974a, Isolation and structure of two prostaglandin endoperoxides that cause platelet aggregation, *Proc. Nat. Acad. Sci. U.S.A.* **71**:345.

Hamberg, M., Svensson, J., and Samuelsson, B., 1974b, Prostaglandin endoperoxides. A new concept concerning the mode of action and release of prostaglandins, *Proc. Nat. Acad. Sci. U.S.A.* **71**:3824.

Hamberg, M., Svensson, J., and Samuelsson, B., 1975, Thromboxanes: A new group of biologically active compounds derived from prostaglandin endoperoxides, *Proc. Nat. Acad. Sci. U.S.A.* **72**:2994.

Hanson, J. P., Repke, D. I., Katz, A. M., and Aledort, L. M., 1973, Calcium ion control of platelet thrombosthenin ATPase activity, *Biochim. Biophys. Acta* **314**:382.

Harbury, C. B., Hershgold, J. E., and Schrier, S. L., 1972, Requirements for aggregation of washed human platelets suspended in buffered salt solutions, *Thromb. Diath. Haemorrh.* **28**:1.

Harper, E., Simons, E. R., Chesney, C. McI., and Coleman, R. W., 1975, The effect of chemical or enzymatic modifications upon the ability of collagen to form multimers and to initiate platelet aggregation, *Thromb. Res.* **7**:113.

Haslam, R. J., 1973, Interactions of the pharmacological receptors of blood platelets with adenylate cyclase, *Ser. Hematol. VI* **3**:333.

Haslam, R. J., and McClenaghan, M. D., 1974, Effects of collagen and of aspirin on the concentration of guanosine 3':5'-cyclic monophosphate in human platelets: Measurement by a prelabelling technique, *Biochem. J.* **138**:317.

Haslam, R. J., and Taylor, A., 1971, Role of cyclic 3',5'-adenosine monophosphate in platelet aggregation, *in Platelet Aggregation* (J. Caen, ed.), p. 85, Masson, Paris.

Haslam, R. J., 1975, Roles of cyclic nucleotides in platelet function, *in Biochemistry and Pharmacology of Platelets,* Ciba Foundation Symposium 35, (New Series) pp. 121–151, Elsevier, Amsterdam.

Jaffe, R. M., 1977, Platelet interaction with connective tissue, in *Cellular Reactions of Blood Platelets* (J. Gordon, ed.), p. 261.

Jaffe, R., and Deykin, D., 1974, Evidence for a structural requirement for the aggregation of platelets by collagen, *J. Clin. Invest.* **53**:875.

Jamieson, G. A., 1974a, Glycosyltransferases in platelet adhesion, *Thromb. Diath. Haemorrh.* **LX** (Suppl.):111.

Jamieson, G. A., 1974b, Biochemical events in platelet–collagen adhesion, *in Platelets and Thrombosis* (S. Sherry and A. Scriabine, eds.), p. 139, University Park Press, Baltimore, Maryland.

Jamieson, G. A., Urban, C. L., and Barber, A. J., 1971, Enzymatic basis for platelet:collagen adhesion as the primary step in haemostasis, *Nature New Biol.* **234**:5.

Kang, A. H., Beachey, E. H., and Katzman, R. L., 1974, Interaction of an active glycopeptide from chick skin collagen ($\alpha$1-CB5) with human platelets, *J. Biol. Chem.* **249**:1054.

Kaplan, K. L., and Nachman, R. L., 1975, The interaction of platelets and concanavalin A, *Thromb. Res.* **7**:847.

Katzman, R. L., Kang, A. H., and Beachey, E. H., 1973, Collagen-induced platelet aggregation: Involvement of an active glycopeptide fragment ($\alpha$1-CB5), *Science* **181**:670.

Kloeze, J., 1967, Influence of prostaglandins on platelet adhesiveness and platelet aggregation, *in Prostaglandins* (S. Bergstrom and B. Samuelsson, eds.), p. 241, Wiley-Interscience, New York.

Laskowski, M., Jr., and Sealock, R. W., 1971, Protein-proteinase inhibitors—Molecular aspects, *Enzymes* **3**:376.

Lis, H., and Sharon, N., 1973, The biochemistry of plant lectins (phytohemagglutinins), *Annu. Rev. Biochem.* **42**:541.

Lucas, R. C., Gallagher, M., and Stracher, A., 1977, *Actin and Actin Binding Protein in Platelets*, Symposium on Contractile Systems in Non-Muscle Tissues, pp. 31–39, North Holland-Elsevier, Amsterdam.

Lyons, R. M., Stanford, N., and Majerus, P. W., 1975, Thrombin-induced protein phosphorylation in human platelets, *J. Clin. Invest.* **56**:924.

Magnusson, S., 1971, Thrombin and prothrombin, *Enzymes* **3**:277.

Malik, M. N., Abramowitz, J., Detwiler, T. C., and Stracher, A., 1974a, Enzymatic properties of platelet actomyosin, *Arch Biochem. Biophys.* **161**:268.

Malik, M. N., Detwiler, T. C., and Stracher, A., 1974b, Allosteric regulation of platelet actomyosin, *Biochem. Biophys. Res. Commun.* **55**:912.

Malik, M. N., Rosenberg, S., Detwiler, T. C., and Stracher, A., 1974c, Role of $Ca^{2+}$ in the allosteric regulation of platelet actomyosin, *Biochem. Biophys. Res. Commun.* **61**:1071.

Malmsten, C., Granstrom, E., and Samuelsson, B., 1976, Cyclic AMP inhibits synthesis of prostaglandin endoperoxide ($PGG_2$) in human platelets, *Biochem. Biophys. Res. Commun.* **68**:569.

Marcus, A. J., 1969, Platelet function, *N. Engl. J. Med.* **280**:1213, 1278, 1330.

Marcus, A. J., and Zucker, M. B., 1965, *The Physiology of Blood Platelets*, Grune & Stratton, New York.

Marcus, A. J., Ullman, H. L., and Safier, L. B., 1969, Lipid composition of subcellular particles of human blood platelets, *J. Lipid Res.* **10**:108.

Martin, B. M., Feinman, R. D., and Detwiler, T. C., 1975, Platelet stimulation by thrombin and other proteases, *Biochemistry* **14**:1308.

Martin, B. M., Wasiewski, W., Fenton, J. W., II, and Detwiler, T. C., 1976, The equilibrium binding of thrombin to platelets, *Biochemistry* **15**:4886.

Massini, P., and Luscher, E. F., 1974, Some effects of ionophores for divalent cations on blood platelets. Comparison with the effects of thrombin, *Biochim. Biophys. Acta* **372**:109.

McDonald, J. W. D., and Stuart, R. K., 1973, Regulation of cyclic AMP levels and aggregation in human platelets by prostaglandin $E_1$, *J. Lab. Clin. Med.* **81**:839.

Michal, F., and Born, G. V. R., 1971, Effect of rapid shape change of platelets on the transmission and scattering of light through plasma, *Nature (London)* **231**:220.

Mills, D. C. B., and MacFarlane, D. E., 1974, Stimulation of human platelet adenylate cyclase by prostaglandin $D_2$, *Thromb. Res.* **5**:401.

Mills, D. C. B., and MacFarlane, D. E., 1975, The effects of ATP on platelets: Evidence against the central role of released ADP in primary aggregation, *Blood* **46**:309.

Mohammed, S. F., Whitworth, C., Chuang, H. Y. K., Lundblad, R. L., and Mason, R. G., 1976, Multiple active forms of thrombin: Binding to platelets and effects on platelet function, *Proc. Nat. Acad. Sci. U.S.A.* **73**:1660.

Muggli, R., and Baumgartner, H. R., 1973, Collagen-induced platelet aggregation: Requirements for tropocollagen multimers, *Thromb. Res.* **3**:715.

Murer, E. H., 1969, Thrombin-induced release of calcium from blood platelets, *Science* **166**:623.

Mustard, J. F., and Packham, M. A., 1970, Factors influencing platelet function: Adhesion, release, and aggregation, *Pharmacol. Rev.* **22**:97.

Mustard, J. F., Packham, M. A., Perry, D. W., Guccione, M. A., and Kinlough-Rathbone, R. L., 1975, Enzyme activities on the platelet surface in relation to the action of adenosine diphosphate, *in Biochemistry and Pharmacology of Platelets*, Ciba Foundation Symposium 35 (New Series), p. 47, Elsevier, Amsterdam.

Muszbek, L., Fesus, L., Olveti, E., and Szabo, T., 1976, Cleavage of thrombosthenin A by thrombin. Evidence for the existence of two types of bovine platelet actin, *Biochim. Biophys. Acta* **427**:171.

Nachman, R. L., 1975, Binding of adensine diphosphate by human platelet membrane, *in Biochemistry and Pharmacology of Platelets*, Ciba Foundation Symposium 35 (New Series), pp. 23–37, Elsevier, Amsterdam.

Nachman, R. L., and Ferris, B., 1972, Studies on the proteins of human platelet membranes, *J. Biol. Chem.* **247**:4468.

Nachman, R. L., and Ferris, B., 1974, Binding of adenosine diphosphate by isolated membranes from human platelets, *J. Biol. Chem.* **249**:704.

Nachman, R. L., and Kaplan, K. L., 1975, The interaction of platelets and concanavalin A, *Thromb. Res.* **7**:847.

Nachman, R. L., Marcus, A. J., and Safier, L. B., 1967, Platelet thrombosthenin: Subcellular localization and function, *J. Clin Invest.* **46**:1380.

Nachman, R. L., Hubbard, A., and Ferris, B., 1973, Iodination of the human platelet membrane, *J. Biol. Chem.* **248**:2928.

Niederman, R., and Pollard, T. D., 1975, Human platelet myosin. II. *In vitro* assembly and structure of myosin filaments, *J. Cell Biol.* **67**:72.

Nugteren, D. H., and Hazelhof, E., 1973, Isolation and properties of intermediates in prostaglandin biosynthesis, *Biochim. Biophys. Acta* **326**:448.

Pepper, D. S., and Jamieson, G. A., 1969, Studies on glycoproteins. III. Isolation of sialoglycopeptides from human platelet membranes, *Biochemistry* **8**:3362.

Phillips, D. R., 1972, Effect of trypsin on the exposed polypeptides and glycoproteins in the human platelet membrane, *Biochemistry* **11**:4582.

Phillips, D. R., 1974, Thrombin interaction with human platelets. Potentiation of thrombin-induced aggregation and release by inactivated thrombin, *Thromb. Diath. Haemorrh.* **32**:207.

Phillips, D. R., and Agin, P. P., 1974, Thrombin substrates and the proteolytic site of thrombin action on human platelet plasma membranes, *Biochim. Biophys. Acta* **352**:218.

Phillips, D. R., Jenkins, C. S. P., Luscher, E. F., and Larrieu, M.-J., 1975, Molecular differences of exposed surface proteins on thrombasthenic platelet plasma membranes, *Nature (London)* **257**:599.

Piper, P. J., and Vane, J. R., 1969, Release of additional factors in anaphylaxis and its antagonism by anti-inflammatory drugs, *Nature (London)* **223**:29.

Pollard, T. D., 1975, Functional implications of the biochemical and structural properties of cytoplasmic contractile proteins, *in Molecules and Cell Movement* (S. Inoue and R. E. Stephens, eds.), pp. 259–285, Raven Press, New York.

Pollard, T. D., and Weihing, R. R., 1974, Actin and myosin and cell movement, *Crit. Rev. Biochem.* **2**:1.

Pollard, T. D., Thoms, S. M., and Niederman, R., 1974, Human platelet myosin. I. Purification by a rapid method applicable to other nonmuscle cells, *Anal. Biochem.* **60**:258.

Pressman, B. C., 1973, Properties of ionophores with broad range of cation selectivity, *Fed. Proc.* **32**:1698.

Probst, E., and Luscher, E. F., 1972, Studies on thrombosthenin A, the actin-like moiety of the contractile protein from blood platelets. I. Isolation, characterization and evidence for two forms of thrombosthenin A, *Biochim. Biophys. Acta* **278**:577.

Puszkin, E., Puszkin, S., and Aledort, L. M., 1971, Colchicine-binding protein from human platelets and its effect on muscle myosin and platelet myosin-like thrombosthenin-M, *J. Biol. Chem.* **246**:271.

Puszkin, S., Kochwa, S., Puszkin, E. G., and Rosenfield, R. E., 1975, A solid–liquid biphasic model for characterization of properties of muscle and platelet contractile proteins, *J. Biol. Chem.* **250**:2085.

Rasmussen, H., Goodman, D. B. P., and Tenenhouse, A., 1972, The role of cyclic AMP and calcium in cell activation, *CRC Crit. Rev. Biochem.* **1**:95.

Robblee, L. S., Shepro, D., and Belamarich, F. A., 1973a, Calcium uptake and associated adenosine triphosphatase activity of isolated platelet membranes, *J. Gen. Physiol.* **61**:462.

Robblee, L. S., Shepro, D., Belamarich, F. A., and Towle, C., 1973b, Platelet calcium flux and the release reaction, *Ser. Haematol.* **6**:311.

Ross, R., Glomset, J., Kariya, B., and Harker, L., 1974, A platelet-dependent serum factor that stimulates the proliferation of arterial smooth muscle cells *in vitro, Proc. Nat. Acad. Sci. U.S.A.* **71**:1207.

Rubin, R. P., 1974, *Calcium and the Secretory Process,* Plenum Press, New York.

Rutherford, R. B., and Ross, R., 1976, Platelet factors stimulate fibroblasts and smooth muscle cells quiescent in plasma serum to proliferate, *J. Cell. Biol.* **69**:203.

Salzman, E. W., 1976, Prostaglandins and platelet function, *in Advances in Prostaglandin and Thromboxane Research* (Samuelsson and Paoletti, eds.), p. 767, Raven Press, New York.

Salzman, E. W., and Neri, L. L., 1969, Cyclic 3',5'-adenosine monophosphate in human blood platelets, *Nature (London)* **224**:609.

Sato, T., Herman, L., Chandler, J. A., Stracher, A., and Detwiler, T. C., 1975, Localization of a thrombin-sensitive calcium pool in platelets, *J. Histochem. Cytochem.* **23**:103.

Sekhar, N. C., 1970, Effect of eight prostaglandins on platelet aggregation, *J. Med. Chem.* **13**:39.

Shuman, M. A., and Majerus, P. W., 1975, The perturbation of thrombin binding to human platelets by anions, *J. Clin. Invest.* **56**:945.

Silver, M. J., Smith, J. B., Ingerman, C., and Kocsis, J. J., 1973, Arachidonic acid-induced human platelet aggregation and prostaglandin formation, *Prostaglandins* **4**:863.

Simons, E. R., Chesney, C. McI., Coleman, R. W., Harper, E., and Samberg, E., 1975, The effect of the conformation of collagen on its ability to aggregate platelets, *Thromb. Res.* **7**:123.

Singer, S. J., and Nicolson, G. L., 1972, The fluid mosaic model of the structure of cell membranes, *Science* **175**:720.

Smith, J. B., and Macfarlane, D. E., 1974, Platelets, *in The Prostaglandins,* (P. Ramwell, ed.), p. 293, Plenum Press, New York.

Smith, J. B., and Willis, A. L., 1970, Formation and release of prostaglandins by platelets in response to thrombin, *Br. J. Pharmacol.* **40**:545.

Smith, J. B., and Willis, A. L., 1971, Aspirin selectively inhibits prostaglandin production in human platelets, *Nature (London)* **231**:235.

Smith, J. B., Ingerman, C., Kocsis, J., and Silver, M., 1973, Formation of prostaglandins during the aggregation of human blood platelets, *J. Clin. Invest.* **52**:965.

Smith, J. B., Ingerman, C. M., and Silver, M. J., 1975, Prostaglandins and precursors in platelet function, *in Biochemistry and Pharmacology of Platelets,* Ciba Foundation Symposium 35 (New Series), p. 23, Elsevier, Amsterdam.

Smith, J. B., Ingerman, C. M., and Silver, M. J., 1976a, Platelet prostaglandin production and its implications, *in Advances in Prostaglandin and Thromboxane Research* (Samuelsson and Paoletti, eds.), p. 747, Raven Press, New York.

Smith, J. B., Ingerman, C. M., and Silver, M. J., 1976b, Malondialdehyde formation as an indicator of prostaglandin production by human platelets, *J. Lab. Clin. Med.* **88**:167.

Sobieszek, A., and Small, J. V., 1976, Myosin-linked calcium regulation in vertebrate smooth muscle, *J. Mol. Biol.* **101**:75.

Spudich, J. A., 1972, Effects of cytochalasin B on actin filaments, *Cold Spring Harbor Symp. Quant. Biol.* **37**:585.

Statland, B. E., Heagan, B. M., and White, J. G., 1969, Uptake of calcium by platelet relaxing factor, *Nature (London)* **223**:521.

Steiner, M., 1973, Effect of thrombin on the platelet membrane, *Biochim. Biophys. Acta* **323**:653.

Sutherland, E. W., and Rall, T. W., 1960, The relation of adenosine-3',5'-cyclic monophosphate and phosphorylase to the actions of catecholamines and other hormones, *Pharmacol. Rev.* **12**:265.

Tanner, M. J. A., and Boxer, D. H., 1974, A set of surface proteins common to the circulating human platelet and lymphocyte, *Biochem. J.* **141**:909.

Tilney, L. G., 1975, The role of actin in nonmuscle cell motility, *in Molecules and Cell Movement* (S. Inoue and R. E. Stephens, eds.), pp. 339–388, Raven Press, New York.

Tollefsen, D. M., and Majerus, P. W., 1976, Evidence for a single class of thrombin-binding sites on human platelets, *Biochemistry* **15**:2144.

Tollefsen, D. M., Feagler, J. R., and Majerus, P. W., 1974a, The binding of thrombin to the surface of human platelets, *J. Biol. Chem.* **249**:2646.

Tollefsen, D. M., Feagler, J. R., and Majerus, P. W., 1974b, Induction of the platelet release reaction by phytohemagglutinin, *J. Clin. Invest.* **53**:211.

Tollefsen, D. M., Jackson, C. M., and Majerus, P. W., 1975, Binding of the products of prothrombin activation to human platelets, *J. Clin. Invest.* **56**:241.

Weiss, H. J., 1976, Platelet physiology and abnormalities of platelet function, *N. Engl. J. Med.* **293**:531, 580.

Weiss, H. J., and Aledort, L. M., 1967, Impaired platelet/connective-tissue reaction in man after aspirin ingestion, *Lancet* **ii**:495.

Weissmann, G., and Claiborne, R. (eds.), 1975, *Cell Membranes: Biochemistry, Cell Biology and Pathology*, HP Publishing Co., New York.

White, J. G., 1971, Platelet morphology, *in The Circulating Platelet* (S. Johnson, ed.), pp. 45–121, Academic Press, New York.

White, J. G., 1972, Interaction of membrane systems in blood platelets, *Am. J. Pathol.* **66**:295.

White, J. G., Goldberg, N. D., Estensen, R. D., Haddox, M. K., and Rao, G. H. R., 1973, Rapid increase in platelet cyclic 3',5'-guanosine monophosphate (cGMP) levels in association with irreversible aggregation, degranulation, and secretion, *J. Clin. Invest.* **52**:89 (Abstract).

White, J. G., Rao, G. H. R., and Gerrard, J. M., 1974, Effects of the ionophore A23187 on blood platelets. I. Influence on aggregation and secretion, *Am. J. Pathol.* **77**:135.

Willis, A. L., and Kuhn, D., 1973, A new potential mediator of arterial thrombosis whose biosynthesis is inhibited by aspirin, *Prostaglandins* **4**:127.

Willis, A. L., Vane, F. M., Kuhn, D. C., Scott, C. G., and Petrin, M., 1974, An endoperoxide aggregator (LASS) formed in platelets in response to thrombotic stimuli, *Prostaglandins* **8**:453.

Wilner, G. D., Nossel, H. L., and LeRoy, E. C., 1968, Aggregation of platelets by collagen, *J. Clin. Invest.* **47**:2616.

Zucker-Franklin, D., 1969, Microfibrils of blood platelets: Their relationship to microtubules and the contractile protein, *J. Clin. Invest.* **48**:165.

Zucker-Franklin, D., 1970, The submembranous fibrils of human blood platelets, *J. Cell Biol.* **47**:293.

Zucker-Franklin, D., and Grusky, G., 1972, The actin and myosin filaments of human and bovine blood platelets, *J. Clin. Invest.* **51**:419.

# Significance of Platelet Volume Measurements

## Simon Karpatkin

## 15.1. Summary

Extreme density populations of platelets have been separated with differential centrifugation techniques, employing various suspending media. The heavy population is enriched with large platelets having an average volume greater than the lighter population. These large platelets have been termed megathrombocytes. The heavy fraction has been shown to be more metabolically active. This population is also more resistant to osmotic stress and lipid peroxidation.

Kinetic studies with a cohort label, [$^{75}$Se]selenomethionine, in humans and rabbits have revealed that the heavy platelet population enriched with megathrombocytes is preferentially labeled with isotope during the first 24–48 hr following isotope administration, indicating that megathrombocytes and other heavy platelets are young platelets relative to the light platelet population. Thrombopoietic studies with thrombopoietic stimuli in guinea pigs and rabbits have revealed enhanced megathrombocyte production over basal values as elucidated by Coulter Counter analysis.

Clinical studies with EDTA-peripheral smears and/or electronic platelet volume distribution analysis have revealed increased percent megathromobocytes (2.6- to 3.6-fold over basal value) during thrombocytopenias associated with increased platelet turnover such as autoimmune

SIMON KARPATKIN • New York University Medical School, New York, New York 10016.

thrombocytopenic purpura (ATP), systemic lupus erythematosus, drug-induced immunologic thrombocytopenias, disseminated intravascular coagulation (DIC), and hypersplenism. This was associated with a 2.3- to 4.2-fold increase in megakaryocyte number and excellent correlation coefficient ($r = 0.7$, $P < 0.001$).

A compensated thrombocytolytic state could be predicted in patients with normal platelet counts and increased megathrombocyte number. This was demonstrated with in vivo [$^{32}$P]DFP (diisopropyl fluorophosphate) platelet survival studies in seven patients. The possibility of a compensated thrombocytolytic state was further explored in several other clinical disorders with normal platelet counts. Increased megathrombocytes were noted in 47% of patients with ATP in apparent remission, 48% of patients with severe rheumatic heart disease (RHD), 20% of patients with RHD and prosthetic heart valves, 52% of patients with DIC, and 30% of patients with diabetes mellitis and retinopathy.

The megathrombocyte-rich population has also been shown to be functionally more active with respect to macroscopic platelet aggregation with ADP, thrombin, and epinephrine and release of adenine nucleotide. Recent studies with platelet aggregometry have demonstrated a significant correlation between platelet aggregation velocity (slope) and platelet volume parameters as determined with a Coulter Counter. The best correlation was obtained with number of large platelets or megathrombocytes ($r = 0.6$, $P < 0.001$). An inverse correlation was obtained with platelet count and volume ($r = -0.53$, $P < 0.001$).

Megathrombocytes are preferentially sequestered by the spleen and rapidly mobilized (2–6 min) by epinephrine and/or exercise. The splenic platelet pool was estimated to be 40% of total platelets, compared to a splenic megathrombocyte pool of 52% ($P < 0.05$).

It is proposed that megathrombocytes are a subpopulation of young and/or stress platelets with greater functional capacity than the remainder of the population. These correlate with increased megakaryocyte number and usually indicate increased platelet turnover. It is conceivable that some megathrombocytes fragment into two or more platelets in the peripheral circulation.

Severe autoimmune thrombocytopenias are also associated with a "small" particle peak noted on platelet volume distribution analysis. The "microcytic" peaks could be simulated in rabbits given antiplatelet antibody intravenously. Similar peaks could be simulated in unwashed human platelet fractions isolated from PRP via differential centrifugation. Recent electron microscopic data indicate the presence of red blood cell fragments as well as platelet fragments in PRP from ATP patients with "microcytic" peaks, suggesting mild red blood cell hemolysis with antibody also directed against cells other than platelets.

## 15.2. Introduction

Early studies on the heterogeneity of human platelets led to the isolation of two extreme density populations via differential centrifugation techniques employing various suspending media. The heavy population was enriched with large platelets (termed megathrombocytes), whereas the lighter population was enriched with smaller platelets. The heavy fraction was more metabolically active (Fig. 1), more resistant to osmotic stress (Fig. 2), more resistant to lipid peroxidation (Table I), and had greater functional capacity (Karpatkin, 1969a,b; Karpatkin and Charmatz, 1970; Karpatkin and Strick, 1972). When all 11 enzymes of the Embden–Meyerhof pathway plus five related enzymes were examined in platelet lysates from total, heavy and light, platelet populations, heavy platelets contained approximately twofold greater enzyme activity (per

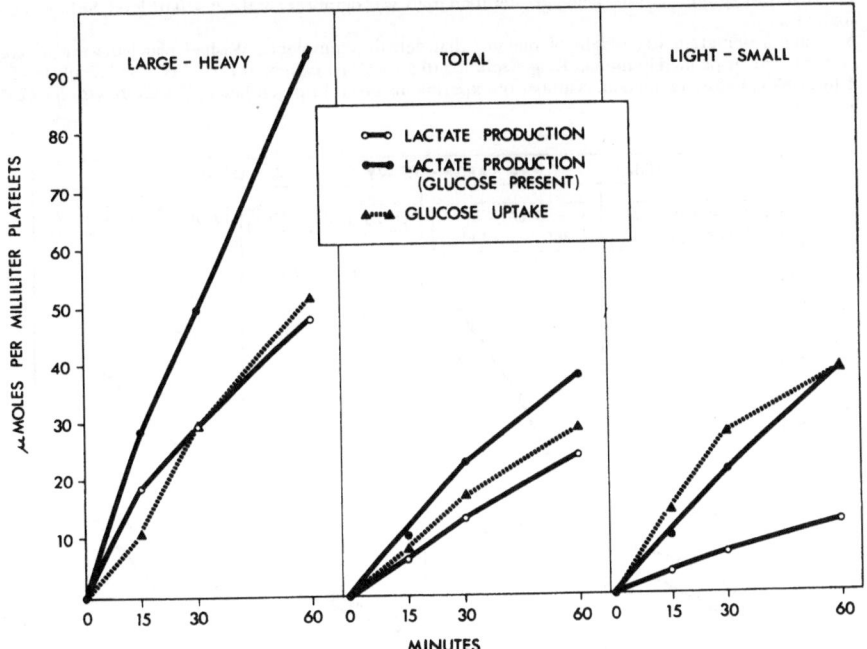

**Fig. 1.** Lactate production and glucose uptake of separate platelet populations. Human platelets were separated into extreme density populations and incubated at 37°C for 15, 30, and 60 min. Large–heavy platelets, 25% of total volume; light–small platelets, 17% of total volume; and a total population, 100% of total volume, are compared. The platelet volume ratio of large–heavy to light–small platelets was 1.9. Data are expressed as micromoles per milliliter packed platelets. Each point represents a minimum of five experiments, incubated in duplicate and assayed in triplicate. SEM was less than 10%. (*J. Clin. Invest.*, **48**:1073, 1969.)

**Table I.**  Reductive Capacity and Resistance to Lipid Peroxidation of Different Platelet Populations

| | Heavy | Total | Light | Heavy/light[a] ratio | Heavy[b] incubation |
|---|---|---|---|---|---|
| GSH (5)[c] | 10.2 | 7.20 | 5.42 | 1.9 | 6.29 |
| DPNH (4) | 0.049 | 0.035 | 0.029 | 1.7 | 0.036 |
| TPNH (4) | 0.069 | 0.063 | 0.057 | 1.2 | 0.062 |
| | | | | Light/heavy[d] ratio | |
| Lipid peroxidation (4)[e] | 2.19 | | 3.95 | 1.8 | 3.85 |
| +FeCl₃ (5) | 5.39 | | 12.94 | 2.4 | |

[a]Probability of heavy/light ratio being greater than unity was significant at the $P < 0.01$ level. SEM was less than 10%.

[b]Heavy platelets were suspended in plasma (0.5 vol %) and incubated for 1 hr (GSH) or 17 hr (DPNH, TPNH, lipid peroxidation) at 37°C, before extraction.

[c]Micromoles per gram wet weight of initially extracted GSH, DPNH, and TPNH of various platelet populations; number of experiments given in parentheses.

[d]Probability of light/heavy ratio being greater than unity was significant at the $P < 0.01$ level. SEM was less than 10%.

[e]Nanomoles per gram wet weight of malonyl dialydehyde equivalents. Washed platelets were initially extracted, or suspended in human Ringer solution (0.5 vol %) containing 0.1 mol $FeCl_3$ and incubated for 1 hr at 37°C before extraction. Number of experiments given in parentheses. (*J. Clin. Invest.*, **51**:1235, 1972.)

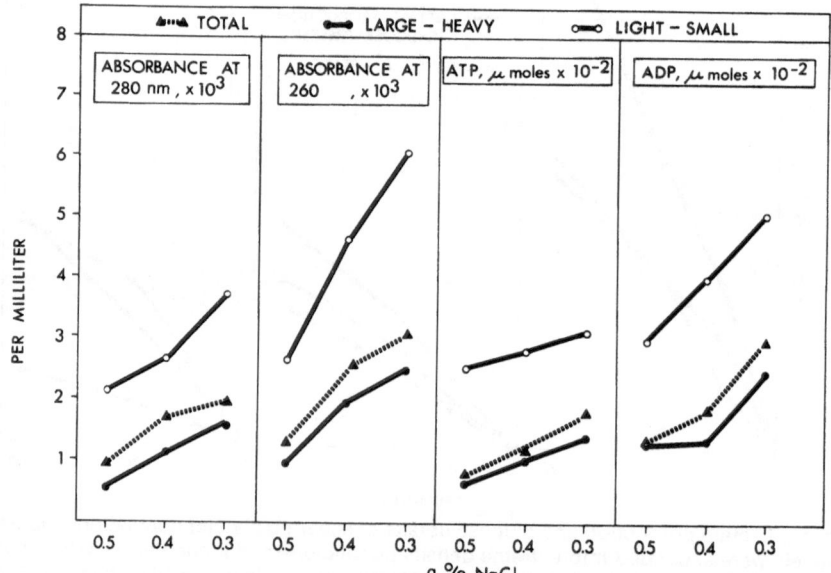

**Fig. 2.**  Resistance of separate platelet populations to osmotic shock. A 5 vol % platelet suspension was exposed to 0.3, 0.4, and 0.5 g/100 NaCl containing 5 mmol glucose for 5 min at 37°C. Release of material into the extracellular solution was measured with respect to 280 and 260 nm absorbance and with respect to ATP and ADP release. Data are expressed per milliliter of extracellular fluid. To obtain data per milliliter of platelets or per gram wet weight, divide by 0.05. Data represent four different experiments assayed in triplicate. SEM was less than 10%. (*J. Clin. Invest.*, **48**:1073, 1969.)

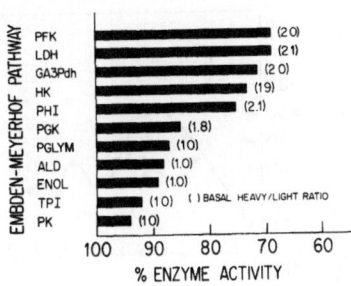

**Fig. 3.** *In vitro* incubation of heavy platelets for 17 hr at 37°C. Empirical $V_{max}$ was measured at zero time and after 17 hr of sterile incubation in plasma with 0.5 vol % platelet suspension. The percentage of remaining enzyme activity is compared with initial heavy/light ratio. Data represent the average of four incubation experiments. (*J. Clin. Invest.*, 51:1235, 1972.)

gram wet weight) than light platelets for 7 of the 11 enzymes (Fig. 3), which included the three rate-limiting enzymes: hexokinase, phosphofructokinase, and glyceraldehyde-3-phoshate dehydrogenase. *In vitro* senescence was simulated by sterile incubation of heavy platelets for 17 hr. This resulted in a significant loss of enzyme activity for the elevated seven enzymes when compared with the remainder, indicating greater *in vitro* lability for some of the Embden–Meyerhof pathway enzymes. This was associated with increased lipid peroxidation of incubated platelets and could be reversed with reducing agents such as dithiothreitol, GSH, or ascorbic acid (Karpatkin and Strick, 1972), suggesting evidence for oxidative stress during *in vitro* senescence. It was tempting to speculate that this could result from loss of glycolytic "rate limiting" enzyme activity. This could contribute to lower energy stores, i.e., glycogen and adenine nucleotide content, since the platelet is dependent to an appreciable extent on the Embden–Meyerhof pathway for its energy requirement (Karpatkin and Langer, 1968). Any impairment in energy storage or utilization could be disadvantageous to the cell with respect to viability.

These data led to the suggestion that the heavy fraction was enriched with younger–lighter platelets, the lighter fraction with smaller–older platelets; and that platelet senescence might be a function of conversion of heavy–larger platelets to lighter–smaller platelets (Karpatkin, 1969a,b; Karpatkin and Charmatz, 1970; Karpatkin and Strick, 1972).

## 15.3. *In Vivo* Kinetic Studies during Basal Conditions

This was supported by kinetic studies (Fig. 4A) performed in human volunteers (Amorosi *et al.*, 1971) with the *in vivo* cohort isotopic label, [$^{75}$Se]selenomethionine, which does not label circulating platelets but does label megakaryocytes. A critical concentration of injected isotope leads to its complete removal from the circulation by platelet precursors, other protein-synthesizing tissue, and excretion. There is insignificant *in vitro* incorporation of isotope into peripheral platelets (young platelets). The

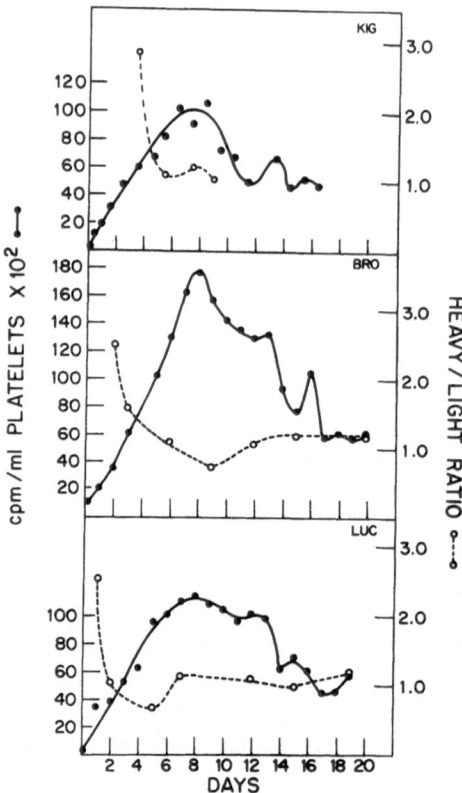

**Fig. 4A.** *In vivo* [$^{75}$Se]selenomethionine platelet survival curves on subjects Kig, Bro, and Luc. Data are expressed as cpm per milliliter of packed platelets (●). At varying time intervals, one unit of platelet-rich plasma was removed from the subject, processed into "heavy" and "light" platelet populations, and assayed for radioactivity and PCV. Data are expressed as just described. The heavy/light ratio is plotted as ○. (*Br. J. Haematol.*, 21:227, 1971.)

isotope is thought to be an irreversible label (although some reutilization does appear to take place) (Amorosi *et al.*, 1971). These properties make it possible to follow a platelet from birth to death. A theoretical senescent curve should provide an ascending limb, plateau, and descending limb. The approximation obtained *in vivo* is apparent in Fig. 4A. The time interval between the 50% ascending limb and 50% descending limb is equivalent to the platelet survival, 10–12 days. Following injection of the cohort label, platelets were harvested at various time intervals during the platelet survival (red blood cells, white blood cells, and residual plasma returned to the subject) and separated into heavy–large and light–small populations via centrifugation in inert density oils. An increase in the heavy/light specific activity ratio on early days of the survival, followed by a decrease in this ratio on later days, is consistent with the concept that heavy–large platelets are young platelets which progress with age to lighter–smaller platelets. Similar observations were obtained in rabbits (Charmatz and Karpatkin, 1974), employing a discontinuous albumin gradient (Fig. 4B) for separation of extreme heavy and light platelet populations (Fig. 4C).

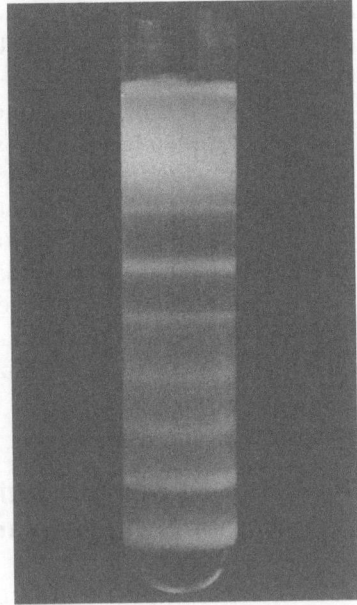

**Fig. 4B.** Photograph of albumin density gradient separation of various platelet populations. A discontinuous albumin density gradient with specific gravities ranging from 1.040 on top to 1.080 at bottom with increments of 0.005 was employed. (*Thromb. Diath. Haemorrh., 31*:485, 1974.)

These kinetic considerations, however, do not indicate that heavy–large platelets are the only young platelets. The data are also consistent with the concept that all platelets, regardless of initial size, become lighter and smaller with time. Alternatively, it is also conceivable that large–heavy platelets might be derived from megakaryocyte precursors which are more metabolically active with respect to incorporation of the cohort label and hence produce platelets which appear preferentially labeled on days 1–2 in the peripheral circulation. This has been proposed by Penington *et al.* (1976a), who recently confirmed our data in rats with reference to the platelet volume–density relationship and the decrease in heavy/light ratio with time. They suggest that heavy–large platelets are released indepen-

**Fig. 4C.** *In vivo* [$^{75}$Se]selenomethionine platelet survival curve. Six rabbits were injected intravenously on day 0 with approximately 15 $\mu$Ci/K/g of [$^{75}$Se]selenomethionine. Each rabbit represented one time point in the kinetic protocol. Data represent the average of two experiments and are expressed as cpm per packed platelets (●——●). The heavy/light ratio (○– – –○) was calculated by dividing cpm per milliliter of packed platelets obtained from the heavy platelet population isolated by cpm per milliliter of packed platelets obtained from the light platelet population. (*Thromb. Diath. Haemorrh., 31*:485, 1974.)

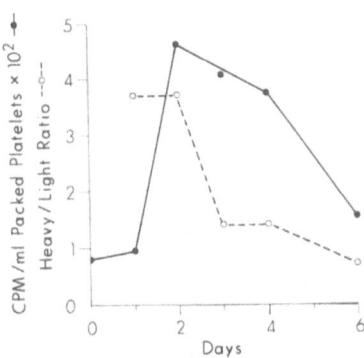

dently of lighter–smaller platelets by different bone marrow megakaryocytes (Penington *et al.,* 1976b) and that heavy platelets do not become lighter platelets. However, this would not explain the decline of the heavy/ light ratio with time unless one further postulates that metabolically active heavy–large platelets have a shorter survival than the remainder of the population, which is unlikely. Penington *et al.* (1976a) attempt to explain this decline by suggesting that heavy platelets selectively lose protein, not density, with time compared to lighter–smaller platelets. However, Penington *et al.* (1976a) do believe that platelets become smaller with age and that megathrombocytes, on the average, are younger platelets. Needless to say, both hypotheses are not mutually exclusive. Specific megakaryocytes could give rise to specific density–size platelets, which could become lighter and smaller with time, regardless of their density–size at birth.

## 15.4. Kinetic Studies during Thrombopoietic Stress ("Thrombopoietin" Injection)

Further support that large platelets (probably large–heavy platelets) or megathrombocytes are young platelets was obtained from the experiments of Weiner and Karpatkin (1972) who employed a thrombopoietic stimulus (injection of plasma from thrombocytopenic guinea pigs into recipient animals) and noted a 2.7-fold increase in megathrombocyte number (as determined by volume analysis with a Coulter Counter; see below for methodology) compared to a 1.5-fold increase in platelet count following a 4- to 5-day lag period (Fig. 5A). These observations were confirmed in another species by Weintraub and Karpatkin (1974) who employed the same thrombopoietic stimulus in rabbits and noted a twofold rise in megathrombocyte number compared to a 1.4-fold rise in

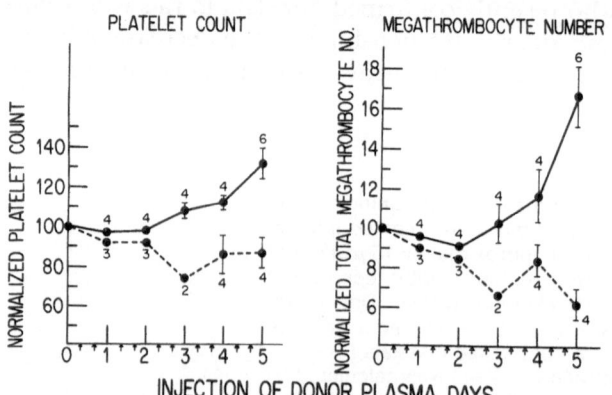

**Fig. 5A.** Platelet count and megathrombocyte number in recipient animals injected twice daily, intraperitoneally, with 1 ml of test donor plasma (•——•) or control donor plasma (○– – – ○). Arrows refer to injections. SEM and number of experiments are given. (*Thromb. Diath. Haemorrh., 28*:24, 1975.)

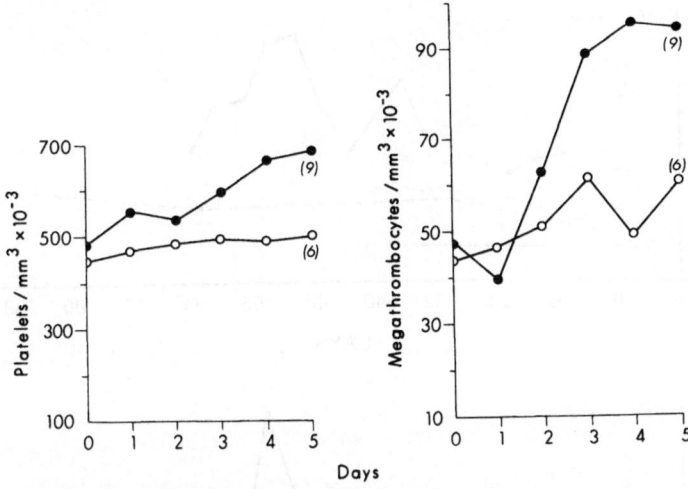

**Fig. 5B.** Platelet and megathrombocyte response to a thrombopoietic stimulus. Test animals (●) were injected intravenously twice daily for 4 days with 5 ml of plasma obtained from animals made thrombocytopenic with guinea pig anti-rabbit platelet antibody. Control animals (○) were similarly injected with plasma obtained from normal rabbits. (*J. Lab. Clin. Med.*, **83**:896, 1974.)

platelet count (Fig. 5B). However, two of their nine animals had a poor to absent rise in megathrombocyte number despite a rise in platelet count, suggesting that megathrombocytes might not be the only young platelets.

## 15.5. Kinetic Studies during Thrombopoietic Stress Induced by Blood Loss and/or Iron Deficiency

The mechanism of blood-loss-induced thrombopoiesis was also studied by measuring thrombocyte and megathrombocyte (young platelet) kinetics in guinea pigs made thrombocytotic by acute or chronic blood loss or by iron deficiency diet (Karpatkin *et al.*, 1974). Chronic blood loss alone, or iron-deficient diet alone, led to a thrombocytosis of 1.4-fold above basal values (Fig. 6). However, chronic blood loss plus replacement of iron lost via blood loss led to a 2.5-fold thrombocytosis. Of interest were the changes in megathrombocyte number or "young platelet" production (Fig. 6). Chronic blood loss alone was associated with a 1.7-fold rise in megathrombocyte number, which was 1.2-fold greater than the rise in platelet count; and chronic blood loss plus iron replacement was associated with a 3.8-fold rise in megathrombocyte number, which was 1.5-fold greater than the rise in platelet count. The thrombocytosis as a result of an iron-deficient diet was associated with a 1.4-fold rise in megathrombocyte number which was no greater than the rise in platelet count. Thus iron replacement was associated with the greatest rise in megathrombocyte

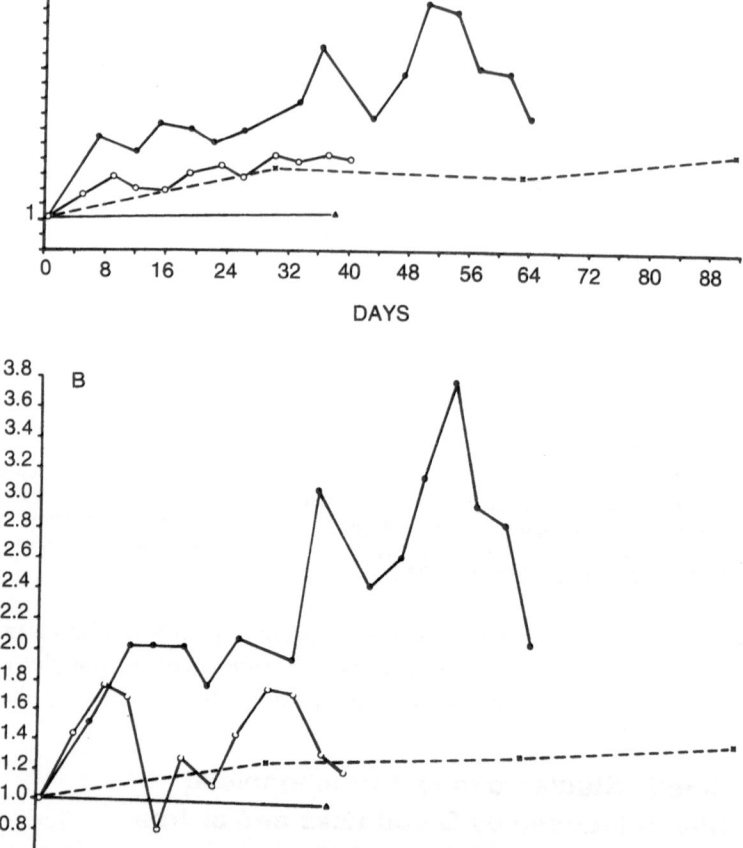

**Fig. 6.** Effect of chronic blood loss (○), chronic blood loss plus iron replacement (●), and iron deficiency diet (×) on thrombocyte (A) and megathrombocyte (B) kinetics. Guinea pigs (nine in each group) were either chronically bled by cardiac puncture, 2 ml every 3–4 days, or sham-manipulated as in control group (▲) or iron-deficient diet group (×). The amount of iron replaced (Imferon) was equivalent to the amount of iron lost in the blood removed. Abscissa refers to changes from values normalized to 1 on day 0. (*Am. J. Med.*, 57:521, 1974.)

number as well as platelet count. In acute studies (Fig. 7), acute blood loss was associated with a rise in platelet count of 1.2-fold over basal values. Acute blood loss plus iron replacement resulted in a 2.1-fold rise in platelet count. However, acute blood loss while on an iron-deficient diet resulted in no rise in platelet count. The megathrombocyte response was also of interest (Fig. 7). Whereas animals on an acute blood loss regimen increased their megathrombocyte number 1.6-fold, animals on an acute

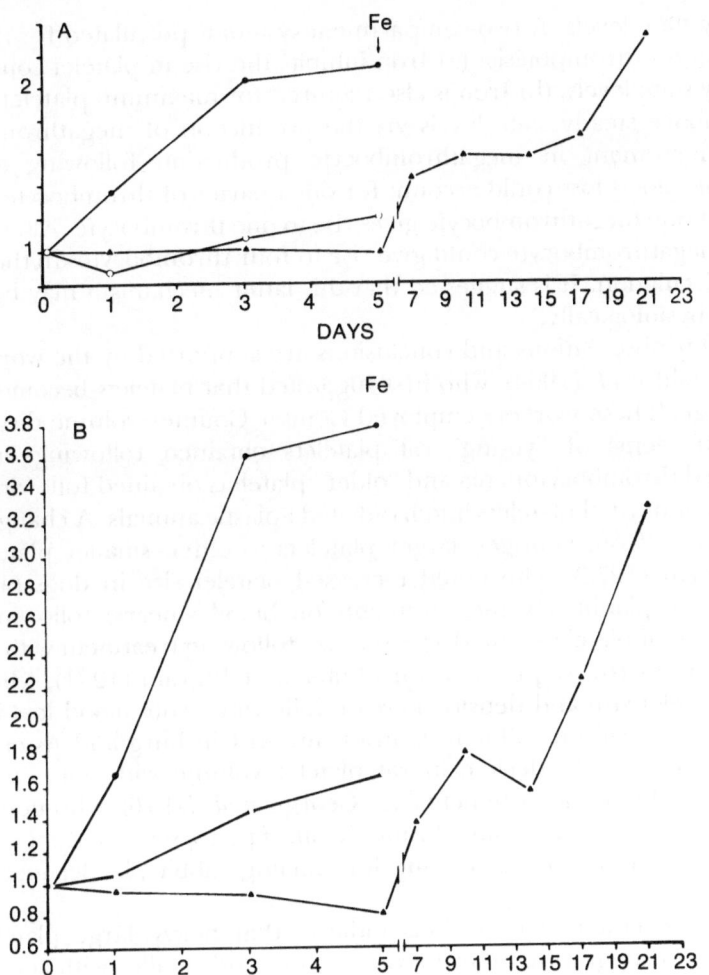

**Fig. 7.** Effect of acute blood loss (○), acute blood loss plus iron replacement (●), and acute blood loss while maintained on iron-deficient diet (▲) on thrombocyte (A) and megathrombocyte (B) kinetics. Guinea pigs (six in each group) were acutely bled, 2 ml every 2 days. On day 5 an injection of 2 mg of iron was given to the (▲) group, which was also placed on a regular diet. (*Am. J. Med.*, **57**:521, 1974.)

blood loss plus iron replacement regimen increased their megathrombocyte number 3.8-fold. However, animals acutely bled while maintained on an iron-deficient diet did not raise their megathrombocyte number. These data clearly indicate that iron is required for the production of platelets and megathrombocytes. The association of maximum platelet production with maximum megathrombocyte rise suggests that megathrombocyte production may be required for maximum platelet production above steady state levels. A two-compartment system is postulated for the effect of iron on thrompoiesis: (a) Iron inhibits the rise in platelet count above steady state levels. (b) Iron is also required for maximum platelet production above steady state levels via the production of megathrombocytes. The increment in megathrombocyte production following acute or chronic blood loss could account for one-quarter of thrombocyte production, if one megathrombocyte gives rise to one thrombocyte. Alternatively, one megathrombocyte could give rise to four thrombocytes in the peripheral circulation. It is suggested that this latter mechanism may be important physiologically.

Our observations and conclusions are supported by the work of: (1) McDonald *et al.* (1964), who first suggested that platelets become smaller with age. These workers employed Coulter Counter volume distribution measurements of "young" rat platelets obtained following antibody-induced thrombocytopenia and "older" platelets obtained following transfusion of normal platelets into irradiated aplastic animals. A change in size was noted from younger–larger platelets to older–smaller platelets. (2) Kraytman (1973), who noted increased platelet size in dogs (as determined by planimetry measurements on blood smears) following acute depletion of platelets, and decreased size following treatment with antimycin C, a marrow depressant. (3) Minter and Ingram (1971), who noted that platelet size and density increase following acute blood loss in dogs, employing a silicone oil density gradient. (4) Ginsburg and Aster (1972), who noted a 22% decline in rat platelet volume with age, employing Coulter volume measurements. (5) George *et al.* (1976), who noted preferential loss of platelet membrane during *in vivo* senescence, employing an isotopic iodination technique for labeling rabbit platelet membranes (Fig. 8).

These kinetic observations indicate that heavy–large platelets are young and suggest that they become lighter and smaller with age. Minter and Ingram (1971) have proposed that large–heavy platelets obtained from acutely bled dogs are "stress" platelets with a normal life span. Ebbe *et al.* (1968) as well as Harker and Finch (1969) have noted an increase in megakaryocyte volume following the stress of acute thrombocytopenia. It is conceivable that those megakaryocytes could give rise to "stress" megathrombocytes. Indeed, the studies of McDonald *et al.* (1964), Kraytman (1973), and Ginsburg and Aster (1972) were also performed with "stress" platelets. However, Amorosi and co-workers (1971) and Charmatz and Karpatkin (1974) noted early preferential isotopic labeling of megathrombocytes under basal conditions in which thrombopoietic stress was not present. It is therefore possible that both situations obtain: one in which young megathrombocytes are produced normally, the other in which "stress" megathrombocytes are produced following acute platelet depletion.

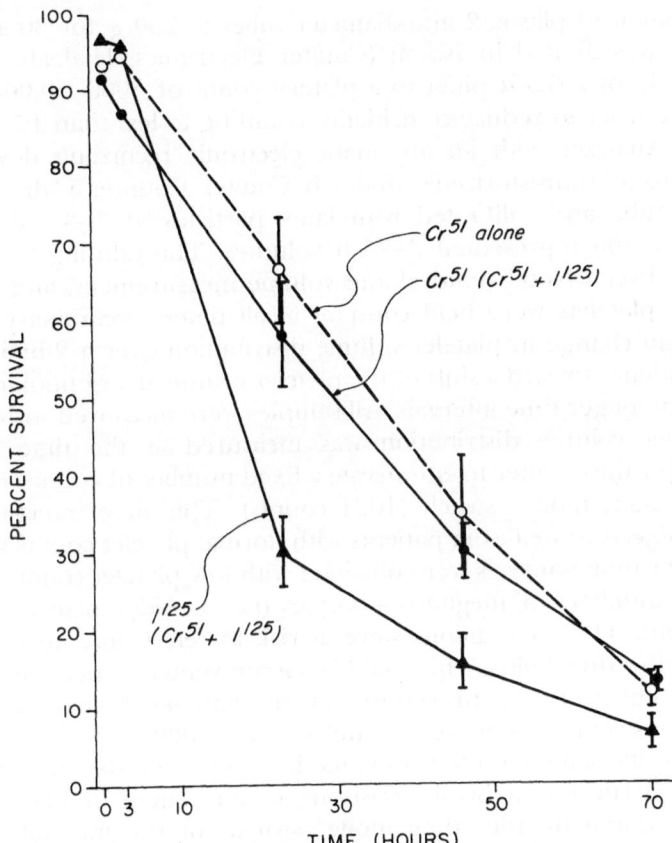

**Fig. 8.** *In vivo* survival of singly and doubly labeled platelets. Data from 11 rabbits are shown, four studied with platelets labeled by $^{51}Cr$ alone and seven studied with platelets labeled simultaneously by $^{51}Cr$ and diazotized [$^{125}I$]diiodosulfanilic acid ($DD^{125}ISA$). The point of maximal *in vivo* recovery of each isotope, which occurred at 30 min or 3 hr after injection, was assigned a value of 100%. Mean values ± SE are plotted. There was no difference among any of the values at 30 min and 3 hr and no difference between the rate of subsequent disappearance of $^{51}Cr$ of singly labeled platelets (open circles) and doubly labeled platelets (solid circles) ($P > 0.2$). The difference between the $^{51}Cr$ (solid circles) and $DD^{125}ISA$ (solid triangles) disappearance from the doubly labeled platelets was significant at 23 hr ($P < 0.002$), 46 hr ($P < 0.02$), and 70 hr ($P < 0.05$). Statistical comparisons were made using the *t* test. (J. N. George *et al.*, *J. Lab. Clin. Med.*, **88**:247, 1976.)

## 15.6. Clinical Methodology for Platelet Volume Distribution Analysis of Human Platelets

Whole blood was drawn into EDTA-anticoagulated Vacutainer tubes (Becton, Dickinson and Co., Rutherford, New Jersey). All operations were performed at room temperature. Platelet-rich plasma was obtained by centrifugation in plastic 2-mm-diameter tubes at 250 $g$ for 30 sec. The specimen was diluted in Isoton (Coulter Electronics, Hialeah, Florida) with the aid of a 3.3-$\mu$ pipet to a platelet count of 5000–10,000/0.1-ml volume in order to reduce coincidence counting to less than 1%. A P-64 Channel Analyzer with an automatic electronic recording device was attached to a "transistorized" Model B Coulter Counter with a 70-$\mu$m aperture tube and calibrated with latex particles of 3–3.5 fl so that windows 4–100 represented 2–25 fl volumes. The diluting fluid, time interval between blood removal and volume measurement, and concentration of platelets were held constant at all times. Preliminary studies revealed no change in platelet volume distribution over a 2-hr interval, with a tendency toward a shift of the platelet volume distribution curve to the right at longer time intervals. All samples were measured within 2 hr.

Platelet volume distribution was measured at the time interval required for the counter to enumerate a fixed number of counts, employing the "count mode" switch (1024 counts). This time interval in 20 normal subjects as well as in patients with normal platelet counts was 7–8 sec. Longer time intervals were obtained with low platelet counts or with increased numbers of megathrombocytes (i.e., a wider platelet volume distribution). These conditions were at risk to "electronic noise" at the lower window thresholds. This could be circumvented to negligible interference by either of three procedures: (a) addition of sufficient platelets to the isoton cuvette to achieve a platelet count 5000–10,000/0.1 ml; (b) monitoring the sample on the "time mode," and fixing this interval at 10 sec; and (c) running a blank consisting of an aliquot of platelet-poor plasma in isoton on the "time mode" switch for the interval of time required to count the platelets with the "count mode" switch. Under these conditions, significant "electronic noise" interference did not occur until time intervals of approximately 30–45 sec. The introduction of significant noise was rarely encountered and when found was not included in the studies. All measurements were made in duplicate. The aperture tube was kept clear by continual monitoring of the oscilloscope screen for "interference" distribution patterns. Background counts, as determined on the Coulter Model B, were kept at below 50 prior to use of the P-64 Channel Analyzer.

Twenty healthy laboratory personnel were employed to determine the mean platelet volume distribution scan and platelet volume parameters given in Fig. 9. Note the skewing to the right. The shaded area represents $\pm 2$ standard deviations (SD) from the mean. Microthrombocytes and/or platelet fragments were arbitrarily defined by a mean $\pm$ 2SD, $L_{50}$ value. The $L_{50}$ represents the 50 percentile point on the ascending limb (left side) of the platelet volume distribution curve where it intercepts the horizontal axis ($L_{50} = 8.38 \pm 3.18$). The megathrombocyte index was

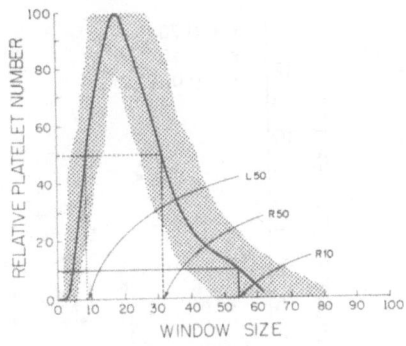

**Fig. 9.** Mean platelet volume distribution curve and platelet volume parameters for 20 normal subjects ± 2SD. An aliquot of platelet-rich plasma was diluted in isoton and then monitored on a Coulter Model B Counter attached to a P64 Channel Analyzer with automatic electronic recorder, employing a 70-μm aperture tube. Each window was calibrated to equal 0.25 fl. (*Br. J. Haematol.*, **31**:449, 1975.)

similarly arbitrarily defined by a mean ± 2SD, $R_{10}$ value. The $R_{10}$ represents the tenth percentile point on the descending limb (right side) of the platelet volume distribution curve where it intercepts the horizontal axis ($R_{10} = 55.1 \pm 15.7$). The mean peak value, or mode, was similarly obtained ± 2SD (mode = $17.5 \pm 5.64$). The mean volume was estimated by averaging the $R_{50}$ and $L_{50}$ horizontal coordinate (mean = $19.8 \pm 2.6$). Percent megathrombocytes was also arbitrarily defined as the percent total platelets having a volume of 12.5 fl or greater (i.e., all platelets enumerated between windows 50 and 100 divided by all platelets enumerated between windows 4 and 100, multiplied by 100). The standard deviation for 10 replicated measurements of these parameters obtained from a single sample cuvette varied from 0.5 to 2%.

## 15.7. Clinical Significance of Megathrombocyte Measurements

Regardless of whether megathrombocytes are normally produced or stress produced, they may be conveniently employed to predict megakaryocyte number, and hence platelet turnover (Garg *et al.*, 1971). An excellent correlation was found between the number of megakaryocytes in the bone marrow and the percentage of megathrombocytes in the peripheral blood in most clinical situations with normal or low platelet counts, $r = 0.70$, $P < 0.001$ (Fig. 10). In disorders of increased peripheral destruction or utilization of platelets, such as autoimmune thrombocytopenic purpura (ATP/ITP), drug-induced immunologic thrombocytopenic purpura, systemic lupus erythematosus (SLE), and disseminated intravascular coagulation (DIC), megathrombocyte number was increased 2.6- to 3.6-fold over basal levels. This was associated with a 2.3- to 4.2-fold increase in megakaryocyte number. In hypersplenism megathrombocyte and megakaryocyte numbers were increased 2.5- and 2.4-fold respectively. In aplas-

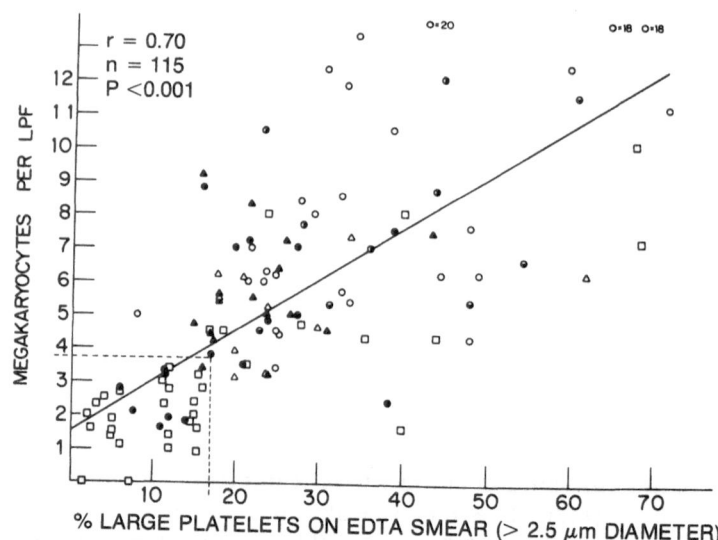

**Fig. 10.** Correlation between the percentage of large platelets on EDTA peripheral smear (diameter greater than 2.5 μm) and the number of megakaryocytes per low power field of bone marrow aspirate (100×). The open circles refer to ITP, the closed circles to SLE, the horizontal half-crossed circles to DIC, the vertical half-closed circles to drug-induced thrombocytopenia, the open triangles to hypersplenism, the closed triangles to iron deficiency anemia (normal to low platelet count), and the open boxes to other disorders. The dashed lines include +2SD of the "control mean" (95% upper confidence limit). (*N. Engl. J. Med.*, **284**:11, 1971.)

tic anemia megathrombocyte and megakaryocyte numbers were decreased to 0.35- and 0.29-fold respectively.

A compensated thrombocytolytic state could be postulated in patients with increased megathrombocytes in the peripheral blood and a normal platelet count (Garg *et al.*, 1971; Karpatkin *et al.*, 1971). This was demonstrated with *in vivo* [³²P]DFP platelet survival studies in seven patients: one with a history of easy bruising, five with SLE (Fig. 11), and one subject

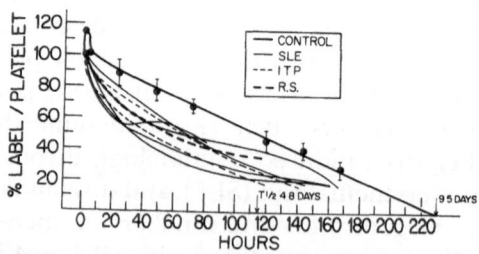

**Fig. 11.** *In vivo* [³²P]DFP platelet survival studies in 10 control subjects compared with 8 subjects having increased numbers of megathrombocytes and normal platelet counts. (*Am. J. Med.*, **51**:1, 1971.)

screened from 105 healthy volunteers with a persistent elevation of megathrombocyte number (Fig. 12). The possibility of a compensated thrombocytolytic state was further explored in several other clinical disorders with normal platelet counts, where this might be predicted (Garg *et al.*, 1972): (a) chronic autoimmune thrombocytopenic purpura (ATP) in "remission"; (b) increased utilization of platelets, such as disseminated intravascular coagulation (DIC); (c) increased mechanical destruction such as rheumatic heart disease (RHD) with abnormal heart valves and/or prosthetic devices, or small vessel angiopathies such as diabetes mellitus and retinitis, or vasculitis. Megathrombocyte elevation was noted in 47% of patients with ATP in apparent "remission," 48% of patients with severe RHD, 20% of patients with RHD and prosthetic valves, 52% of patients with DIC, and 30% of patients with diabetes mellitus and retinopathy (Fig. 13).

Patients with ATP in apparent remission are of particular interest in illustrating the compensated thrombocytolytic state. Twelve such patients with previous history of thrombocytopenia were studied during an apparent spontaneous recovery phase or an apparent recovery while on steroids. Figure 14 illustrates the marked shift to the right in their platelet volume distribution curve (dashed line) compared to the normal curve (Fig. 9), indicating increased megathrombocytes as well as other large platelets. Eight of these 12 patients eventually shifted their platelet volume distribution curves to normal patterns (solid line, Figs. 9 and 14). A negative linear relationship has recently been demonstrated for platelet count and platelet volume in normal subjects (von Behrens, 1975; Karpat-

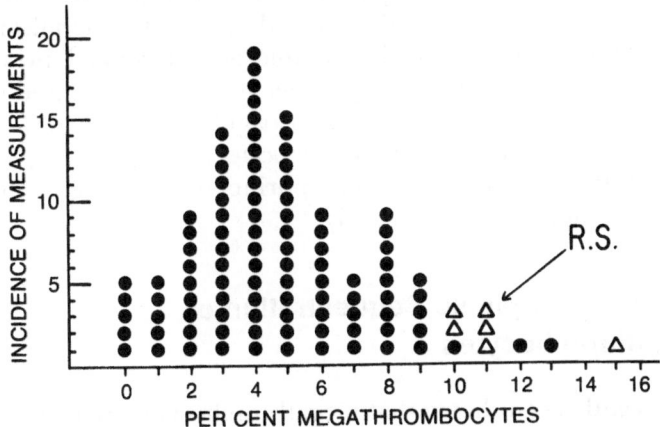

**Fig. 12.** The percentage of megathrombocytes determined by Coulter Counter in 105 normal laboratory personnel with normal platelet counts. (*Am. J. Med.,* **51**:1, 1971.)

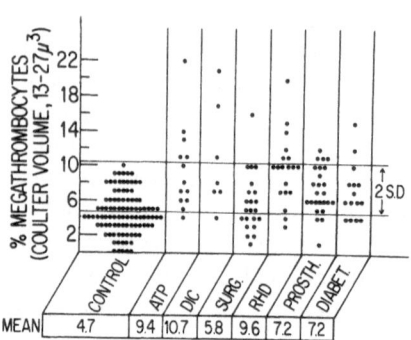

**Fig. 13.** Distribution of the percentage of megathrombocytes, as measured by a Coulter Counter, in 96 control subjects and 101 patients with normal platelet counts. These included 13 patients with chronic autoimmune thrombocytopenic purpura (ATP), 7 patients with disseminated intravascular coagulation (DIC), 22 patients studied 2 hr after surgery, 19 patients with rheumatic heart disease (RHD), 25 patients with rheumatic heart disease and prostheses (PROSTH), and 15 patients with diabetes mellitus and retinopathy (DIABET). The two thin horizontal lines refer to the mean control measurement + 2SD. Values were rounded off to the nearest whole number. (*Ann. Intern. Med.*, **77**:361, 1972.)

kin, 1976) as well as patients with various clinical disorders (O'Brien, 1974). This "normal physiologic pattern" could not explain the marked shift in platelet volume distribution for patients A, B, F, G, where no significant change in platelet count was noted.

## 15.8. Functional Capacity of Megathrombocytes

Recent studies with more sensitive techniques have revealed that large platelets are more functionally active than smaller platelets (Karpatkin, 1969a), confirming previous observations (Karpatkin, 1969b) of more rapid macroscopic aggregation as well as greater platelet release of adenine nucleotides from heavy compared to light populations exposed to thrombin, ADP, or epinephrine. Recent studies indicate a significant ($P <$ 0.001) correlation between platelet volume as determined by Coulter Counter volume measurements and platelet velocity as measured with an aggregometer in platelet-rich plasma anticoagulated with 0.38% sodium citrate. The correlation of megathrombocyte index with aggregation velocity for ADP-, collagen-, and epinephrine-induced aggregation was $r = +0.62, 0.59$, and 0.53, respectively.

## 15.9. Preferential Splenic Sequestration of Megathrombocytes

It has recently been shown that megathrombocytes are preferentially sequestered by the spleen and rapidly mobilized by epinephrine (Freedman and Karpatkin, 1975a,b) and/or exercise (Freedman and Karpatkin,

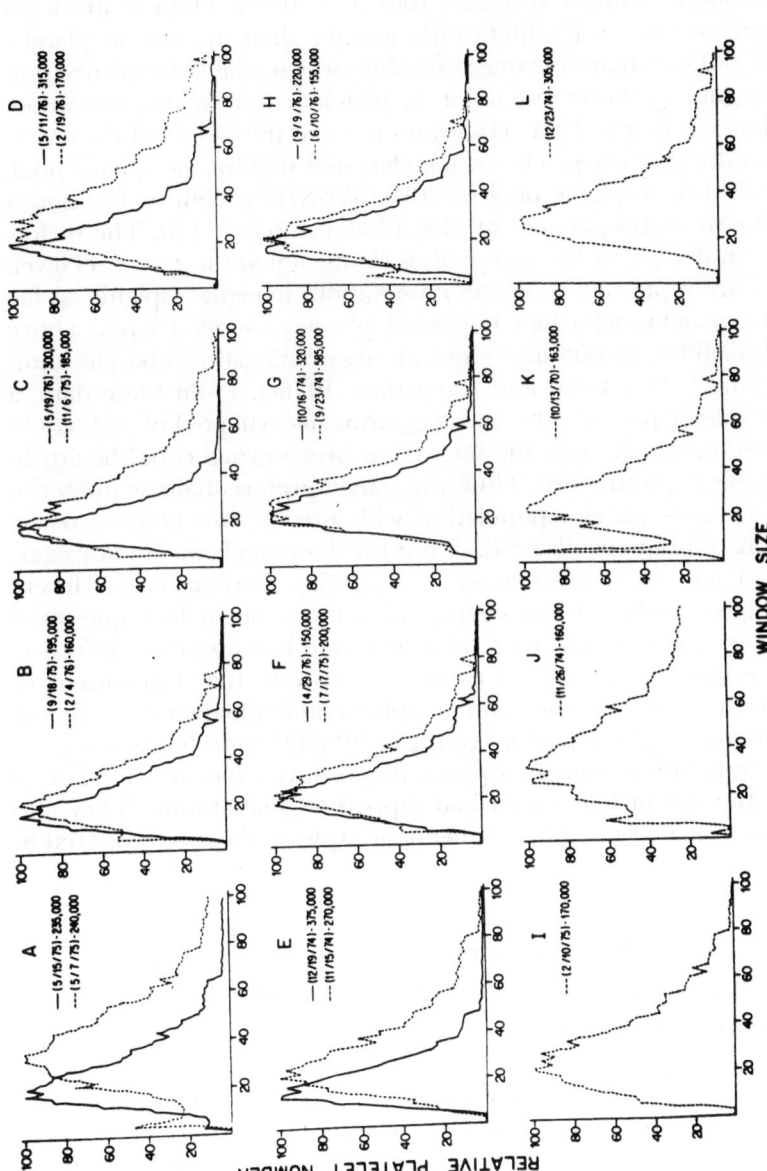

**Fig. 14.** Platelet volume distribution curves from 12 patients with autoimmune thrombocytopenic purpura in remission following a spontaneous recovery phase or recovery following treatment. Dashed curve refers to a transient shift of the platelet volume distribution curve toward the right, suggesting a compensated thrombocytolytic state. Solid curve refers to a return of the platelet volume distribution curve toward normal.

1976). Thus, following splenic blockade with phenylhydrazine treatment in rabbits, the platelet count rose 1.85-fold ($P < 0.01$) whereas the megathrombocyte number rose 2.24-fold ($P < 0.01$). The rise in megathrombocyte number was significantly greater than the rise in platelet count ($P < 0.05$). When the same procedure was repeated in splenectomized rabbits, no significant rise in either platelet count or megathrombocyte number was noted (Table II). Assuming that the source of the rise in platelet count was newly produced platelets destined for the splenic pool, one can calculate a splenic pool of 40% (378/378 + 556) $\times$ 100 and a splenic megathrombocyte pool of 52% (68/68 + 63) $\times$ 100. The difference between the size of the two pools is significant at the $P < 0.05$ level. These data are supported by recent observations in eight "asplenic" sickle cell anemia patients who had increased platelet counts 1.7-fold above normal (438,000 $\pm$ 86,000 mm$^3$) and increased megathrombocyte numbers of 2.3-fold (Freedman and Karpatkin, 1975c). From these data, a theoretical splenic pool of 40% and megathrombocyte pool of 56% could be calculated (assuming that the increment over normal could be attributed to splenic sequestration). Thus, the spleen preferentially sequesters a relatively younger platelet population with greater functional capacity which can be rapidly mobilized (2–6 min) with epinephrine and/or exercise. It is of interest that Shulman et al. (1969), employing a different approach, also concluded that young platelets are normally sequestered by the spleen and that only these platelets were hemostatically effective. Their experimental approach was to demonstrate that transfusion of platelets from a normal donor into an aplastic individual gave a bleeding time of 10 min despite a platelet count of 300,000 mm$^3$ in the recipient whereas a transfusion from an asplenic donor gave a bleeding time of 10 min only after the platelet count had dipped to 50,000 mm$^3$. They also noted better clot retraction in recipients of asplenic donors compared to normal donors.

## 15.10. Platelet and Red Blood Cell Fragmentation in Severe Autoimmune Thrombocytopenia

Platelet volume distribution curves obtained in 21 patients with autoimmune thrombocytopenic purpura revealed a striking microcytic peak (Khan et al., 1975) as well as megathrombocytes in 86% of patients studied on one or more occasion, particularly in the presence of severe thrombocytopenia, i.e., <60,000 mm$^3$ (Fig. 15). The platelet volume distribution curves revealed a shift to the left as well as right. The shift to the left was demonstrable as either a separate peak distinguishable from

**Table II.** Platelet Count and Megathrombocyte Number in Intact and Splenectomized Rabbits Following Phenylhydrazine[a]

| Day | Increment in platelet count | | | Increment in megathrombocyte number | | |
|---|---|---|---|---|---|---|
| | Intact | Splenectomy | Difference | Intact | Splenectomy | Difference |
| 0 | 556 ± 31 | 556 ± 58 | — | 63 ± 20 | 63 ± 7 | — |
| 1 | 668 ± 42 | 556 ± 71 | 112 | 79 ± 29 | 65 ± 8 | 14 |
| 2 | 840 ± 65 | 638 ± 96 | 202 | 87 ± 12 | 97 ± 27 | — |
| 3 | 1024 ± 86 | 659 ± 82 | 365 | 146 ± 29 | 68 ± 18 | 78 |
| 4 | 1036 ± 90 | 646 ± 70 | 390 | 136 ± 46 | 78 ± 17 | 58 |
| Average 3 + 4 | | | 378 | | | 68 |

[a]Sixteen intact and nine splenectomized animals were injected intramuscularly for 4 days with 1 ml of 2.5% phenylhydrazine. The mean platelet count and megathrombocyte number is given × 10⁹/liter, with SEM. The platelet count and megathrombocyte number for the splenectomized rabbits have been normalized to the same parameters for intact animals on day 0. The true platelet count and megathrombocyte number for splenectomized animals were 653 and 69 × 10⁹/liter. (*Br. J. Haematol.*, **31**:255, 1975.)

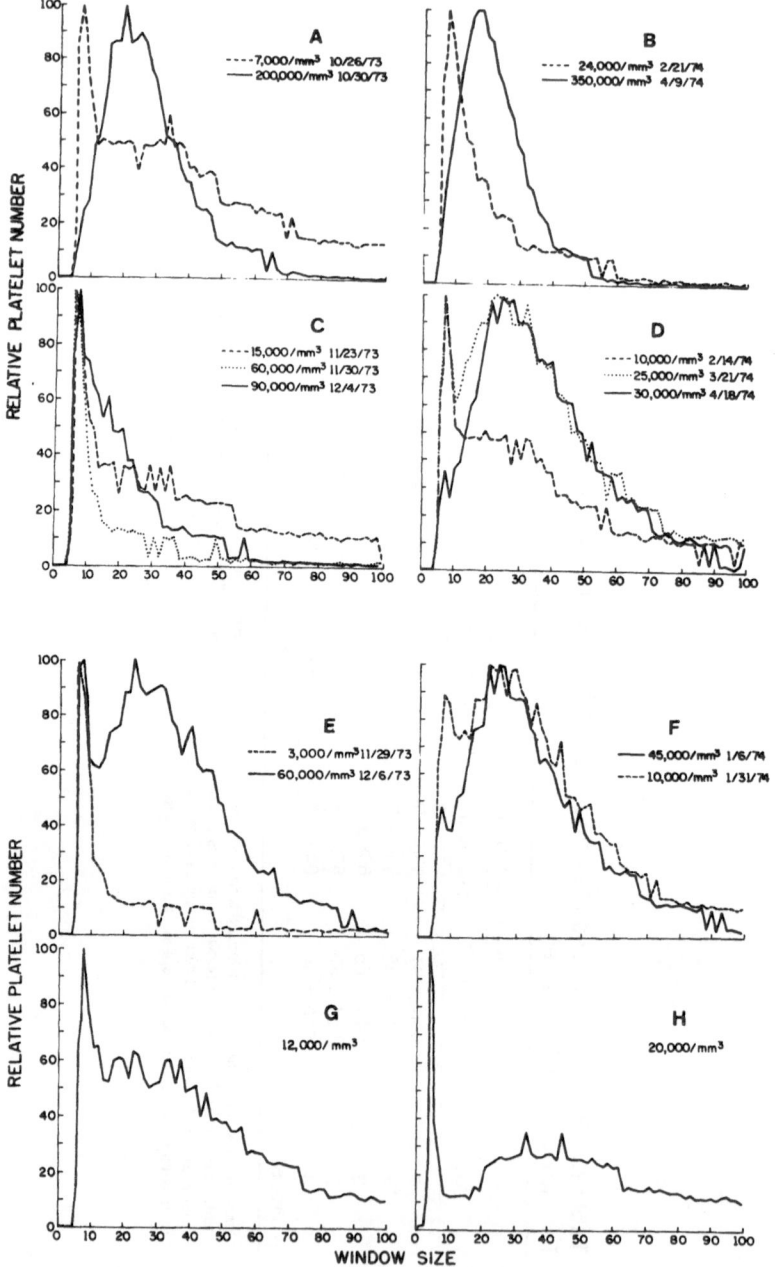

**Fig. 15.** Platelet volume distribution curves obtained in eight patients with autoimmune thrombocytopenic purpura at different time intervals with varying platelet counts. (*Br. J. Haematol.*, **31**:449, 1975.)

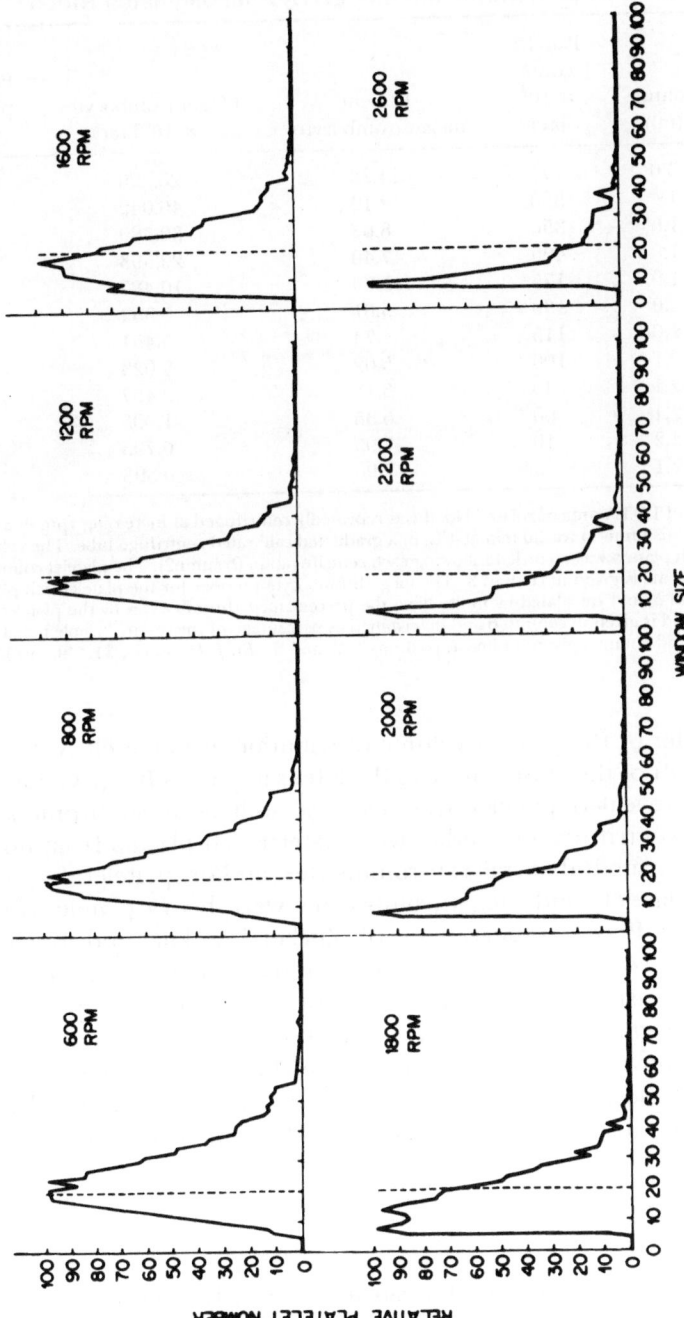

**Fig. 16.** Platelet volume distribution curves from EDTA-anticoagulated blood of a normal subject following repeated centrifugation at increasing rpm of the "residual" platelet-rich plasma in a Sorvall RC3 centrifuge at 4°C. See Table III for further details.

**Table III.**  Differential Centrifugation of EDTA-Anticoagulated Blood[a]

| RPM | Volume (ml) | Platelet count $\times 10^9/$ liter | Percent megathrombocytes | Megathrombocytes $\times 10^9/$liter | Percent platelet yield |
|---|---|---|---|---|---|
| W.B. | 5.0 | 175 | 14.98 | 26.220 | 100.0 |
| 600 | 1.4 | 380 | 12.12 | 46.042 | 60.8 |
| 800 | 1.6 | 350 | 8.68 | 30.380 | 64.0 |
| 1000 | 1.8 | 400 | 7.40 | 29.593 | 82.3 |
| 1200 | 1.9 | 175 | 5.99 | 10.487 | 38.0 |
| 1400 | 2.0 | 130 | 5.81 | 7.552 | 29.7 |
| 1600 | 2.0 | 115 | 4.74 | 5.451 | 26.3 |
| 1800 | 2.1 | 100 | 5.02 | 5.023 | 24.0 |
| 2000 | 2.1 | 40 | 6.14 | 2.457 | 9.6 |
| 2200 | 2.1 | 60 | 6.35 | 1.905 | 7.2 |
| 2400 | 2.2 | 10 | 7.95 | 0.795 | 2.5 |
| 2600 | 2.1 | 5 | 7.96 | 0.398 | 1.2 |

[a]Five milliliters of EDTA-anticoagulated blood was repeatedly centrifuged at increasing rpm in a Sorvall RC3 centrifuge (column 1) for 20 min at 4°C, in a graduated calibrated centrifuge tube. The volume of the platelet-rich plasma was recorded following each centrifugation (column2). The platelet count of the platelet-rich plasma is given in column 3. The megathrombocyte number for the platelet-rich plasma is given in column 5, and calculated by multiplying the percent megathrombocytes by the platelet count. The platelet yield is given in column 6 and determined as percentage of the original whole blood (W.B.) platelet count and volume, given on line 1, columns 1, 2, and 3. (*Br. J. Haematol.*, **31**:449, 1975.)

the remainder of the platelet volume distribution as in panels A, D, E, G, H, or as a shift of the entire curve to the left as in panels B and C. Electron microscopy revealed platelet fragments as well as megathrombocytes. Differential centrifugation studies with platelet-rich plasma from normal subjects confirmed that microthrombocytes and/or platelet fragments were light platelets and megathrombocytes were heavy platelets (Table III, Fig. 16). Recent observations of Zucker-Franklin and Karpatkin (1976) have also revealed the presence of red blood cell fragments in platelet-rich plasmas from 12 of 15 patients with microcytic peaks, suggesting mild red blood cell hemolysis. One might speculate that this could result from autoantibody directed against red blood cells and other tissues as well as platelets. Indeed, weak complement sensitization of red blood cells was noted in 8 of 14 patients tested with microcytic peaks.

# References

Amorosi, E. L., Garg, S. K., and Karpatkin, S., 1971, Heterogeneity of human platelets. IV. Identification of a young platelet population with [75]Se-seleno-methionine, *Br. J. Haematol.* **21**:227.

Charmatz, A., and Karpatkin, S., 1974, Heterogeneity of rabbit platelets. I. Employment of an albumin density gradient for separation of a young platelet population identified with $^{75}$Se-selenomethionine, *Thromb. Diath. Haemorrh.* **31**:485.

Ebbe, S., Stohlman, F., Jr., Overcash, J., Donovan, J., and Howard, D., 1968, Megakaryocyte size in thrombocytopenic and normal rats, *Blood* **32**:383.

Freedman, M. L., and Karpatkin, S., 1975a, Heterogeneity of rabbit platelets. IV. Thrombocytosis with absolute megathrombocytosis in phenylhydrazine-induced hemolytic anemia in rabbits, *Thromb. Diath. Haemorrh.* **33**:335.

Freedman, M. L., and Karpatkin, S., 1975b, Heterogeneity of rabbit platelets. V. Preferential splenic sequestration of megathrombocytes, *Br. J. Haematol.* **31**:255.

Freedman, M. L., and Karpatkin, S., 1975c, Elevated platelet count and megathrombocyte number in sickle cell anemia, *Blood* **46**:579.

Freedman, M. L., and Karpatkin, S., 1976, Evidence for a nonsplenic platelet pool, *Clin. Res.* **24**:308A.

Garg, S. K., Amorosi, E. L., and Karpatkin, S., 1971, Use of the megathrombocyte as an index of megakaryocyte number, *N. Engl. J. Med.* **284**:11.

Garg, S. K., Lackner, H., and Karpatkin, S., 1972, The increased percentage of megathrombocytes in various clinical disorders, *Ann. Intern. Med.* **77**:361.

George, J. N., Lewis, P. C., and Sears, D. A., 1976, Studies on platelet plasma membranes. 11. Characterization of surface proteins of rabbit platelets *in vitro* and during circulation *in vivo* using diazotized [$^{125}$I]diiodosulfanilic acid as a label, *J. Lab. Clin. Med.* **88**:247.

Ginsburg, A. D., and Aster, R. H., 1972, Changes associated with platelet aging, *Thromb. Diath. Haemorrh.* **27**:407.

Harker, L. A., and Finch, C. A., 1969, Thrombokinetics in man, *J. Clin. Invest.* **48**:963.

Karpatkin, S., 1969a, Heterogeneity of human platelets. I. Metabolic and kinetic evidence suggestive of young and old platelets, *J. Clin. Invest.* **48**:1073.

Karpatkin, S., 1969b, Heterogeneity of human platelets. II. Functional evidence suggestive of young and old platelets, *J. Clin. Invest.* **48**:1083.

Karpatkin, S., 1976, Evidence that megathrombocyte number determines platelet function, *Clin. Res.* **24**: 440A.

Karpatkin, S., and Charmatz, A., 1970, Heterogeneity of human platelets. III. Glycogen metabolism in platelets of different sizes, *Br. J. Haematol.* **19**:135.

Karpatkin, S., and Langer, R. M., 1968, Biochemical energetics of simulated platelet plug formation. Effect of thrombin, adenosine diphosphate and epinephrine on intra- and extracellular adenine nucleotide kinetics, *J. Clin. Invest.* **47**:2158.

Karpatkin, S., and Strick, N., 1972, Heterogeneity of human platelets. V. Differences in glycolytic and related enzymes with possible relation to platelet age, *J. Clin. Invest.* **51**:1235.

Karpatkin, S., Garg, S. K., and Siskind, G. W., 1971, Autoimmune thrombocytopenic purpura and the compensated thrombocytolytic state, *Am. J. Med.* **51**:1.

Karpatkin, S., Garg, S. K., and Freedman, M. L., 1974, Role of iron as a regulator of thrombopoiesis, *Am. J. Med.* **57**:521.

Khan, I., Zucker-Franklin, D., and Karpatkin, S., 1975, Microthrombocytosis and platelet fragmentation associated with idiopathic/autoimmune thrombocytopenic purpura, *Br. J. Haematol.* **31**:449.

Kraytman, M., 1973, Platelet size in thrombocytopenias and thrombocytosis of various origin, *Blood* **41**:587.

McDonald, T. P., Odell, T. T., Jr., and Gosslee, D. G., 1964, Platelet size in relation to platelet age, *Proc. Soc. Exp. Biol. Med.* **115**:684.

Minter, F. M., and Ingram, M., 1971, Platelet volume: Density relationships in normal and acutely bled dogs, *Br. J. Haematol.* **20**:55.

O'Brien, J. R., 1974, A relationship between platelet volume and platelet number, *Thromb. Diath. Haemorrh.* **31**:363.

Penington, D. G., Lee, N. Y. T., Roxburgh, A. E., and McGready, J. E., 1976a, Platelet density and size: The interpretation of heterogeneity, *Br. J. Haematol.* **34**:365.

Penington, D. G., Streatfield, K., and Roxburgh, A. E., 1976b, Megakaryocytes and the heterogeneity of circulating platelets, *Br. J. Haematol.* **34**:639.

Shulman, N. R., Watkins, S. P., Jr., Itscoitz, S. B., and Students, A. B., 1969, Evidence that the spleen retains the youngest and hemostatically most effective platelets, *Trans. Assoc. Am. Physicians* **81**:302.

von Behrens, W. E., 1975, Mediterranean macrothrombocytopenia, *Blood* **46**:199.

Weiner, M., and Karpatkin, S., 1972, Use of the megathrombocyte to determine thrombopoietin, *Thromb. Diath. Haemorrh.* **28**:24.

Weintraub, A., and Karpatkin, S., 1974, Heterogeneity of rabbit platelets. II. Use of the megathrombocyte to demonstrate a thrombopoietic stimulus, *J. Lab. Clin. Med.* **83**:896.

Zucker-Franklin, D., and Karpatkin, S., 1976, Subclinical erythrocyte fragmentation in idiopathic/autoimmune thrombocytopenic purpura, *Clin. Res.* **24**:481A.

# Mechanisms of Polycythemia

## John W. Adamson

## 16.1. Introduction

Polycythemia in man is defined as an increase in the hematocrit and hemoglobin concentration above accepted normal values. As such, the finding of polycythemia implies the increased production of erythrocytes. Since red cell production is governed normally by interaction of oxygen ($O_2$) availability, the elaboration of the regulatory hormone, erythropoietin, and marrow function, it is not surprising that derangements in these interrelationships account for virtually all causes of polycythemia. This chapter summarizes briefly various aspects of the regulation of red cell production and focuses on those identified mechanisms which lead to polycythemia.

## 16.2. Oxygen Transport and Erythropoietin Production in Normal Man

The primary function of the hemoglobin molecule is $O_2$ transport, and abnormalities in this function, brought about either by a reduction in hemoglobin mass or molecular disorders, result in altered erythropoiesis.

JOHN W. ADAMSON • Division of Hematology, Department of Medicine, University of Washington School of Medicine and the Veterans Administration Hospital, Seattle, Washington.

Oxygen transport in mammals is complex and the adequate tissue delivery of molecular $O_2$, sufficient to meet metabolic requirements, is the sum of a number of factors. These include $O_2$ availability, cardiac and pulmonary function, regional blood flow, red cell mass, and the structure and function of molecular hemoglobin (Finch and Lenfant, 1972). In normal man, these various components are adjusted so as to maintain normal capillary $O_2$ tension and normal cell function. When tissue oxygenation is inadequate, symptoms and signs are produced which are relevant to the organ or system involved. This may result in specific localized problems (myocardial infarction, stroke, etc.) or more generalized ones (fatigue, muscular cramping, breathlessness). A number of compensatory factors are available to the host to combat tissue hypoxia but the one which is dealt with here is the erythropoietic response.

It is now widely held that the hormone, erythropoietin (ESF), regulates both steady state and accelerated erythropoiesis in animals and man. The production of ESF is governed by $O_2$ availability to the kidney (Gordon et al., 1967). The exact nature of the biogenesis of ESF and its cellular site of origin are uncertain, and essentially two major mechanisms have been proposed. The first suggests that the erythropoietically active principle, ESF, arises through the interaction of a renal-released enzyme, the renal erythropoietic factor (or erythrogenin), with a plasma substrate protein (Gordon et al., 1967). However, others contend that the kidney elaborates ESF intact (Erslev, 1975) or else in an inactive form which is somehow modified in circulation to become active (Peschle and Condorelli, 1975). It is not likely that the final understanding of the mechanisms of ESF synthesis, release, and possible modification will be known until more acceptably pure hormone preparations and specific assays are available. Nevertheless, studies of the relationship of ESF to red cell production continue to provide useful information about the regulation of erythropoiesis.

In man, an inverse relationship between the $O_2$-carrying capacity of the blood and ESF excretion has been established (Adamson, 1968). This type of analysis rests on the availability of assays capable of quantitating ESF excretion in normal subjects (Adamson et al., 1966; Alexanian, 1966). Such studies have demonstrated the excretion of 2–6 International Reference Preparation (IRP) units/day in the urine of normal males and 1–3 IRP units/day for normal females. The advantages of the assay of urine concentrates in studies of erythropoietic regulation are twofold: (a) the ability to measure ESF activity in normal human urine permits definition of absent or subnormal levels, measurements still not possible with normal serum; (b) the urine can be collected over a 24-hr period and aliquoted, thus providing average values which smooth differences due to diurnal variations in ESF production (Adamson et al., 1966).

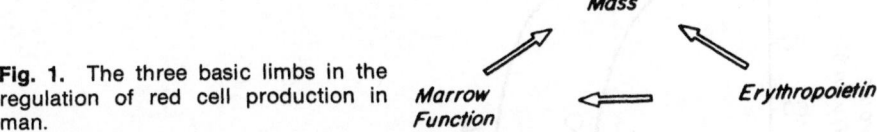

**Fig. 1.** The three basic limbs in the regulation of red cell production in man.

The physiological usefulness of this approach is documented by appropriate changes in both red cell production and hormone excretion which accompany perturbations of the $O_2$-carrying capacity. If normal subjects are bled in a controlled fashion, there is a logarithmic increase in ESF excretion which is inversely related to the hematocrit or hemoglobin concentration (Adamson, 1968). Similarly, hypertransfusion results in the reduction of both ESF excretion and reticulocyte production (Adamson, 1968). Clearly, then, ESF production is directly linked to alterations in $O_2$ availability and changes in ESF production are followed by changes in red cell production until a new equilibrium between $O_2$ supply and tissue requirements is achieved. With prolonged ESF stimulation the red cell mass enlarges to normalize $O_2$ delivery.

The physiological relationships, shown in Fig. 1, among $O_2$ transport (represented by the red cell mass), ESF production, and marrow function, can be used to define the mechanisms which result in polycythemia. This simplified scheme also provides the framework for the physiological classification of these disorders in man.

## 16.3. Definition and Classification of Polycythemia

The laboratory definition of polycythemia is an increased concentration of red cells which is reflected by an elevated hemoglobin or hematocrit. However, since these are values which depend on measurements of concentration, there is only a likelihood or "probability" of an abnormal value representing a true increase in red cell production and red cell mass. In population analyses, values for hemoglobin and hematocrit are normally distributed and the "probability" of polycythemia, based on routine laboratory data, is as shown in Fig. 2 (Hillman and Finch, 1972). Thus, a male with a hemoglobin of 17 g % has about a 65% chance of being "normal," that is, having no increase in red cell mass. A similar experience has been reported by Berlin (1975).

Consequently, because of the variability of these laboratory values, the definition of polycythemia requires both an increased hemoglobin concentration and hematocrit, as well as an increase in red cell mass. The method of choice in quantitating the red cell mass employs the dilution of

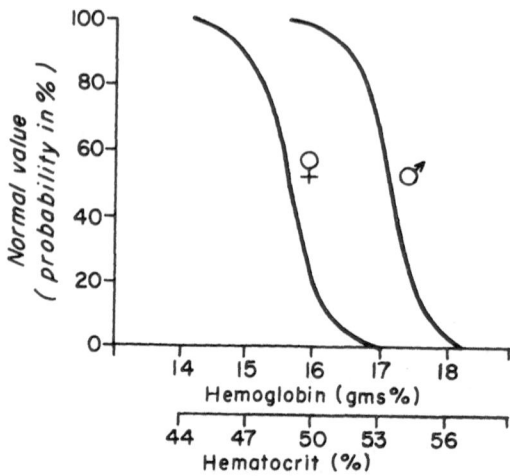

**Fig. 2.** The likelihood of a hemoglobin or hematocrit value being within the normal range. Approximately half of all men with a hemoglobin value of 17 g % will be hematologically normal. (Reproduced from Hillman and Finch, 1972, with permission of the authors and the publisher.)

[51]Cr-labeled autologous red cells. Care must be taken to wash the cells throughly in order to remove unbound isotope which would spuriously increase the result. It should also be noted that an increased mixing time may be required in patients with marked splenomegaly due to the disproportionate volume of red cells trapped in that organ (Mollison, 1972). With this technique, the normal ranges for adult males and females are 27–35 and 23–32 ml/kg, respectively. Since reliable values for red cell mass are not always available and alterations in body habitus may invalidate the expression of the results, the total clinical picture must be considered whenever such patients are evaluated.

## 16.3.1. Normal Red Cell Mass

The finding of an elevated hemoglobin and hematocrit in the absence of a corresponding increase in red cell mass is most commonly referred to as stress, relative, or "spurious" polycythemia (Weinreb and Shih, 1975). In making this diagnosis it is important to be sure there is no coexistent iron deficiency so as not to interpret the red cell mass data incorrectly. "Stress" polycythemia is most often seen in middle-aged men with mild hypertension or in heavy smokers. Although this condition frequently exists as a chronic finding, it may be found transiently as the result of several factors which include hypertension, protein loss in the urine or via the gastrointestinal tract, diuretic therapy, and dehydration.

When chronic, this condition has been felt to be benign (Brown *et al.,* 1971). However, recent analyses of survival data in patients with this diagnosis suggest otherwise. Thus, a decreased life expectancy was observed in patients with a substantially reduced plasma volume whereas patients with a red cell mass at the upper limits of normal and only a marginal reduction in plasma volume had a normal life expectancy (Weinreb and Shih, 1975). The numbers in this analysis are small and require confirmation. In any event, this diagnosis, by definition, excludes an increase in red cell production and thus requires no therapeutic intervention directed toward erythropoiesis.

### 16.3.2. Increased Red Cell Mass

A documented increase in red cell mass represents increased red cell production and requires explanation. Based on the major limbs of hematopoietic regulation outlined in Fig. 1, one can physiologically classify the mechanisms resulting in polycythemia in a meaningful way. These are (a) tissue hypoxia, (b) autonomous or "fixed" erythropoietin production, and (c) autonomous marrow function.

## 16.4. Tissue Hypoxia

Chronic abnormalities of $O_2$ transport evoke polycythemia by stimulating ESF production. Such abnormalities in $O_2$ transport can be further subclassified as loading, transport, and unloading defects.

### 16.4.1. $O_2$ Loading Defects

#### 16.4.1.1. Inability to Get $O_2$ to the Hemoglobin Molecule

*16.4.1.1a. Low Ambient $pO_2$.* If the partial pressure of $O_2$ in the atmosphere falls, systemic hypoxemia occurs. This is most typically seen in high-altitude dwellers. In general, there is an inverse correlation between hemoglobin–$O_2$ saturation and hemoglobin concentration in such individuals (Hurtado, 1960) (Fig. 3).

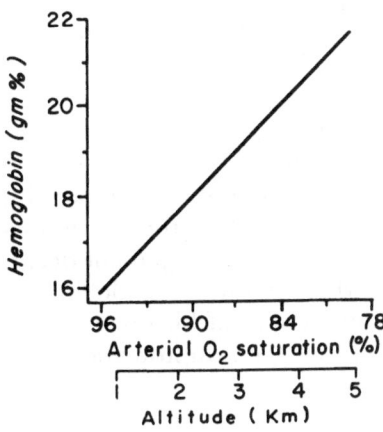

**Fig. 3.** The relationship between $O_2$–hemoglobin saturation and hemoglobin concentration in man. Such a relationship characterizes high-altitude dwellers and individuals with congenital cyanotic heart disease. (Reproduced from Hillman and Finch, 1972, with permission of the authors and the publisher.)

*16.4.1.1b. Cardiac Disease.* Heart disease alone may result in dramatic polycythemia due to shunting of blood from the right to left side of the circulation. This typically is manifested by cyanosis and most commonly results from congenital abnormalities. Similar to the situation in high-altitude dwellers, the hemoglobin concentration is directly related to the degree of arterial desaturation.

*16.4.1.1c. Chronic Pulmonary Disease with Inadequate Gas Exchange.* Clinically, polycythemia associated with chronic pulmonary disease is very common but the association may be difficult to document. In general, the relationship of erythropoiesis to $O_2$ transport is best defined by the red cell mass and hemoglobin–$O_2$ saturation (Weil *et al.*, 1968; Balcerzak and Bromberg, 1975). General correlations also exist between hemoglobin/hematocrit and $O_2$ saturation but are less significant due to the frequent abnormalities of plasma volume seen with chronic lung disease. Owing to the complex nature of the $O_2$–hemoglobin dissociation curve, predictable increases in red cell mass do not occur until the $pO_2$ falls below 65 mm Hg (Weil *et al.*, 1968). These analyses suggest that the hemoglobin saturation is the most accurate determinant of the erythropoietic response. A possible mechanism which might explain this relationship is that ESF production is regulated by renal interstitial or intracellular $pO_2$, rather than arterial $pO_2$ (Weil *et al.*, 1968). As will be seen later, similar conclusions are reached by studies of marrow regulation in patients with $O_2$ unloading defects.

Documentation of chronic pulmonary dysfunction as the etiology of polycythemia may prove difficult because of the variety of factors which subtly influence $O_2$ transport. Blood gas analysis of a single arterial blood sample often correlates poorly with the degree of polycythemia. This may be due to a number of factors, including stimulation of ventilatory activity during the time of sampling, or desaturation which occurs only during sleep, recumbancy, or physical exercise. Until blood gases are obtained under the latter circumstances, intermittent systemic hypoxemia cannot be excluded. Other factors which significantly modify $O_2$ exchange include acid–base changes affecting hemoglobin–$O_2$ affinity, complicating infections, and iron deficiency. In spite of these variables, the critical diagnostic test permitting definition of this group of disorders is the measurement of arterial blood gases, drawn under controlled conditions.

The goals of therapy in this group of patients are poorly defined. In general, the management decision in patients with hypoxic polycythemia is whether the hemoglobin concentration is optimal for the decreased amount of available $O_2$. The only practical way to make this judgment is to evaluate the symptomatic status of the patient before and after phlebotomy. If phlebotomy ameliorates symptoms, then such treatment should be continued. It should be noted, however, that phlebotomy-induced iron deficiency may result in its own symptoms of fatigability and decreased exercise tolerance due to an abnormality of mitochondrial $O_2$ transport imposed by the iron lack (Finch *et al.*, 1976).

### 16.4.1.2. Inability to Get $O_2$ on the Hemoglobin Molecule

Certain inert forms of hemoglobin are unable to transport $O_2$ physiologically. In these instances, iron is in the ferric ($Fe^{3+}$) state or is liganded with a molecule which has a higher affinity for hemoglobin than does $O_2$.

*16.4.1.2a. Hemoglobins M (M Boston; M Iwate, etc.).* In the structure of normal hemoglobin, histidines near the heme play an important role in stabilizing the iron molecule. Substitutions of tyrosine for histidine at these sites result in methemoglobin formation. These abnormalities are functionally generally mild and the degree of polycythemia, when present, is limited. The abnormality is inherited in an autosomal dominant manner and the clinical presentation is usually one of dramatic but unusual (slate gray) cyanosis (Heller *et al.*, 1962; Ranney, 1970).

*16.4.1.2b. Methemoglobin Reductase Deficiency.* In the absence of this enzyme system, about 2% of circulating hemoglobin is oxidized daily until about 20–30% of the hemoglobin within the red cells is found as methemoglobin. Nonspecific reductants are sufficient to keep the iron in the remaining hemoglobin in the ferrous ($Fe^{2+}$) state. If the condition is stable, mild polycythemia results (Sievers and Ryon, 1945; Eder *et al.*, 1949; Jaffé, 1966).

*16.4.1.2c. Carboxyhemoglobin.* Carbon monoxide (CO) binds tightly to hemoglobin. Recently, reports have appeared of polycythemia in heavy smokers associated with elevated CO–hemoglobin levels (Sagone *et al.*, 1973; Sagone and Balcerzak, 1975). Such individuals frequently smoked three or more packs of cigarettes daily and CO–hemoglobin levels of 15% were recorded. Red cell mass values were clearly elevated and the abnormalities subsided when the individuals stopped smoking.

The key to the diagnosis of CO–hemoglobinemia as the cause of polycythemia is the *direct* measurement of hemoglobin saturation. Ordinarily, this determination is calculated indirectly based on arterial blood $pO_2$ and the assumption of a normally positioned $O_2$–hemoglobin dissociation curve. Thus, such measurements will miss significant levels of inert hemoglobins.

## 16.4.2. O₂ Transport Defects Due to Impaired Flow

A variety of abnormalities in regional blood flow lead to critical impairment of $O_2$ delivery to sites within the kidney which regulate ESF production. Because the kidney is the organ primarily responsible for ESF production, occasional lesions which reduce either total or regional blood flow to a critical degree result in increased ESF production and polycythemia. These disorders, although physiologically comprehensible, occur very rarely. They may be seen with the following conditions.

### 16.4.2.1. Renal Artery Stenosis

Only two well-documented cases have demonstrated an association of of polycythemia with renal artery stenosis. Both of the patients reported also had hypertension and these complications of the vascular insufficiency disappeared with corrective surgery (Luke *et al.*, 1965; Hudgson *et al.*, 1967). Studies in animals, however, have confirmed the pathogenetic significance of this mechanism (Fisher *et al.*, 1965; Fisher and Samuels, 1967). Ordinarily, the kidney is relatively insensitive to changes in blood flow since reduction in flow is associated with reduced $O_2$ consumption (Finch and Lenfant, 1972). However, when overall flow falls to 25–30% of normal, renal hypoxia occurs and ESF elaboration rises.

A specialized association of polycythemia and renal vascular insufficiency has been observed recently following renal transplantation and, in some, as a consequence of rejection phenomena (Nies *et al.*, 1965; Denny *et al.*, 1966; Westerman *et al.*, 1967; Hoffman, 1968). It is believed that damage of smaller arteries and arterioles, perhaps immunologically mediated, results in sufficient ischemia to increase ESF levels.

### 16.4.2.2. Hydronephrosis

In rare instances in man (Krantz and Jacobson, 1970; Thorling, 1972; Hammond and Winnick, 1974) and in appropriately studied animal models (Mitus *et al.*, 1964; Toyama and Mitus, 1966), the increased intrapelvic pressure due to partial or near-total constriction of the ureter results in compression of surrounding renal tissue and increased ESF production. This may occur unilaterally or bilaterally. However, the increase in intrapelvic pressure is only effective within a critical range. If the pressure is too low, no polycythemia occurs and if too great, infarction of the compressed renal tissue is seen and, again, polycythemia is not.

### 16.4.2.3. Renal Cysts

Single or multiple cysts of either one or both kidneys may result in compression of surrounding renal tissue and increased ESF production.

The mechanism appears to be analogous to that outlined for hydrone-phrosis. The cyst fluid may contain high levels of ESF, but the previous belief that the lining cells of the cyst secreted ESF is probably not patho-physiologically important. Several instances of either resection or simple percutaneous drainage of the cyst have documented complete resolution of the polycythemia (Rosse *et al.*, 1963; Krantz and Jacobson, 1970; Hammond and Winnick, 1974).

Since the disorders summarized here have in common impaired general or regional renal blood flow, the diagnostic tests of choice are renal contrast studies, including intravenous pyelography and renal arteriography.

### 16.4.3. $O_2$ Unloading Defects

Abnormalities in the function of molecular hemoglobin which result in polycythemia have assumed increasing recognition and importance over the past 12 years. These defects are characterized by increased affinity of the hemoglobin molecule for $O_2$ and provide examples of disease pathogenesis defined at the molecular level.

The first report of such an abnormal hemoglobin resulting in polycy-themia appeared in 1966 (Charache *et al.*, 1966). Mild polycythemia was found in multiple members of three generations in a single family and correctly linked to the increased $O_2$ affinity which characterized the mutant, Hb Chesapeake. The $O_2$–hemoglobin dissociation curve was shifted to the left of normal and the shape of the curve was altered from the normal sigmoid form to a more hyperbolic one, signifying decreased heme–heme interaction.

To date, at least 25 such mutants have been described with associated polycythemia, and several examples of identical mutations in apparently unrelated families have been reported. The discovery and unraveling of the $O_2$ transport properties of these mutants have contributed signifi-cantly to the understanding of the structure–function relationships of the hemoglobin molecule. Since these relationships have been the subject of several recent reviews (Perutz and Lehmann, 1968; Nagel and Bookchin, 1974; Adamson and Finch, 1975; Bellingham, 1976) they are only sum-marized here.

The hemoglobin molecule functions normally in a tetrameric form composed of dimers of like chains. The tetramer is held together and stabilized by a number of important interactions including electrostatic bonds, chemical bonds, and van der Waals forces. The most important contacts are found at the interfaces between chains ($\alpha_1\beta_1$ and $\alpha_1\beta_2$). It has been proposed by Perutz (1970, 1972) that hemoglobin has two quaternary structures, the oxygenated (liganded) form and the deoxygenated (constrained) form.

As molecular $O_2$ is loaded, a number of important spatial changes occur in the hemoglobin molecule. These changes are associated with the rupturing of a number of chemical bonds, shifts in the relationships of certain subunits to one another, and progressive alteration of $O_2$ affinity (so-called heme–heme interactions). Thus, with oxygenation, the hemoglobin molecule behaves as an allosteric enzyme, after the model of Monod (Monod *et al.*, 1965). The initial events in oxygenation are believed to involve the heme ring of a given globin chain and its proximal histidine. First, there is a shift in the position of the iron atom relative to the heme plate and an area of the surrounding globin chain. This results in displacement of a helical segment of one of the globin chains and results in the squeezing of a "pocket" between the F and H helices. Normally the penultimate tyrosines reside in this pocket when hemoglobin is in the deoxygenated state. As these tyrosines are displaced, the nearby terminal residues of the chains are pulled along, leading to the disruption of important constraining bonds which stabilize the structure of the hemoglobin molecule. As these constraints are lost, the molecular equilibrium shifts from the deoxygenated to the oxygenated configuration. When this occurs, certain of the hemoglobin subunits rotate on one another, particularly at the interface between unlike chains ($\alpha_1\beta_2$). Thus, in the deoxy form, the hydrogen bond joining the aspartate of $\beta99$ and the tyrosine at $\alpha42$ "shifts" with oxygenation to $\alpha94$ aspartate and $\beta102$ asparagine (Perutz and TenEyck, 1971). As oxygenation of the molecule progresses, stabilizing bonds become weaker, and the quaternary structure of the molecule changes to the oxy configuration. Amino acid substitutions at critical sites within the hemoglobin molecule alter the ease with which it undergoes "respiratory" motion and thus significantly change its oxygen binding properties. If substitutions produce changes which stabilize the oxy form of hemoglobin, an increased affinity results, and the $O_2$–hemoglobin dissociation curve shifts to the left, resulting in a decreased $p50_{std}$.*

Thus, hemoglobins Chesapeake ($\alpha92$ arginine $\rightarrow$ leucine), Yakima ($\beta99$ aspartate $\rightarrow$ histidine), and Kempsey ($\beta99$ aspartate $\rightarrow$ asparagine) are all examples of substitutions at, or near, the important $\alpha_1\beta_2$ interface. The mutations at these sites may influence hemoglobin $O_2$ affinity by stabilizing the molecule in the oxy form and restricting its respiratory motion. Almost half the stable mutants described to date affect this important region of the molecule.

*The $p50_{std}$ is a simplified method to characterize the position of the $O_2$–hemoglobin dissociation curve. It is defined by the partial pressure of $O_2$ at which 50% of hemoglobin is saturated under standard conditions of temperature and pH.

Other substitutions of the molecule involve residues near the carboxy terminus of the globin chains and lead to increased affinity by other mechanisms. In two such mutants (Hbs Bethesda and Rainier), the loss of the $\beta145$ tyrosine renders the deoxy form of hemoglobin unstable. Normally, in the deoxygenated state these tyrosines fit into an interhelical "pocket" within the hemoglobin molecule and are held by various constraining bonds. With substitutions of these tyrosines, stabilization of the deoxy form is less favored, either because of the limitations of physical size of the amino acid substitution or of charge incompatibilities between the new residue and the pocket's environment. Thus, normally occurring stabilizing bonds may not form, weakening the deoxy configuration (Hayashi and Stamatoyannopoulos, 1972).

In addition, $O_2$ affinity may be influenced by amino acid substitutions which affect the interaction of the hemoglobin molecule with the intracellular organic phosphate, 2,3-diphosphoglycerate (DPG). The important regulatory role of this molecule in $O_2$ exchange is reviewed in detail by Oski and McMillan in Chapter 3 of this volume. DPG reacts only with deoxy hemoglobin and, by binding the $\beta$ chains together, stabilizes this form of the hemoglobin molecule. Sites on the $\beta$ chain which interact with DPG include 1 valine, 143 histidine, and 82 lysine. Substitutions at or near these positions might impair DPG binding and thus favor the oxy or liganded form, leading to a left shift in the $O_2$–hemoglobin dissociation curve. An example of a mutant having altered DPG binding properties is Hb Little Rock ($\beta143$ histidine $\rightarrow$ glutamine) (Bromberg et al., 1973).

Whatever the contribution of the loss of DPG interaction, however, all the mutants thus far described also demonstrate increased affinity for $O_2$ in hemolysate free of DPG. Thus the amino acid substitution itself alters the inherent liganding properties of the molecule. In addition, a reduction in heme–heme interaction is usually seen.

The importance of DPG in maintaining normal $O_2$ delivery is also seen in individuals with reduced red cell levels of DPG on an inherited basis. Thus, mild polycythemia was found in affected members of one family with reduced DPG and elevated ATP. Although detailed measurements of hemoglobin function or red cell mass were not provided, it is likely that the biochemical lesion resulted in increased $O_2$ affinity and a compensatory rise in hemoglobin concentration (Zürcher et al., 1965).

The molecular substitutions at functionally critical sites on the globin chain result in a variable increase in hemoglobin–$O_2$ affinity. The implication of such increased affinity is that over the physiologic range of $O_2$ tension, less $O_2$ is available to tissue for metabolic requirements. Thus, a state of relative tissue hypoxia exists at normal hemoglobin concentrations (Fig. 4).

Studies of $O_2$ transport in individuals with high affinity hemoglobin

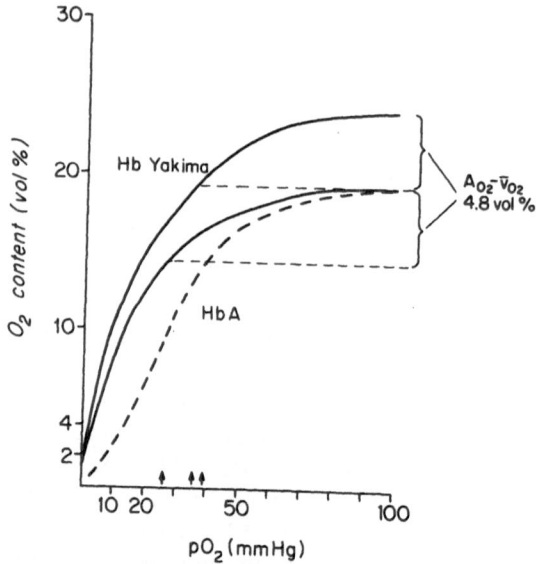

**Fig. 4.** The $O_2$ dissociation characteristics of Hb A (dashed line) and Hb Yakima (solid lines), a mutant with increased $O_2$ affinity. In this figure, the $O_2$ content of whole blood is plotted for different $O_2$ tensions. The dissociation curves of Hb Yakima are shifted to the left of normal and do not display the usual sigmoid shape. The figure also shows the effects of differences in hemoglobin concentration on the $VpO_2$ (indicated by the upright arrows along the horizontal axis). Under conditions of normal $O_2$ consumption ($A_{O2} - \bar{V}_{O2}$), the $\bar{V}pO_2$ in carriers of Hb A is 37–40 mm Hg. An individual with Hb Yakima and with a hemoglobin concentration of 15 g %, would have a $\bar{V}pO_2$ of about 26 mm Hg. In the presence of polycythemia, the $\bar{V}pO_2$ is about 36 mm Hg, nearly normal. (Reproduced from Adamson, 1975, with permission of the publisher.)

mutants have provided insight into the regulation of ESF production. According to the Fick principle, if the $O_2$ dissociation curve is shifted to the left at a normal hemoglobin concentration, the mixed venous $pO_2$ ($\bar{V}pO_2$) must fall if $O_2$ consumption ($VO_2$) and cardiac output remain normal (Fig. 4). Since studies of $\bar{V}O_2$ and cardiac output have been normal when tested in this setting, the major physiologic response to the tissue hypoxia caused by the displaced hemoglobin–$O_2$ dissociation curve is an increase in red cell mass.

The effect of changes in $O_2$ content and $O_2$ dissociation characteristics on the $\bar{V}pO_2$ is shown in Fig. 4. When equilibrium is achieved at the higher hematocrit, the $\bar{V}pO_2$ is nearly normal. Thus, the adequacy of tissue oxygen supply may be closely gauged by the $\bar{V}pO_2$, and "compensation" is defined by the near normality of this value (Finch and Lenfant, 1972).

In studies of patients with hemoglobin mutants having altered $O_2$ affinity, compensation is also defined by near-normal values of ESF excretion. However, as $O_2$ delivery is reduced by phlebotomy, increased ESF excretion is found along with a subsequent rise in reticulocyte production (Fig. 5). Further information concerning the regulation of ESF production is provided by the fact that the arterial $O_2$ content of the blood of affected individuals is above normal. Thus, the renal cellular site which is sensitive to alterations in $O_2$ availability is likely to be in the postarterial limb of the vascular tree.

The clinical expression in affected individuals with a hemoglobin mutant having increased $O_2$ affinity is a varying degree of polycythemia. White cell and platelet counts are not elevated and splenomegaly is not seen. In general, the degree of polycythemia parallels the severity of the shift in the dissociation curve although within families the degree of hemoglobin rise is less marked in females and children. Thus, the blood $O_2$-carrying capacity is matched to the increased $O_2$ affinity. Although the degree of polycythemia is generally modest, considerable variation of hemoglobin and hematocrit is seen between individuals within the same family, implying modification of $O_2$ transport by other factors.

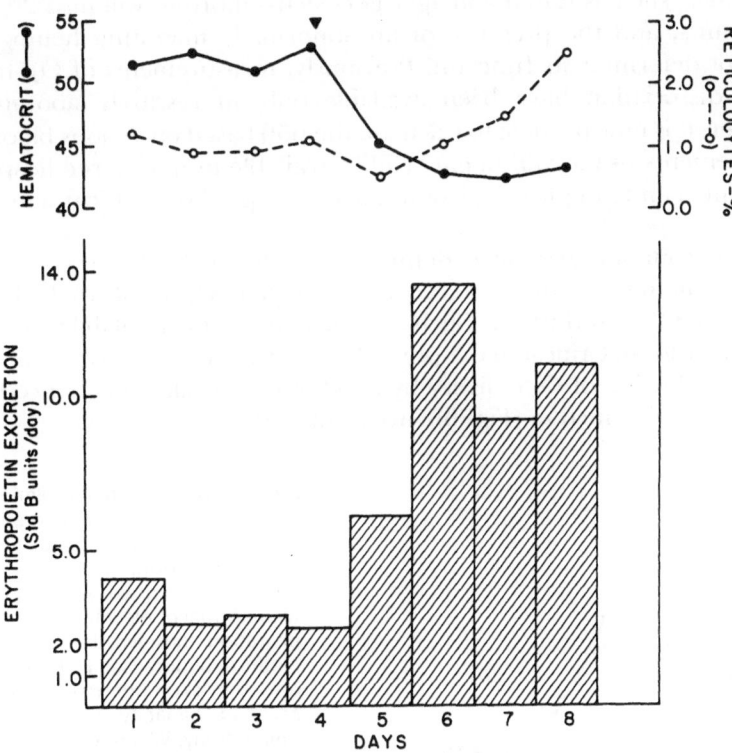

**Fig. 5.** Pre- and postphlebotomy (▼) measurements of daily ESF excretion, hematocrit, and corrected reticulocyte count in a patient with polycythemia associated with a hemoglobin mutant (Hb Rainier) with increased $O_2$ affinity. In response to the fall in hematocrit, ESF excretion and red cell production increased. (Reproduced from Adamson, 1975, with permission of the publisher.)

High affinity hemoglobin mutants are inherited in an autosomal dominant fashion and are probably more common than appreciated because of the generally mild degree of polycythemia seen. For the most part, the elevated blood values in affected individuals are well tolerated, required for normal tissue $O_2$ delivery, and the increased viscosity attending this form of polycythemia is not associated with obvious deleterious effects. Although critical long-term studies of the influence of the elevated red cell mass on life span are not available, a number of affected individuals live to an advanced age. Therapy, rarely indicated in polycythemia of this type, should consist only of occasional phlebotomies to provide symptomatic relief when necessary.

Critical to the definition of an $O_2$ unloading defect is the characterization of the $O_2$–hemoglobin dissociation curve. Hemoglobin electrophoresis is not to be relied upon exclusively since even highly specialized techniques, such as starch and agar gel electrophoresis, will miss 20–25% of mutants, and the presence of an abnormally migrating hemoglobin does not determine its function. Previously, measurements of $O_2$–hemoglobin dissociation have been available only in research laboratories. However, it is now possible to calculate the p50 based on venous blood gas measurements using equipment readily available in most large hospitals; the formula and sample calculations have been published (Lichtman *et al.*, 1976).

The common *functional* definition of all the $O_2$ transport defects which result in polycythemia is that an inadequate $O_2$ supply to the kidney stimulates ESF production. Such impairment of $O_2$ availability may be systemic or local. Critical to the physiology of the definition is the fact that further reduction of $O_2$ delivery by phlebotomy results in enhanced ESF and red cell production (Fig. 6) (Adamson, 1968).

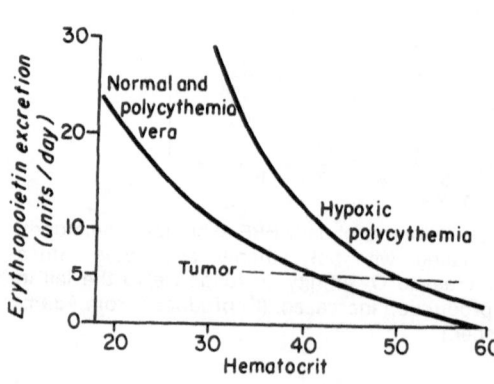

**Fig. 6.** The schematic relationship of hematocrit to ESF excretion in normal and polycythemic man. All secondary forms of polycythemia thus far described are associated with normal or elevated rates of ESF excretion. In polycythemia vera, the plethora suppresses ESF excretion; however, excretion rises as the $O_2$-carrying capacity is reduced by phlebotomy. Where polycythemia is associated with neoplasms, ESF excretion is fixed at a level and is independent of blood $O_2$ content, at least over the normal range. (Reproduced from Hillman and Finch, 1972, with permission of the authors and publisher.)

## 16.5. Autonomous Erythropoietin Production

### 16.5.1. Neoplasms

Occasionally, and often dramatically, polycythemia may be associated with various malignancies, and this association has been reviewed in detail (Krantz and Jacobson, 1970; Thorling, 1972; Hammond and Winnick, 1974). A number of mechanisms have been proposed to account for this association, including (a) production of ESF or one of the putative proforms of the hormone; (b) decreased catabolism of ESF; (c) local hypoxia due to tissue compression by renal tumors; and (d) production by the tumor of erythropoietically active substances other than ESF. The latter might include androgen-producing tumors. Of these mechanisms, however, only the first is supported by experimental evidence and must be considered of importance.

In the exhaustive review by Thorling (1972) of the more than 250 cases of polycythemia associated with neoplasms, nearly half were due to tumors arising in the kidney—almost all hypernephromas. The incidence of polycythemia as a manifestation of hypernephroma has been variably estimated from about 1% (Lawrence and Donald, 1959), to nearly 11% (Smith and Riches, 1963).

Other renal neoplasms associated much less frequently with polycythemia include adenomas, hemangiomas, sarcomas, and Wilm's tumor. These associations are not surprising because of the kidney's unique role in ESF production.

Other sites and neoplasms which have been convincingly associated with polycythemia include the liver (hepatoma, hemartoma), cerebellum (hemangioblastoma), and uterus (leiomyoma). Nearly 70 cases of hepatoma have been reported with polycythemia, and it has been estimated that between 5 and 10% of all hepatomas are associated with polycythemia. Almost as many cases of cerebellar hemangioblastomas associated with polycythemia have been reported; here the coexistence may be as great as 15%. Of interest, this tumor frequently resembles the hypernephroma histologically.

A number of other neoplasms have occasionally been reported with polycythemia, but Thorling (1972) believes these associations to be of dubious significance. Thus, other possible explanations should be sought when polycythemia is associated with tumors of the lung, stomach, prostate, and ovary.

The association of polycythemia with pheochromocytoma, although interesting, may be considered more often than is justified. Most commonly, the elevated hemoglobin concentration which is seen results from the catecholamine-induced contraction of the plasma volume, and there is no increase in red cell mass.

It is currently believed that when polycythemia occurs in association with neoplasms it is because the tumor is releasing or stimulating the production of ESF or ESF-like material. Virtually all earlier studies which failed to demonstrate this association employed assays of serum ESF activity which were insensitive to normal or even modestly elevated levels of the hormone. Whenever measurable erythropoietic activity from serum or tumor extracts has been tested in the presence of antibodies to ESF, neutralization of the stimulating activity has been observed. Thus, the erythropoietically active principles appear chemically similar to normal ESF, although strict identity is not possible to prove.

In terms of the proposed mechanisms of ESF biogenesis, it is conceivable that either erythrogenin or the plasma substrate protein might be produced in excess. In fact, both mechanisms have been suggested as resulting in polycythemia in cases of hypernephroma, where erythrogenin is said to be increased (Peschle and Condorelli, 1971), and hepatomas, where increased substrate production by the tumor has been proposed (Gordon *et al.*, 1970). However, since noncontroversial details of ESF biochemistry and biogenesis are not available, the real and possibly varied roles of neoplasms in producing polycythemia remain to be precisely defined.

Studies of urinary ESF carried out in patients with neoplasms have documented inappropriately elevated levels. However, ESF excretion, and presumably production of the hormone, is not linked to $O_2$ transport. Consequently, there is no change in ESF excretion in response to phlebotomy (Adamson, 1968). Thus, the elaboration of erythropoietically active material appears autonomous. This pattern of ESF excretion is schematized in Fig. 6.

The critical diagnostic test for this type of polycythemia is a renal contrast study. For all practical purposes, the neoplasm most likely to present with polycythemia as the initial clue is hypernephroma. Since this neoplasm is potentially curable, all patients with unexplained polycythemia should have such a diagnostic study. The other neoplasms capable of producing this syndrome are either not curable (hepatoma), are relatively benign (uterine leiomyoma), or else present with other associated clinical sequelae which assist in diagnosis (cerebellar tumor).

Therapy of the polycythemia associated with tumors is simple phlebotomy and is almost never of primary importance. Obviously, treatment, when possibly effective, should be directed at the underlying neoplasm and hematologic intervention is secondary.

## 16.5.2. Recessively Inherited Polycythemia

Detailed reviews of familial forms of polycythemia have recently been published (Stamatoyannopoulos, 1972; Adamson, 1975). In a number of the reports, polycythemia is confined to multiple individuals within a single generation. The hemoglobin and hematocrit values are usually markedly elevated and the polycythemia is noted in childhood. Platelet and leukocyte counts are not elevated. Genetic analysis of such families suggests that this form of polycythemia is inherited in an autosomal recessive fashion. Hematologically, the parents are normal or only a mild elevation of the hemoglobin concentration is seen. The offspring of affected individuals are also hematologically normal. Where data are available, the findings at autopsy of affected individuals do not provide an explanation for the polycythemia (Adamson, unpublished observations).

Although the exact mechanism responsible for the polycythemia in such individuals is not defined, certain facts are known. First, no detectable abnormality in $O_2$ transport or hemoglobin function has been found to date. Studies of whole blood p50 in members of five affected families (Stamatoyannopoulos and Adamson, unpublished observations) were normal. Second, no abnormalities of cardiac or pulmonary function have been found. Finally, the renal microvasculature was normal (Stamatoyannopoulos, 1972; Adamson et al., 1973).

Physiological studies of the relationship of ESF to $O_2$-carrying capacity have provided insight into the defect. In three families studied to date, ESF excretion has been above normal, demonstrating that the marrow is under hormonal stimulation. Phlebotomy of affected individuals failed to stimulate ESF production and, thus, ESF production and $O_2$ transport are not reciprocally related, in contrast to normal. This pattern of marrow regulation is similar to that seen with neoplasms, in which an elevated fixed level of ESF production is seen, unrelated to tissue $O_2$ requirements. The findings of these family studies suggest that the regulatory abnormality resides in the mechanism or site of ESF production and is not primary to the marrow.

The clinical features of recessively expressed disease are more accentuated than the polycythemia inherited as a dominant trait—i.e., the polycythemia seen with mutant hemoglobins. In the recessive form there is more obvious involvement in early life, the hemoglobin and hematocrit are higher, and splenomegaly may be seen. Recent experience, in fact, suggests that this condition may not be benign and the potential risks of hyperviscosity and vascular occlusion are underestimated (Adamson et al., 1973). Therefore, after these patients have been carefully evaluated, phlebotomy therapy should be instituted to reduce the hemoglobin to the normal range.

There are no precise diagnostic tests for this category of polycythemia. Certainly the young age, lack of family history, and extreme degree of erythrocytosis which may be observed dictate that a most careful search for all possible mechanisms be carried out. Without the ready availability of an ESF bioassay of demonstrated clinical usefulness, the diagnosis of this type of polycythemia will most often be arrived at by exclusion and without confirmatory data.

## 16.6. Autonomous Marrow Function

### 16.6.1. Pathogenesis

The classical example of a disorder of presumably autonomous marrow function is polycythemia vera. In this disease there is the apparently purposeless proliferation of all marrow elements, including granulocytes and platelets, as well as erythrocytes. Splenomegaly is common and felt to be an important distinguishing point in making the diagnosis. Although the full clinical picture is striking and rarely confused with other causes of polycythemia, subtle cases are seen frequently in which diagnosis is not immediately certain.

The basic hypotheses of the pathogenesis of this disease fall broadly into two categories. In the first, consideration is given to possible stimuli which could account for the marrow proliferation. Initial attention focused on various forms of tissue hypoxia, but such an abnormality would only explain the increase in red cell production and would not account for the leukocytosis and thrombocytosis. In addition, urinary levels of ESF are markedly reduced or absent in patients with this disease, unlike other forms of polycythemia (Adamson and Finch, 1968).

Others have suggested that there is a general "myelostimulatory factor" in polycythemia vera which leads to an increase in the size of the stem cell pool and, thereby, to an increase in hormone-responsive cells (Reisner, 1967; Ward et al., 1974). Observations compatible with this hypothesis have been reported by Zanjani (1976). These studies demonstrated that serum from patients with polycythemia vera produced polycythemia when injected repeatedly into mice. This stimulation was not blocked by antiserum capable of neutralizing ESF. In addition, bone marrow cells from these mice appeared to respond more dramatically to ESF in vitro. However, no analogous changes in granulopoiesis or thrombopoiesis were reported. These types of studies imply that polycythemia vera arises as a proliferative response to an ill-defined "myelostimulatory" factor and that the increase in stem cell pool size, and perhaps in the size of the committed stem cell compartment, leads to an overproduction of all cellular elements.

Further support for this concept was introduced by Ward and Block (1970) who, by indirect morphological assessment of the pattern of tissue involvement in the myeloproliferative disorders, concluded that chronic granulocytic leukemia and polycythemia vera were inherently different. The former, accepted as a hematological malignancy, was characterized by invasive cellular proliferation whereas the proliferative picture of polycythemia vera recapitulated the hematopoietic proliferation characteristic of embryogenesis. The conclusion based on such analysis was that polycythemia vera represented the proliferation of normal stem cells and thus differed in a fundamental way from chronic granulocytic leukemia.

The second major hypothesis suggests that the disease arises from an abnormal stem cell, much like chronic granulocytic leukemia (Gurney, 1965). This has been appealing because of the frequent clinical similarities between the various disorders classified among the myeloproliferative syndromes (Dameshek, 1951).

The first hypothesis of the pathogenesis of polycythemia vera makes the important prediction that the disease has a multicellular origin. The most useful approach to this question takes advantage of a naturally occurring system of cell markers in man, that of the X-chromosome-linked genes for glucose-6-phosphate dehydrogenase (G6PD) (Fialkow, 1974). Such analysis is predicated on the fact that early in embryogenesis in female cells, random inactivation of one of the X chromosomes occurs. This process is irreversible, as far as is known, and, once having occurred within a cell, that cell and all its subsequent progeny will contain the gene products of only one of the X chromosomes. By selecting study patients who are naturally heterozygous for G6PD, the cellular origin of a neoplasm may be analyzed. Tumors of multicellular origin would be expected to contain more than one isoenzyme type whereas neoplasms of unicellular or clonal origin would contain only a single isoenzyme of G6PD.

This type of analysis has recently been applied to polycythemia vera in two G6PD heterozygotes (Adamson et al., 1976). Heterozygosity was established by analysis of skin biopsies and cultured skin fibroblasts. In contrast to the finding of two isoenzyme types in skin cells, peripheral blood red cells, granulocytes, and platelets contained only one isoenzyme type. These results documented the stem cell origin of the disease and strongly suggested its clonal nature; they were in every way similar to studies in chronic granulocytic leukemia. Thus, contrary to the prediction of the model of normal stem cell proliferation in response to a myelostimulatory factor, the increased cellular proliferation in polycythemia vera is most likely due to the proliferation of a single clone. Recently Jacobson and Fialkow (1976) have reported similar findings in patients with agnogenic myeloid metaplasia and myelofibrosis. Thus, there is reason to continue to classify all these myeloproliferative diseases together since all appear to be of clonal origin.

## 16.6.2. Response to Humoral Regulators

The response of polycythemia vera marrow cells to regulatory hormones has been a matter of particular interest and recent attention. In the initial analyses of the relationship of ESF to marrow function in polycythemic states, it was shown that patients with untreated polycythemia vera excreted markedly reduced or unmeasurable quantities of ESF (Adamson and Finch, 1968; Adamson, 1968). However, if the patient was phlebotomized, ESF excretion rose, demonstrating the intactness of this regulatory process (Fig. 6) (Adamson, 1968). In patients who were not iron deficient, the increase in ESF was accompanied by an increase in effective red cell production, as monitored by the reticulocyte index and quantitative ferrokinetics (Adamson, 1970). Thus, at least some marrow cells appeared capable of responding *in vivo* to humoral regulation although whether the cells were part of the abnormal clone remained undetermined.

Recently, the response of polycythemia vera marrow cells to ESF has been demonstrated *in vitro,* both in suspension culture by Golde and Cline (1975) and in semisolid medium using the erythroid colony-forming technique by Prchal and Axelrad (1974). In addition, these latter investigators observed that marrow cells from polycythemia vera patients formed erythroid colonies in the absence of added ESF and suggested that these "independent" colonies arose autonomously, although colony growth could be substantially increased by ESF. These studies clearly demonstrated that cells capable of responding to ESF are present in the marrow. What was unclear was whether the response was due to the abnormal or the residual normal cells.

An alternative explanation of the "independent" erythroid colonies has been advanced by Zanjani and colleagues who have analyzed the behavior of these colonies when exposed to antiserum to ESF (Zanjani, 1976). Such antiserum inhibited the growth of the erythroid colonies, suggesting that their appearance was due to the minute quantities of ESF in the culture medium. Thus, the cellular proliferation in polycythemia vera would result, at least in part, from the heightened sensitivity of various precursors to humoral regulators. Presumably, this would account for the granulocytic and megakaryocytic hyperplasia as well. Although the properties of the polycythemia vera clone are of considerable interest, some other initial event must occur which results in the expression of a clonal disorder.

The nature of the cells responding to ESF *in vitro* has been studied using marrow cultures from G6PD heterozygotes with polycythemia vera (Prchal *et al.,* 1976b). The analysis took advantage of the fact that each colony arises from a single cell and that the G6PD isoenzyme type for single colonies could be determined by electrophoresis (Prchal *et al.,* 1976a). As expected, all of the so-called independent erythroid colonies contained the isoenzyme type of characteristic of the polycythemia vera clone. As the concentration of ESF was increased *in vitro,* however, colonies appeared which did not contain the clonal isoenzyme type.

Statistical analysis of the ratio of the colonies bearing the two isoenzyme types led to the conclusion that both normal and abnormal cells are capable of responding to ESF. These findings in polycythemia vera parallel previous observations of *in vitro* granulocytic colony growth in chronic granulocytic leukemia. In addition to the fact that both diseases are clonal in origin, myelosuppression-induced clinical remission is not characterized by the appearance of normal cells in circulation. Thus, clinical remission is associated with the reappearance of response to and control by normal regulators, without the requirement for the ascension of normal stem cell lines. The studies of the regulation of hematopoiesis in these disorders will continue to provide insight into regulatory mechanisms in normal man.

The optimal therapy of polycythemia vera has been debated for several years. For many, treatment with radioactive phosphorus ($^{32}$P) was the choice; however, a significant incidence of leukemia—perhaps as high as 10–15%—was seen in patients treated with this modality, and the incidence of leukemia appeared to be directly related to the cumulative radiation dose (Modan and Lilienfeld, 1965). Although untreated disease is associated with a very short median survival (approximately 18 months), phlebotomy alone will significantly extend life (Videbaek, 1950).

In 1967, the International Polycythemia Vera Study Group was established to prospectively resolve questions of optimal therapy, the incidence of leukemia in patients treated by different regimens, and the relationship of other identifiable features (age, chromosomal abnormalities, spleen size, thrombocytosis, etc.) to disease progress and patient survival. Initial results of this important study have now appeared (Wasserman, 1976). An increased number of cases of leukemia have been seen, particularly in the chemotherapy-treated group, but early survival data fail to demonstrate the advantage of one form of treatment over another, and the median survival of all patients is similar to that of age- and sex-matched controls without polycythemia vera. It has been suggested that not only leukemia but other hematologic complications associated with progessive polycythemia vera, such as myelofibrosis and myeloid metaplasia, will be seen more frequently with myelosuppressive therapy (Silverstein, 1976). This will be of particular importance as the younger patients are followed by the Study Group for a longer period of time. The eventual conclusions from this important study should contribute significantly to both the understanding and rational management of this disorder.

## 16.7. Overview

The definition of mechanisms producing polycythemia in man is becoming increasingly detailed. The elucidation of $O_2$ transport defects at the molecular level of hemoglobin function and studies of the cellular origin of polycythemia vera are examples of such detail. It is virtually predictable that as the knowledge of ESF biochemistry increases, and the interaction of ESF with its marrow target cells is clarified, additional mechanisms of polycythemia will be described which are based on abnormalities at these molecular levels. Until then, however, it seems most rational to continue to approach polycythemic disorders physiologically, in terms of the relationships among $O_2$ transport, ESF production, and marrow proliferation.

Acknowledgments

This work was supported in part by research grants AM-19410 and HL-06242 of the NIH, DHEW, designated research funds of the Veterans Administration, and Research Career Development Award AM-70222 of the NIAMDD. During the preparation of this chapter, the author was supported by a Faculty Scholar Award for 1976–1977 from the Josiah Macy, Jr. Foundation.

## References

Adamson, J. W., 1968, The erythropoietin/hematocrit relationship in normal and polycythemic man: Implications of marrow regulation, *Blood* **32**:597.

Adamson, J. W., 1970, The regulation of erythropoiesis in polycythemia vera and related myeloproliferative disorders, in *Myeloproliferative Disorders in Animals and Man* (W. J. Clark, E. B. Howard, and P. L. Hackett, eds.), p. 440, U.S. Atomic Energy Commission, Washington, D.C.

Adamson, J. W., 1975, Familial polycythemia, *Semin. Hematol.* **12**:383.

Adamson, J. W., and Finch, C. A., 1968, Erythropoietin and the polycythemias, *Ann. N.Y. Acad. Sci.* **149**:560.

Adamson, J. W., and Finch, C. A., 1975, Hemoglobin function, oxygen affinity, and erythropoietin, *Annu. Rev. Physiol.* **37**:351.

Adamson, J. W., Alexanian, R., Martinez, C., and Finch, C. A., 1966, Erythropoietin excretion in normal man, *Blood* **28**:354.

Adamson, J. W., Stamatoyannopoulos, G., Kontras, S., Lascari, A., and Detter, J., 1973, Recessive familial erythrocytosis: Aspects of marrow regulation in two families, *Blood* **41**:641.

Adamson, J. W., Fialkow, P. J., Murphy, S., Prchal, J. F., and Steinmann, L., 1976, Polycythemia vera: Stem cell and probable clonal origin of the disease, *N. Engl. J. Med.* **295**:913.

Alexanian, R., 1966, Urinary excretion of erythropoietin in normal men and women, *Blood* **28**:344.

Balcerzak, S. P., and Bromberg, P. A., 1975, Secondary polycythemia, *Semin. Hematol.* **12**:353.

Bellingham, A. J., 1976, Hemoglobins with altered oxygen affinity, *Br. Med. Bull.* **32**:234.

Berlin, N. I., 1975, Diagnosis and classification of polycythemia, *Semin. Hematol.* **12**:339.

Bromberg, P. A., Alben, J. O., and Bare, G. H., 1973, Haemoglobin Little Rock ($\beta^{143}$his → gln; H21): A high oxygen affinity haemoglobin variant with unique properties, *Nature New Biol.* **243**:177.

Brown, S. M., Gilbert, H. S., Krauss, S., and Wasserman, L. R., 1971, Spurious (relative) polycythemia. A nonexistent disease, *Am. J. Med.* **50**:200.

Charache, S., Weatherall, D. J., and Clegg, J. B., 1966, Polycythemia associated with a hemoglobinopathy, *J. Clin. Invest.* **45**:813.

Dameshek, W., 1951, Some speculations on the myeloproliferative syndromes, *Blood* **6**:372.

Denny, W. F., Flanigan, W. J., and Zukoski, C. F., 1966, Serial erythropoietin studies in patients undergoing renal homotransplantation, *J. Lab. Clin. Med.* **67**:386.

Eder, H. A., Finch, C. A., and McKee, R. W., 1949, Congenital methemoglobinemia. A clinical and biochemical study of a case, *J. Clin. Invest.* **28**:265.

Erslev, A. J., 1975, Renal biogenesis of erythropoietin, *Am. J. Med.* **58**:25.

Fialkow, P. J., 1974, The origin and development of human tumors studied with cell markers, *N. Engl. J. Med.* **291**:26.

Finch, C. A., and Lenfant, C., 1972, Oxygen transport in man, *N. Engl. J. Med.* **286**:407.

Finch, C. A., Miller, L. R., Inamder, A. R., Person, R., Seiler, K., and Mackler, B., 1976, Iron deficiency in the rat. Physiological and biochemical studies of muscle dysfunction, *J. Clin. Invest.* **58**:447.

Fisher, J. W., and Samuels, A. I., 1967, Relationship between renal blood flow and erythropoietin production in dogs, Proc. Soc. Exp. Biol. Med. **125**:482.

Fisher, J. W., Schofield, R., and Porteous, D. D., 1965, Effects of renal hypoxia on erythropoietin production, *Br. J. Haematol.* **11**:382.

Golde, D. W., and Cline, M. J., 1975, Erythropoietin responsiveness in polycythemia vera, *Br. J. Haematol.* **29**:567.

Gordon, A. S., Cooper, G. W., and Zanjani, E. D., 1967, The kidney and erythropoiesis, *Semin. Hematol.* **4**:337.

Gordon, A. S., Zanjani, E. D., and Zalusky, R., 1970, A possible mechanism for the erythrocytosis associated with hepatocellular carcinoma in man, *Blood* **35**:151.

Gurney, C. W., 1965, Polycythemia vera and some pathogenetic mechanisms, *Annu. Rev. Med.* **16**:169.

Hammond, D., and Winnick, S., 1974, Paraneoplastic erythrocytosis and ectopic erythropoietin, *Ann. N.Y. Acad. Sci.* **230**:219.

Hayashi, A., and Stamatoyannopoulos, G., 1972, Role of Penultimate tyrosine in haemoglobin $\beta$ subunit, *Nature New Biol.* **235**:70.

Heller, Pl, Weinstein, H. G., and Yakulis, V. J., 1962, Hemoglobin M Kankakee, a new variant of hemoglobin M, *Blood* **20**:287.

Hillman, R. S., and Finch, C. A., 1972, *Red Cell Manual,* Davis, Philadelphia, Pennsylvania.

Hoffman, G. C., 1968, Human erythropoiesis following kidney transplantation, *Ann. N.Y. Acad. Sci.* **149**:504.

Hudgson, P., Pearce, J. M. S., and Yeates, W. K., 1967, Renal artery stenosis with hypertension and high hematocrit, *Br. Med. J.* **i**:18.

Hurtado, A., 1960, Some clinical aspects of life at high altitudes, *Ann. Intern. Med.* **53**:247.

Jacobson, R. J., and Fialkow, P. J., 1976, Idiopathic myelofibrosis: Stem cell abnormality and probable neoplastic origin, *Clin. Res.* **24**:439A.

Jaffé, E. R., 1966, Hereditary methemoglobinemias associated with abnormalities in the metabolism of erythrocytes, *Am. J. Med.* **41**:786.

Krantz, S. B., and Jacobson, L. O., 1970, *Erythropoietin and the Regulation of Erythropoiesis,* University of Chicago Press, Chicago.

Lawrence, J. H., and Donald, G., 1959, Polycythemia and hydronephrosis or renal tumors, *Ann. Intern. Med.* **50**:959.

Lichtman, M. A., Murphy, M. S., and Adamson, J. W., 1976, Detection of mutant hemoglobins with altered affinity for oxygen, *Ann. Intern. Med.* **84**:517.

Luke, R. G., Kennedy, A. C., Stirling, W. B., and McDonald, G. A., 1965, Renal artery stenosis, hypertension and polycythemia, *Br. Med. J.* **i**:164.

Mitus, W. J., Galbraith, P., Gollerkeri, M., and Toyama, K., 1964, Experimental erythrocytosis. I. Effects of pressure and vascular interference, *Blood* **24**:343.

Modan, B., and Lilienfeld, A. M., 1965, Polycythemia vera and leukemia—The role of radiation treatment: A sudy of 1222 patients, *Medicine* **44**:305.

Mollison, P. L., 1972, *Blood Transfusion in Clinical Medicine,* 5th ed., Blackwell, Oxford.

Monod, J., Wyman, J., and Changeux, J.-P., 1965, On the nature of allosteric transitions: A plausible model, *J. Mol. Biol.* **12**:88.

Nagel, R. L., and Bookchin, R. M., 1974, Human hemoglobin mutants with abnormal oxygen binding, *Semin. Hematol.* **11**:385.

Nies, B. A., Cohn, R., and Schrier, S. L., 1965, Erythremia after renal transplantation, *N. Engl. J. Med.* **273**:785.

Perutz, M. F., 1970, Stereochemistry of cooperative effects in haemoglobin, *Nature (London)* **228**:726.

Perutz, M. F., 1972, Nature of haem–haem interaction, *Nature (London)* **237**:495.

Perutz, M. F., and Lehmann, H., 1968, Molecular pathology of human haemoglobin, *Nature (London)* **219**:902.

Perutz, M. F., and TenEyck, L. F., 1971, Stereochemistry of cooperative effects in hemoglobin, *Cold Spring Harbor Symp. Quant. Biol.* **36**:295.

Peschle, C., and Condorelli, M., 1971, Mechanisms underlying erythrocytosis associated with kidney adenocarcinoma, *Blood* **38**:829.

Peschle, C., and Condorelli, M., 1975, Biogenesis of erythropoietin: Evidence for proerythropoietin in a subcellular fraction of kidney, *Science* **190**:910.

Prchal, J. F., and Axelrad, A. A., 1974, Bone marrow response in polycythemia vera, *N. Engl. J. Med.* **289**:1382.

Prchal, J. F., Adamson, J. W., Fialkow, P. J., and Steinmann, L., 1976a, Evidence for the clonal origin of human erythroid colonies, *J. Cell. Physiol.* **89**:489.

Prchal, J. F., Adamson, J. W., Murphy, S., Steinmann, L., and Fialkow, P. J., 1976b, Polycythemia vera: Demonstration of normal and abnormal stem cells and characterization of the *in vitro* response to erythropoietin, *Clin. Res.* **24**:442A.

Ranney, H. M., 1970, Clinically important variants of human hemoglobin, *N. Engl. J. Med.* **282**:144.

Reisner, E. H., Jr., 1967, Tissue culture of bone marrow. III. Myelostimulatory factors in serum of patients with myeloproliferative diseases, *Cancer* **20**:1679.

Rosse, W. F., Waldmann, T. A., and Cohen, P., 1963, Renal cysts, erythropoietin and polycythemia, *Am. J. Med.* **34**:76.

Sagone, A. L., Jr., and Balcerzak, S. P., 1975, Smoking as a cause of polycythemia, *Ann. Intern. Med.* **82**:512.

Sagone, A. L., Jr., Lawrence, T., and Balcerzak, S. P., 1973, Effect of smoking on tissue oxygen supply, *Blood* **41**:845.

Sievers, R. F., and Ryon, J. B., 1945, Congenital idiopathic methemoglobinemia: Favorable response to ascorbic acid therapy, *Arch. Intern. Med.* **76**:299.

Silverstein, M., 1976, The evolution into and the treatment of late stage polycythemia vera, *Semin. Hematol.* **13**:79.

Smith, H., and Riches, H., 1963, Hemoglobin values in renal carcinoma, *Lancet* **284**:1017.

Stamatoyannopoulos, G., 1972, Familial erythrocytosis, in *Birth Defects,* Vol. 8, Original Article Series, Part XIV, *Blood* (D. Bergsma, ed.), p. 39, Williams & Wilkins for the National Foundation, March of Dimes, Baltimore, Maryland.

Thorling, E. B., 1972, Paraneoplastic erythrocytosis and inappropriate erythropoietin production. A review, *Scand. J. Haematol.* Suppl. 17, 11–166.

Toyama, K., and Mitus, W. J., 1966, Experimental renal erythrocytosis. III. Relationship between the degree of hydronephrotic pressure and the production of erythrocytosis, *J. Lab. Clin. Med.* **68**:740.

Videbaek, A., 1950, Polycythemia vera: Course and prognosis, *Acta Med. Scand.* **138**:179.

Ward, H. P., and Block, M. H., 1970, The natural history of agnogenic myeloid metaplasia (AMM) and a critical evaluation of its relationship with the myeloproliferative syndrome, *Medicine* **50**:357.

Ward, H. P., Vautrin, R., and Kurnick, J., 1974, Presence of a myeloproliferative factor in patients with polycythemia vera and agnogenic myeloid metaplasia. I. Expansion of the erythropoietin-responsive stem cell compartment, *Proc. Soc. Exp. Biol. Med.* **147**:305.

Wasserman, L. R., 1976, The treatment of polycythemia vera, *Semin. Hematol.* **13**:57.

Weil, J. V., Jamieson, G., Brown, D. W., Grover, R. F., 1968, The red cell mass-arterial oxygen relationship in normal man, *J. Clin. Invest.* **47**:1627.

Weinreb, N.J., and Shih, C.-F., 1975, Spurious polycythemia, *Semin. Hematol.* **12**:397.

Westerman, M. P., Jenkins, J. L., Dekker, A., Kreutner, A., and Fisher, B., 1967, Significance of erythrocytosis and increased erythropoietin secretion after renal transplantation, *Lancet* **ii**:755.

Zanjani, E. D., 1976, Hematopoietic factors in polycythemia vera, *Semin. Hematol.* **13**:1.

Zürcher, C., Loos, J. A., and Prins, H. K., 1965, Hereditary high ATP content of human erythrocytes, *Folia Haematol. Leipzig* **83**:366.

# 17

# Nutritional Anemias Overview; Megaloblastic Anemias

## Victor Herbert, Neville Colman, and Elizabeth Jacob

## 17.1. Nutritional Anemias Overview

Nutritional anemia is defined as a condition in which the hemoglobin content of the blood is lower than normal as a result of deficiency of one or more essential nutrients, regardless of the cause of such deficiency (WHO Scientific Group on Nutritional Anemias, 1968). To delineate that a given anemia is due to deficiency of a nutrient, two criteria must be met: First, it must be demonstrated that lack of the nutrient will produce the anemia, and second, that providing the nutrient will correct the anemia (Herbert, 1970). By these two criteria, there are only three unequivocal true nutritional anemias: those due to lack of the mineral iron and those due to lack of the vitamins folate (folic acid) and vitamin $B_{12}$.

Although it is true that the anemia of copper deficiency meets the two criteria for nutritional origin, namely that its cure requires the administration of copper, and it can be produced in infants given a copper-deficient

VICTOR HERBERT, NEVILLE COLMAN, and ELIZABETH JACOB • Department of Medicine, State University of New York Downstate Medical Center, Brooklyn, New York 11209, and Veterans Administration Hospital, Bronx, New York 10468.

milk diet, these two criteria are only met when the infant's congenital copper stores are simultaneously depleted by diarrhea (Cordano et al., 1966).

The anemia of protein deficiency, like the anemia of hypothyroidism (Herbert, 1977a), appears to be largely a physiologic response to decreased oxygen need associated with decreased tissue mass and therefore decreased oxygen consumption (Finch, 1975). However, amino acids are the building blocks for protein, and the generation of hemoglobin obviously requires that there be protein feeding in order to have adequate response of the anemia of protein deficiency. As Viteri et al. (1968) have noted, the moderate degree of anemia that is usual in protein–calorie malnutrition appears to be primarily an adaptation phenomenon to decreased body mass to which various deficiencies and disease states can add their own characteristic changes. Thus, there is a distinction in protein–calorie malnutrition between *apparent* anemia, which is a fall in red cell mass because of a lower oxygen need due to the sharp fall in lean body mass, and *true* anemia, in which the level of the total circulating red cell mass is below the corresponding loss in the body mass. *True* anemia appears to occur when deficiencies of the mineral iron and the vitamins folate and $B_{12}$ are associated with the protein–calorie malnutrition, which itself may lead to intestinal atrophy (Brunser et al., 1968; Tandon et al., 1968) and, therefore, subnormal nutrient absorption.

It has not yet been demonstrated that withdrawal of vitamin E will produce anemia in humans. However, there is evidence that vitamin E deficiency anemia may occur in infants receiving potential oxidant compounds such as iron with the simultaneous administration of relatively large quantities of polyunsaturated fatty acids, which require vitamin E for their metabolism (Williams et al., 1975), and that this anemia responds to vitamin E therapy (or to therapy by reducing the feeding of large quantities of polyunsaturated fatty acids and oxidant compounds such as iron). Thus, the situation is perhaps better characterized as a nutrient-responsive anemia, rather than a nutrient deficiency anemia.

The distinction between a nutrient *deficiency* anemia and a nutrient-*responsive* anemia is not an idle one. Lack of either vitamin $B_{12}$ or of folate produces a nutrient *deficiency* anemia. However, the anemia of vitamin $B_{12}$ deficiency is *responsive* to therapy with folate, and folate deficiency anemia is *responsive* to therapy with vitamin $B_{12}$. Failure to make this crucial distinction between nutrient *deficiency* anemia and nutrient-*responsive* anemia has led in the past to patients with anemia due to lack of vitamin $B_{12}$ being treated with the wrong agent, namely folate, to which they are *responsive*. Such patients often experience marked hematologic improvement because of the biochemical interrelationships between vitamin $B_{12}$ and folic acid in actions on the hematopoietic system, but they suffer progressive neurologic damage because folate has no known positive biochemical interrelation with vitamin $B_{12}$ in the neurologic system, where only vitamin $B_{12}$ will arrest the gradual progression of the neurologic damage.

Some of the sideroblastic anemias appear to have some relation to vitamin $B_6$, and to respond to therapy with this vitamin. However, it has not yet been demonstrated either that deprivation of vitamin $B_6$ will produce anemia in man or that supplying this vitamin will produce complete return to normality. Therefore, not only are those sideroblastic anemias which respond to vitamin $B_6$ appropriately designated as nutrient-*responsive* anemias rather than nutrient *deficiency* anemias, but also it is an open question as to whether, when we treat a sideroblastic anemia which is pyridoxine responsive with vitamin $B_6$ and improve the anemia, we may be allowing progression of other facets of the disease, due to our failure to attack unknown or unrecognized underlying etiologic factors.

It has been demonstrated that men given a riboflavin-deficient diet plus the riboflavin antagonist, galactoflavin, develop a severe anemia which is reversed by the administration of riboflavin (Alfrey and Lane, 1970). Thus, this is not a "pure" nutritional anemia, in that it is not produced by simple dietary deprivation without superimposition of a second factor (i.e., galactoflavin). In this need for an additional factor for anemia to develop, it is similar to the anemia of copper deficiency, which requires not only that the diet be inadequate in copper but also that there be diarrhea to wipe out copper stores. Since a number of nutrient antagonists may be present in various possible bizarre diets (Committee on Food Protection, 1973), it is possible there may be a number of other as yet unrecognized situations of anemia induced by nutrient depletion plus a nutrient antagonist. It is probable that blockade of the function of any of a variety of vitamins or minerals could result in anemia; such possibilities have not yet been clearly demonstrated, and it is possible that large quantities of nutrient antagonists present in a given bizarre diet might produce deaths at the same time as they are producing anemia.

Since the distribution of hemoglobin concentrations in anemic persons overlaps that in persons with normal hemoglobin concentrations, the presence of mild anemia resulting from a nutritional deficiency can frequently be disclosed only by demonstrating increases in the hemoglobin concentration following therapy (Garby *et al.*, 1969; WHO Group of Experts, 1972). Mild or moderate anemia cannot be equated with hypoxia at ordinary levels of activity, but it does reduce maximum oxygen transport (Andersen and Barkve, 1970).

Nutritional anemias due to lack of iron, folate, and vitamin $B_{12}$ are prevalent throughout the world (WHO Scientific Group, 1968; WHO Group of Experts, 1972).

Understanding and management of the nutritional anemias require adequate diagnosis and appropriate therapy. The basic diagnostic tools include the various laboratory tests, both old and new, by which the existence of a nutrient deficiency may be adequately defined, and appropriate therapy is based on adequate evaluation of which of the various six possible etiologic factors underlying any nutritional deficiency are the culprits. These six possible etiologic factors, one or more of which must underlie any nutritional deficiency, include inadequate ingestion, inadequate absorption, inadequate utilization, increased excretion, increased requirement, and increased destruction of nutrient. Thus, a great deal of research in the nutritional anemia field is related to iron, folate, and vitamin $B_{12}$ form and content in various foodstuffs, factors inhibiting and enhancing their absorption from foods, and mechanisms affecting their transport, distribution, metabolic roles, catabolism, and excretion.

Nutritional anemia due to lack of iron, folate, or vitamin $B_{12}$ reflects an important nutritional problem affecting large population groups, particularly the poverty-stricken and those under metabolic stress regardless of degree of affluence. Iron deficiency and folate deficiency are more common in women because of two forms of metabolic stress peculiar to women: the monthly blood loss in the childbearing years and the drain on maternal nutrient stores imposed by pregnancy. The fetus will take from the mother whatever it needs in order to be born normal, even if this produces severe nutrient deficiency in the mother (Committee on Maternal Nutrition, 1970). Since anemia is a relatively late manifestation of nutritional deficiency, those patients diagnosed as having nutritional anemia are the "tip of the iceberg"—part of a larger group suffering from nutrient depletion of more moderate degree which is not yet manifest by unequivocal anemia. The metabolic stress of menstrual blood loss is increased by the use of some intrauterine contraceptive devices (Medical Letter, 1974, 1975), and decreased by the use of oral contraceptives (Medical Letter, 1973).

The high frequency of iron and folate deficiency in American women in the childbearing years makes a reasonable case for giving iron and folic acid supplements throughout pregnancy, and for increasing the existing iron fortification of American flour (Herbert, 1977c). The need for public health programs to supply adequate iron and folate to American women in the childbearing years has seemed clear for almost a decade (Herbert, 1970), but we still do not have such a program on a national basis. Hopefully, individual physicians will stimulate local and regional programs, using various diagnostic tests to define the frequency of the problem in various population groups in their own areas of the country. To provide ammunition for this work, the sections on deficiency of folate and $B_{12}$ begin with a review of the frequency of such deficiency in Americans.

## 17.2. Folate (Folic Acid) Deficiency

### 17.2.1. Frequency

The reported frequency of folate deficiency has varied greatly according to the diagnostic criteria used. The serum folate level is a labile index that cannot be used as the sole test for deficiency because it falls to low levels after a few weeks of folate deprivation, while folate stores may still be adequate (Herbert, 1962). The red cell folate level provides a good measure of tissue stores (Herbert and Zalusky, 1962; Chanarin, 1969) and has been shown to correlate closely with folate levels in the main storage organ, the liver (Wu et al., 1975).

Pregnant and lactating women comprise the major target group for folate deficiency. Recent surveys of low-income pregnant women in the United States indicate that 30% have red cell folate levels suggestive of deficiency (Herbert et al., 1975) and that about two-thirds have low serum folate levels (Herbert et al., 1975; Jacob et al., 1976). Women who receive inadequate supplements during pregnancy and lactation may remain folate deficient for several years thereafter (Colman et al., 1975a). Although the Ten-State Survey of nutritional status of Americans did not indicate in its final report the actual incidence of folate deficiency (USDHEW, 1972), data from Massachusetts workers participating in that survey revealed red cell folate levels suggestive of deficiency in a quarter of 1087 low-income women (Edozien, 1972).

### 17.2.2. Diagnostic Aspects

There are essentially three clinically discernible stages in the development of folate deficiency. As stated, serum folate levels fall to below 3 ng/ml after about 3 weeks of negative folate balance, and such levels generally reflect circumstances conducive to the development of deficiency. If negative balance is present and persists, tissue folate stores become depleted; this is reflected in a low red cell folate (below 150 ng folate/ml red cells) and inadequate folate for coenzyme function, with bone marrow becoming megaloblastic, the deoxyuridine (dU) suppression test becoming abnormal, and the hemoglobin falling. Each of these stages is identified by a specific test, namely serum folate, red cell folate, and dU suppression test.

Macrocytosis is often the presenting sign in folate deficiency. As recently outlined (Chanarin, 1976), the advent of automatic blood counters which directly size red cells led to a dramatic improvement in the recognition of macrocytosis, which appears before (Herbert, 1962) there is a significant fall in hemoglobin. Such counters have one disability: They do not separate the macroovalocytes which are the red cell hallmark of megaloblastosis from the macrocytes which are not oval and which occur in the many conditions mentioned immediately below. Thus, the examination of red cells in a peripheral blood film remains important. The advisability of investigating subjects with persistently raised mean corpuscular volume is apparent from studies reflecting a narrow range in normal subjects (Silver and Frankel, 1971; England *et al.*, 1972; McPhedran *et al.*, 1973; Croft *et al.*, 1974). Macrocytosis (but not macroovalocytosis) may occur in the absence of $B_{12}$ or folate deficiency in liver disease, aplastic and sideroblastic anemias, hypothyroidism, myeloma, neoplasia, antimetabolite drug therapy, and in any condition associated with reticulocytosis (Chanarin *et al.*, 1973; McPhedran *et al.*, 1973). Macrocytosis in alcoholics and in epileptics on anticonvulsants may be due either to folate deficiency associated with the use of these agents or to an apparent direct effect of alcohol or anticonvulsant drug in the absence of folate deficiency (Wu *et al.*, 1975; Wickramasinghe *et al.*, 1975).

Following examination of the peripheral blood for macroovalocytes, hypersegmentation of granulocyte nuclei, and giant platelets, a bone marrow aspirate is examined for evidence of morphologic and biochemical megaloblastosis. Biochemical megaloblastosis is studied using the dU suppression test (Metz *et al.*, 1968; Herbert *et al.*, 1973; Das and Herbert, 1976b), which compares the incorporation of tritiated thymidine into DNA in the absence and in the presence of nonradioactive dU. In the presence of normal folate coenzyme function, thymidylate synthetase converts dU to thymidine, resulting in a decreased proportion of the thymidine pool which is radioactive and a consequent "suppression" of the amount of radioactivity incorporated into DNA. Vitamin $B_{12}$ function is tested indirectly because it is an essential component in one of the reactions which convert the circulating form of folate, 5-methyltetrahydrofolate, into 5,10-methylenetetrahydrofolate, which is involved in thymidine synthesis. Addition of the missing nutrient affords specific diagnosis in the presence of an abnormal dU suppression test due to folate or $B_{12}$ deficiency. Morphologic megaloblastosis in the presence of a normal dU suppression test may occur with the use of antitumor drugs which inhibit DNA synthesis, and has been reported in patients taking anticonvulsants (Wickramasinghe *et al.*, 1975).

The potential use of lymphocyte culture in the dU suppression test (Das and Hoffbrand, 1970) is currently being developed as a test for prior folate and $B_{12}$ deficiency despite treatment making the bone marrow dU suppression test normal (Das and Herbert, 1976a).

Red cell folate levels are low not only in folate deficiency but also in $B_{12}$ deficiency, the latter because marrow folate uptake is decreased in $B_{12}$ deficiency and corrected by $B_{12}$ addition (Tisman and Herbert, 1973).

Measurement of folate levels originally required microbiologic assay (Herbert, 1961), but radioisotopic assays recently became available using the techniques of competitive inhibition (Waxman *et al.*, 1971) and sequential saturation (Waxman *et al.*, 1971; Rothenberg *et al.*, 1972; Rothenberg and da Costa, 1976). A series of improvements have resulted in the development of a practical reliable folate radioassay, which capitalizes on the availability of radioiodinated folate and on the fact that at pH 9.3 milk folate binder is unable to differentiate stable folic acid from unstable methyl folate (Longo and Herbert, 1976); heat is used to separate serum folate from the small amount of endogenous binder for it (Colman and Herbert, 1976; Colman *et al.*, 1976).

### 17.2.3. Metabolic Aspects

Figure 1 presents a flow chart of folate metabolism.

The suggestion that a falling serum potassium during therapy may contribute to early mortality in megaloblastic anemia (Lawson *et al.*, 1972) has been challenged by evidence that hypokalemia is rarely significant and does not require potassium supplements (Hesp *et al.*, 1975).

The interrelationships between vitamin $B_{12}$ and folate metabolism have been reviewed elsewhere (Das and Herbert, 1976b). The interrelationships between iron and folate deficiency are being elucidated as studies proceed to identify the reasons why erythroid megaloblastosis may be masked in iron deficiency. Thymidine incorporation into DNA is decreased in iron deficiency (Hershko *et al.*, 1970) or by *in vitro* addition of penicillamine (Tisman and Herbert, 1971) or desferrioxamine to normal marrow (van der Weyden *et al.*, 1972), and is corrected by the addition of iron-dextran (Longo and Herbert, 1975). In general, the changes in the dU suppression test in iron deficiency are opposite to those in folate deficiency (van der Weyden *et al.*, 1972), providing a biochemical corollary to the morphological effects. Studies of the effects of desferrioxamine and iron deficiency on nucleotide pools in stimulated lymphocytes have been interpreted as supporting the concept that altered DNA synthesis in iron deficiency may be mediated by defective ribonucleotide reductase function rather than by direct effects on folate-dependent pathways (Hoffbrand *et al.*, 1976). This hypothesis was further supported by the concurrent demonstration that *in vitro* addition of the iron chelating agent inhibited ribonucleotide reductase activity.

The possibility that folate deficiency may cause neurological changes has once again been raised in a number of reports, including one which describes 10 cases of folate-responsive neuropathy (Manzoor and Runcie, 1976). A specific role for folate in biogenic amine metabolism has been proposed (Banerjee and Snyder, 1973), and challenged (Meller *et al.*,

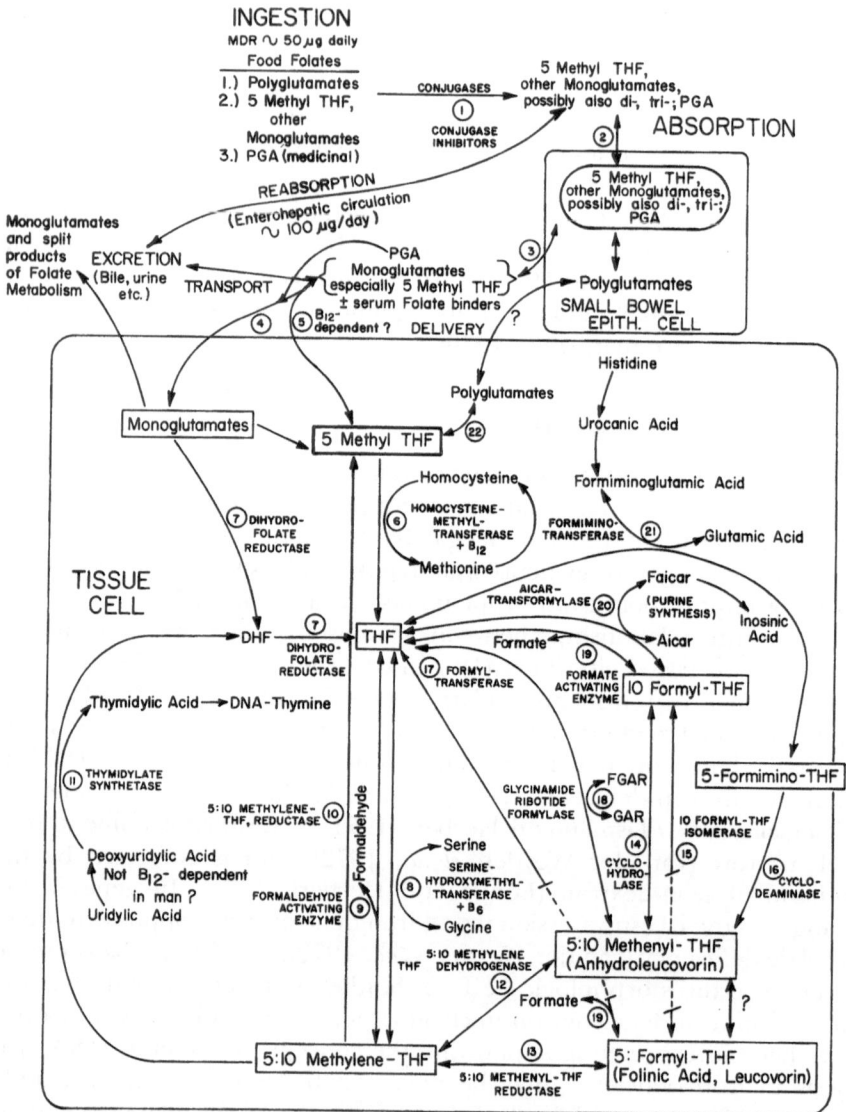

**Fig. 1.** Flow chart of folate metabolism. Circled numbers identify individual steps in folate metabolism. THF, tetrahydrofolate; DHF, dihydrofolate; MDR, adult minimal daily requirement from exogenous sources to sustain normality. (From Herbert, 1975a, by courtesy of W. B. Saunders.)

1975). The contradictory reports in this field have recently been reviewed by one of the prominent investigators involved (Reynolds, 1976), who favors the possibility that folate deficiency may produce neuropathy in adults. Further study in this area is clearly indicated, particularly study aimed at defining the existence of a specific biochemical or morphologic lesion in the neurologic system due to folate deficiency in the adult. No such lesion has yet been reported, and until it is, allegations of neurologic damage due to folate deficiency in adults will continue to be treated skeptically.

## 17.2.4. Clinical Aspects

Appropriate management of nutritional deficiency states involves both specific replacement therapy and treatment of the underlying cause. There are some 50 recognized causes of folate deficiency, outlined in detail elsewhere (Herbert, 1975a) and classifiable into the six broad categories listed in Section 17.1. Three of these categories include the vast majority of folate-deficient megaloblastic anemias; these are inadequate ingestion, inadequate absorption, and increased utilization. Recent studies have expanded our knowledge in each of these three areas.

The mechanism whereby ingested foods may mediate the development of folate deficiency has long been recognized as dependent not only on their folate content but also on the availability of that content from the specific foods concerned (Herbert, 1963). It has generally been assumed that variations in the availability of food folate are due to "a wide range of availability of the polyglutamate form" (Food and Nutrition Board, 1974). Two known ways in which polyglutamate availability may be altered by foods, both involving inhibition of the intestinal conjugase enzyme which removes extra glutamate residues, are inhibition by lowering intestinal pH as occurs with acidic foods such as orange juice (Tamura et al., 1976); and the presence of a heat-stable heat-activated conjugase inhibitor, such as occurs in beans and other pulses (Krumdieck et al., 1973), with properties which suggest it as a causative factor in folate deficiency (Butterworth et al., 1974). In addition, emerging evidence strongly suggests that the availability of not only polyglutamate but also monoglutamate in different foods differs widely, since the availability of synthetic pteroylmonoglutamate added to different foods is variable, depending on the food studied (Tamura and Stokstad, 1973; Colman et al., 1975b). The factors that determine monoglutamate availability are largely unknown.

The mechanisms of folate absorption have been clarified by studies using pure folate polyglutamates synthesized by a method that allows radioactive labeling of a preselected glutamate residue (Krumdieck and Baugh, 1969). Studies using these compounds suggest there are three main steps in folate absorption: the uptake of both monoglutamate and polyglutamate by the mucosal cell, removal of glutamate residues by intracellular conjugase, and passage of monoglutamate into the portal blood without further enzymatic conversion (Butterworth and Krumdieck, 1975; Rosenberg, 1976).

The finding that glucose enhances folic acid absorption (Gerson et al., 1971) appears critical to triple lumen tube in vivo gastroenterologic studies of folate malabsorption. Independent studies indicate that in tropical sprue, the gastrointestinal disease most often characterized by folate deficiency, the existing folate malabsorption is only detectable when adequate glucose or galactose is added to the ingested material; absorption is similar in patients and controls in the absence of the monosaccharides (Gerson *et al.*, 1974; Corcino *et al.*, 1975, 1976).

Increased utilization of folate appears to be the critical factor in a newly recognized syndrome of megaloblastic anemia developing rapidly in subjects receiving intensive therapy. The first recognition of this association in subjects on hyperalimentation therapy appears to be that of Ballard and Lindenbaum (1974). A series of subsequent reports and letters on this subject (Wardrop *et al.*, 1975a,b; Ibbotson *et al.*, 1975a,b; Saary and Hoffbrand, 1976) indicate that this anemia develops too rapidly to be wholly attributable to inadequate ingestion, that alcohol in the infusion fluid may be an important factor but is not essential to the genesis of the syndrome, and that there may be a link between this syndrome and one of megaloblastic anemia with bizarre features (dyserythropoiesis, gigantoblasts, multinuclearity) reported in seriously ill patients (Saary *et al.*, 1975).

Megaloblastic anemia has been reported in women taking oral contraceptives. Controlled trials of the effects of these agents on folate in serum and red cells suggest that the mean serum and red cell folate are lower in subjects taking them than in controls (Smith *et al.*, 1975; Prasad *et al.*, 1975). It is not yet clear that folate supplementation is needed by women taking such products (Medical Letter, 1973; Lindenbaum *et al.*, 1975). Animal studies provide evidence that the complex regulation of tissue folate metabolism is subject to mediation by female sex hormones (Krumdieck *et al.*, 1976).

## 17.3. Vitamin $B_{12}$ Deficiency

Of the three true nutritional anemias vitamin $B_{12}$ deficiency is the least common in Americans generally (Herbert, 1977b), although it is prominent in certain special groups of subjects such as dietary faddists and those suffering from diseases of the stomach or small intestine, as discussed in detail later. The reasons for this low prevalence are related to the high intake of animal protein and therefore of vitamin $B_{12}$ in the average American diet (Chung *et al.*, 1961), the ease with which normal subjects absorb the vitamin (Mollin *et al.*, 1957), the small daily requirement (Sullivan and Herbert, 1965), and the relatively large body stores

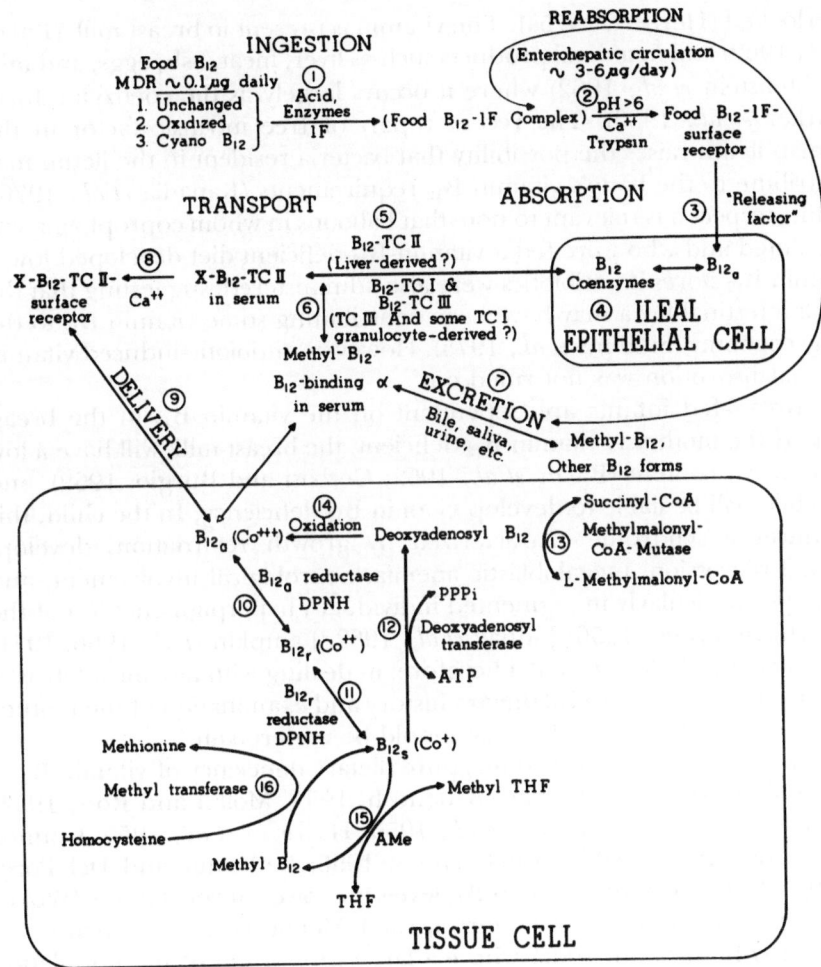

**Fig. 2.** Flow chart of vitamin $B_{12}$ metabolism. MDR, adult minimum daily requirement from exogenous sources to sustain normality. (From Herbert, 1975a, by courtesy of W. B. Saunders.)

which tide over temporary periods of decreased intake of the vitamin or increased requirements for it. Figure 2 presents a flow chart of vitamin $B_{12}$ metabolism.

## 17.3.1. Inadequate Ingestion

Human requirements of vitamin $B_{12}$ are usually thought to be met exclusively by the vitamin $B_{12}$ content of the diet; the major contribution from reabsorption of vitamin $B_{12}$ excreted in the bile has been largely overlooked (Herbert, 1975a). The vitamin is present in breast milk (Baker *et al.*, 1962) and in animal products such as liver, meat, fish, eggs, and milk (Lichtenstein *et al.*, 1962) where it occurs largely as the coenzyme form (Barker *et al.*, 1960). The recent report of free intrinsic factor in the human ileum raises the possibility that bacteria resident in the ileum may contribute to the body's vitamin $B_{12}$ requirements (Kapadia *et al.*, 1976). In this respect it is relevant to note that baboons in whom coprophagia was prevented and who were fed a vitamin-$B_{12}$-deficient diet developed lower vitamin $B_{12}$ stores if antibiotics were also administered, suggesting that the small-intestinal flora may have been contributing some vitamin $B_{12}$ to the body economy (Siddons *et al.*, 1975). However, antibiotic-induced vitamin $B_{12}$ malabsorption was not ruled out.

Breast-fed infants are dependent on the vitamin $B_{12}$ in the breast milk. If the mother is vitamin $B_{12}$ deficient, the breast milk will have a low vitamin $B_{12}$ content (Baker *et al.*, 1962; Gerbasi and Burgio, 1962), and the child will be liable to develop vitamin $B_{12}$ deficiency. In the child, this produces a syndrome characterized by growth retardation, developmental regression, megaloblastic anemia, neurological involvement, and perhaps, particularly in pigmented individuals, hyperpigmentation of the skin (Burgio *et al.*, 1956; Jadhav *et al.*, 1962, Lampkin *et al.*, 1966, 1971; Srikantia and Reddy, 1967). Therefore, in dealing with any megaloblastic anemia in infants, a careful dietary history and examination of the mother to exclude vitamin $B_{12}$ deficiency should be undertaken.

In older children and adults, pure dietary deficiency of vitamin $B_{12}$ is seen only in strict vegetarians (Badenoch, 1954; Mollin and Ross, 1954; Wokes *et al.*, 1955; Pollycove *et al.*, 1956; Harrison *et al.*, 1956; Connor and Pirola, 1963; Habib, 1964; Hines, 1966; Ledbetter and Del Pozo, 1969). Although serum vitamin $B_{12}$ levels are lower in vegetarians (Wokes *et al.*, 1955; Banerjee and Chatterjea, 1960; Mehta *et al.*, 1964; Armstrong *et al.*, 1974), in South India where a large proportion of the population are vegetarian, pure dietary deficiency of vitamin $B_{12}$ is an uncommon cause of megaloblastic anemia (Baker and Mathan, 1971). In this situation, the vitamin $B_{12}$ requirement appears to be met to a significant degree by the small amounts of the vitamin arising by contamination of the food and water with fecal and other animal matter (Baker, personal communication). It has been reported from North India that in pregnancy serum vitamin $B_{12}$ levels are frequently reduced (Sood *et al.*, 1967).

Ingested vitamin $B_{12}$ is normally liberated from the food by digestion. The liberated vitamin $B_{12}$ combines with intrinsic factor (IF) secreted by the gastric parietal cells (Hoedemaeker *et al.*, 1964; Taylor, 1965; Jacob and Glass, 1969, 1971a). The intrinsic factor–vitamin $B_{12}$ complex then passes down the intestine to the ileum (Booth and Mollin, 1959), where, in

**Table I.** Factors Interfering with Vitamin $B_{12}$ Absorption

Structural or functional damage affecting:
1. Stomach:
    Hereditary abnormality of IF molecule; congenital deficiency of IF secretion (congenital pernicious anemia); gastric atrophy (loss of acid and enzymes reduce ability to free vitamin $B_{12}$ from food); pernicious anemia (acquired); gastritis; gastrectomy; secondary to vitamin $B_{12}$ deficiency
2. Small bowel:
    Fish tapeworm infestation; stagnant bowel syndrome; coeliac disease; tropical sprue; congenital vitamin $B_{12}$ malabsorption (Imerslund–Gräsbeck syndrome); intestinal resection and short circuits; secondary to vitamin $B_{12}$ deficiency
3. Pancreas:
    Inadequate bicarbonate secretion; inadequate enzyme (trypsin?) secretion; inadequate ionic calcium?
4. Ingested or injected substances:
    Drugs: neomycin; colchicine; $p$-aminosalicylic acid (PAS); slow release potassium chloride; metformin; ethanol; methotrexate

the presence of calcium (Herbert, 1959a), it attaches to the receptors of the ileal enterocytes (Herbert, 1959b; Nieweg *et al.*, 1957). The vitamin is then transported through the epithelial cell and enters the circulation, where it combines with the vitamin $B_{12}$ transport protein transcobalamin II, which takes it to the liver, bone marrow, and other tissues (Allen, 1975). This absorption mechanism may be interfered with at any one of a number of points (Table I).

## 17.3.2. Stomach

### 17.3.2.1. Hereditary Abnormality of IF Molecule

Katz *et al.* (1972) described a 13-year-old boy who developed vitamin $B_{12}$ deficiency due to a physiologically abnormal intrinsic factor, quantitatively inefficient in facilitating vitamin $B_{12}$ absorption even though it was immunologically indistinguishable from normal intrinsic factor. His parents were first cousins and it was shown by immunological studies that they and his sister had 50% of abnormal intrinsic factor, indicating an autosomal recessive type of genetic transmission (Katz *et al.*, 1974).

### 17.3.2.2. Congenital Deficiency of IF Secretion

Mollin *et al.* (1955) described a patient who, although he had normal acid and pepsin secretion and a histologically normal gastric mucosa, had only a very small amount of intrinsic factor in his gastric juice. Chanarin

(1969) reviewed over 30 cases of this syndrome from the literature. Parietal cell and intrinsic factor antibodies have not been found in these subjects (Herbert *et al.*, 1964). Although congenital deficiency and hereditary abnormality of intrinsic factor are rare, they should be borne in mind in all cases of vitamin $B_{12}$ deficiency anemia in children (Cooper, 1976).

### 17.3.2.3. Pernicious Anemia

There is increasing evidence that classical pernicious anemia, i.e., vitamin $B_{12}$ deficiency anemia due to reduced or absent intrinsic factor secretion, associated with atrophy of the gastric mucosa, has both a genetic and an autoimmune (Herbert, 1967) component in its etiology. This evidence has recently been reviewed (Baker, 1975; Herbert, 1975; Taylor, 1976). Although parietal cell and intrinsic factor antibodies are common in patients with pernicious anemia, and both types of antibodies have been shown to fix complement (Jacob and Glass, 1969, 1971a,b), their role in the production of the gastric atrophy is not clear. Two types of intrinsic factor antibody have been described (Roitt *et al.*, 1964; Garrido-Pinson *et al.*, 1966; Schade *et al.*, 1967): that which reacts only with native intrinsic factor and prevents binding of vitamin $B_{12}$, termed "blocking antibody," and that which combines with the intrinsic factor molecule even after vitamin $B_{12}$ is attached to it, termed "binding antibody." Binding antibody has also been demonstrated in plasma cells in gastric mucosa (Baur *et al.*, 1968).

The diagnosis of pernicious anemia depends on the demonstration of a vitamin-$B_{12}$-responsive anemia and the lack of intrinsic factor secretion. The latter can be confirmed by doing vitamin $B_{12}$ absorption tests, showing subnormal absorption when the vitamin is given alone, which is normalized when the vitamin is given with added intrinsic factor. (It should be noted, however, that in severe vitamin $B_{12}$ deficiency, the addition of intrinsic factor may fail to normalize absorption—see Section 17.3.3.7.) Lack of intrinsic factor can also be demonstrated by direct assay of gastric juice following appropriate stimulation (histalog or pentagastrin). The assay can be carried out in a number of ways, including the coated charcoal procedure and the use of the "blocking antibody" (Gottlieb *et al.*, 1965) and the zirconium gel assay using the "binding antibody" (Jacob and O'Brien, 1972).

### 17.3.2.4. Gastritis

Gastritis, from whatever cause, if severe and chronic enough, can produce a reduction in intrinsic factor secretion and malabsorption of vitamin $B_{12}$ (Glass, 1963). Such cases will clinically resemble classic pernicious anemia, and indeed classic pernicious anemia may include cases with this pathogenesis of the gastric lesion.

### 17.3.2.5. Gastrectomy

Reduction in parietal cell mass by gastrectomy will reduce intrinsic factor secretion proportionately. Complete removal of the parietal cell mass, as in total gastrectomy, results in complete absence of intrinsic factor and the eventual development of severe vitamin $B_{12}$ deficiency (Swendseid et al., 1953). Such patients should therefore receive regular parenteral vitamin $B_{12}$ therapy to ensure that they maintain normal body stores of the vitamin.

In subjects who have undergone partial gastrectomy, other factors may also reduce intrinsic factor secretion, such as the development of gastritis in the remaining gastric remnant (MacLean, 1957) and reduced vagal stimulation following vagotomy (Adams et al., 1967).

Finally, it has been shown that subjects who have hypochlorhydria or achlorhydria, including those who have had a partial gastrectomy, may malabsorb food vitamin $B_{12}$ even though they can absorb normally the usual dose of crystalline radioactive vitamin $B_{12}$ when given in the fasting state (Doscherholmen and Swaim, 1973). This suggests that normal gastric acid and enzyme secretion plays an important role in absorption of food $B_{12}$ by liberating the vitamin from its bonds in food. The prevalence of megaloblastic anemia following partial gastrectomy has been reported as occurring in from 1% (MacLean, 1957) to 4% (Hines et al., 1967) of patients. However, low serum vitamin $B_{12}$ concentration occurs more frequently, and a study of 351 patients who had undergone Bilroth II partial gastrectomy revealed serum vitamin $B_{12}$ levels that showed a steady decline for the first 8–10 years following surgery, but plateaued thereafter (Rygvold, 1974). In view of the relatively low prevalence of obvious megaloblastic anemia in these patients, it may not be justified to advise routine prophylactic vitamin $B_{12}$; however, the possiblity of developing vitamin $B_{12}$ deficiency should be borne in mind by the attending physician, who should evaluate yearly for this possibility.

### 17.3.3. Small Bowel

#### 17.3.3.1. Fish Tapeworm Infestation

Infestation with fish tapeworm, Diphyllobothrium latum, is frequently associated with vitamin $B_{12}$ deficiency and megaloblastic anemia (von Bonsdorff, 1947). This occurs in subjects who ingest uncooked or poorly cooked freshwater fish. The worm takes up vitamin $B_{12}$ from the intestinal lumen, rendering it unavailable to the host (von Bonsdorff *et al.*, 1960). Expulsion of the worms may be followed by spontaneous hematological improvement (Nyberg and Saarni, 1964). Such patients should also be treated with parenteral vitamin $B_{12}$ for a short period of time. The disease is disappearing in Finland as the freshwater fish die off due to water pollution (Gräsbeck, personal communication).

### 17.3.3.2. Stagnant Bowel Syndrome

A variety of lesions of the gastrointestinal tract may be accompanied by stasis of luminal content and resultant overgrowth of intestinal bacteria. Such lesions include gastroenterostomy, small-intestinal diverticula, short circuits, blind loops, and strictures. These conditions are frequently associated with malabsorption of vitamin $B_{12}$ which is not corrected by supplying extra intrinsic factor, but is frequently corrected, at least temporarily, by antibiotics (Mollin and Baker, 1955; Cooke *et al.*, 1963a; Donaldson, 1965). This suggests that the vitamin $B_{12}$ malabsorption is related to the presence of the intraluminal bacteria. However, the mechanism by which the bacteria produce this malabsorption is not clear. It has been suggested that it may be related to bacterial toxins (Drexler, 1958; Dawson and Isselbacher, 1960; Faulk and Farrar, 1964). However, it has not been possible to demonstrate such an effect in an animal model (Schjönsby, 1974). More probably the bacteria take up the intrinsic factor–vitamin $B_{12}$ complex, thus rendering the vitamin $B_{12}$ unavailable to the host (Donaldson *et al.*, 1962; Schjönsby *et al.*, 1970; Schjönsby, 1974).

The stagnant bowel syndrome should always be considered, particularly in subjects who have had a previous history of abdominal surgery and in subjects who appear to have pernicious anemia but who have normal amounts of intrinsic factor in their gastric juice or whose absorption of vitamin $B_{12}$ is not normalized by the addition of added intrinsic factor when vitamin $B_{12}$ deficiency has been corrected. A full and careful radiological examination of the gastrointestinal tract is essential in such patients.

### 17.3.3.3. Coeliac Disease

Vitamin $B_{12}$ malabsorption occurs in some patients with coeliac disease. This appears to be caused by interference with ileal uptake of vitamin $B_{12}$ due to the toxic effect of wheat gluten (Rubin *et al.*, 1962). The reported prevalence of vitamin $B_{12}$ malabsorption in this condition varies from 10% (Cooke *et al.*, 1963b) to 80% (Oxenhorn *et al.*, 1958), but the latter figure probably is due to inclusion of New York Puerto Rican patients with tropical sprue. However, pure vitamin $B_{12}$ deficiency megaloblastic anemia seems to be unusual in this condition (Mollin *et al.*, 1959).

### 17.3.3.4. Tropical Sprue

Vitamin $B_{12}$ malabsorption is almost a universal finding in patients with tropical sprue (Baker, 1972). In about a third of cases this is associated with a gastric lesion causing reduced to absent intrinsic factor secretion (Baker and Mathan, 1968). However, usually the defect is not corrected by additional intrinsic factor. In a number of cases, broad spectrum antibiotics will cure the vitamin $B_{12}$ absorptive defect (Baker, 1972), suggesting that it is related to the presence of luminal bacteria. It has been shown that the defect is not related to uptake by intestinal bacteria or to alterations in the intrinsic factor–vitamin $B_{12}$ complex as it passes down the intestine (Kapadia *et al.*, 1975). Therefore, the bacteria must in some way interfere either with the uptake of the vitamin by the ileal receptors or its transport through the ileal enterocytes. Klipstein *et al.* (1973) and Corcino (1975) have implicated ethanol-producing bacteria in the Puerto Rico variety of tropical sprue. Since the lesion of tropical sprue may be present for a number of years, vitamin $B_{12}$ deficiency megaloblastic anemia is not unusual in this condition. Anyone who presents with a megaloblastic anemia who has been in a region such as Southeast Asia or the Caribbean, where this condition is endemic, must be investigated to exclude it, particularly if they were born in such a region. The disease may manifest itself years after leaving the tropics (Booth and Mollin, 1964).

### 17.3.3.5. Congenital Vitamin $B_{12}$ Malabsorption (Imerslund–Gräsbeck Syndrome)

A condition of megaloblastic anemia due to vitamin $B_{12}$ malabsorption with normal intrinsic factor secretion and proteinuria was first described by Najman and Brausil (1952). Further cases were described by Imerslund (1960) and Gräsbeck *et al.* (1960), and the condition is frequently called the Imerslund–Gräsbeck syndrome. To date, at least 49 such cases have been described (Mohamed *et al.*, 1966; Ben-Bassat *et al.*, 1969; Gräsbeck, 1969, 1972; Khakee *et al.*, 1974). In one subject with this condition, the intrinsic factor–vitamin $B_{12}$ complex was shown to reach the ileum in normal amounts and to be immunologically reactive (Jacob, Kapadia, Baker, unpublished observations, 1972). In another case, MacKenzie *et al.*, (1972) could not demonstrate any abnormality in intrinsic factor–vitamin $B_{12}$ uptake by the ileal receptors from an ileal biopsy, and electron microscopy of the ileal enterocytes was normal. Thus the defect in this condition may be related to defective transport through the ileal mucosal cells.

### 17.3.3.6. Intestinal Resection and Short Circuits

Since physiological absorption of vitamin $B_{12}$ in man occurs exclusively in the ileum, resection or short-circuiting of the ileum results in vitamin $B_{12}$ malabsorption and vitamin $B_{12}$ deficiency (McIntyre *et al.*, 1956; Mollin *et al.*, 1957; Booth and Mollin, 1957, 1959; Sherman and May, 1963; Booth *et al.*, 1964). With the popularity of jejunoileal bypass for the treatment of intractable obesity, the importance of this condition as a cause of vitamin $B_{12}$ deficiency needs to be reemphasized. A comparatively short length of terminal ileum may be enough to ensure adequate vitamin $B_{12}$ absorption (Sherman and May, 1963). However, Hippe *et al.* (1974) found that some patients subjected to this type of surgery developed a bacterial overgrowth in the lumen of the small intestine, suggesting that the situation may be further complicated by the development of a stagnant bowel syndrome. Therefore, any individual who has had an ileal resection should be given regular prophylactic parenteral vitamin $B_{12}$, and subjects with an ileojejunal bypass should be tested at appropriate intervals to ensure that they are not developing vitamin $B_{12}$ malabsorption or vitamin $B_{12}$ deficiency.

### 17.3.3.7. Vitamin $B_{12}$ Deficiency "Vicious Cycle"

In some subjects with vitamin $B_{12}$ deficiency, there is an interference with absorption of vitamin $B_{12}$ which is corrected by treating the vitamin $B_{12}$ deficiency (Haurani *et al.*, 1964; Brody *et al.*, 1966; Carmel and Herbert, 1967; Lampkin and Mauer, 1967). This transient (reversible) vitamin $B_{12}$ malabsorption may be the result of secondary damage to stomach or ileum by $B_{12}$ deficiency caused by primary damage to the other organ (Herbert, 1972a). It may play a role in aggravating vitamin $B_{12}$ deficiency once it has developed, thereby producing a vicious cycle. Since the diagnosis of pernicious anemia is usually based on the demonstration of failure to absorb labeled vitamin $B_{12}$ given alone and correction of this malabsorption by intrinsic factor, it must be realized that secondary intestinal malabsorption of vitamin $B_{12}$ may occur in up to 40% of cases, thus misleadingly suggesting a diagnosis of primary small-intestinal disease. Thus, before concluding from radioactive-labeled $B_{12}$ absorption studies that intestinal malabsorption is primary, the test must be repeated 1 or 2 months after the start of vitamin $B_{12}$ therapy (Herbert, 1969, 1972b; Lindenbaum *et al.*, 1974).

### 17.3.4. Pancreas

Malabsorption of vitamin $B_{12}$, as measured with the radioactive-labeled vitamin given alone or with IF, has been demonstrated in some subjects with pancreatic insufficiency (McIntyre *et al.*, 1956; Veeger *et al.*, 1962; Perman *et al.*, 1960; Toskes *et al.*, 1971, 1973) and it has been corrected by supplying bicarbonate or pancreatic extract (Toskes *et al.*, 1973). Henderson *et al.* (1972) demonstrated in some cases, that although there was malabsorption of vitamin $B_{12}$ when given alone, when the vitamin was given with food, absorption was normal. The occasional occurrence of vitamin $B_{12}$ malabsorption in chronic pancreatitis is an interesting observation which may prove of importance as a diagnostic test for suspected chronic pancreatitis (Herbert, 1972b; Toskes *et al.*, 1973).

It has been demonstrated *in vitro* that calcium is required for the binding of vitamin $B_{12}$–IF complex to the intestinal mucosa (Herbert, 1959a). However, there is no evidence that calcium deficiency per se produces a megaloblastic anemia.

### 17.3.5. Drugs

Several drugs have been described which, when administered to man, may be associated with vitamin $B_{12}$ malabsorption. These include neomycin (Jacobson *et al.*, 1960), colchicine (Webb *et al.*, 1968), *p*-aminosalicylic acid (PAS) (Heinivaara *et al.*, 1964; Toskes and Deren, 1972), slow release potassium chloride (Solakannel *et al.*, 1970; Palva *et al.*, 1972), metformin (Berchtold *et al.*, 1969; Tomkin *et al.*, 1971), and ethanol (Roggin *et al.*, 1969; Lindenbaum and Lieber, 1969). When these agents are administered for a short period of time, the vitamin $B_{12}$ malabsorption is not of clinical significance. However, PAS and, particularly, antidiabetic agents may be administered for long periods of time and could then result in significant deficiency of the vitamin. Two cases of megaloblastic anemia in subjects receiving PAS therapy for tuberculosis were reported by Heinivaara and Palva (1964). However, other investigators have not been able to demonstrate a decline in serum vitamin $B_{12}$ levels in patients on long-term PAS therapy (Markkanen *et al.*, 1967). It therefore seems probable that administration of this drug is not an important cause of vitamin $B_{12}$ deficiency. In 71 subjects receiving long-term (mean 4–6 years) metformin therapy, 30% were found to have low vitamin $B_{12}$ absorption, though only four patients had evidence of vitamin $B_{12}$ deficiency (Tomkin *et al.*, 1971). This topic has been reviewed (Herbert, 1972c). The mechanism of malabsorption is not clear, but absorption is not normalized by intrinsic factor and is presumably related to a lesion of the ileal uptake or transport mechanism. In view of these findings, diabetic patients maintained on metformin therapy should be checked at regular intervals to ensure that they are not developing vitamin $B_{12}$ deficiency.

## 17.3.6. Inadequate Utilization

In man, vitamin $B_{12}$ is known to function in the isomerization of methylmalonic CoA to succinyl CoA and in the conversion of homocysteine to methionine. These vitamin-$B_{12}$-dependent enzymatic reactions have been reviewed by Das and Herbert (1976b). Several inherited metabolic defects of vitamin-$B_{12}$-related pathways have been described (Mahoney and Rosenberg, 1970). There are two types of methylmalonic aciduria in which there is a block in the conversion of methylmalonyl CoA to succinyl CoA: one type, which is vitamin $B_{12}$ unresponsive, is due to a defect in the methylmalonyl CoA mutase apoenzyme, and the other, which is vitamin $B_{12}$ responsive, is caused by a defect in the metabolism of 5-deoxyadenosyl vitamin $B_{12}$ coenzyme. Patients with this latter disorder may benefit from treatment with pharmacological doses of vitamin $B_{12}$ (Nyhan, 1975). This may be considered as an example of defective utilization of the vitamin, although the condition is not associated with megaloblastic anemia.

Three infants have been described who had a deficiency of the vitamin $B_{12}$ binding protein, transcobalamin II (Hakami *et al.*, 1971; Scott *et al.*, 1972; Hitzig *et al.*, 1974; Gompert *et al.*, 1975), the transport and delivery protein for vitamin $B_{12}$. This condition was associated with a severe neonatal megaloblastic anemia, failure of growth, diarrhea, and repeated infections. Serum vitamin $B_{12}$ levels were within normal limits, but transcobalamin II was completely absent from the serum. The patients did not respond to small amounts of vitamin $B_{12}$ but did respond to pharmacological doses (1000 $\mu$g/week).

## 17.3.7. Increased Excretion

There is normally an enterohepatic circulation of vitamin $B_{12}$ (Okuda *et al.*, 1958; Reizenstein, 1959). This topic has been reviewed by Ardeman *et al.* (1965). When vitamin $B_{12}$ absorption is interfered with due to inadequate secretion of intrinsic factor, or ileal or pancreatic dysfunction, the percentage of biliary vitamin $B_{12}$ reabsorbed is decreased, resulting in vitamin $B_{12}$ deficiency (Herbert, 1975b). Failure to reduce biliary excretion of vitamin $B_{12}$ adequately as the body stores diminish also plays a role in the accelerated development of vitamin $B_{12}$ deficiency in these subjects (Herbert, 1975b) as compared to persons who eat no animal protein and hence eat no vitamin $B_{12}$.

### 17.3.8. Increased Requirement

Since vitamin $B_{12}$ is needed for DNA synthesis, conditions which are associated with rapid cell multiplication, such as pregnancy, will increase the demand for the vitamin. Because of the relatively large stores usually present in the body these conditions are not usually associated with overt vitamin $B_{12}$ deficiency, but if body stores are low, there may be overt deficiency. This has been described in pregnant women in South India (Baker *et al.*, 1962). There is also evidence that in thyrotoxicosis, requirement for vitamin $B_{12}$ may be increased (Ziffer *et al.*, 1957; Alperin *et al.*, 1970).

### 17.3.9. Increased Destruction

Two patients who were receiving megadoses of vitamin C to maintain an acid urine had unexplained low serum vitamin $B_{12}$ concentrations (Jacob *et al.*, 1973). Megaloblastosis was observed by Hines (1975) in two patients who had been taking megadoses of vitamin C for more than 3 years. Investigations to determine the cause of this phenomenon showed that vitamin C added to food caused significant reduction in the amount of assayable vitamin $B_{12}$ (Herbert and Jacob, 1974). This study has been attacked by Newmark *et al.* (1976) and defended subsequently (Herbert *et al.*, 1977). *In vivo*, the feeding of a large dose of vitamin C produced a significant reduction in the amount of vitamin $B_{12}$ assayable in bile and *in vitro*, addition of ascorbate to bile also reduced the amount of vitamin $B_{12}$ recoverable from bile (Jacob and Herbert, 1974). These observations suggest that megadoses of vitamin C may cause destruction of vitamin $B_{12}$ and, in some individuals, when continued for a long period of time, may produce vitamin $B_{12}$ deficiency. This possibility should be borne in mind in dealing with anyone receiving such therapy.

## References

Adams, J. F., Cox, A. G., Kennedy, E. H., and Thompson, J., 1967, Effect of medical and surgical vagotomy on intrinsic factor secretion, *Br. Med. J.* **3**:473.

Alfrey, C. P., and Lane, M., 1970, The effect of riboflavin deficiency on erythropoiesis, *Semin. Hematol.* **3**:49.

Allen, R. H., 1975, Human vitamin $B_{12}$ transport proteins, *Prog. Hematol.* **9**:57–84.

Alperin, J. B., Haggard, M. E., and Haynie, T. P., 1970, A study of vitamin $B_{12}$ requirements in a patient with pernicious anemia and thyrotoxicosis: Evidence of an increased need for vitamin $B_{12}$ in the presence of hyperthyroidism, *Blood* **36**:632.

Andersen, H. H., and Barkve, H., 1970, Iron deficiency and muscular work performance. An evaluation of the cardio-respiratory function of iron-deficient subjects with and without anaemia, *Scand. J. Clin. Lab. Invest.* **114** (Suppl.):1.

Ardeman, S., Chanarin, I., and Berry, V., 1965, Studies on human gastric intrinsic factor. Observations on its possible absorption and enterohepatic circulation, *Br. J. Haematol.* **11**:11.

Armstrong, B. K., Davis, R. E., Nicol, D. J., van Merwyk, A. J., and Lariwood, C. J., 1974, Hematological vitamin $B_{12}$ and folate studies in Seventh-day Adventist vegetarians, *Am. J. Cl. Nutr.* **27**:712.

Badenoch, J., 1954, The use of labelled vitamin $B_{12}$ and gastric biopsy in the investigation of anaemia, *Proc. Roy. Soc. Med.* **47**:426.

Baker, S. J., 1972, Vitamin $B_{12}$ and tropical sprue, *Br. J. Haematol.* **23** (Suppl.):135.

Baker, S. J., 1975, Nutrition and diseases of the blood: The megaloblastic anemias, *Prog. Food Nutr. Sci.* **1**:421.

Baker, S. J., and Mathan, V. I., 1968, Syndrome of tropical sprue in South India, *Am. J. Clin. Nutr.* **21**:984.

Baker, S. J., and Mathan, V. I., 1971, Tropical sprue in Southern India, *in Tropical Sprue and Megaloblastic Anemia,* Wellcome Trust Collaborative Study, 1961–1969, Churchill Livingstone, Edinburgh and London.

Baker, S. J., Jacob, E., Rajan, K. T., and Swaminathan, S. P., 1962, Vitamin $B_{12}$ deficiency in pregnancy and the puerperium, *Br. Med. J.* **1**:1658.

Ballard, H. S., and Lindenbaum, J., 1974, Megaloblastic anemia complicating hyperalimentation therapy, *Am. J. Med.* **56**:740.

Banerjee, D. K., and Chatterjea, J. B., 1960, Serum vitamin $B_{12}$ in vegetarians, *Br. Med. J.* **ii**:992.

Banerjee, S. P., and Snyder, S. H., 1973, Methyltetrahydrofolic acid mediates *N*- and *O*-methylation of biogenic amines, *Science* **182**:74.

Barker, H. A., Smyth, R. D., Weissbach, H., Toohey, J. I., Ladd, J. N., and Volcani, B. E., 1960, Isolation and properties of crystalline cobamide coenzymes containing benzimidazole or 5,6-dimethylbenzimidizole, *J. Biol. Chem.* **235**:480.

Baur, S., Fisher, J. M., Strickland, R. G., and Taylor, K. B., 1968, Autoantibody-containing cells in the gastric mucosa in pernicious anemia, *Lancet* **ii**:887.

Ben-Bassat, I., Feinstein, A., and Ramot, B., 1969, Selective vitamin $B_{12}$ malabsorption with proteinuria in Israel, *Israel J. Med. Sci.* **5**:62.

Berchtold, P., Bolli, P., Arbenz, U., and Keiser, G., 1969, Intestinale Absorptionsstorung infolge Metformin behandling (Zur Frage der Wirkungsweise der Biguanide), *Diabetologia* **5**:405.

Booth, C. C., and Mollin, D. L., 1957, Importance of the ileum in the absorption of vitamin $B_{12}$, *Lancet* **ii**:1007.

Booth, C. C., and Mollin, D. L., 1959, The site of absorption of vitamin $B_{12}$ in man, *Lancet* **i**:18.

Booth, C. C., and Mollin, D. L., 1964, Chronic tropical sprue in London, *Am. J. Dig. Dis.* **9**:770.

Booth, C. C., MacIntyre, I., and Mollin, D. L., 1964, Nutritional problems associated with extensive lesions of the distal small intestine in man, *Q. J. Med.* **33**:401.

Brody, E. A., Estren, S., and Herbert, V., 1966, Coexistent pernicious anemia and malabsorption in four patients including one whose malabsorption disappeared with vitamin $B_{12}$ therapy, *Ann. Int. Med.* **64**:1246.

Brunser, O., Reid, A., Monckeberg, F., Maccioni, A., and Contreras, I., 1968, Jejunal mucosa in infant malnutrition, *Am. J. Clin. Nutr.* **21**:976.

Burgio, G. R., Russo, G., and Jacono, F. L., 1956, Die hämatologische Reaktion auf kleine peronale Dosen von Vitamin $B_{12}$ bei der perniziosiformen Anämie des Säuglings (Gerbasi), *Arch. Kinderheilk.* **152**:109.

Butterworth, C. E., and Krumdieck, C. L., 1975, Intestinal absorption of folic acid monoglutamates and polyglutamates: A brief review of some recent developments, *Br. J. Haematol.* **31** (Suppl.):111.

Butterworth, C. E., Newman, A. J., and Krumdieck, C. L., 1974, Tropical sprue: A consideration of possible etiologic mechanisms with emphasis on pteroylpolyglutamate metabolism, *Trans. Am. Clin. Climatol. Assoc.* **86**:11.

Carmel, R., and Herbert, V., 1967, Correctable intestinal defect of vitamin $B_{12}$ absorption in pernicious anemia, *Ann. Int. Med.* **67**:1201.

Chanarin, I., 1969, *The Megaloblastic Anaemias*, Davis, Philadelphia.

Chanarin, I., 1976, Investigation and management of megaloblastic anemia, *Clin. Haematol.* **5**:747.

Chanarin, I., England, J. M., and Hoffbrand, A. V., 1973, Significance of large red blood cells, *Br. J. Haematol.* **25**:351.

Chung, A. S., Pearson, W. N., Darby, W. J., Miller, O. N., and Goldsmith, G. A., 1961, Folic acid, vitamin $B_6$, pantothenic acid, and vitamin $B_{12}$ in human dietaries, *Am. J. Clin. Nutr.* **9**:573.

Colman, N., and Herbert, V., 1976, Total folate binding capacity of normal human plasma, and variations in uremia, cirrhosis, and pregnancy, *Blood* **48**:911.

Colman, N., Barker, E. A., Barker, M., Green, R., and Metz, J., 1975a, Prevention of folate deficiency by food fortification. IV. Identification of target groups in addition to pregnant females in an adult rural population, *Am. J. Clin. Nutr.* **28**:471.

Colman, N., Green, R., and Metz, J., 1975b, Prevention of folate deficiency by food fortification. II. Absorption of folic acid from fortified staple foods, *Am. J. Clin. Nutr.* **28**:459.

Colman, N., Longo, D., and Herbert, V., 1976, Folate radioassay and crude milk binder, *Blood* **48**:626.

Committee on Food Protection, 1973, *Toxicants Occurring Naturally in Foods*, National Academy of Sciences, Washington, D.C.

Committee on Maternal Nutrition, 1970, *Maternal Nutrition and the Course of Pregnancy*, National Academy of Sciences, Washington, D.C.

Connor, P. M., and Pirola, R. C., 1963, Nutritional vitamin $B_{12}$ deficiency, *Med. J. Aust.* **2**:451.

Cooke, W. T., Cox, E. V., Fone, D. J., Meynell, M. J., and Gaddie, R., 1963a, The clinical and metabolic significance of jejunal diverticula, *Gut* **4**:115.

Cooke, W. T., Fone, D. J., Cox, E. V., Meynell, M. J., and Gaddie, R., 1963b, Adult coeliac disease, *Gut* **4**:279.

Cooper, B. A., 1976, Megaloblastic anaemia and disorders affecting utilization of vitamin $B_{12}$ and folate in childhood, *Clin. Haematol.* **5**:631.

Corcino, J. J., 1975, Recent advances in tropical sprue, in *Intestinal Absorption and Malabsorption* (T. Z. Csaky, ed.), pp. 285–299, Raven Press, New York.

Corcino, J. J., Coll, G., and Klipstein, F. A., 1975, Pteroylglutamic acid malabsorption in tropical sprue, *Blood* **45**:577.

Corcino, J. J., Reisenaur, A. M., and Halsted, C. H., 1976, Jejunal perfusion of simple and conjugated folates in tropical sprue, *J. Clin. Invest.* **58**:298.

Cordano, A., Placko, R. P., and Graham, G. G., 1966, Hypocupremia and neutropenia in copper deficiency, *Blood* **28**:280.

Croft, R. F., Streeter, A. M., and O'Neill, B. J., 1974, Red cell indices in megaloblastosis and iron deficiency, *Pathology* **6**:107.

Das, K. C., and Herbert, V., 1976a, Use of the lymphocyte deoxyuridine (dU) suppression test and lymphocyte chromosome study for retrospective diagnosis of vitamin $B_{12}$ and/or folate deficiency despite "shotgun" treatment, *Clin. Res.* **24**:480A.

Das, K. C., and Herbert, V., 1976b, Vitamin $B_{12}$–folate interrelations, *Clin. Haematol.* **5**:697.

Das, K. C., and Hoffbrand, A. V., 1970, Lymphocyte transformation in megaloblastic anemia. Morphology and DNA synthesis, *Br. J. Haematol.* **9**:459.

Dawson, A. M., and Isselbacher, K. J., 1960, Studies on lipid metabolism in the small intestine with observations on the role of bile salts, *J. Clin. Invest.* **39**:730.

Donaldson, R. M., 1965, Studies on the pathogenesis of steatorrhea in the blind loop syndrome, *J. Clin. Invest.* **44**:1815.

Donaldson, R. M., Corrigan, H., and Natsios, G., 1962, Malabsorption of [60]Co-labeled cyanocobalamin in rats with intestinal diverticula: II. Studies on contents of diverticula, *Gastroenterology* **43**:282.

Doscherholmen, A., and Swaim, W. R., 1973, Impaired assimilation of egg [57]Co vitamin $B_{12}$ in patients with hypochlorhydria and achlorhydria and after gastric resection, *Gastroenterology* **64**:913.

Drexler, J., 1958, Effect of indole compounds on vitamin $B_{12}$ utilization, *Blood* **13**:239.

Edozien, J. C., May 1972, National Nutrition Survey, Massachusetts, July 1969–June 1971, Report of the Survey Director to the Commissioner for Public Health, Commonwealth of Massachusetts, Boston, Massachusetts (kindly supplied to us by Derek Robinson, M.D., Director, Division of Community Operations, Department of Public Health, Commonwealth of Massachusetts).

England, J. M., Walford, D. M., and Waters, D. A. W., 1972, Reassessment of the reliability of the hematocrit, *Br. J. Haematol.* **23**:247.

Faulk, E. A., and Farrar, W. E., 1964, Diverticulosis of the small intestine and megaloblastic anemia, *Am. J. Med.* **37**:473.

Finch, C. A., 1975, Erythropoiesis in protein–calorie malnutrition, *in Protein–Calorie Malnutrition* (R. E. Olson, ed.), pp. 247–256, Academic Press, New York.

Food and Nutrition Board, 1974, *Recommended Dietary Allowances*, 8th ed., National Academy of Sciences, Washington, D.C.

Garby, L., Irnell, L., and Werner, I., 1969, Iron deficiency in women of fertile age in a Swedish community. III. Estimation of prevalence based on response to iron supplementation, *Acta Med. Scand.* **185**:113.

Garrido-Pinson, G. C., Turner, M. D., Crookston, J. H., Samloff, I. M., Miller, U., and Segal, H. L., 1966, Studies of human intrinsic factor autoantibodies, *J. Immunol.* **97**:897.

Gerbasi, M., and Burgio, G. R., 1962, Megaloblastic anaemias, *Pediatr. Clin. N. Am.* **9**:727.

Gerson, C. D., Cohen, N., Hepner, G. W., Brown, N., Herbert, V., and Janowitz, H. D., 1971, Folic acid absorption in man: Enchancing effect of glucose, *Gastroenterology* **61**:224.

Gerson, C. D., Cohen, N., Brown, N., Lindenbaum, J., Hepner, G. W., and Janowitz, H. D., 1974, Folic acid and hexose absorption in sprue, *Dig. Dis.* **19**:911.

Glass, G. B. J., 1963, Gastric intrinsic factor and its function in the metabolism of vitamin $B_{12}$, *Physiol. Rev.* **43**:529.

Gompert, E., Jakob, M., and Hitzig, W. H., 1975, Vitamin $B_{12}$ transport in blood. 1. Congenital deficiency of transcobalamin II, *Blood* **45**:71.

Gottlieb, C., Lau, K.-S., Wasserman, L. R., and Herbert, V., 1965, Rapid charcoal assay for intrinsic factor (IF), gastric juice unsaturated $B_{12}$ binding capacity, antibody to IF, and serum unsaturated $B_{12}$ binding capacity, **25**:875.

Gräsbeck, R., 1969, Intrinsic factor and the other vitamin $B_{12}$ transport proteins, *Prog. Hematol.* **6**:233.

Gräsbeck, R., 1972, Familial selective vitamin $B_{12}$ malabsorption, *N. Engl. J. Med.* **287**:358.

Gräsbeck, R., Gordin, R., Kantero, I., and Kuhlback, B., 1960, Selective vitamin $B_{12}$ malabsorption and proteinuria in young people, *Acta Med. Scand.* **167**:289.

Habib, G. G., 1964, Nutritional vitamin $B_{12}$ deficiency among Hindus, *Trop. Geogr. Med.* **16**:206.

Hakami, N., Neiman, P. E., Canellos, G. P., and Lazerson, J., 1971, Neonatal megaloblastic anemia due to inherited transcobalamin II deficiency in two siblings, *N. Engl. J. Med.* **285**:1163.

Harrison, R. J., Booth, C. C., and Mollin, D. L., 1956, Vitamin $B_{12}$ deficiency due to defective diet, *Lancet* **1**:727.

Haurani, F., Sherwood, W., and Goldstein, F., 1964, Intestinal malabsorption of vitamin $B_{12}$ in pernicious anemia, *Metabolism* **13**:1342.

Heinivaara, O., and Palva, I. P., 1964, Malabsorption of vitamin $B_{12}$ during treatment with *p*-aminosalicylic acid, *Acta Med. Scand.* **175**:469.

Heinivaara, O., Palva, I., Siurala, M., and Pelkoner, R., 1964, Selectivity of the PAS-induced malabsorption of vitamin $B_{12}$, *Ann. Med. Int. Fenn.* **53**:75.

Henderson, J. T., Simpson, J. D., Warwick, R. R. G., Shearman, D. J. C., 1972, Does malabsorption of vitamin $B_{12}$ occur in chronic pancreatitis? *Lancet* **2**:241.

Herbert, V., 1959a, Mechanism of intrinsic factor action in everted sacs of rat small intestine, *J. Clin. Invest.* **38**:102.

Herbert, V., 1959b, Studies on the role of intrinsic factor in vitamin $B_{12}$ absorption, transport, and storage. *Am. J. Clin. Nutr.* **7**:433.

Herbert, V., 1961, The assay and nature of folic acid activity in human serum, *J. Clin. Invest.* **40**:81.

Herbert, V., 1962, Experimental nutritional folate deficiency in man, *Trans. Assoc. Am. Physicians* **75**:307.

Herbert, V., 1963, A palatable diet for producing experimental folate deficiency in man, *Am. J. Clin. Nutr.* **12**:17.

Herbert, V., 1967, Immunologic factors in pernicious anemia, *Postgrad. Med.* **42**:298.

Herbert, V., 1969, Transient (reversible) malabsorption of vitamin $B_{12}$, *Br. J. Haematol.* **17**:213.

Herbert, V., 1970, Introduction to the nutritional anemias, *Semin. Hematol.* **7**:2.

Herbert, V., 1972a, Malabsorption syndrome secondary to $B_{12}$ deficiency, *in Hematopoietic and Gastrointestinal Investigations with Radionuclides* (A. J. Gilson, W. M. Smoak III, and M. B. Weinstein, ed.), pp. 287–293, Charles C. Thomas, Springfield, Illinois.

Herbert, V., 1972b, Detection of malabsorption of vitamin $B_{12}$ due to gastric or intestinal dysfunction, *Semin. Nucl. Med.* **2**:220.

Herbert, V., 1972c, Metformin and $B_{12}$ malabsorption, *Ann. Intern. Med.* **76**:140.

Herbert, V., 1975a, Megaloblastic anemias, *in Textbook of Medicine,* 14th ed. (P. B. Beeson and W. McDermott, eds.), pp. 1404–1413, Saunders, Philadelphia.

Herbert, V., 1975b, Drugs effective in megaloblastic anemias: Vitamin $B_{12}$ and folic acid, *in The Pharmacological Basis of Therapeutics,* 5th ed. (L. S. Goodman and A. Gilman, eds.), pp. 1324–1349, Macmillan, New York.

Herbert, V., 1977a, The blood in hypothyroidism, *in The Thyroid* (S. C. Werner and S. H. Ingbar, ed.), Harper & Row, New York, in press.

Herbert, V., 1977b, Anemias, *in Nutritional Disorders of American Women* (M. Winick, ed.), pp. 79–89, Wiley, New York.

Herbert, V., 1977c, Folic acid requirements in adults (including pregnant and lactating females), *in Folic Acid: Biochemistry and Physiology in Relation to the Human Folate Requirement. Proceedings of a Workshop on Human Folate Requirement* (Food and Nutrition Board), National Academy of Science, Washington, D.C.

Herbert, V., and Jacob, E., 1974, Destruction of vitamin $B_{12}$ by ascorbic acid, *JAMA* **230**:241.

Herbert, V., and Zalusky, R., 1962, Interrelations of vitamin $B_{12}$ and folate metabolism: Folic acid clearance studies, *J. Clin. Invest.* **41**:1263.

Herbert, V., Streiff, R. R., and Sullivan, L. W., 1964, Notes on vitamin $B_{12}$ absorption, autoimmunity and childhood pernicious anaemia; relation of intrinsic factor to blood group substance. *Medicine* **43**:679.

Herbert, V., Tisman, G., Go, L. T., and Brenner, L., 1973, The dU suppression test using $^{125}$IUdR to define biochemical megaloblastosis, *Br. J. Haematol.* **24**:713.

Herbert, V., Colman, N., Spivack, M., Ocasio, E., Ghanta, V., Kimmel, K., Brenner, L., Freundlich, J., and Scott, J., 1975, Folic acid deficiency in the United States: Folate assays in a prenatal clinic, *Am. J. Obstet. Gynecol.* **123**:175.

Herbert, V., Jacob, E., and Wong, K.-T. J., 1977, Destruction of vitamin $B_{12}$ by vitamin C (Letter to the Editor), *Am. J. Clin. Nutr.* **30**:297.

Hershko, C. H., Karsai, A., Eylon, L., and Izak, G., 1970, The effect of chronic iron deficiency on some biochemical functions of the human hemopoietic tissue, *Blood* **36**:321.

Hesp, R., Chanarin, I., and Tait, C., 1975, Potassium changes in megaloblastic anaemia, *Clin. Sci. Mol. Med.* **49**:77.

Hines, J. D., 1966, Megaloblastic anemia in an adult vegan, *Am. J. Clin. Nutr.* **19**:260.

Hines, J. D., 1975, Ascorbic acid and vitamin $B_{12}$ deficiency (Letter to the Editor), *JAMA* **234**:24.

Hines, J. D., Hoffbrand, A. V., and Mollin, D. L., 1967, The hematologic complications following partial gastrectomy, *Am. J. Med.* **43**:555.

Hippe, E., Juhl, E., Bruusgaard, A., Korner, B., Quaade, F., and Baden, H., 1974, Malabsorption of vitamin $B_{12}$ in obese patients treated with jejunoileal shunt, *Scand. J. Gastroenterol.* **9** (Suppl. 29):81.

Hitzig, W. H., Dohmann, U., Pluss, H. J., and Vischer, D., 1974, Hereditary transcobalamin II deficiency: Clinical findings in a new family, *J. Pediatr.* **85**:622.

Hoedemaeker, P. J., Abels, J., Wachters, J. J., Arends, A., and Nieweg, H. O., 1964, Investigations about the site of production of Castle's gastric intrinsic factor, *Lab. Invest.* **13**:1394.

Hoffbrand, A. V., Ganeshaguru, K., Hooton, J. W. L., and Tattersall, M. H. N., 1976, Effect of iron deficiency and desferrioxamine on DNA synthesis in human cells, *Br. J. Haematol.* **33**:517.

Ibbotson, R. M., Colvin, B. T., and Colvin, M. P., 1975a, Folic acid deficiency during intensive therapy, *Br. Med. J.* **4**:145.

Ibbotson, R. M., Colvin, B. T., and Colvin, M. P., 1975b, Folic acid deficiency during intensive therapy, *Br. Med. J.* **4**:522.

Imerslund, O., 1960, Idiopathic chronic megaloblastic anemia in children, *Acta Paediatr.* Suppl. 119.

Jacob, E., and Glass, G. B. J., 1969, The participation of complement in the parietal cell antigen–antibody reaction in pernicious anaemia and atrophic gastritis, *Clin. Exp. Immunol.* **5**:141.

Jacob, E., and Glass, G. B. J., 1971a, Localization of intrinsic factor and complement fixing intrinsic factor–intrinsic factor antibody complex in parietal cell of man, *Clin. Exp. Immunol.* **8**:517.

Jacob, E., and Glass, G. B. J., 1971b, Separation of intrinsic factor antibodies from parietal cell antibodies in pernicious anemia serum by gel filtration, *Proc. Soc. Exp. Biol. Med.* **137**:243.

Jacob, E., and O'Brien, H. A. W., 1972, A simple assay of intrinsic factor–vitamin $B_{12}$ complex employing the binding intrinsic factor antibody, *J. Clin. Pathol.* **25**:320.

Jacob, E., Scott, J., Brenner, L., and Herbert, V., 1973, Apparent low serum vitamin $B_{12}$ levels in paraplegic veterans taking ascorbic acid, *in Proceedings of the 16th Annual Meeting, American Society of Hematology, Chicago, December 4, 1973*, p. 125.

Jacob, M., Hunt, I. F., Dirige, O., and Swendseid, M. E., 1976, Biochemical assessment of the nutritional status of low-income pregnant women of Mexican descent, *Am. J. Clin. Nutr.* **29**:650.

Jacobson, E. D., Chodos, R. B., and Faloon, W. W., 1960, An experimental malabsorption syndrome induced by neomycin, *Am. J. Med.* **28**:524.

Jadhav, M., Webb, J. K. G., Vaishnava, S., and Baker, S. J., 1962, Vitamin $B_{12}$ deficiency in Indian infants. A clinical syndrome, *Lancet* **2**:903.

Kapadia, C. R., Bhat, P., Jacob, E., and Baker, S. J., 1975, Vitamin $B_{12}$ absorption—A study of intraluminal events in control subjects and patients with tropical sprue, *Gut* **16**:988.

Kapadia, C. R., Mathan, V. I., and Baker, S. J., 1976, Free intrinsic factor in the small intestine of man, *Gastroenterology* **70**:704.

Katz, M., Lee, S. K., and Cooper, B. A., 1972, Vitamin $B_{12}$ malabsorption due to a biologically inert intrinsic factor, *N. Engl. J. Med.* **287**:425.

Katz, M., Mehlman, C. S., and Allen, R. H., 1974, Isolation and characterization of an abnormal human intrinsic factor, *J. Clin. Invest.* **53**:1274.

Khakee, S., Stachewitsch, A., and Katz, M., 1974, Selective vitamin $B_{12}$ malabsorption in two siblings, *Can. Med. Assoc. J.* **110**:53.

Klipstein, F. A., Holdeman, L. V., Corcino, J. J., and Moore, W. E. C., 1973, Enterotoxigenic intestinal bacteria in tropical sprue, *Gastroenterology* **79**:632.

Krumdieck, C. L., and Baugh, C. M., 1969, The solid phase synthesis of polyglutamates of folic acid, *Biochemistry* **8**:1568.

Krumdieck, C. L., Newman, A. J., and Butterworth, C. E., 1973, A naturally occurring inhibitor of folic acid conjugase (pteroylpolyglutamate hydrolase) in beans and other pulses, *Am. J. Clin. Nutr.* **26**:460.

Krumdieck, C. L., Boots, L. R., Cornwell, P. E., and Butterworth, C. E., 1976, Cyclic variations in folate composition and pteroylpolyglutamyl hydrolase (conjugase) activity of the rat uterus, *Am. J. Clin. Nutr.* **29**:288.

Lampkin, B. C., and Mauer, A. M., 1967, Congenital pernicious anemia with coexistent transitory intestinal malabsorption of vitamin $B_{12}$, *Blood* **30**:495.

Lampkin, B. C., Shore, N. A., and Chadwick, D., 1966, Megaloblastic anemia of infancy secondary to maternal pernicious anemia, *N. Engl. J. Med.* **21**:1168.

Lampkin, B. C., Pyesmany, A., Hyman, C. B., and Hammond, D., 1971, Congenital familial megaloblastic anemia, *Blood* **37**:615.

Lawson, D. H., Murray, R. M., and Parker, J. L. W., 1972, Early mortality in the megaloblastic anemias, *Q. J. Med.* **41**:1.

Ledbetter, R. B., Jr., and Del Pozo, E., 1969, Severe megaloblastic anemia due to nutritional vitamin $B_{12}$ deficiency, *Acta Haematol.* **42**:247.

Lichtenstein, H., Beloiam, A., and Murphy, E. W., 1962, Vitamin $B_{12}$ microbiological assay methods and distribution in selected foods, Res. Rep. USDA Home Econ. No. 13, cited in *Nutr. Abstr. Rev.* **32**:431.

Lindenbaum, J., and Lieber, C. S., 1969, Alcohol-induced malabsorption of vitamin $B_{12}$ in man, *Nature (London)* **224**:806.

Lindenbaum, J., Pezzumenti, J. F., and Shea, N., 1974, Small intestinal function in vitamin $B_{12}$ deficiency, *Ann. Intern. Med.* **80**:326.

Lindenbaum, J., Whitehead, N., and Reyner, F., 1975, Oral contraceptive hormones, folate metabolism, and the cervical epithelium. *Am. J. Clin. Nutr.* **28**:346.

Longo, D. L., and Herbert, V., 1975, Iron and DNA synthesis: Inhibition of $^3$H-TdR incorporation into DNA by an iron chelating agent and enhancement by iron dextran, *Clin. Res.* **23**:278A.

Longo, D. L., and Herbert, V., 1976, Radioassay for serum and red cell folate, *J. Lab. Clin. Med.* **87**:138.

Mackenzie, I. L., Donaldson, R. M., Jr., Trier, J. S., and Mathan, V. I., 1972, Ileal mucosa in familial selective vitamin $B_{12}$ malabsorption, *N. Engl. J. Med.* **286**:1021.

MacLean, L. D., 1957, Incidence of megaloblastic anemia after subtotal gastrectomy, *N. Engl. J. Med.* **257**:262.

Mahoney, M. J., and Rosenberg, L. E., 1970, Inherited defects of $B_{12}$ metabolism, *Am. J. Med.* **48**:584.

Manzoor, M., and Runcie, J., 1976, Folate-responsive neuropathy: Report of ten cases, *Br. Med. J.* **1**:1176.

Markkanen, T., Levanto, A., Sallinen, V., and Virtanen, S., 1967, Folic acid and vitamin $B_{12}$ in tuberculosis, *Scand. J. Haematol.* **4**:283.

McIntyre, P. A., Sachs, M. V., Krevans, J. R., and Conley, C. L., 1956, Pathogenesis and treatment of macrocytic anemia, *Arch. Intern. Med.* **96**:541.

McPhedran, P., Barnes, M. G., Weinstein, J. S., and Robertson, J. S., 1973, Interpretation of electronically determined macrocytosis, *Ann. Intern. Med.* **78**:677.

Medical Letter, 1973, Feminins and other vitamin–mineral supplements for women taking oral contraceptives, *Med. Lett.* **15**:81.

Medical Letter, 1974, Topical and systemic contraceptive agents, *Med. Lett.* **16**:37.

Medical Letter, 1975, Cu-7, a copper containing IUD, *Med. Lett.* **17**:26.

Mehta, B. M., Rege, D. V., and Satoskar, R. S., 1964, Serum vitamin $B_{12}$ and folic acid activity in lactovegetarian and nonvegetarian healthy adult Indians, *Am. J. Clin. Nutr.* **15**:77.

Meller, E., Rosengarten, H., Friedhoff, A. J., Stebbins, R. D., and Silber, R., 1975, 5-Methyltetrahydrofolic acid is not a methyl donor for biogenic amines—Enzymatic formation of formaldehyde, *Science* **187**:171.

Metz, J., Kelly, A., Swett, V. C., Waxman, S., and Herbert, V., 1968, Deranged DNA synthesis by bone marrow from vitamin $B_{12}$-deficient humans, *Br. J. Haematol.* **14**:575.

Mohamed, S. D., McKay, E., and Galloway, W. H., 1966, Juvenile familial megaloblastic anaemia due to selective malabsorption of vitamin $B_{12}$, *Q. J. Med.* **35**:433.

Mollin, D. L., and Baker, S. J., 1955, The absorption and excretion of vitamin $B_{12}$ in man, *Biochem. Soc. Symp.* **13**:52.

Mollin, D. L., and Ross, G. I. M., 1954, Vitamin $B_{12}$ deficiency in the megaloblastic anaemias, *Proc. Roy. Soc. Med.* **47**:428.

Mollin, D. L., Baker, S. J., and Doniach, I., 1955, Addisonian pernicious anaemia without gastric atrophy in a young man, *Br. J. Haematol.* **1**:278.

Mollin, D. L., Booth, C. C., and Baker, S. J., 1957, The absorption of vitamin $B_{12}$ in control subjects in Addisonian pernicious anaemia and in the malabsorption syndrome, *Br. J. Haematol.* **3**:412.

Mollin, D. L., Booth, C. C., and Chanarin, I., 1959, The pathogenesis of deficiency of vitamin $B_{12}$ and folic acid in idiopathic steatorrhoea, *in Proceedings of the*

*World Congress on Gastroenterology, 1958,* pp. 483–490, Williams & Wilkins, Baltimore, Maryland.

Najman, E., and Brausil, B., 1952, Megaloblastishe Anämie mit Relapsen ohne Achylia gastrica im Kindesalter, *Ann. Paediatr. Basel* **178**:47.

Newmark, H. L., Scheiner, J., Marcus, M., and Prabhudesai, M., 1976, Stability of vitamin $B_{12}$ in the presence of ascorbic acid, *Am. J. Clin. Nutr.* **29**:645.

Nieweg, H. O., Shen, S. C., and Castle, W. B., 1957, Mechanism of intrinsic factor action in the gastrectomized rat, *Proc. Soc. Exp. Biol. Med.* **94**:223.

Nyberg, W., and Saarni, M., 1964, Calculations on the dynamics of vitamin $B_{12}$ in fish tapeworm carriers spontaneously recovering from vitamin $B_{12}$ deficiency. *Acta Med. Scand.* **412** (Suppl.):65.

Nyhan, W. L., 1975, Prenatal treatment of methylmalonic acidemia, *N. Engl. J. Med.* **293**:353.

Okuda, K., Gräsbeck, R., and Chow, B. F., 1958, Bile and vitamin $B_{12}$ absorption, *J. Lab. Clin. Med.* **51**:17.

Oxenhorn, S., Estren, S., Wasserman, L. R., and Adlersberg, D., 1958, Malabsorption syndrome: Intestinal absorption of vitamin $B_{12}$, *Ann. Intern. Med.* **48**:30.

Palva, I. P., Salskannel, S. J., Timanen, T., and Palva, H. L. A., 1972, Drug-induced malabsorption of vitamin $B_{12}$, *Acta Med. Scand.* **191**:355.

Perman, G., Gullberg, R., Reizenstein, P. G., Snellman, B., and Allgen, L. G., 1960, A study of absorbtion patterns in malabsorption syndromes, *Acta Med. Scand.* **168**:117.

Pollycove, M., Apt, L., and Colbert, M. J., 1956, Pernicious anemia due to dietary deficiency of vitamin $B_{12}$. *N. Engl. J. Med.* **255**:164.

Prasad, A. S., Lei, K. Y., Oberleas, D., Moghissi, K. S., and Stryker, J. C., 1975, Effect of oral contraceptive agents on nutrients. II. Vitamins, *Am. J. Clin. Nutr.* **28**:385.

Reizenstein, P. G., 1959, Excretion of nonlabelled vitamin $B_{12}$ in man, *Acta Med. Scand.* **165**:313.

Reynolds, E. H., 1976, Neurologic aspects of folate and vitamin $B_{12}$ metabolism, *Clin. Haematol.* **5**:661.

Roggin, G. M., Iber, F. L., Krater, R. M. H., and Tobon, F., 1969, Malabsorption in the chronic alcoholic, *Johns Hopkins Med. J.* **125**:321.

Roitt, I. M., Doniach, D., and Shapland, C., 1964, Intrinsic factor autoantibodies, *Lancet* **2**:469.

Rosenberg, I. H., 1976, Absorption and malabsorption of folates, *Clin. Haematol.* **5**:589.

Rothenberg, S. P., and DaCosta, M., 1976, Folate binding proteins and radioassay for folate, *Clin. Haematol.* **5**:569.

Rothenberg, S. P., DaCosta, M., and Rosenberg, Z., 1972, A radioassay for serum folate: Use of a two-phase sequential-incubation, ligand-binding system, *N. Engl. J. Med.* **286**:1335.

Rubin, C. E., Brandborg, L. L., Flick, A. L., Phelps, P., Parmentier, C., and van Niel, S., 1962, Studies of celiac sprue: III, The effect of repeated wheat installation into the proximal ileum of patients on a gluten-free diet, *Gastroenterology* **43**:621.

Rygvold, O., 1974, Hypovitaminosis $B_{12}$ following partial gastrectomy by the Bih II method, *Scand. J. Gastroenterol.* **9** (Suppl. 29):57.

Saary, M., and Hoffbrand, A. V., 1976, Folic acid deficiency during intensive therapy, *Br. Med. J.* **1**:461.

Saary, M., Sissons, J. G. P., Davies, W. A., and Hoffbrand, A. V., 1975, Unusual megaloblastic anaemia with multinucleate erythroblasts: Two cases with septicaemia and acute renal failure, *J. Clin. Pathol.* **28**:324.

Schade, S. C., Abels, J., Schilling, R. F., Feick, P., and Muckerheide, M., 1967, Studies on antibody to intrinsic factor, *J. Clin. Invest.* **46**:615.

Schjönsby, H., 1974, The absorption of vitamin $B_{12}$ in the blind loop syndrome, *Scand. J. Gastroenterol.* **9** (Suppl. 29):65.

Schjönsby, H., Peters, T. J., Hoffbrand, A. V., and Tabaqchali, S., 1970, The mechanism of vitamin $B_{12}$ malabsorption in the blind loop syndrome, *Gut* **11**:371.

Scott, C. R., Hakami, N., Teng, C. C., and Sagerson, R. N., 1972, Hereditary transcobalamin II deficiency: The role of transcobalamin II in vitamin $B_{12}$-mediated reactions, *J. Pediatr.* **81**:1106.

Sherman, C. D., and May, A. G., 1963, The lieum, site of vitamin $B_{12}$ absorption, *Arch. Surg.* **86**:187.

Siddons, R. C., Spence, J. A., and Dayan, A. D., 1975, Experimental vitamin $B_{12}$ deficiency in the baboon, in *Advances in Neurology,* Vol. 10 (B. S. Meldrum and C. D. Marsden, eds.), Raven Press, New York.

Silver, H., and Frankel, S., 1971, Normal values for mean corpuscular volume as determined by the Model S Coulter Counter, *Am. J. Clin. Pathol.* **55**:438.

Smith, J. L., Goldsmith, G. A., and Lawrence, J. D., 1975, Effects of oral contraceptive steroids on vitamin and lipid levels in serum, *Am. J. Clin. Nutr.* **28**:377.

Solakannel, S. J., Palva, L. P., and Tukkunen, J. T., 1970, Malabsorption of vitamin $B_{12}$ during treatment with slow-release potassium chloride, *Acta Med. Scand.* **187**:431.

Sood, S. K., Banerjee, L., and Ramalingaswami, V., 1967, Pathogenesis of nutritional anemia of pregnancy in northern India (Delhi area), *in Fourth Congress of the Asian and Pacific Society of Haematology, New Delhi, India,* E10, p. 70, Pfizer, Bombay.

Srikantia, S. G., and Reddy, V., 1967, Megaloblastic anaemia of infancy and vitamin $B_{12}$, *Br. J. Haematol.* **13**:949.

Sullivan, L. W., and Herbert, V., 1965, Studies on the minimum daily requirement for vitamin $B_{12}$, *N. Engl. J. Med.* **272**:340.

Swendseid, M. E., Halstead, J. A., and Libby, R. L., 1953, Excretion of cobalt-60-labeled vitamin $B_{12}$ after total gastrectomy, *Proc. Soc. Exp. Biol. Med.* **82**:226.

Tamura, T., and Stokstad, E. L. R., 1973, The availability of food folate in man, *Br. J. Haematol.* **25**:513.

Tamura, T., Shin, Y. S., Buehring, K. U., and Stokstad, E. L. R., 1976, The availability of folates in man: Effect of orange juice supplement on intestinal conjugase, *Br. J. Haematol.* **32**:123.

Tandon, B. N., Magotra, M. L., Saraya, A. K., and Ramalingaswami, V., 1968, Small intestine in protein malnutrition, *Am. J. Clin. Nutr.* **21**:813.

Taylor, K. B., 1965, The localisation of gastric intrinsic factor, *Gastroenterology* **48**:853.

Taylor, K. B., 1976, Immune aspects of pernicious anaemia and atrophic gastritis, *Clin. Haematol.* **5**:497.

Tisman, G., and Herbert, V., 1971, Inhibition by penicillamine of DNA synthesis by human bone marrow *in vitro, Fed. Proc.* **30**:518.

Tisman, G., and Herbert, V., 1973, $B_{12}$ dependence of cell uptake of serum folate: An explanation for high serum folate and cell folate depletion in $B_{12}$ deficiency, *Blood* **41**:465.

Tomkin, G. H., Hadden, D. R., Weaver, J. A., and Montgomery, D. A. D., 1971, Vitamin $B_{12}$ status of patients on long-term metformin therapy, *Br. Med. J.* **2**:685.

Toskes, P. P., and Deren, J. J., 1972, Selective inhibition of vitamin $B_{12}$ absorption by paraaminosalicylic acid, *Gastroenterology* **62**:1232.

Toskes, P. P., Hansell, J., Cerda, J., and Deren, J. J., 1971, Vitamin $B_{12}$ malabsorption in chronic pancreatic insufficiency. Studies suggesting the presence of a pancreatic "intrinsic factor," *N. Eng. J. Med.* **284**:627.

Toskes, P. P., Deren, J. J., and Conrad, M. E., 1973, Trypsin-like nature of the pancreatic factor that corrects vitamin $B_{12}$ malabsorption associated with pancreatic dysfunction, *J. Clin. Invest.* **52**:1660.

U.S. Department of Health, Education and Welfare, 1972, *Ten-State Nutrition Survey 1968–1970*, DHEW Publications No (HSM) 72-8130–72-8134.

van der Weyden, M., Rother, M., and Firkin, B., 1972, Megaloblastic maturation masked by iron deficiency: A biochemical basis, *Br. J. Haematol.* **22**:299.

Veeger, W., Abels, J., Hellemans, N., and Nieweg, H. O., 1962, Effect of sodium bicarbonate and pancreatin on the absorption of Vitamin $B_{12}$ and fat in pancreatic insufficiency, *N. Eng. J. Med.* **257**:1341.

Viteri, F. E., Alvarado, J., Luthringer, D. G., and Wood, R. P., 1968, Hematological changes in protein calorie malnutrition, *Vitam. Horm.* **26**:573.

von Bonsdorff, B., 1947, The site of infestation with fish tapeworm determined by means of intestinal intubation: *Diphyllobothrium latum* and pernicious anaemia, *Acta Med. Scand.* **129**:213.

von Bonsdorff, B., Nyberg, W., and Gräsbeck, R., 1960, Vitamin $B_{12}$ deficiency in carriers of the fish tapeworm, *Diphyllobothrium latum, Acta Haematol.* **24**:15.

Wardrop, C. A. J., Heatley, R. V., Tennant, G. B., and Hughes, L. E., 1975a, Acute folate deficiency in surgical patients on amino acid/ethanol intravenous nutrition, *Lancet* **2**:640.

Wardrop, C. A. J., Heatley, R. V., Williams, R. H. P., Lewis, M. H., Tennant, G. B., and Hughes, L. E., 1975b, Folic acid deficiency during intensive therapy, *Br. Med. J.* **4**:344.

Waxman, S., Schreiber, C., and Herbert, V., 1971, Radioisotopic assay for measurement of serum folate levels, *Blood* **38**:219.

Webb, D. I., Chodos, R. B., Mahar, C. Q., and Faloon, W. W., 1968, Mechanism of vitamin $B_{12}$ malabsorption in patients receiving colchicine, *N. Engl. J. Med.* **279**:845.

WHO Group of Experts, 1972, *Nutritional Anaemias*, WHO Technical Report Ser. #503, Geneva.

WHO Scientific Group, 1968, *Nutritional Anemias,* WHO Tech. Rep. Ser. 405, pp. 1–37. (Available for $1.00 from World Health Organization, Distribution and Sales Unit, Geneva, Switzerland).

Wickramasinghe, S. N., Williams, G., Saunders, J., and Durston, J., 1975, Megaloblastic erythropoiesis and macrocytosis in patients on anticonvulsants, *Br. Med. J.* **4**:136.

Williams, M. L., Shott, R. J., O'Neal, P. L., and Oski, F., 1975, Role of dietary iron and fat on vitamin E deficiency anemia of infancy, *N. Engl. J. Med.* **292**:887.

Wokes, F., Badenoch, J., and Sinclair, H. M., 1955, Human dietary deficiency of vitamin $B_{12}$, *Am. J. Clin. Nutr.* **3**:375.

Wu, A., Chanarin, I., Slavin, G., and Levi, A. J., 1975, Folate deficiency in the alcoholic—Its relationship to clinical and haematological abnormalities, liver disease and folate stores, *Br. J. Haematol.* **29**:469.

Ziffer, H., Gutman, A., Pasher, I., Sabotka, H., and Baker, H., 1957, Vitamin $B_{12}$ in thyrotoxicosis and myxedema, *Proc. Soc. Exp. Biol. Med.* **96**:229.

# Index

583